PEDIATRIC NEUROPSYCHOLOGY

THE SCIENCE AND PRACTICE OF NEUROPSYCHOLOGY
A Guilford Series

Robert A. Bornstein, *Series Editor*

APHASIA AND LANGUAGE: THEORY TO PRACTICE
Stephen E. Nadeau, Leslie J. Gonzalez Rothi, and Bruce A. Crosson, *Editors*

COGNITIVE AND BEHAVIORAL REHABILITATION:
FROM NEUROBIOLOGY TO CLINICAL PRACTICE
Jennie Ponsford, *Editor*

DEVELOPMENTAL MOTOR DISORDERS:
A NEUROPSYCHOLOGICAL PERSPECTIVE
Deborah Dewey and David E. Tupper, *Editors*

THE HUMAN FRONTAL LOBES:
FUNCTIONS AND DISORDERS, SECOND EDITION
Bruce L. Miller and Jeffrey L. Cummings, *Editors*

NEUROPSYCHOLOGY OF EVERYDAY FUNCTIONING
Thomas D. Marcotte and Igor Grant, *Editors*

PEDIATRIC NEUROPSYCHOLOGY:
RESEARCH, THEORY, AND PRACTICE, SECOND EDITION
Keith Owen Yeates, M. Douglas Ris, H. Gerry Taylor, and Bruce F. Pennington, *Editors*

Pediatric Neuropsychology

Research, Theory, and Practice

SECOND EDITION

Edited by
KEITH OWEN YEATES
M. DOUGLAS RIS
H. GERRY TAYLOR
BRUCE F. PENNINGTON

Series Editor's Note by Robert A. Bornstein

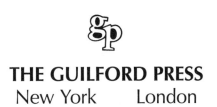

THE GUILFORD PRESS
New York   London

© 2010 The Guilford Press
A Division of Guilford Publications, Inc.
72 Spring Street, New York, NY 10012
www.guilford.com

Printed in the United States of America

This book is printed on acid-free paper.

Last digit is print number: 9   8   7   6   5   4   3   2   1

Library of Congress Cataloging-in-Publication Data

Pediatric neuropsychology: research, theory, and practice / editors, Keith Owen Yeates . . .
[et al.]. — 2nd ed.
        p. cm.
    Includes bibliographical references and index.
    ISBN 978-1-60623-465-5 (alk. paper)
    1. Pediatric neuropsychology.   I. Yeates, Keith Owen.
    RJ486.5.P435 2010
    618.92′8—dc22

                                                                          2009032255

About the Editors

Keith Owen Yeates, PhD, ABPP-CN, is Professor in the Departments of Pediatrics, Psychology, and Psychiatry at The Ohio State University in Columbus. He is also Director of the Center for Biobehavioral Health at The Research Institute and Chief of the Department of Psychology at Nationwide Children's Hospital. Dr. Yeates is a Fellow of the American Psychological Association (APA) and has served as President of the Division of Clinical Neuropsychology of the APA and of the Association of Postdoctoral Programs in Clinical Neuropsychology (APPCN). In 2004, he was named the Canadian Association of Child Neurology John Tibbles Lecturer by the Royal College of Physicians and Surgeons of Canada and was a Visiting Fellow of the Australian Psychological Society. Dr. Yeates has received over $10 million in grant funding for research that focuses on the neurobehavioral outcomes of childhood brain injuries and disorders and is a recipient of an Independent Scientist Career Development Award from the National Institutes of Health (NIH).

M. Douglas Ris, PhD, ABPP-CN, is Professor and Head of the Psychology Section in the Department of Pediatrics, Baylor College of Medicine. He is also Chief of the Psychology Service at Texas Children's Hospital in Houston. Previously, he founded and directed the Neuropsychology Program and the Pediatric Neuropsychology Postdoctoral Program at Cincinnati Children's Hospital Medical Center. Dr. Ris has held several leadership positions in the Division of Clinical Neuropsychology of the APA, the American Board of Clinical Neuropsychology, the International Neuropsychological Society, and the APPCN. As a clinical researcher, he has been awarded major funding from the National Institute of Environmental Health Sciences for his research on the neurodevelopmental effects of exposure to environmental lead and from the National Cancer Institute for his research on late effects in pediatric brain tumors.

H. Gerry Taylor, PhD, ABPP-CN, is Professor of Pediatrics at Case Western Reserve University and Rainbow Babies and Children's Hospital, University Hospitals of Cleveland. Dr. Taylor is a pediatric neuropsychologist with a background in clinical assessment of children. His research aims to better understand the effects of early neurological risks on the child and family, the neurological basis of developmental problems, and the influences of social and environmental factors on outcome. Dr. Taylor has conducted NIH-funded research on the outcomes of childhood neurological conditions, including traumatic brain injury and low birthweight, for more than 20 years. He is a past member of NIH review panels in behavioral medicine and maternal and child health, a past or present member of several journal editorial boards, currently associate editor for the *Journal of the International Neuropsychological Society*, and advisor or director of fellowship training programs in pediatric neuropsychology, pediatric psychology, and behavioral pediatrics.

Bruce F. Pennington, PhD, is a John Evans Professor of Psychology at the University of Denver, where he heads the Developmental Cognitive Neuroscience Program. He has conducted research for over 30 years on the genetics and neuropsychology of developmental disorders, including dyslexia, attention-deficit/hyperactivity disorder, autism, and intellectual disability syndromes. His honors include the Research Scientist, MERIT, and Fogarty awards from the National Institute of Mental Health; the Samuel T. Orton Award from the International Dyslexia Association; the Emanuel Miller Memorial Lecture from the British Association for Child and Adolescent Mental Health; and selection as a Fellow by the American Association for the Advancement of Science. Dr. Pennington has been the primary research supervisor for 35 doctoral and postdoctoral students, many of whom are now pursuing their own research on developmental disorders. In addition to his work as a researcher and a research mentor, he is also a child clinical neuropsychologist and has been active in clinical training and practice throughout his career.

Contributors

Richard Abbey, PhD, Child and Adolescent Psychiatry Clinic, Stanford University Medical Center, Stanford, California

Vicki Anderson, PhD, Department of Psychology, Royal Children's Hospital, Parkville, Australia

Marcia A. Barnes, PhD, Children's Learning Institute, Department of Pediatrics, University of Texas Health Science Center, Houston, Texas

Ida Sue Baron, PhD, ABPP-CN, Department of Pediatrics, Inova Fairfax Hospital for Children, Falls Church, Virginia

Anna W. Byars, PhD, Department of Pediatrics, Cincinnati Children's Hospital Medical Center, Cincinnati, Ohio

Benjamin J. Deery, PhD, Department of Psychology, Royal Children's Hospital, Parkville, Australia

Maureen Dennis, PhD, Department of Psychology and Research Institute, The Hospital for Sick Children, Toronto, Ontario, Canada

Kim N. Dietrich, PhD, Department of Environmental Health, University of Cincinnati College of Medicine, Cincinnati, Ohio

Linda Ewing-Cobbs, PhD, Children's Learning Institute, Department of Pediatrics, University of Texas Health Science Center, Houston, Texas

Janet E. Farmer, PhD, ABPP-RP, Thompson Center for Autism and Neurodevelopmental Disorders, University of Missouri–Columbia, Columbia, Missouri

Jack M. Fletcher, PhD, Department of Psychology, University of Houston, Houston, Texas

Lynn S. Fuchs, PhD, Department of Special Education, Vanderbilt University, Nashville, Tennessee

Maureen O'Kane Grissom, PhD, Thompson Center for Autism and Neurodevelopmental Disorders, University of Missouri–Columbia, Columbia, Missouri

Marianna E. Hayiou-Thomas, PhD, Department of Psychology, University of York, York, United Kingdom

Rani Jacobs, PhD, Department of Psychology, Royal Children's Hospital, Parkville, Australia

Angela E. John, MA, Department of Psychological and Brain Sciences, University of Louisville, Louisville, Kentucky

Stephen M. Kanne, PhD, ABPP-CN, Thompson Center for Autism and Neurodevelopmental Disorders, University of Missouri–Columbia, Columbia, Missouri

Andrew J. Kornberg, MB, Department of Psychology, Royal Children's Hospital, Parkville, Australia

Susan C. Levine, PhD, Department of Psychology, University of Chicago, Chicago, Illinois

Sarah N. Mattson, PhD, Department of Psychology, San Diego State University, San Diego, California

Carolyn B. Mervis, PhD, Department of Psychological and Brain Sciences, University of Louisville, Louisville, Kentucky

Pamela Moses, PhD, Department of Psychology, San Diego State University, San Diego, California

Ruth D. Nass, MD, Department of Neurology, New York University Medical Center, New York, New York

Sally Ozonoff, PhD, Department of Psychiatry and M.I.N.D. Institute, University of California Davis Medical Center, Sacramento, California

Bruce F. Pennington, PhD, Department of Psychology, University of Denver, Denver, Colorado

Robin L. Peterson, MA, Department of Psychology, University of Denver, Denver, Colorado

Judy S. Reilly, PhD, Department of Psychology, San Diego State University, San Diego, California

M. Douglas Ris, PhD, ABPP-CN, Department of Pediatrics, Baylor College of Medicine, Houston, Texas

Margaret J. Snowling, PhD, Department of Psychology, University of York, York, United Kingdom

Joan Stiles, PhD, Department of Cognitive Science, University of California, San Diego, California

H. Gerry Taylor, PhD, ABPP-CN, Department of Pediatrics, Case Western Reserve University, Cleveland, Ohio

Linnea Vaurio, MS, Department of Psychology, San Diego State University, San Diego, California

Michael Westerveld, PhD, ABPP-CN, Medical Psychology Associates, Florida Hospital, Orlando, Florida

Erik G. Willcutt, PhD, Department of Psychology and Neuroscience, University of Colorado, Boulder, Colorado

Keith Owen Yeates, PhD, ABPP-CN, Department of Pediatrics, The Ohio State University, and Center for Biobehavioral Health, The Research Institute at Nationwide Children's Hospital, Columbus, Ohio

Series Editor Note

The second edition of *Pediatric Neuropsychology: Research, Theory, and Practice* reflects the continuing growth of our understanding of the neuropsychological consequences of medical and neurodevelopmental disorders that affect children. This edition, as the first, reflects the vital integration among theory, research, and practice, which is fundamental to all disciplines that focus on the study of brain–behavior relationships. It contains a completely new section, as well as chapters written by new authors on topics similar to those in the first edition. The two editions share only four chapters written by the same authors on the same subjects. Thus, this is in many ways a companion volume to the original edition.

Yeates, Ris, Taylor, and Pennington present a fresh perspective on several topics from the first edition. In the coverage of medical disorders, the chapters on very low birthweight (Taylor), epilepsy (Westerveld), and brain tumors (Ris and Abbey) are written by new authors. Comparing these new chapters with the first edition affords the reader an opportunity to appreciate the different perspectives of leaders in these fields. This section also includes chapters on several disorders that are frequently not included in texts on pediatric neuropsychology including stroke (Stiles, Nass, Levine, Moses, and Reilly); tuberous sclerosis (Byars); encephalomyelitis and multiple sclerosis (Anderson, Deery, Jacobs, and Kornberg); and fetal alcohol (Mattson and Vaurio). The chapters on spina bifida and hydrocephalus (Fletcher and Dennis); brain injury (Yeates); and environmental toxicants (Dietrich) have all been updated to include the most recent research. The second edition also includes a completely new section on neurodevelopmental disorders, some of which are rarely incorporated in pediatric neuropsychology books. This section includes chapters on reading disability (Peterson and Pennington); language impairment (Snowling and Hayiou-Thomas); attention disorders (Willcutt); autism spectrum disorders (Ozonoff); math disabilities (Barnes, Fuchs, and Ewing-Cobbs); and intellectual disability (Mervis and John). There also is a new chapter on interventions (Kanne, Grissom, and Farmer) and one on an integrated theoretical structure for pediatric neuropsychological evaluations (Baron).

This volume is the sixth in The Guilford Press series *The Science and Practice of Neuropsychology*. The goal of this series is to integrate the scientific foundations and clinical applications of knowledge of brain–behavior relationships. The expansion of knowledge in pediatric neuropsychology and the appreciation that some disorders have different manifestations in children and adults have provided the basis for an increasingly science-based practice in pediatric neuropsychology. The contributors to this book are the leaders in their fields and exemplify this integration of theory and research into clinical practice.

—ROBERT A. BORNSTEIN, PhD

Preface

In the preface to the first edition of this book, which was published in 2000, the three of us serving as the original editors (Keith Owen Yeates, M. Douglas Ris, and H. Gerry Taylor) noted the need for a book that would provide an overview of neurological and medical conditions frequently seen in the practice of pediatric neuropsychology. At that time, few books focused on the neuropsychology of pediatric neurological and medical conditions. We felt that a book describing these conditions, reviewing their neuropsychological outcomes, critiquing the existing research, suggesting avenues for future exploration, and discussing the clinical implications of the existing knowledge base would make a valuable and unique contribution to the field, particularly for students and trainees seeking to become pediatric neuropsychologists.

To judge by the enthusiastic reception that the first edition received, our impression was correct. Nearly a decade later, we decided to undertake a second edition. The decision to do so reflected the tremendous growth that has occurred in pediatric neuropsychology since the first edition and the need to update the book to reflect this burgeoning knowledge base. However, we were also impressed that despite this growth, no other text was available that explored the boundaries of current research, theory, and practice by highlighting lacunae in the existing knowledge base for a broad range of childhood disorders. Several excellent texts are now available that focus on neuropsychological evaluation of children (Anderson, Northam, Hendy, & Wrennall, 2001; Baron, 2004; Baron, Fennell, & Voeller, 1995; Pennington, 2009), disturbances in neurocognitive functions in children (Reid & Warner-Rogers, 2008), or the treatment of neuropsychological disorders in children (Farmer, Donders, & Warschausky, 2006; Hunter & Donders, 2007). But the present book's emphasis on comprehensive reviews and scientific critiques of the empirical literature across the spectrum of pediatric neuropsychology remains unique.

The second edition differs from the first in several ways. Perhaps most significantly, the book continues to focus on summarizing the state of the art in neuropsychology research for childhood medical and neurological disorders, but we have added an entirely new section on developmental disorders. The decision to add this section was a response to reviews of the first edition that bemoaned the absence of chapters on common developmental disorders, such as reading disability. Reflecting this change is our addition of a fourth editor, Bruce F. Pennington, whose expertise in developmental disorders has been critical to the development of this new edition.

More than half of the chapters are new to the second edition. We have made significant changes to the list of medical/neurological disorders, excising 10 chapters on medical disorders that were in the previous edition (i.e., meningitis, neurofibromatosis, metabolic and neurodegenerative disorders, Turner syndrome, phenylketonuria, acute lymphoblastic leukemia, sickle cell disease, diabetes, end-stage renal disease, and human immunodeficiency virus) and adding 4 new chapters on other medical disorders (i.e., acute disseminated encephalomyelitis and childhood multiple sclerosis, tuberous sclerosis complex, perinatal stroke, and fetal alcohol spectrum disorders). The changes reflect our impression that some disorders have received relatively little research attention since the first edition and could therefore be dropped or that some disorders not covered in the first edition warranted coverage in the second. We have also added 6 new chapters on developmental disorders (i.e., math disabilities, reading disability, specific language impairment, attention-deficit/hyperactivity disorder, autism spectrum disorders, and intellectual disability syndromes). In sum, we have dropped 13 chapters from the first edition and added 11.

Our plan for the present book, as with the original, was to combine reviews of research on specific disorders with discussions of theoretical issues and clinical applications. Most of the conditions we have selected for inclusion are common in clinical practice, although we have again included a few that are less common or even unusual. All of the disorders have been foci of research that addresses critical issues regarding the neurobehavioral outcomes associated with childhood medical illnesses and neurodevelopmental disorders. Thus, although this book is not exhaustive, it encompasses a broad range of disorders, all of which have been the subjects of attention from pediatric neuropsychologists.

To ensure that the chapters on specific disorders would provide similar types of information, we again asked the authors to follow a common format. Most chapters begin with a section describing the condition's epidemiology, as well as its associated neural substrate or neuropathology and pathophysiology. The next section includes a description of the neurobehavioral outcomes associated with the disorder, as well as a critique of the existing research from both conceptual and methodological perspectives. The chapters generally conclude with a discussion of future directions for research on the disorder in question.

The book is divided into three parts. Part I contains 10 chapters devoted to specific neurological or other medical conditions. Part II consists of 6 chapters focusing on neurodevelopmental disorders. Finally, Part III concludes with 2 chapters focusing on the clinical implications of the knowledge base described in the preceding chapters, with one concerning neuropsychological evaluation and the other intervention. Although the book is not intended as a "how-to" guide to neuropsychological assessment or treatment, we believe it appropriate to include some consideration of how research on the neuropsychological consequences of medical conditions and developmental disorders is brought to bear on clinical practice.

In comparing the chapters in the second edition to those in the first, we are struck by several themes that have characterized the growth of pediatric neuropsychology over the past decade. First, the range of outcomes examined in research has broadened. Although neuropsychological research in the past tended to focus almost exclusively on cognitive functioning, in recent times a growing emphasis has been placed on noncognitive outcomes, such as social functioning, psychiatric disorder, adaptive behavior, and broader aspects of quality of life. Another theme consists of the tremendous advances in neuroimaging and their growing application to common childhood disorders. Both structural and functional imaging techniques are helping to deepen our understanding of the neural substrates of these disorders, as well as to raise interesting questions about the nature of brain–behavior relationships in childhood. In a related fashion, research in pediatric neuropsychology has increasingly begun to incorporate methods and theories drawn from the broader domain of neuroscience. A fourth theme is the growing recognition that the outcomes of childhood brain disorders are inherently multidetermined. Research on the determinants of outcomes has begun increasingly to reflect complex models that incorporate both biological and social predictors. A final theme is the increasing recognition of the importance of development in understanding outcomes. Development would seem to be the sine qua non of research in pediatric neuropsychology, yet most past studies have utilized cross-sectional designs that do not permit an examination of how development moderates outcomes. The growth of longitudinal studies that base comparisons on age at insult or onset and examine children's functioning across time has fostered a greater appreciation for the role of development in childhood brain disorders.

In contrast to these advances, the chapters in the new edition also reflect some themes that have not yet received much attention, but are likely to become topics of research in the future. Most neuropsychological research remains largely descriptive in nature. More research is needed that attempts to delineate the mechanisms accounting for the outcomes of childhood brain disorders. Future studies that investigate causal mechanisms will need to draw on theoretical models of brain–behavior relationships, developmental approaches to the outcomes of childhood brain disorders, and experimental paradigms based in part on brain injury research in animals. In this regard, neuropsychological research also has not tended to incorporate broader developmental theories. A rapprochement between developmental neuroscience and developmental psychology would help to advance the field. More generally, research needs to become interdisciplinary, incorporating multiple levels of analysis, and more translational, promoting the application of knowledge to clinical care. The scientific advances that have occurred over the past 10 years are not likely to affect the clinical management of children with brain disorders until efforts are made to empirically test interventions and treatments based on this knowledge. Our hopes are that this volume will help to push the field in that direction.

In summary, we believe that the new edition continues to provide a unique contribution to the field of pediatric neuropsychology. It spans a wide range of medical, neurological, and developmental conditions, and it provides current, in-depth reviews of empirical research on those conditions. The chapters have been written by recognized experts in the field of pediatric neuropsychology who have been actively involved in research on their chapter topics. Finally, and perhaps most important, the book continues to push the boundaries of current research, theory, and practice not only by highlighting what we know, but also by identifying areas in which further investigation is needed. Thus, the book not only reflects the tremendous growth in pediatric neuropsychology that has occurred in recent decades, but also foreshadows the scientific and professional journey to come. In so doing, it helps to ensure that we do not reach beyond our scientific boundaries in our clinical work with children. Indeed, the book presents principles of assessment and intervention precisely to encourage a closer examination of these practices in light of the existing knowledge base.

The book should be of interest to a wide audience of scientists and practitioners, including neuropsychologists, developmental neuroscientists, pediatric and child clinical psychologists, school psychologists, pediatric neurologists, child psychiatrists, behavioral–developmental pediatricians, and speech pathologists. It should also be of interest to graduate students, predoctoral psychology interns, and postdoctoral residents in neuropsychology. It is intended for use both as a primary text in graduate courses on pediatric neuropsychology, and as a resource on medical and neurodevelopmental conditions for the broad range of health care professionals who provide care to children.

The book could not have been completed without the help of many individuals, all of whom deserve our gratitude. First, we would like to thank the authors for their contributions. We appreciate the time and energy that they devoted to writing their chapters and their willingness to respond to our editorial suggestions for revisions. We would also like to thank our former and current students, interns, and postdoctoral fellows for the inspiration that they provided to undertake a second edition. Our editor at The Guilford Press, Rochelle Serwator, who has shepherded the book toward completion with just the right blend of encouragement and exhortation, deserves our thanks as well. Finally, we want to thank our friends and families for their ongoing support and understanding.

REFERENCES

Anderson, V., Northam, E., Hendy, J., & Wrennall, J. (2001). *Developmental neuropsychology: A clinical approach.* Hove, UK: Psychology Press.

Baron, I. S. (2004). *Neuropsychological evaluation of the child.* New York: Oxford University Press.

Baron, I. S., Fennell, E. B., & Voeller, K. S. (1995). *Pediatric neuropsychology in the medical setting.* New York: Oxford University Press.

Farmer, J. E., Donders, J., & Warschausky, S. (Eds.). (2006). *Treating neurodevelopmental disabilities: Clinical Research and Practice.* New York: Guilford Press.

Hunter, S. J., & Donders, J. (Eds.). (2007). *Pediatric neuropsychological intervention.* New York: Cambridge University Press.

Pennington, B. F. (2009). *Diagnosing learning disorders: A neuropsychological framework* (2nd ed.). New York: Guilford Press.

Reid, J., & Warner-Rogers, M. (Eds.). (2008). *Child neuropsychology: Concepts, theory, and practice.* Chichester, UK: Wiley–Blackwell.

Contents

PART II. NEURODEVELOPMENTAL DISORDERS

PART III. CLINICAL ASSESSMENT AND INTERVENTION

PEDIATRIC NEUROPSYCHOLOGY

PART I

MEDICAL DISORDERS

PART I

MEDICAL DISORDERS

CHAPTER 1

Spina Bifida and Hydrocephalus

JACK M. FLETCHER
MAUREEN DENNIS

S pina bifida meningomyelocele (SBM) is a major, disabling neurodevelopmental disorder. Over the last 20 years, knowledge about SBM has advanced on many fronts, allowing a fuller description of the condition. Of more importance, knowledge has been accrued in a way that associates outcomes for groups and individuals with multiple sources of variability that can be modeled in a principled manner in relation to genetic variation, structural anomalies of brain development, and cognitive function. The new knowledge about the complex interrelations among gene, brain, and behavior in SBM is proving to be relevant to a broader understanding of neurodevelopmental disorders. In this chapter, we review current understanding of outcomes in SBM, organized around five ideas:

1. SBM is one of a cluster of neurodevelopmental disorders that have hydrocephalus as a common complication.
2. Neurobehavioral outcomes of SBM can be modeled in a principled manner as a function of primary and secondary types of brain anomalies, genetic factors, and environmental factors.
3. There exists a modal cognitive profile in SBM that involves within-domain processing strengths and weaknesses, not cross-domain deficits or competencies.
4. Variability in outcomes around the modal cognitive profile can also be modeled in a principled manner as a function of primary and secondary types of brain anomalies, genetic factors, and environmental factors.
5. A limited number of core deficits underlie the modal profile.

HYDROCEPHALUS AS A COMMON FACTOR IN A CLUSTER OF NEURODEVELOPMENTAL DISORDERS

Hydrocephalus is a condition in which the ventricles fill with cerebrospinal fluid (CSF) and become enlarged. Although hydrocephalus is not a disease entity, it is the final common path of several neurodevelopmental conditions that have specific and measurable effects on the brain. Some of these effects are primary or congenital, and reflect the brain malformations that cause hydrocephalus, but also directly influence outcomes. Other effects are secondary, such as the destructive effects of hydrocephalus on the development of gray and white matter.

Gene–environment interactions cause the central nervous system (CNS) malformations underlying congenital hydrocephalus, most of which are prenatal. In addition, postnatal environmental factors (poverty, nutrition, and parenting) affect the development of a child with hydrocephalus. An adequate understanding of neuropsychological outcomes in different etiologies of early hydrocephalus requires consideration of each of these sources of variability, for outcomes are heterogeneous and varied. As we argued in the first edition of this book (Fletcher, Dennis, & Northrup, 2000), any investigation of neurobehavioral outcomes after early hydrocephalus should focus on the variability as well as the modal outcomes. There is a modal neurocognitive profile, but the departures from modal outcomes may be just as illuminating as the presence of the modal pattern.

Acquired hydrocephalus can occur at any age. In an adult, it may be associated with dementia-like conditions; in either a child or an adult, it may be associated with trauma, infections, tumors, or hemorrhages of the brain. In all these conditions of *acquired* hydrocephalus, the age of onset will vary unsystematically, so hydrocephalus is a secondary phenomenon that is less important in determining functional outcome than the primary traumatic, infectious, neoplastic, or hemorrhagic disorder.

Early Hydrocephalus

Hydrocephalus is commonly identified and treated before the first birthday, often within the first days of life. The principal etiologies of early-onset hydrocephalus involve congenital conditions that occur in association with neural tube defects (NTDs), essentially SBM and aqueductal stenosis (AS). In addition, intraventricular hemorrhage (IVH) associated with prematurity can cause hydrocephalus, along with Dandy–Walker syndrome (DWS). Although we focus on SBM in this chapter as the most common and best-understood form of early hydrocephalus, it is helpful to briefly consider other disorders associated with early hydrocephalus.

Less Frequent Etiologies of Early Hydrocephalus

AS develops because of a congenital narrowing of the cerebral aqueduct (Barkovich, 2005). It occurs in approximately 1 per 17,000 live births and is generally observed only in the presence of symptomatic hydrocephalus (Menkes, 1995). In contrast to SBM (and DWS), the cerebellum is generally normal, although some downward extension of the cerebellum may be present because of pressure effects from hydrocephalus. The only other neural anomalies involve partial callosal dysgenesis, along with the effects of hydrocephalus on brain development. Of all congenital etiologies of hydrocephalus, AS tends to have the most positive (Fletcher, Brookshire, Bohan, Brandt, & Davidson, 1995; Fletcher et al., 2004).

DWS is quite rare, occurring in about 1 per 30,000 live births (Menkes, 1995). The primary defining characteristic is the presence of a large cystic fourth ventricle, with partial to complete agenesis of the cerebellar vermis. The posterior fossa is enlarged, with substantial dilation of the fourth ventricle, which is usually treated by draining the cyst. Although the ventricular dilation could be characterized as hydrocephalus, it is really a cystic malformation that often requires shunting around the blockage created by the cyst (Chuang, 1986). Because of its rarity, and also because of the complexity of accurate diagnosis, we know relatively little about outcomes in DWS.

Children with prematurity-associated IVH develop hydrocephalus because of a hemorrhage of the germinal matrix shortly after birth. The presence of IVH is clearly related to perinatal asphyxia, with the hemorrhage occurring as part of a complex sequence of events involving problems with cerebral blood flow and perfusion. The germinal matrix hemorrhage bleeds into the ventricles and can obstruct the flow of CSF. Shunting is sometimes necessary, but arrested hydrocephalus is also a more common outcome in children with prematurity-associated IVH. Although prematurity-associated IVH was once estimated to occur in about half of all preterm infants, the incidence has been declining dramatically, and the condition now occurs infrequently in premature infants (Volpe, 2001). The presence of shunted hydrocephalus is clearly associated with more adverse outcomes in premature infants (Fletcher et al., 1997), but there is no specific neurobehavioral pattern. Neurobehavioral outcomes are influenced by many other factors associated with premature birth.

SBM: An Overview

In contrast to AS, DWS, and IVH, much more has become known about SBM—especially over the last decade, as studies have been flourishing in several domains of inquiry. Spina bifida (literally, "bifurcated spine") receives its name because of a defining defect in the closure of the neural tube at the spinal end that leads to a lesion along the spinal cord. It has a post-dietary-fortification rate of 0.3–0.5 per 1,000 live births; the decline over the past 20 years has been widely attributed to the emphasis on dietary supplementations of folate acid and Vitamin B (Williams, Rasmussen, Flores, Kirby, & Edmonds, 2005). Meningomyelocele is the most common form of spina bifida, representing an open lesion in the spinal cord through which the meninges protrude into a fluid-filled sac. Less common spinal defects include meningocele, a lesion in which the spinal cord is basically normal, but the meninges have herniated through the spinal opening. Like other less common forms of spina bifida, which involve fatty tumors (lipomas) and anatomic abnormalities of the spine (diastomyelia, occulta), meningoceles are not generally associated with neuropsychological deficits, although any form of spina bifida can impair ambulation and bladder control (Reigel & Rotenstein, 1994).

Despite the reduction in incidence, spina bifida is still the most common nonlethal NTD. Anencephaly, a lethal failure of the neural tube to close on the head end that results in an absence of the forebrain, has a roughly equal prevalence. Although spina bifida is defined by the presence of the spinal lesion, meningomyelocele is usually associated with a malformation of the cerebellum and hindbrain referred to as the Chiari II malformation, which causes hydrocephalus. The mechanism underlying the Chiari II malformation and hydrocephalus is essentially brain development in a small posterior fossa (McLone & Knepper, 1989), which leads to other anomalies, especially in the midbrain. Callosal dysgenesis, which is not caused by the Chiari II malformation, is also common. Not surprisingly, neurobehavioral outcomes are variable. Over the past two decades, neuropsychological studies have identified the major outcome domains affected by SBM, and have provided a picture of the prototypical impairments in children with this condition.

In the remainder of this chapter, we focus on SBM, presenting a model of outcomes in SBM. We expand on the arguments from our chapter in the first edition (Fletcher et al., 2000), which emphasize that multiple sources of variability affect outcomes in hydrocephalus and that these sources of variability can be modeled in a principled manner in relation to structural anomalies of brain development. However, we expand this modeling to consider primary and secondary types of brain anomalies, genetic and environmental factors, and core deficits that cut across traditional outcome domains and underlie domain-specific strengths and weaknesses. We present the model and then summarize the literature pertaining to the different components. We use the model as a context for understanding complicated neurogenetic disorders like SBM; we hope that this provides a more integrative account of neurobehavioral outcomes and their multiple sources of variability.

A MODEL OF NEUROBEHAVIORAL OUTCOMES IN SBM

Figure 1.1 presents a model of outcomes in SBM that begins at the level of gene–environment interactions and ends in a modal cognitive phenotype that is variably expressed, depending on the relation of associative and assembled processing (Dennis, Landry, Barnes, & Fletcher, 2006). The model begins with gene–environment interactions because NTDs like SBM are themselves the products of these interactions. Interactions at this level determine how the neural tube will be disrupted, which will include the type of NTD (e.g., anencephaly, spina bifida); the type of spinal lesion (meningocele, meningomyelocele); and the location of the defining defect, which can occur anywhere on the spinal cord. It is also likely that these factors influence the manifestations of the other primary brain malformations (e.g., severity of Chiari II malformation, presence and severity of callosal dysgenesis). It is also possible that some genetic factors more directly influence outcomes, although these are not depicted in Figure 1.1; such factors include the presence of genetic constellations associated with mental retardation, attention-deficit/hyperactivity disorder, and other outcomes. In addition, as Figure 1.1 shows, the nature of the environment influences the genetic expression of SBM.

SBM is a disorder with multiple phenotypes—neural, physical, and cognitive. These phenotypes are addressed in different parts of Figure 1.1, which distinguishes primary CNS insults to the spine (physical phenotype) and brain (neural phenotype) from secondary insults to the brain that involve hydrocephalus and its treatment (neural phenotype). These phenotypes vary within individuals with SBM and are not independent, because a more severe physical phenotype is usually associated with more severe brain dysmorphology (Fletcher et al., 2005). As Figure 1.1 shows, the cognitive phenotype is ultimately depen-

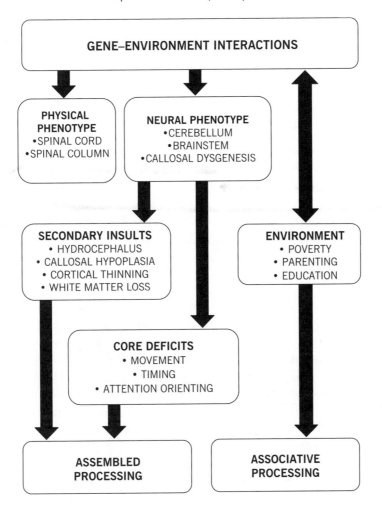

FIGURE 1.1. A model of spina bifida showing the links of gene-environment interactions with the physical and neural phenotypes, environmental factors, and the resultant cognitive phenotype.

dent not only on the neural and physical phenotypes, but also on factors involving the environment that influence postnatal development (e.g., poverty, parenting).

Physical Phenotype

SBM is usually identified at birth or through prenatal ultrasonography because of the spinal lesion and sometimes because of hydrocephalus. The spinal lesion almost always leads to impairment of the lower extremities, a neurogenic bladder and incontinence, and other orthopedic abnormalities. The orthopedic impairments, including paraplegia, vary with spinal lesion level: The higher the lesion, the greater the orthopedic impairment (and corresponding severity of brain malformations). In addition, higher lesions are associated with poorer cognitive and motor outcomes, most likely because the neural phenotype is more severe (Fletcher et al., 2005).

Neural Phenotype

Primary CNS Insults

At the level of the brain, most children with SBM have the Chiari II malformation; this involves herniation of a compressed cerebellum through the exits of the fourth ventricle, and causes obstruction of the flow of CSF in the fourth and/or third ventricles. Partial dygenesis of the corpus callosum is commonly observed in children with SBM, representing a congenital defect that occurs as a result of the disruption in neuroembryogensis characteristic of NTDs (Barkovich, 2005). Finally, abnormalities of the midbrain (e.g., tectal beaking) occur in about 65% of children (Fletcher et al., 2005). These abnormalities occur because the posterior fossa is too small to promote normal growth and causes compression. Each of these primary CNS anomalies occurs during gestation and can be shown to directly affect neurobehavioral outcomes.

Secondary Effects of Hydrocephalus

Secondary CNS effects reflect the variable impact of hydrocephalus, which has significant consequences for brain development (Aoyama, Kinoshita, Yokota, & Hamada, 2006; Del Bigio, 1993, 2004). The effects are most visibly apparent in the degree to which the corpus callosum is thinned, although recent studies based on radiological review (Miller, Widjaja, Blaser, Dennis, & Raybaud, 2008) and diffusion tensor imaging (DTI) are showing that the extent of white matter alteration extends far beyond the corpus callosum and is likely not due just to hydrocephalus (Hasan et al., 2008a, 2008b; Vachha, Adams, & Rollins, 2006). There is significant volume loss of both cerebral gray and white matter, which tends to be greater in posterior regions of the cerebral hemispheres.

Regardless of etiology, hydrocephalus is always due to an obstruction that blocks the flow of CSF (Raimondi, 1994). The site of the blockage varies, depending in part on the etiology. In addition, the condition may be progressive or arrested. The former often requires aggressive neurosurgical intervention, such as the insertion of a shunt to divert the flow of CSF around the obstruction. *Arrested* hydrocephalus, also referred to as *compensated* or *nonprogressive* hydrocephalus, indicates the presence of large ventricles with pressure effects from the accumulation of CSF. In arrested hydrocephalus, the relations of CSF production and absorption were obstructed but then became balanced, leaving residual dilation of the ventricles, or ventriculomegaly (McCullough, 1990). The interventions themselves can contribute to variability in outcomes as shunts become obstructed or infected, leading to additional neurosurgical interventions.

Cognitive Phenotype

In depicting the nature of neurobehavioral outcomes in SBM, Figure 1.1 makes a distinction between core deficits in assembled and associative processing. We argue that a modal neurocognitive profile associated with SBM can be described in terms of strengths and weaknesses within each of a set of content domains (see Figure 1.2). Thus neuropsychological research studies using psychometric tests have differentiated preserved and impaired functions within a number of cognitive and academic domains.

ASSOCIATIVE PROCESSING
- Data- or stimulus-driven
- Involves formation of associations
- Adaptive changes in response to stimulus repetition
- Categorization of stimulus information

ASSEMBLED PROCESSING
- Model- or concept-driven
- Involves assembly of models of input
- Requires dissociation, suppression, disengagement, and contingent relations

Domain	ASSETS	DEFICITS
MOTOR	Adaptation (e.g., mirror drawing)	Online control (e.g., tracking)
PERCEPTION	Categories (e.g., face recognition)	Relations (e.g., mental rotations)
MEMORY	Implicit (e.g., priming)	Explicit (e.g., episodic recall)
LANGUAGE	Stipulation (e.g., word definitions)	Construction (e.g., inferences)
READING	Decoding (e.g., word recognition)	Comprehension (e.g., text meaning)
MATH	Numbers (e.g., exact calculation)	Algorithms (e.g., estimations)

FIGURE 1.2. The relation of assembled and associative processing and domain-specific functional assets and deficits that make up the cognitive phenotype.

Cross-Domain Comparisons

As a group, children with SBM and lower-level spinal lesions (lumbar and sacral) are stronger in language and weaker in perceptual and motor skills, as demonstrated through many comparisons of Verbal and Performance IQ scores (Dennis et al., 1981; Fletcher et al., 1992; Raimondi & Soare, 1974). Within the language domain, children with SBM use and understand single words with some skill; however, many of these children have significant problems with language at the level of text and discourse—in other words, an inability to use and understand language in a flexible and adaptive manner (Barnes & Dennis, 1992, 1998; Dennis, Jacennik, & Barnes, 1994). These problems with language integration also interfere with reading comprehension (Barnes & Dennis, 1998). In terms of academic competencies, math is commonly impaired relative to word recognition skills, and writing problems are common (Barnes et al., 2002; Dennis & Barnes, 2002). Studies involving memory and learning functions show significant problems on different indices of short-term memory, especially list learning, in groups with SBM (Scott et al., 1998; Yeates, Enrile, Loss, Blumenstein, & Delis, 1995). Some attention and executive regulation skills may also be impaired (Brewer, Fletcher, Hiscock, & Davidson, 2001; Fletcher et al., 1996), but, as with memory, skills within this domain are not uniformly impaired. Behavioral studies generally show higher rates of adjustment difficulties, but specific types of adjustment difficulties have not been identified, other than a higher rate of internalized than externalized difficulties (Greenley, Holmbeck, Zuckerman, & Buck, 2006) and an elevated rate of inattention (Burmeister et al., 2005).

Core Deficits Underlying Cross-Domain Cognitive Assets and Deficits

We propose, first, that core processing deficits involving movement, timing, and attention orientation underlie these content domain assets and deficits; and, second, that the modal cognitive phenotype is not domain-specific, but represents manifestations of unobservable constructs involving assembled and associative processing. *Assembled* cognitive processes involve the ability to construct and integrate information, whereas *associative* cognitive processes involve the ability to activate or categorize information. Assembled processing directly reflects the impact of the primary and secondary CNS factors on core deficits involving movement, timing, and attention orienting that cut across content domains. Associative processes would be preserved in children with SBM, were it not for the secondary CNS insults and environmental factors (e.g., poverty, parenting, and education) that lead to reduced capabilities subsumed by this construct. The preservation of strengths in associative processing, and thus the presence of both strengths and weaknesses, depend in part on the severity of the CNS deficits in SBM and in part on the impact of the environment.

Processing differences have long been identified as dichotomies, such as holistic–analytic and global–local. Historically, the holistic–analytic distinction has been linked strongly to hemispheric lateralization (e.g., holistic to right-hemisphere and analytic to left-hemisphere function), and the global–local distinction to processing within the spatial content domain. No form of neural or cognitive processing is strictly parallel or serial; rather, each has elements of both. In characterizing the differences between the kinds of tasks individuals with SBM can and cannot perform, we need terms that are not tied to hemispheric asymmetry or to particular content domains, and that are congruent with current thinking about cognitive processing across content domains and materials.

We have adopted the terms *assembled processing* and *associative processing* to characterize functional outcome for individuals with SBM, which involves assets in stimulus-driven associative processing and deficits in model-driven assembled processing. Figure 1.2 provides definitions of these constructs and examples of assets and deficits within each content domain.

In the next sections of this chapter, we expand on selected portions of the model, beginning with an examination of gene–environment interactions in SBM and focusing on lesion level as a phenotypic factor tied to expressions of the genotype and both the neural and cognitive phenotypes. We then examine studies of the impact of the primary CNS insults on the core deficits in movement, timing, and attention orienting, highlighting their impact on assembled processing. A review of secondary CNS events that moderate outcomes associated with assembled processing, and of environmental factors that moderate outcomes related to associative processing, is then provided. The chapter concludes with a discussion of relations with other disorders and other models of outcomes in SBM.

GENE–ENVIRONMENT INTERACTIONS

SBM is a heterogeneous disorder with a multifactorial etiology involving genetic and environmental factors. There is a very early disruption of neuroembryogensis that is variable, suggesting that many genes may be involved, and that their influence is also modified by the environment and therefore related to variations in the physical and neural phenotypes associated with spina bifida. Understanding these factors in SBM requires an appreciation of the factors that produce NTDs, the second most common congenital birth defects (after conditions affecting the heart) in North America (Detrait et al., 2005). NTDs occur at a rate of about 1 per 1,000 births in North America (mostly SBM and anencephaly), but rates are much higher in some part of the world.

Spina bifida and its different types (meningomyelocele, meningocele, occulta, lipoma) represent just one kind of NTD. Anencephaly occurs at rates that are comparable to meningomyelocele, representing a failure of the neural tube to close at the caudal end. This produces a child with essentially no cerebral cortex and is usually a lethal defect. Like SBM, anencephaly can be considered an "open" NTD, whereas other NTDs occur under the surface of the skin and do not protrude as in anencephaly and SBM.

The NTDs that result in different types of spina bifida occur in the first month of gestation, during the process of primary neurulation (see Detrait et al., 2005, for a summary of neurulation). Although the process that leads to the abnormalities of the neural tube is well understood, less clear is how the neural tubes are fused, which is the last stage of development (Detrait et al., 2005). Different models propose single-site theories, in which fusion occurs at a single site and proceeds up and down the neural tube, or multisite theories (van Allen et al., 1993). Multisite theories propose that the neural folds are fused in multiple locations, and that where on the neural tube fusion is disrupted may explain different kinds of NTDs. van Allen et al. (1993) have proposed two points at which closure occurs, one cervical and the other a lower site with a proposed meeting point at L_1–L_2. Other research has suggested alternative closure sites (Detrait et al., 2005), but the point is that multisite models yield hypotheses that help explain the variable presentation of lesion level in SBM (Northrup & Volcik, 2000).

Genetic factors are clearly involved in NTDs and specifically in SBM. The genotype is almost certainly multifactorial (Detrait et al., 2005; Kirkpatrick & Northrup, 2003). NTDs, including SBM, are commonly seen in a variety of syndromes with known genetic causes. Within families, the recurrence risk rises with increases in the number of affected family members, almost doubling with the birth of each additional affected child (Toriello & Higgins, 1983). Children with an affected sibling have a risk of 2–5%, which is 25–50 times the population risk. For a third-degree relative, the risk is reduced to that of the general population (Elwood, Little, & Elwood, 1992).

Specific-gene-searching studies are based on animal models of NTDs as well as human studies. According to Detrait et al. (2005), animal models implicate over 80 mutations and over 100 genes in NTDs. These findings are not strongly linked to human findings, which focus on genes involved in neural growth and development, folate metabolism, and glucose metabolism. Genes related to folate metabolism are interesting because of the evidence that prenatal supplementation of the diet with folate and Vitamin B reduces the incidence of NTDs by 50–70% (Northrup & Volcik, 2000). Women with affected children have elevations of homocysteine, which may occur in association with problems with the metabolism of folate acid. A number of genes related to folate metabolism have been identified as risk factors for SBM (Kirkpatrick & Northrup, 2003; Rozen, 1997). Mutations of these genes vary across ethnic groups in much the same way as differences in the rates of NTDs do: common among Hispanics and whites, and rare in blacks (Botto, Moore, Khoury, & Erickson, 1999). Glucose genes are implicated because of the elevated rates of NTDs in diabetic mothers, while growth factor genes relate to early neural development.

Various environmental factors are also involved in NTDs and may moderate the expression of different genes (Kirkpatrick & Northrup, 2003). The most significant factors involve diet. Surveillance reports from the Centers for Disease Control and Prevention indicate that the incidence of NTDs has decreased by about 20% for NTDs since the initiation of food fortification began in the United States (Centers for Disease Control and Prevention, 1993; Honein, Paulozzi, Mathews, Erickson, & Wong, 2001). How folate prevents NTDs is not well understood.

Maternal diabetes and obesity are also associated with an increased risk of NTDs. Independent of folate intake and family history of NTDs, maternal obesity prior to pregnancy increases risk for an NTD (Northrup & Volcik, 2000). For mothers with diabetes, the risk of NTDs is two to three times higher than in the general population (Northrup & Volcik, 2000). These findings are usually related to issues involving mutations affecting glucose metabolism.

Other environmental risk factors include environmental teratogens, as well as radiation exposure and anticonvulsants (Shurtleff & Lemire, 1995). The former is commonly observed in polluted areas of the world, while the latter reflects the increased risk of NTDs (about 10 times the rate of the general population) in mothers with epilepsy who use anticonvulsants in early pregnancy (Northrup & Volcik, 2000). Maternal illness and exposure to hyperthermia early in fetal development because of hot baths, fever, and saunas also increase NTD risk (Botto et al., 1999). The mechanisms by which these factors affect neurulation and result in NTDs are not well understood.

The clearest link of how variability at the level of gene–environment interactions influences the multiple phenotypes in SBM comes from an examination of lesion level. To reiterate, the type of NTD—and, in the case of SBM, the location of the spinal lesion— are products of gene–environment interactions. But lesion level varies from lower sacral levels to the upper thoracic level. Genetic heterogeneity in SBM accounts for variations in lesion level, with some research showing variations in the genotype even within ethnic groups (Northrup & Volcik, 2000). In terms of the classifications derived from genetic studies, lesion level is also associated with variability in the physical, neural, and cognitive phenotypes. To understand the neuropsychological outcomes associated with spina bifida, we must reliably classify the nature of the spinal lesion and its location, and also take into account the socioeconomic status (SES) and ethnicity of the family. The latter are important clinical markers of heterogeneity, although most existing studies of the neuropsychological outcomes of spina bifida are based on European American populations with lower-level lesions.

At some point, extrapolations from the genotype to the neural and cognitive phenotypes may be possible. For now, we turn to relations of the neural phenotype with the physical and cognitive phenotypes.

PRIMARY CNS INSULTS AND CORE DEFICITS

At the heart of the model in Figure 1.1 is a hypothesized link between primary CNS insults and core deficits involving timing, attention orienting, and movement. The primary CNS insults are direct products of gene–environment interactions, including the type and level of the spinal lesion, the Chiari II malformation, midbrain defects, and callosal dysgenesis. *Core deficits* are defined as impairments that (1) emerge early in development and persist into adulthood; (2) are apparent in tasks that invoke different assembled processes; (3) appear over a range of ability levels (i.e., are not simply a product of general cognitive functioning); (4) are weakly related to other core deficits; (5) are correlated with assessments of the primary brain insults; and (6) demonstrate little functional plasticity in relation to age. Elsewhere (Dennis et al., 2006), we and our colleagues have reviewed the evidence for both the primary CNS insults and the basis for identifying core deficits in timing, attention, and movement. In the discussion that follows, we examine this evidence.

Spinal Lesion

The strongest evidence linking genotype and phenotype is from research showing that genetic heterogeneity accounts for variations in spinal lesion level in the expression of NTDs (e.g., King et al., 2007; Volcik et al., 2000). This link can also be generalized from relations of lesion level and both the neural and cognitive phenotypes, although not directly from the genotype to the neural and cognitive phenotypes. This is a topic of active investigation. However, as noted earlier, lesion level is related to neural and cognitive outcomes: The higher the lesion, the lower the level of cognitive functions and the greater the number of neural anomalies (Badell-Ribera, Shulman, & Riddock, 1966; Fletcher et al., 2005; Lonton, 1977).

As we have also indicated above, there are several types of spinal lesions, the most common of which is a meningomyelocele. Identifying the type of spinal lesion is important, because only meningomyelocele is associated with changes in the neural phenotype. Other spinal lesions (meningocele, lipoma, diastomyelia) account for fewer than 20% of cases of spina bifida (Menkes, 1995). Although all spinal lesions affect orthopedic and urological function to some degree, depending on the level of the lesion, the impairment is more severe in meningomyelocele (Norman, McGillivray, Kalousek, Hill, & Poskitt, 1995).

To illustrate, in our sample of 323 children with spina bifida (Fletcher et al., 2004), 295 have meningomyelocele; 93% (n = 276) of those with SBM are shunted for hydrocephalus. Of the other 7% without shunts, 5% (n = 15) have magnetic resonance imaging (MRI) evidence of arrested hydrocephalus, and 2% (n = 6) have no evidence of ventricular dilation. Of the 28 children with meningocele and other spinal lesions, 2 are shunted for hydrocephalus. Neither has a Chiari II malformation, and both probably have hydrocephalus due to AS. Of the other 26, 6 have arrested hydrocephalus, and 20 have no hydrocephalus. Other than the 2 cases with shunted hydrocephalus due to AS and the 6 with arrested hydrocephalus, the MRIs of children with other spinal lesions were read with virtually no abnormalities (e.g., cerebellum and corpus callosum were normal). Even at the level of ambulation, half of the children with SBM and shunts use wheelchairs; this is true for only 5% of the mixed group with evidence of arrested hydrocephalus, and none of the children with other spinal lesions and no hydrocephalus. For research purposes, adding children who do not have SBM and are not shunted for hydrocephalus to a sample reduces the neural morbidity and the likelihood of cognitive difficulties. An interesting issue is the current trend in some neurosurgical centers toward avoiding shunting of children with SBM for as long as possible. This trend will make it even more important to examine lesion type, since only meningomyelocele is consistently associated with congenital brain anomalies (Reigel & Rotenstein, 1994).

Lesion level is clearly related to the core deficit in movement that characterizes children with SBM from birth. Infants with SBM have poorer upper- and lower-limb movement quality (Landry, Lomax-Bream, & Barnes, 2003). Movement deficits vary in severity but are lifelong, and are likely to contribute to cognitive deficits because of the restrictions in environmental search and play present from birth. Deficits in movement and visual–motor control are apparent in children and adolescents with SBM (Dennis, Fletcher, Rogers, Hetherington, & Francis, 2002; Hetherington & Dennis, 1999). The physical limitations on movement of the lower limbs extend to the eyes (Biglan, 1995) and the upper limbs, although these limitations are probably related to the effects of the cerebellum on upper-extremity movement and of the cerebellum, midbrain, and hydrocephalus on ocular control (Salman et al., 2005).

Cerebellum

The Chiari II malformation is a congenital deformity of the brainstem and cerebellum that occurs in virtually all births involving meningomyelocele (Barkovich, 2005; Reigel & Rotenstein, 1994). In a study of qualitative coding of structural MRIs in a sample of 191 children with SBM (Fletcher et al., 2004), 96% of children with spinal lesions at T_{12} and higher met criteria for a Chiari II malformation; 90% of children with SBM and spinal lesions below T_{12} met Chiari II criteria. In both groups, only 4 children had normal cerebellums. Cerebellar deficits lead to difficulties with control of motor movements, including truncal and axial movement (Miall, Reckess, & Imamizu, 2001), and, along with the midbrain, to problems with control of eye movements (Leigh & Zee, 1999).

The cerebellar impairments extend to a variety of cognitive functions because of their effects on timing, another core deficit. In this context, *timing* refers to a person's capacity to process temporal information that permits the synchronization of sensation and movement across small (half-second or less) time intervals. The cerebellum acts like a timer of perceptual experiences, which helps generate predictions about the consequences of movement. Infants with SBM show less synchronous and more poorly organized upper-limb coordination (Landry et al., 2003). Children and adolescents with SBM have deficits in short-duration timing on both perceptual and motor timing tasks (Dennis et al., 2004). Within the perceptual domain, these children and adolescents show deficits on a timing discrimination task (judging durations of about 400 ms) although not on a pitch discrimination task (judging frequencies at about 3,000 Hz), showing that the deficit is specific to timing and not a result of a general perceptual impairment. Within the motor domain, children with SBM can tap along in synchrony with a computerized beat, but are unable to maintain the tapping when the beat stops (Dennis et al., 2004). Relative to controls, children with SBM show significantly small cerebellar volumes on quantitative MRI studies (Fletcher et al., 2005). In school-age children with SBM, perceptual and motor timing deficits are correlated with these reductions in cerebellar volume (Dennis et al., 2004).

Early motor development includes aspects of timing and contributes to cognitive development (Bushnell & Boudreau, 1993; Gibson, 1982; Thelen & Smith, 1994). In infants with SBM, early deficits in the regulation of motor movements predict subsequent abilities involving visual search and memory (Landry et al., 2003). Many tasks involving eye–hand coordination require synchrony of sensation and movement, which in turn requires ongoing, online integration of temporal information (Hore, Ritchie, & Watts, 1999).

Brainstem and Midbrain

The Chiari II malformation includes a small posterior fossa, which results in distortion of the posterior fossa contents and their herniation through the foramen magnum. Because of the small posterior fossa, many individuals with SBM have abnormalities of the brainstem, such as tectal beaking. In the Fletcher et al. (2005) study, 96% of those with upper-level lesions and 80% with lower-level lesions had tectal beaking, and about 60% of both groups had other midbrain anomalies.

The midbrain is partly responsible for control of eye movements, which are impaired in children with SBM (Salman et al., 2005). The midbrain, including the superior colliculus, is part of a brain circuit that orients attention to salient aspects of the environment, which we have defined as a core deficit. Children with SBM and abnormalities of the midbrain and tectum are impaired on a variety of paradigms assessing attention orienting, including tasks requiring overt shifts of eye movement, and covert shifts of attention. These impairments in attention orienting are more apparent in those with tectal beaking, including more difficulties orienting to salience (Dennis et al., 2005a) and a more attenuated inhibition of return response in the vertical plane (Dennis et al., 2005b). Infants with SBM show reduced orienting to salient faces and take longer than similar-age peers to shift from a perceptually salient stimulus (a beeping light) to a second, face stimulus (Taylor, Landry, Cohen, Barnes, & Swank, 2008). The deficit in attention orienting is selective, as children with SBM do not have difficulty orienting to cognitively interesting stimuli that are under goal-directed, top-down control (Dennis et al., 2005a). Thus, given the evidence for two attention systems in the brain (Posner & Raichle, 1994)—one involving a stimulus-driven, automatic response to salience, and the other a goal-directed engagement based on the regulatory influences of knowledge and expectations of cognitively engaging stimuli—children with SBM have difficulty with the former. The nature of the difficulty is consistent with the brainstem and midbrain pathology characteristic of many individuals with SBM.

Callosal Dysgenesis

About half of children with SBM show partial dysgenesis of the corpus callosum, reflecting further disruption of neuroembryogensis during the period (7–20 weeks gestational age) corresponding to the development of the corpus callosum (Barkovich, 2005; Hannay, 2000). These anomalies are considered congenital because the ends of the corpus callosum (rostrum, splenium) are most commonly missing; the destructive effects of hydrocephalus usually affect the middle structures, often stretching and thinning the entire corpus callosum. In the Fletcher et al. (2004) study, 4% had a normal corpus callosum, 52% had dysgenesis usually in association with hypoplasia, and 44% had only hypoplasia. There were no cases of complete dysgenesis.

The relation of callosal dysgenesis to core deficits is less direct than the relation of other primary CNS insults to timing, attention-orienting, and movement deficits. Three general patterns are available. First, area measurements of the corpus callosum have been correlated with measures of fine motor skills and spatial processing (Fletcher et al., 1996), most likely representing a marker for more general disturbances of neural connectivity.

Second, patterns of aberration are related to performance on measures of interhemispheric communication. Hannay et al. (2008) administered a dichotic listening test to 90 children with SBM and 28 normal controls. Typically developing controls demonstrated the expected right-ear advantage (REA). Children with SBM who were right-handed, had a normal/hypoplastic splenium, and/or had lower-level lesions were more likely to show the expected REA. Children with splenial dysgenesis did not show the REA. In other analyses not reported by Hannay et al., the area measurement of the corpus callosum was correlated significantly ($r = .40$) with the number of stimuli correctly identified on the first trial in the right ear. Thus interhemispheric transfer is impaired in children with SBM, but the extent of this compromise depends on the integrity of the corpus callosum, as well as handedness and lesion level.

Primary CNS insults are linked to assembled processing. Huber-Okrainek, Blaser, and Dennis (2005) found that children with SBM had difficulty integrating context to determine the meaning of an idiom, especially those who had dysgenesis of the splenium of the corpus callosum. Corpus callosum dysgenesis is a marker for reduced connectivity across the brain, consistent with MRI DTI studies of disrupted integrity of white matter and association fibers in SBM (Hasan et al., 2008a).

SECONDARY CNS INSULTS AND ASSEMBLED PROCESSES

Figure 1.1 shows that primary CNS insults cause secondary CNS insults. This link reflects mostly the connection of the Chiari II malformation and hydrocephalus, which thins the brain in a posterior–anterior direction. Hydrocephalus destroys cerebral gray matter and stretches and thins the white matter. Thus, in the Fletcher et al. (2005) study, voxel-based MRI morphometry of the cerebral cortex (excluding the cerebellum and brainstem) of children with SBM showed significant reductions in gray matter and white matter in regions marked by the corpus callosum—essentially those regions subtending the corpus callosum (pericallosal) and posterior to the splenium (retrocallosal). There was little reduction in areas anterior to the genu (precallosal). Relative to controls, the reductions amounted to a volume loss of about 2.3% in gray matter and 2.6% in white matter, and a corresponding increase in CSF (total volume about 8.7% vs. 3.9% in controls).

These reductions are related to a variety of cognitive and motor skills. Correlations between the CSF measure within the group with SBM (Spearman's rho) and tasks involving verbal reasoning, visual–spatial skills (a composite of Stanford–Binet Visual/Abstract Reasoning and the Beery Developmental Test of Visual–Motor Integration), fine motor skills, word recognition, and math computations revealed a pattern of weak but consistent relationships. There were no significant correlations with precallosal CSF. Pericallosal CSF and postcallosal CSF were correlated with all these measures except word identification ($p < .0006$; range $= -.34$ to $-.50$). Since CSF volumes are crude indices of the degree of hydrocephalus (after shunting), these results show effects on motor tasks involving movement and timing, as well as on other tasks that invoke assembled processing at the level of functional deficits—but not on word identification, which is a strong marker of associative processing. A weakness of this prediction is the evidence that complications related to shunting (e.g., infections) and other problems (e.g., seizures) have a weak but generalized effect on the brain and on cognition (Dennis et al., 1981).

ENVIRONMENTAL FACTORS AND ASSOCIATIVE PROCESSING

Poverty is associated with restricted diets and exposures to environmental teratogens that increase risk for NTDs (Kirkpatrick & Northrup, 2003). In addition, the relation of poverty to language/achievement is well established and holds in SBM. The Fletcher et al. (2005) study found clear evidence of generalized relations between poverty and performance on neurocognitive tests. Similarly, Lomax-Bream, Barnes, Copeland, Taylor, and Landry (2007a), in a study of infants with SBM and typically developing controls from birth to 3 years, found a main effect of SES on mental and motor outcomes, but no interactions. Similarly, in a study of school-age children with SBM, Holmbeck et al. (2003) reported that SES and SBM were additive in increasing risk for psychosocial difficulties, relative to the effects of just lower SES or SBM alone.

There are also links between specific psychosocial factors and outcomes. Lomax-Bream et al. (2007b) found that higher-quality parenting was associated with higher performance on assessments of mental development and language in infants with spina bifida and controls followed from 6 to 36 months. However, on daily living skills, an interaction of parenting and group indicated that higher-quality parenting was not associated with higher levels of performance in the group with spina bifida—only for the typically developing children. This finding is different from studies of other groups of high-risk infants (e.g., premature children), where parenting is a significant moderator of development. In another study, Seefeldt, Holmbeck, Belvedere, Gorey-Ferguson, and Hudson (1997) also evaluated parenting in a sample of families with a school-age child with SBM and controls. They found that lower-SES families with a child with SBM were much more likely to show autocratic parenting styles, compared to families with only one of these risk factors.

Children with SBM are clearly at risk for psychosocial difficulties because of the problems associated with the physical phenotype. Varying degrees of ambulatory difficulties as well as the bladder and bowel problems put them at risk for peer issues, familial stress, and other negative societal reactions. Learning to catheterize and independently manage the bowel/bladder problems reduces this risk. In addition, children with SBM also experience many surgical and medical procedures related to their orthopedic problems (spinal cord, hips, back) and to shunting. Finally, SBM leads to cognitive difficulties that could potentially affect the development of social skills, family functioning, peer relations, and response to schooling—all of which have an impact on children's overall adjustment.

To illustrate, psychosocial factors in SBM have been researched in a series of studies by Holmbeck and associates, bolstered by a recent review of the literature (Holmbeck, Greenley, Coakley, Greco, & Hagstrom, 2006). Across studies, Holmbeck et al. (2006) found that relatively few families with a child with SBM exhibit family dysfunction at clinically significant levels, with rates of about 12%. The authors also noted that families tend to be resilient. However, many parents exhibit significant psychological distress, particularly internalizing difficulties. The parents of children with SBM often feel less confident and less optimistic about the future. Findings of marital dysfunction are inconsistent, but may be predicted by the quality of the marital relationship prior to the birth of the affected child. Siblings do not seem to show major adjustment problems specific to SBM. On average, parents tend to exercise more control and can be overprotective of their affected child, but this is influenced by cognitive ability. Lower-functioning children with SBM tend to have parents who feel the need to exercise more control and provide less fostering of autonomy. Holmbeck et al. (2006) noted that families with multiple adjustment issues may be at higher risk for psychosocial difficulties. Altogether, Holmbeck et al. (2006) concluded that "spina bifida appears to disrupt some aspect of family and parent functioning for many families, but such families also tend to demonstrate considerable resilience across other adjustment domains" (p. 253).

FUNCTIONAL ASSETS AND DEFICITS

At this point in the model, we begin to deal with traditional neuropsychological outcomes. These are typically portrayed in terms of the pervasive weaknesses that children and adults with SBM display in motor and perceptual skills, and the strengths they demonstrate in language and reading. But as the examples of language and reading make clear, the dissociation depends on the extent to which the outcome task draws upon associative and assembled processing. It is likely that a child with SBM will show stronger performance on measures of language vocabulary and word decoding than on measures involving the comprehension of narrative discourse or on reading comprehension tasks (Figure 1.2). The latter demand processes that are integrated and constructive (which we have portrayed as associative processes), whereas the former demand processes that are more encapsulated and modular (which we have depicted as assembled processes). Whether an individual child with SBM displays the specific set of functional assets within the language and reading domains depends on the severity of the child's Chiari II malformation and the associated hydrocephalus; on treatment factors related to shunt revisions, infections, and other sources of diffuse injury; and on environmental factors like poverty. Thus one of the more commonly reported discrepancies in outcomes attributed to SBM—the discrepancy in Verbal and Performance IQ—is most apparent in European Americans of middle-class origins who have lower spinal lesions and fewer shunt revisions/infections. Such a pattern is less apparent in children with SBM and upper-level lesions, or in Hispanics. As a group, Hispanics with SBM are more likely to have upper-level spinal lesions, and in North America thy are also more likely to grow up in families of lower SES.

Although much has been learned from comparisons across domains in SBM, we believe that the value of examining variability within domains is apparent not only from the examples from the language and reading domains we have provided, but also from other domains. As Figure 1.2 demonstrates, although the motor and spatial processing problems of children with SBM are well known, several studies demonstrate preservation of skills involved in motor learning (Colvin, Yeates, Enrile, & Coury, 2003; Edelstein et al., 2004). This dissociation emerges not only for the hand, but also for the eye. Similarly, in the spatial domain, facial recognition and simple match-to-sample skills are preserved in comparison to any type of visual-perceptual skills involving figure–ground distinctions, line orientation, or online representations of space (Dennis et al., 2002). But not all children with SBM demonstrate these dissociations. The question then is this: What factors cut across domains to explain why some children show the dissociation and others do not? Is motor learning preserved because of sparing or compensatory development of the basal ganglia? Does word recognition proceed because of compensatory development of the frontal components of the normative neural network, which typically includes prominent involvement of the temporal and parietal areas of the left hemisphere? Can preservation be predicted according to the nature and severity of the primary and secondary CNS insults and specific environmental factors?

Figure 1.2 provides additional specific examples of domain-specific dissociations involving more complex domains of memory, attention, and behavior. These examples (also outlined in Dennis et al., 2006) help illustrate the importance of creating experimental tasks that permit an evaluation of these dissociations, as well as the risks attendant on cross-domain comparisons, especially in domains characterized by factorially confounded constructs like executive functions. Such tasks invariably confound associative and assembled processes, so that children with SBM will inevitably show difficulties on these measures. But tasks that are less confounded may also be more sensitive to specific neural and environmental variations that help explain variability around the modal phenotype.

RELEVANCE TO OTHER NEURODEVELOPMENTAL DISORDERS

Perhaps another advantage of model building in pediatric neuropsychology is the extrapolation across disorders. Certainly children with Williams syndrome, velocardiofacial syndrome, and other disorders show similarities to the modal profile of SBM. But it is not simply a matter of comparing, for example, motor, spatial, and math skills versus language skills; all these groups share impairment in the former domains and are stronger on average in the latter domain. Rather, the question is the specific mechanisms that lead to these impairments. Disorders like SBM have multidetermined outcomes and modal profiles. But examining averages and extrapolating to all cases do not have strong explanatory value. Indeed, a strong model explains the variable outcomes associated with complex disorders. In the case of SBM, a label like *attention disorder* or *nonverbal learning disability* (NLD) is too general and leads to simplistic inferences about pathophysiology. Describing SBM as a white matter disorder does not do justice to the pattern of dysmorphology that affects gray and white matter, stretching tracts and destroying cells across the brain, but in a principled fashion that can be modeled and related to variability in outcomes. Labeling outcomes as related to executive functions, spatial deficits, or inattention does not adequately characterize the different systems that are variably affected, or characterize the underlying cognitive dimensions that help explain consistency and inconsistency across domains.

IMPLICATIONS FOR INTERVENTIONS

Another issue with broad labels like NLD or general cross-domain comparisons is that these classifications do not dictate any specific type of principled intervention, and phenotypes are not uniform. Although both SBM and Asperger syndrome are deemed exemplars of NLD, their cognitive phenotypes are radically different. For example, how can being too social (SBM) and being socially avoidant (Asperger syndrome) both be manifestations of the same NLD condition? Entirely different interventions are required, and the mechanisms of learning may also be different.

Beyond these musings, where the lack of empirical studies is of great concern, let us consider some of the ways in which the model in Figures 1.1 and 1.2 might be applied to interventions. One goal should be to bolster assembled processing and prevent the adverse effects of associative processing as early in development as possible. The psychosocial findings suggest obvious sorts of ways in which some of the adverse outcomes associated with SBM could potentially be ameliorated. In particular, early work on parenting in ways that are designed to increase the promotion of autonomy may be particular useful both for promoting children's cognitive development and for improving their psychosocial adjustment (Lomax-Bream et al., 2007b). In addition, families that experience distress should receive attention as early as possible, to prevent the development of maladaptive patterns of behavior. Interventions may also represent another environmental factor that moderates the expression of cognitive outcomes through the associative processing route. For example, a family that has higher expectations for autonomy may do more to promote flexible use of language and expectations for independent movement early in development. This may reduce the impact of core deficits, lead to the development of strengths in language, and maximize potential within the motor area.

To ameliorate the impact of core deficits on assembled processing environments that support movement and opportunities to learn how movement and attention orientation are linked with changes in environmental contingencies should be provided. Parents of children who do things for the children, such as moving desired toys to them or responding to simple imitation, can be taught to view these situations as opportunities for the children to influence the environment through movement, attention, or higher-order language.

In academic domains, reading and listening comprehension are obvious targets for a general focus on higher-order language skills, including strategies for inferencing, activating background knowledge, and connecting different parts of a conversation or text. This can be accomplished by using explicit instructional methods developed for children with learning disabilities (Fletcher, Lyon, Fuchs, & Barnes, 2007, Ch. 7). It is helpful in teaching to understand the general principle of working on assembled processing in context and not allowing excessive reliance on associative learning processes, to which children with SBM naturally gravitate. In math, the breakdowns often occur before higher-order skills can be taught, so an early focus on concepts involving numbers may be helpful. Explicit teaching of more algorithmic, procedural math operations may best proceed in a verbal, step-by-step manner that is rehearsed. Since there is usually little generalization from process-based instruction to academic outcomes (Fletcher et al., 2007), teaching general principles across academic contexts may facilitate the development of these higher-level skills essential to promoting independence.

Obviously, not all children with SBM are the same, and interventions will need to be tailored to each child. There is little research on intervention specific to children with SBM, and initial efforts to determine the extent to which evidence-based methods used in other domains apply to children with SBM are encouraged. Researchers making these efforts, however, may find the principles in this model useful, especially the focus on core deficits and processes that cut across domains.

LIFESPAN ISSUES

Throughout this chapter, we have emphasized the origins of core deficits in infancy and their continuity into school age for children with SBM. Less is known about continuity into adulthood and adult outcomes in general. This question is critical, because the improvements in medical and surgical techniques have produced a cohort of individuals with SBM who now range in age from young adulthood to middle age. The cross-domain cognitive phenotype of children with SBM is apparent in adults (higher Verbal IQ than Performance IQ, and better reading than mathematics; Hetherington, Dennis, Barnes, Drake, & Gentile, 2006; Hommet et al., 1999). Even within domains, patterns (e.g., facility with words but deficits with texts) appear to persist into adulthood. Finally, in adults with SBM, spinal lesion level affects motor skills such as speech production (Huber-Okrainec, Dennis, Brettschneider, & Speigler, 2002) and motor independence (Hetherington et al., 2006), although not cognitive/academic function (Dennis & Barnes, 2002; Hetherington et al., 2006). The number of lifetime shunt revisions—a marker for the stability of hydrocephalus—is negatively related to memory, functional numeracy, independent living, and employment (Dennis et al., 2007; Dennis & Barnes, 2002; Hetherington et al., 2006; Hunt, Oakeshott, & Perry, 1999).

Although we may find evidence for continuity of core deficits and associative/assembled processing strengths and weaknesses into adulthood, there may also be new issues that emerge for adults with SBM. One concern is that adult life appears to bring exacerbated memory problems. Adult survivors of SBM with hydrocephalus have poorer memory than adults with occult spina bifida (Barf et al., 2003). Dennis et al. (2007) studied different forms of memory in 29 young adults with SBM; they found preserved nondeclarative and semantic memory, but impaired working memory, poor prospective memory, and poor episodic memory. Memory status was positively correlated with functional independence, an important component of quality of life. More research is clearly needed on adult outcomes, which will lead to a lifespan understanding of SBM.

CONCLUSIONS

SBM is the product of gene–environment interactions that reflect a multifactorial inheritance and differential environmental effects, some of which are related to the environment. It has physical, neural, and cognitive phenotypes that are linked through the influence of primary and secondary CNS insults and effects of the postnatal environment. By understanding variability and its associations, we can begin to development an understanding of SBM that will lead to interventions maximizing the potential of the people affected by this relatively common developmental disorder.

REFERENCES

Aoyama, Y. H., Kinoshita, Y. H., Yokota, A. H., & Hamada, T. H. (2006). Neuronal damage in hydrocephalus and its restoration by shunt insertion in experimental hydrocephalus: A study involving the neurofilament-immunostaining method. *Journal of Neurosurgery, 104,* 332–339.

Badell-Ribera, A., Shulman, K., & Riddock, N. (1966). Relationship of non-progressive hydrocephalus to intellectual functioning in children with spina bifida cystica. *Pediatrics, 37,* 787–793.

Barf, H. A., Verhoef, M., Jennekens-Schinkel, A., Post, M. W. M., Gooskens, R. H. J. M., & Prevo, A. J. H. (2003). Cognitive status of young adults with spina bifida. *Developmental Medicine and Child Neurology, 45*, 813–820.

Barkovich, A. J. (2005). *Pediatric neuroimaging* (4th ed.). Philadelphia: Lippincott Williams & Wilkins.

Barnes, M. A., & Dennis, M. (1992). Reading in children and adolescents after early onset hydrocephalus and in normally developing age peers: Phonological analysis, word recognition, word comprehension, and passage comprehension skills. *Journal of Pediatric Psychology, 17*, 445–465.

Barnes, M. A., & Dennis, M. (1998). Discourse after early-onset hydrocephalus: Core deficits in children of average intelligence. *Brain and Language, 61*, 309–334.

Barnes, M. A., Pengelly, S., Dennis, M., Wilkinson, M., Rogers, T., & Faulkner, H. (2002). Mathematics skills in good readers with hydrocephalus. *Journal of the International Neuropsychology Society, 8*, 72–82.

Biglan, A. W. (1995). Strabismus associated with meningomyelocele. *Journal of Pediatric Ophthalmology and Strabismus, 32*, 309–314.

Botto, L. D., Moore, C. A., Khoury, M. J., & Erickson, J. D. (1999). Neural-tube defects. *New England Journal of Medicine, 34*, 1509–1519.

Brewer, V. R., Fletcher, J. M., Hiscock, M., & Davidson, K. C. (2001). Attention processes in children with shunted hydrocephalus versus attention deficit/hyperactivity disorder. *Neuropsychology, 15*, 185–198.

Burmeister, R., Hannay, H. J., Copeland, K., Fletcher, J. M., Boudousquie, A., & Dennis, M. (2005). Attention problems and executive functions in children with spina bifida and hydrocephalus. *Child Neuropsychology, 11*, 265–283.

Bushnell, E. W., & Boudreau, J. P. (1993). Motor development and the mind: The potential role of motor abilities as a determinant of aspects of perceptual development. *Child Development, 64*, 1005–1021.

Centers for Disease Control and Prevention. (1993). Recommendations for use of folic acid to reduce the number of spina bifida cases and other neural tube defects. *Journal of the American Medical Association, 269*, 1233, 1236–1238.

Chuang, S. (1986). Perinatal and neonatal hydrocephalus: Part 1. Incidence and etiology. *Perinatal Neonatology, 10*, 8–19.

Colvin, A. N., Yeates, K. O., Enrile, B. G., & Coury, D. L. (2003). Motor adaptation in children with myelomeningocele: Comparison to children with ADHD and healthy siblings. *Journal of the International Neuropsychological Society, 9*, 642–652.

Del Bigio, M. R. (1993). Neuropathological changes caused by hydrocephalus. *Acta Neuropathologica, 85*, 573–585.

Del Bigio, M. R. (2004). Cellular damage and prevention in spina bifida. *Brain Pathology, 14*, 317–324.

Dennis, M., & Barnes, M. A. (2002). Math and numeracy in young adults with spina bifida and hydrocephalus. *Developmental Neuropsychology, 21*, 141–155.

Dennis, M., Edelstein, K., Copeland, K., Frederick, J., Francis, D. J., Hetherington, R., et al. (2005a). Covert orienting to exogenous and endogenous cues in children with spina bifida. *Neuropsychologia, 43*, 976–987.

Dennis, M., Edelstein, K., Copeland, K., Frederick, J., Francis, D. J., et al. (2005b). Space-based inhibition of return in children with spina bifida. *Neuropsychology, 19*, 456–465.

Dennis, M., Edelstein, K., Hetherington, R., Copeland, K., Frederick, J., Blaser, S. E., et al. (2004). Neurobiology of timing in children with SB: Short duration perceptual timing and isochronous rhythmic tapping in relation to cerebellar volumes. *Brain, 127*, 1–10.

Dennis, M., Fitz, C. R., Netley, C. T., Sugar, J., Harwood-Nash, D. C. F., Hendrick, E. B., et al. (1981). The intelligence of hydrocephalic children. *Archives of Neurology, 38*, 607–715.

Dennis, M., Fletcher, J. M., Rogers, T., Hetherington, R., & Francis, D. (2002). Object-based and action-based visual perception in children with spina bifida and hydrocephalus. *Journal of the International Neuropsychological Society, 8*, 95–106.

Dennis, M., Jacennik, B., & Barnes, M. A. (1994). The content of narrative discourse in children and adolescents after early-onset hydrocephalus and in normally-developing age peers. *Brain and Language, 46*, 129–165.

Dennis, M., Jewell, D., Drake, J., Misakyan, T., Spiegler, B., Hetherington, R., et al. (2007). Prospective, declarative, and non-declarative memory in young adults with spina bifida. *Journal of the International Neuropsychological Society, 13*(2), 312–323.

Dennis, M., Landry, S. H., Barnes, M. H., & Fletcher, J. M. (2006). A model of neurocognitive function in spina bifida over the lifespan: A model of core and functional deficits. *Journal of the International Neuropsychological Society, 12*, 285–296.

Detrait, E. R., George, T. M., Etchevers, H. C., Gilbert, J. R., Vekemans, M., & Speer, M. C. (2005). Human neural tube defects: Developmental biology, epidemiology, and genetics. *Neurotoxicology and Teratology, 27*, 515–524.

Edelstein, K., Dennis, M., Copeland, K., Francis, D., Frederick, J., Brandt, M., et al. (2004). Motor learning in children with spina bifida: Dissociation between performance level and acquisition rate. *Journal of the International Neuropsychological Society, 10*, 877–887.

Elwood, J. M., Little, J., & Elwood, J. H. (1992). *Epidemiology and control of neural tube defects.* Oxford: Oxford University Press.

Fletcher, J. M., Brookshire, B. L., Bohan, T. P., Brandt, M. E., & Davidson, K. C. (1995). Early hydrocephalus. In B. P. Rourke (Ed.), *Syndrome of nonverbal learning disabilities: Neurodevelopmental manifestations* (pp. 206–238). New York: Guilford Press.

Fletcher, J. M., Brookshire, B. L., Landry, S. H., Bohan, T. P., Davidson, K. C., Francis, D. J., et al. (1996). Attentional skills and executive functions in children with early hydrocephalus. *Developmental Neuropsychology, 12*, 53–76.

Fletcher, J. M., Copeland, K., Frederick, J., Hannay, H. J., Brandt, M. E., Francis, D. J., et al. (2005). Spinal lesion level in spina bifida meningomyelocele: A source of neural and cognitive heterogeneity. *Journal of Neurosurgery, 102*, 268–279.

Fletcher, J. M., Dennis, M., & Northrup, H. (2000). Hydrocephalus. In K. O. Yeates, M. D. Ris, & H. G. Taylor (Eds.), *Pediatric neuropsychology: Research, theory and practice* (pp. 25–46). New York: Guilford Press.

Fletcher, J. M., Dennis, M., Northrup, H., Barnes, M. A., Hannay, H. J., Landry, S., et al. (2004). Spina bifida: Genes, brain, and development. In L. Glidden (Ed.), *International review of research in mental retardation* (Vol. 29, pp. 63–117). San Diego: Academic Press.

Fletcher, J. M., Francis, D. J., Thompson, N. M., Brookshire, B. L., Bohan, T. P., Landry, S. H., et al. (1992). Verbal and nonverbal skill discrepancies in hydrocephalic children. *Journal of Clinical and Experimental Neuropsychology, 14*, 593–609.

Fletcher, J. M., Landry, S. H., Davidson, K. C., Brookshire, B. L., Lachar, D., Kramer, L. A., et al. (1997). Effects of intraventricular hemorrhage and hydrocephalus on the long-term neurobehavioral development of premature, very low birthweight children. *Developmental Medicine and Child Neurology, 39*, 596–606.

Fletcher, J. M., Lyon, G. R., Fuchs, L. S., & Barnes, M. A. (2007). *Learning disabilities: From intervention to intervention.* New York: Guilford Press.

Gibson, E. J. (1982). The concept of affordances in development: The renascence of functionalism. In W. A. Collins (Ed.), *Minnesota Symposium on Child Psychology: Vol. 15. The concept of development* (pp. 55–81). Hillsdale, NJ: Erlbaum.

Greenley, R. N., Holmbeck, G. N., Zukerman, J., & Buck, C. (2006). Psychosocial adjustment and family relationships in children and adolescents with spina bifida. In D. Wyszynski (Ed.), *Neural tube defects: From origins to treatment* (pp. 307–324). New York: Oxford University Press.

Hannay, H. J. (2000). Functioning of the corpus callosum in children with early hydrocephalus. *Journal of the International Neuropsychological Society, 6*, 351–361.

Hannay, H. J., Walker, A. M., Dennis, M., Kramer, L., Blaser, S., & Fletcher, J. M. (2008). Auditory interhemispheric transfer in relation to patterns of partial dysgenesis and hypoplasia of the corpus callosum in spina bifida meningomyelocele. *Journal of the International Neuropsychological Society, 14*, 771–781.

Hasan, K. M., Eluvathingal, T. J., Kramer, L. A., Ewing-Cobbs, L., Dennis, M., & Fletcher, J. M. (2008a). White matter microstructural abnormalities in children with spina bifida myelomeningocele and hydrocephalus: A diffusion tensor tractography study of the association pathways. *Journal of Magnetic Resonance Imaging, 27,* 700–709.

Hasan, K. M., Sankar, S., Halphen, C., Kramer, L. A., Ewing-Cobbs, L. Dennis, M., et al. (2008b). Quantitative diffusion tensor imaging and intellectual outcomes in spina bifida. *Journal of Neurosurgery: Pediatrics, 2*(1), 75–82.

Hetherington, R., & Dennis, M. (1999). Motor function profile in children with early onset hydrocephalus. *Developmental Neuropsychology, 15,* 25–51.

Hetherington, R., Dennis, M., Barnes, M., Drake, J., & Gentile, F. (2006). Functional outcome in young adults with spina bifida and hydrocephalus. *Child's Nervous System, 22,* 117–124.

Holmbeck, G. N., Greenley, R. N., Coakley, R. M., Greco, J., & Hagstrom, J. (2006). Family functioning in children and adolescents with spina bifida: An evidence-based review of research and interventions. *Journal of Developmental and Behavioral Pediatrics, 27,* 249–277.

Holmbeck, G. N., Westhoven, V. C., Phillips, W. S., Bowers, R., Gruse, C., Nikolopoulos, T., et al. (2003). A multimethod, multi-informant, and multidimensional perspective on psychosocial adjustment in preadolescents with spina bifida. *Journal of Consulting and Clinical Psychology, 71*(4), 782–796.

Hommet, C., Billard, C., Gillet, P., Barthez, M. A., Lourmiere, J. M., Santini, J. J., et al. (1999). Neuropsychologic and adaptive functioning in adolescents and young adults shunted for congenital hydrocephalus. *Journal of Child Neurology, 14,* 144–150.

Honein, M. A., Paulozzi, L. J., Mathews, T. J., Erickson, J. D., & Wong, L. Y. (2001). Impact of folic acid fortification of the U.S. food supply on the occurrence of neural tube defects. *Journal of the American Medical Association, 285,* 2981–2986.

Hore, J., Ritchie, R., & Watts, S. (1999). Finger opening in an overarm throw is not triggered by proprioceptive feedback from elbow extension or wrist flexion. *Experimental Brain Research, 125,* 302–312.

Huber-Okrainec, J., Blaser, S. E., & Dennis, M. (2005). Idiom comprehension deficits in relation to corpus callosum agenesis and hypoplasia in children with spina bifida myelomeningocele. *Brain and Language, 93,* 349–368.

Huber-Okrainec, J., Dennis, M., Brettschneider, J., & Speigler, B. (2002). Neuromotor speech deficits in children and adults with spina bifida and hydrocephalus. *Brain and Language, 80,* 592–602.

Hunt, G. M., Oakeshott, P., & Kerry, S. (1999). Link between the CSF shunt and achievement in adults with spina bifida. *Journal of Neurology, Neurosurgery and Psychiatry, 67,* 591–595.

King, T., Au, K. S., Kirkpatrick, T. J., Fletcher, J. M., Townsend, I. T., Tyerman, G. H., et al. (2007). The impact of BRCA1 on spina bifida meningomyelocele lesions. *Annals of Human Genetics, 71,* 719–728.

Kirkpatrick, T. J., & Northrup, H. (2003). Genetics of neural tube defects. In D. Cooper (Ed.), *Nature encyclopedia of the human genome.* London: Nature Publishing Group.

Landry, S. H., Lomax-Bream, L., & Barnes, M. (2003). The importance of early motor and visual functioning for later cognitive skills in preschoolers with and without spina bifida. *Journal of the International Neuropsychological Society, 9,* 175.

Leigh, R. J., & Zee, D. S. (1999). *The neurology of eye movements.* New York: Oxford University Press.

Lonton, A. P. (1977). Location of the myelomeningocele and its relationship to subsequent physical and intellectual abilities in children with myelomeningocele associated with hydrocephalus. *Zeitschrift für Kinder-und Jungendpsychiatrie, 22,* 510–519.

Lomax-Bream, L. E., Barnes, M. A., Copeland, K., Taylor, H. B., & Landry, S. H. (2007a). The impact of spina bifida on broad development across the first three years. *Developmental Neuropsychology, 31,* 1–20.

Lomax-Bream, L. E., Taylor, H. B., Landry, S. H., Barnes, M. A., Fletcher, J. M., & Swank, P. (2007b). Role of early parenting and motor skills on development in children with spina bifida. *Journal of Applied Developmental Psychology, 28,* 250–263.

McCullough, D. (1990). Hydrocephalus: Etiology, pathologic effects, diagnosis and natural history. In R. M. Scott (Ed.), *Hydrocephalus* (pp. 180–199). Baltimore: Williams & Wilkins.

McLone, D. G., & Knepper, P. A. (1989). The cause of Chiari II malformation: A unified theory. *Pediatric Neuroscience, 15,* 1–12.

Menkes, J. H. (1995). *Textbook of child neurology* (5th ed.). Baltimore: Williams & Wilkins.

Miall, R. C., Reckess, G. Z., & Imamizu, H. (2001). The cerebellum coordinates eye and hand tracking movements. *Nature Neuroscience, 4,* 638–644.

Miller, E., Widjaja, E., Blaser, S., Dennis, M., & Raybaud, C. (2008). The old and the new: Supratentorial MR findings in Chiari II malformation. *Child's Nervous System, 24,* 563–575.

Norman, M. G., McGillivray, B. C., Kalousek, D. K., Hill, A., & Poskitt K. J. (1995). *Congenital malformations of the brain: Pathologic, embryologic, clinical, radiologic and genetic aspects.* New York: Oxford University Press.

Northrup, H., & Volcik, K. A. (2000). Spina bifida and other neural tube defects. *Current Problems in Pediatrics, 30,* 317–332.

Posner, M. I., & Raichle, M. E. (1994). *Images of mind.* New York: Scientific American Books.

Raimondi, A. J. (1994). A unifying theory for the definition and classification of hydrocephalus. *Child's Nervous System, 10,* 2–12.

Raimondi, A. J., & Soare, P. (1974). Intellectual development in shunted hydrocephalic children. *American Journal of Diseases of Children, 127,* 664–671.

Reigel, D. H., & Rotenstein, D. (1994). Spina bifida. In W. R. Cheek (Ed.), *Pediatric neurosurgery* (3rd ed., pp. 51–76). Philadelphia: Saunders.

Rozen, R. (1997). Genetic predisposition to hyperhomocysteinemia: Deficiency of methylenetetrahydrofolate reductase (MTHFR). *Thrombosis and Haemostatis, 78,* 523–526.

Salman, M. S., Sharpe, J. A., Eizenman, M., Lillakas, L., To, T., Westall, C., et al. (2005). Saccades in children with spina bifida and Chiari Type II malformation. *Neurology, 64,* 2098–2101.

Scott, M. A., Fletcher, J. M., Brookshire, B. L., Davidson, K. C., Landry, S. H., Bohan, T. C., et al. (1998). Memory functions in children with early hydrocephalus. *Neuropsychology, 4,* 578–589.

Seefeldt, T. A., Holmbeck, G. N., Belvedere, M. C., Gorey-Ferguson, L., & Hudson, T. (1997). Socioeconomic status and democratic parenting in families of preadolescents with spina bifida. *Psi Chi Journal of Undergraduate Research, 2*(1), 5–12.

Shurtleff, D. B., & Lemire, R. J. (1995). Epidemiology, etiologic factors, and prenatal diagnosis of open spinal dysraphism. *Neurosurgery Clinics of North America, 6,* 183–1.

Taylor, H. B., Landry, S. H., Cohen, L. B., Barnes, M. A., & Swank, P. (2008). *Early information processing among infants with spina bifida.* Unpublished manuscript.

Thelen, E., & Smith, L. B. (1994). *A dynamic systems approach to the development of cognition and action.* Cambridge, MA: MIT Press.

Toriello, H. V., & Higgins, J. V. (1983). Occurrence of neural tube defects among first-, second-, and third-degree relatives of probands: Results of a United States study. *American Journal of Medical Genetics, 15,* 601–606.

van Allen, M. I., Kalousek, D. K., Chernoff, G. F., Juriloff, D., Harris, M., McGillivray, B. C., et al. (1993). Evidence for multi-site closure of the neural tube in humans. *American Journal of Medical Genetics, 47,* 723–743.

Volcik, K. A., Blanton, S. H., Tyerman, G. H., Jong, S. T., Rott, E. J., Page T. Z., et al. (2000). Methylenetetrahydrofolate reductase and spina bifida: Evaluation of level of defect and maternal genotypic risk in Hispanics. *American Journal of Medical Genetics, 95,* 21–27.

Vachha, B., Adams, R. C., & Rollins, N. K. (2006). Limbic tract anomalies in pediatric myelomeningocele and Chiari II malformation: Anatomic correlations with memory and learning—initial investigation. *Radiology, 240,* 194–202.

Volpe, J. J. (2001). *Neurology of the newborn* (4th ed.). Philadelphia: Saunders.

Williams, L. J., Rasmussen, S. A., Flores, A., Kirby, R. S., & Edmunds, L. D. (2005). Decline in the prevalence of spina bifida and anencephaly by race/ethnicity: 1995–2002. *Pediatrics, 116,* 580–586.

Yeates, K. O., Enrile, B., Loss, N., Blumenstein, E., & Delis, D. C. (1995). Verbal learning and memory in children with myelomeningocele. *Journal of Pediatric Psychology, 20,* 801–812.

CHAPTER 2

Children with Very Low Birthweight or Very Preterm Birth

H. GERRY TAYLOR

Advances made in neonatal intensive care since the 1960s have led to survival of increasing numbers of children with low birthweight (<2,500 g) or preterm birth (<37 weeks gestational age [GA]) (Taylor, Klein, & Hack, 2000a). The steepest increases in survival have been in children with very low birthweight (VLBW, <1,500 g) or very preterm birth (VPTB, <32 weeks GA), and are most dramatic in children with extremely low birthweight (ELBW, <1,000 g) or extremely preterm birth (EPTB, <29 weeks GA) (Fanaroff, Hack, & Walsh, 2003; Hintz, Kendrick, Vohr, Poole, & Higgins, 2005b). Although preterm birth is most directly measured in terms of low GA, GA can be difficult to estimate with precision and is closely related to birthweight for most neonates; hence birthweight is frequently used as a proxy for GA. Both birthweight and GA are considered in studies examining the effects of being born at a weight that is below expected for GA—a condition referred to as *smallness for* GA or *intrauterine growth retardation* (IUGR). Because the majority of studies of outcomes of preterm birth involve samples of children identified on the basis of either VLBW or VPTB, the present chapter focuses on outcomes for this subset of the population with preterm birth/low birthweight (i.e., VLBW/VPTB cohorts).

Interest in the outcomes of VLBW/VPTB relates to the fact that it accounts for a substantial proportion of all congenital neurological morbidity, including cerebral palsy (CP) (Cole, Hagadorn, & Kim, 2002; Goldenberg & Rouse, 1998). Children with VLBW/VPTB are also at much higher risk than term-born children with normal birthweight (NBW) for brain insults and abnormalities in cognitive development, behavior, and learning (Taylor et al., 2000a). Investigations of outcomes is further justified by the need for information on the long-term health, developmental, and family consequences of aggressive efforts to sustain life following VLBW/VPTB, and on ways to accurately identify children at highest risk

26

for adverse outcomes so that they can be closely followed. The neuropsychologist's unique role in assessing outcomes of VLBW/VPTB is to identify associated cognitive impairments and the relations of these impairments to early brain insult and to children's learning and behavior problems. Although VLBW/VPTB can result in generalized cognitive impairments, many children display more subtle deficits. Neuropsychological assessment is widely recognized as a critical aspect of outcome evaluation (Aylward, 2005). Such assessment is sensitive to the sequelae of VLBW/VPTB and is useful in delineating individual variations in outcomes and in furthering knowledge of brain–behavior relationships (Taylor, Burant, Holding, Klein, & Hack, 2002).

The goal of this chapter is to summarize current knowledge regarding infants with VLBW/VPTB and their development. Although the full range of health, behavior, and family consequences is considered, special emphasis is placed on the effects of VLBW/VPTB on cognition, learning, and behavior, and on factors that account for variability in these outcomes. The initial section of the chapter reviews background literature on the prevalence of preterm birth and low birthweight, trends in survival and morbidity, and the effects of more extreme prematurity/low birthweight on the brain. The second section considers the consequences of VLBW/VPTB for child health and development and the family, and the third section reviews predictors of child outcomes. The final sections of the chapter critique existing studies and consider methodological needs and future research directions.

BACKGROUND

Incidence, Correlates, and Survival Rates

According to preliminary data from the National Center for Health Statistics for the year 2005 (Hamilton, Martin, & Ventura, 2006), infants with low birthweight and VLBW, respectively, comprised 8.2% and 1.5% of U.S. live births (from an estimated total of 4,140,419); 12.7% and 2.0% met criteria for preterm birth and VPTB, respectively. These percentages increased only slightly from the final data reported for 2000 (Martin, Hamilton, Ventura, Menacker, & Park, 2002). The latter data also provide incidence rates of 0.7% for ELBW and 0.4% for <750 g birthweight. About 80% of preterm births are spontaneous, with 20% occurring on an elective basis for such conditions as maternal hypertension and fetal growth restriction (Goldenberg & Rouse, 1998).

Medical factors associated with preterm birth include a previous preterm delivery, family history of infertility, multiple gestation, placental abnormalities, uterine abnormalities/infections, and preeclampsia (Alexander & Slay, 2002). Rates of VLBW/VPTB are more than twice as high for non-Hispanic blacks as for whites, and are also higher in single mothers and in those of lower socioeconomic status (SES) (Fiscella, 2005). The reasons for variation in prevalence related to sociodemographic factors remain unclear but are hypothesized to be multifactorial, including the effects of stress on the neuron–endocrine system, smoking and drug use, underutilization of prenatal care, susceptibility to genital tract infections, and the combined effects of low folate intake and gene–environment interactions (Holzman, Lin, Senagore, & Chung, 2007).

The survival rate was 85% for infants with birthweights of 501–1,500 g born from 1997 to 2002 at the 16 participating centers in the National Institute of Child Health and Human Development (NICHD) Neonatal Research Network (Fanaroff et al., 2007). Broken down by birthweight group, survival rates were 55% for infants weighing 501–750 g, 88% for those weighing 751–1,000 g, 94% for those weighing 1,001–1,250 g, and 96% for those weighing 1,251–1,500 g. Survival rates decrease precipitously for infants at the lower end of the VLBW/VPTB spectrum, with females surviving at higher rates than males at the lowest birthweights, and only a small percentage of children living to hospital discharge among those with <500 g birthweight or 21–24 weeks GA (Costeloe et al., 2000; Hintz et al., 2005b). Correspondingly greater costs are incurred in the care and schooling of these high-risk infants (Petrou, 2003; Roth et al., 2004; St. John, Nelson, Cliver, Bishnoi, & Goldenberg, 2000).

Although some variability in survival rates is evident across specialized neonatal treatment centers in the United States (Fanaroff et al., 2007), survival differs markedly between centers that apply different ethical standards in treating the highest-risk infants. In comparing survival rates among infants born at 23–26 weeks GA in the mid-1980s, for example, Lorenz, Paneth, Jetton, den Ouden, and Tyson (2001) found that there were 24.1 additional survivors per 100 live births in the state of New Jersey than in the Netherlands. A major reason for this difference was the almost universal application of aggressive neonatal care in the New Jersey sample, compared with more selective use of these methods in the Netherlands. Consistent with the country's more conservative approach to high-risk care, neonatal care in the Netherlands involved less use of ventilators (1,372 fewer ventilator days per 100 live births), more deaths without assisted ventilation, and fewer cases of CP (7.2 fewer cases per 100 live births).

Historical Trends in Survival and Early Morbidity

The introduction of neonatal intensive care in the 1960s resulted in both increased survival and reduced morbidity in children with VLBW/VPTB (Hack & Fanaroff, 1999). The therapies responsible for these advances included resuscitation, assisted ventilation, drug treatments, intravenous nutrition, and phototherapy for jaundice. During the 1980s, progressively smaller and more premature infants received special obstetrical and delivery room care. Increases in survival continued through the 1990s, with the introduction of surfactant for treatment of immature lungs, antenatal steroids and antibiotics, and high-pressure ventilation (Fanaroff et al., 2003; Hintz et al., 2005b). Changes in survival have been most marked in infants with ELBW, with a 70-fold increase in annual incidence from 1960 to 1983 (Paneth, 1995). To illustrate more recent changes, rates of low birthweight as a percentage of all live births increased only about 1% from 1980 to 2000, while rates of VLBW increased by 12% (Alexander & Slay, 2002).

The major neonatal complications of preterm birth include evidence from neonatal cranial ultrasounds of brain abnormalities (specifically, intraventricular hemorrhage [IVH], periventricular leukomalacia [PVL], and ventricular dilation), pneumothorax (collapsed lung), bronchopulmonary dysplasia (chronic lung disease), patent ductus arteriosis (abnormal opening between the aorta and pulmonary artery), apnea of prematurity (intermittent shallow or arrested breathing), jaundice of prematurity (abnormal accumulation of bilirubin, or hyperbilirubinemia), sepsis (infection), necrotizing enterocolitis or NEC (infection and inflammation of the intestines), retinopathy of prematurity (abnormal growth of blood vessels in the eye), and nutritional disturbances (Cole et al., 2002; Fanaroff et al., 2007).

Common forms of early childhood neurodevelopmental impairments include CP, blindness or deafness, and impaired early cognitive development as measured by the Bayley Scales of Infant Development (original, BSID; second edition, BSID-II).

Research comparing earlier and later birth cohorts of infants with VLBW/VPTB born during the1980s and 1990s indicates that the rates of some neonatal complications, such as more severe grades (grades III–IV) of IVH, declined over this period (Fanaroff et al., 2003; Horbar et al., 2002). For the most part, however, increasing survival was not accompanied by declining morbidity. In fact, Wilson-Costello, Friedman, Minich, Fanaroff, and Hack (2005) reported increases during the 1980s to 1990s in sepsis, PVL, chronic lung disease, and early neurodevelopmental impairment. In their study of infants born at <25 weeks GA, Hintz et al. (2005b) found higher rates of chronic lung disease in infants born in the later 1990s than in those born earlier in that decade. More aggressive efforts to save high-risk infants, along with iatrogenic effects of newer therapies, may have been responsible for these changes (Hack & Fanaroff, 1999; Hack et al., 2000).

A recent study by Wilson-Costello et al. (2007) suggests a more optimistic outlook for the present decade of survivors. Specifically, this study found that children with ELBW from a 2000–2002 birth cohort, compared with those born in the 1990s, had lower rates of IVH (22% vs. 43%) and neurodevelopmental impairment (23% vs. 35%). Factors associated with decreasing morbidity were greater utilization of antenatal steroids (for treatment of immature lungs), more cesarean deliveries, a lower incidence of sepsis and of abnormalities on cranial ultrasounds, and less use of postnatal steroids. Survival rate did not differ for these two cohorts, but the change in morbidity implies a higher rate of survival without impairment.

Neuropathology

The primary processes responsible for brain damage in neonates with VLBW/VPTB are hypoxic ischemia with associated deprivation of oxygen and glucose, and exposure to fetal and maternal infection (Inder & Volpe, 2000). The damage is exacerbated by excitotoxicity due to free radical attack and excess extracellular glutamate, release of proinflammatory cytokines, and suboptimal levels of endogenous protectors (Dammann & Leviton, 1999). Due to underdevelopment of arterial end zones supplying the periventricular white matter, and the vulnerability of immature oligodendrocytes (myelin prescursors) to free radical attack, this structure is particularly susceptible to damage. Brain growth is rapid in the late fetal period and includes substantial increases in total brain volume, proliferation of glial cells and formation of myelin, growth of axonal and dendritic spines, synaptogenesis, and axonal pruning. Disruption of this process and injury to subplate neurons in the periventricular region thus not only lead to immediate damage, but affect early neurogenesis (Allin et al., 2004; Inder et al., 1999a). The infant's fragile medical condition for a period of weeks or months after birth, including recurrent hypoxemia, may further contribute to brain insult (Bass et al., 2004).

Common brain abnormalities in neonates with VLBW/VPTB are PVL, hemorrhagic infarctions associated with germinal matrix IVH, and ventriculomegaly. The brain regions most affected are subcortical structures and circuits connecting these structures to frontal and parietal regions (Lou, 1996). Diffuse reduction in white matter is especially common and is referred to as noncystic PVL or as diffuse excessive high-signal intensity on

T2-weighted magnetic resonance imaging (MRI). This abnormality is believed to represent insult to oligodendroglial precursors of myelin, and thus to set the stage for later white matter impairment (Inder et al., 1999b). Findings from cranial ultrasounds indicate that about 25% of neonates with VLBW have IVH and about 5–15% have PVL (Inder & Volpe, 2000). However, estimates from ultrasounds are insensitive to the smaller lesions and diffuse white matter abnormalities evident in MRI (Inder, Wells, Mogridge, Spencer, & Volpe, 2003); hence reported rates of cystic PVL and IVH underestimate the prevalence of brain insults.

VLBW and VPTB also affect the early development of gray matter and result in cortical atrophy and ischemic/infarctive lesions in the basal ganglia, hippocampus, brainstem, and cerebellum (Inder et al., 1999a). Hypoxic–ischemic insult has less direct effects on cortical gray matter in the premature neonate than in the full-term infant, but is nevertheless linked to reduced cortical volumes (Inder et al., 1999a). Volumetric MRI studies indicate that neonates with VLBW/VPTB have larger ventricular volumes than term-born infants, but smaller volumes for the whole brain, cortical and subcortical gray matter, white matter, and cerebellum (Limperopoulos et al., 2005; Peterson et al., 2003; Srinivasan et al., 2007). Multiple areas of white matter signal changes, less complex cortical folding, and less gray–white matter differentiation are also reported in the neonatal period (Ajayi-Obe, Saeed, Cowan, Rutherford, & Edwards, 2000). Inder et al. (2003) observed a distinct pattern of brain pathology among the least mature neonates on neonatal MRI, characterized by diffuse white matter atrophy, ventriculomegaly, immature development of cortical gyri, and enlarged subarachnoid space.

Structural abnormalities seen in MRI with school-age children and adults with VLBW/VPTB include thinning of the corpus callosum and diffuse reductions in white matter, as well as ventricular dilation, porencephaly, and intraparenchymal cysts secondary to IVH and PVL (Allin et al., 2004; Fearon et al., 2004; Kesler et al., 2004; Nosarti et al., 2002). Some of these abnormalities are illustrated in the images shown in Figure 2.1 of an adolescent participant in our long-term follow-up study of children with ELBW/EPTB. Comparisons of groups with VLBW/VPTB and NBW have additionally identified regionally specific reductions in the temporal, parietal, and occipital lobes, basal ganglia, corpus callosum, amygdala, hippocampus, thalamus, and cerebellum (Allin et al., 2001; Nosarti et al., 2004; Srinivasan et al., 2007). In a study of neonatal MRI by Peterson et al. (2003), reduction of white matter volume was greater in the right hemisphere than in the left. In general, however, neuroimaging findings suggest diffuse effects of VLBW/VLBW on white matter (Gimenez et al., 2006). Factors associated with greater reductions in gray and white matter volumes in VLBW/VPTB samples are lower birthweight, shorter GA, white matter injury, the presence of IVH or PVL, and male sex (Inder, Warfield, Wang, Huppi, & Volpe, 2005; Kesler et al., 2004; Peterson et al., 2000; Reiss et al., 2004).

Other neuroimaging methodologies also reveal brain abnormalities in children with VLBW/VPTB. Several studies have used diffusion tensor imaging to examine fractional anisotropy (FA) in white matter tracts. Better-developed tracts are characterized by higher values of FA, reflecting less water diffusion along the axonal axis. Studies utilizing this technique find lower FA in children with VLBW/VPTB than in controls with NBW in the central white matter, corpus callosum, internal capsules, and superior, middle superior, and inferior fasciculus (Nagy et al., 2003; Skranes et al., 2007). Using functional MRI (fMRI),

(a)

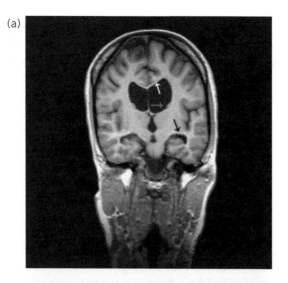

(b)

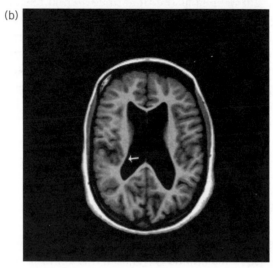

FIGURE 2.1. T1-weighted coronal (a) and axial (b) MP-RAGE magnetic resonance imaging (MRI) scans of a 17-year-old with a birthweight of 640 g and GA of 24 weeks. The coronal scan shows enlarged ventricles, thinning of the corpus callosum (white arrow), small caudate heads (gray arrow), enlarged temporal horns with associated volume reduction in hippocampi (black arrow), and general reduction in cortical volume. The axial scan again reveals large ventricles, as well as reductions in white matter evident in the close proximity of cortical gray matter to the ventricles (white arrow). Although brain abnormalities in most survivors of more extreme low birthweight/low GA are less obvious or may not even be apparent in clinical inspection of scans, this case illustrates the components of neuropathology in the least mature neonates, including diffuse white matter atrophy, ventriculomegaly, maldevelopment of cortical gyri, and enlarged subarachnoid space.

researchers have also found different patterns of cortical activation on tasks involving attentional control, visual matching, sound discrimination, and phonological and semantic processing (Nosarti et al., 2006; Peterson et al., 2002; Rushe et al., 2004; Santhouse et al., 2002). Finally, Groenendaal et al (1997) found that lower ratios of N-acetylaspartate to choline were associated with higher grades of cystic PVL in a study using proton magnetic resonance spectroscopy, a technique with good sensitivity to hypoxic–ischemic perinatal brain insults (Huppi & Inder, 2001).

DEVELOPMENTAL OUTCOMES OF VLBW/VPTB

Early Neurodevelopmental Impairments and Health Consequences

As reported above, the most recent data available document early childhood neurodevelopmental impairments in 23% of a 2000–2002 birth cohort of children with ELBW (Wilson-Costello et al., 2007). The children had reached 20 months corrected age at the time of assessment; *corrected age* is defined as the time since a child reached term-equivalent age (i.e., chronological age minus months of prematurity). The impairments included neurological or sensory disorders (CP, hypotonia, hypertonia, shunt-dependent hydrocephalus, blindness, deafness) in 9% of the sample; impaired mental development (BSID-II Mental Development Index < 70) in 21%; and impaired psychomotor development (BSID-II Psychomotor Development Index < 70) in 15%. In reviewing neurodevelopmental outcomes in the first 2 years among the largest multicenter studies of ELBW born in the 1990s, Msall (2006) reported CP in 8–17% of children, cognitive impairment (BSID indices < 70) in 22–37%, hearing impairment requiring aids in 1–2%, and corrected vision worse than 20/200 in 1–5%.

Other postdischarge health consequences of VLBW/VPTB can include respiratory illnesses (e.g., asthma), rehospitalizations, surgeries, and poor growth attainment (Wilson-Costello, 2007). Hack et al. (1993) found respiratory conditions in 18% of a sample of infants with VLBW, compared to 5% of controls with NBW. The infants with VLBW also had more surgeries of the eyes, ears, nose, and throat, more hernia repairs; and more surgeries to the respiratory, urogenital, and musculoskeletal systems. Our research group has additionally observed higher rates of functional health problems and chronic constipation in samples of school-age children with more extreme degrees of VLBW/VPTB (Cunningham, Taylor, Klein, Minich, & Hack, 2001; Hack et al., 2005a). Measures of growth attainment reveal reduced height, weight, and head circumference in children with VLBW/VPTB compared to children with NBW, as well as incomplete catch-up growth evident in the first years of life (Wood et al., 2003). Peterson, Taylor, Minich, Klein, and Hack (2006) found subnormal head circumference at mean age 6.8 years in 24% of two groups with VLBW (<750 g, 750–1,499 g) but in none of the controls with NBW.

Neuropsychological Consequences

The adverse effects of VLBW/VPTB on children's cognitive abilities are evident early in life. Rose, Feldman, Jankowski, and Van Rossem (2005b) found that 7-month-old infants with <1,750 g birthweight but without neurological deficits at birth performed more poorly than age-matched controls with NBW on tests of memory, processing speed, mental representation of objects, and attention, and that the former group also obtained lower scores at ages 2 and 3 years on the BSID-II Mental Development Index. In this same sample of children with <1,750 g birthweight, Rose, Feldman, and Jankowski (2005a) observed deficits on an elicited imitation task at 1, 2, and 3 years. Similarly, studies by Woodward, Edgin, Thompson, and Inder (2005) and Edgin et al. (2008) documented deficits in working memory and executive function in a cohort with VLBW/VLBW compared to full-term controls. Research findings also indicate deficits in young children with VLBW/VPTB in motor skills, language, and attention (Grunau, Kearney, & Whitfield, 1990; Landry, Fletcher, Denson, & Chapieski, 1993; Miller et al., 1995). Other investigations reveal that preterm children have more limited social and communicative interactions than term-born controls do (Landry, Smith, Miller-Loncar, & Swank, 1997). Many of these studies indicate that early cognitive deficits are more marked among survivors with neonatal complications, including brain abnormalities on ultrasound or chronic lung disease. Nevertheless, deficits in specific skill areas, such as spatial working memory and executive function, are found even in lower-risk children, in those without global cognitive impairment, or when IQ is controlled for (Edgin et al., 2008; Espy et al., 2002; Vicari, Caravale, Carlesimo, Casadei, & Allemand, 2004).

Follow-up studies indicate that children with VLBW/VPTB continue to display pervasive cognitive problems at the age of school entry, with several studies documenting deficits in school readiness skills (Msall, Buck, Rogers, & Catanzaro, 1992; Saigal, Szatmari, & Rosenbaum, 1992; Wolke & Meyer, 1999). Cognitive sequelae persist throughout the school-age years (Saigal, 2000; Taylor, Minich, Klein, & Hack, 2004c). The effect sizes corresponding to differences between VLBW/VPTB samples and NBW controls, as measured by Cohen's d (i.e., difference between group means in units of standard deviation), range from about 0.33 to greater than 1.00 (Anderson, Doyle, & the Victorian Infant Collaborative Study Group, 2003; Johnson, 2007; Saigal, Hoult, Streiner, Stoskopf, & Rosenbaum, 2000b; Schneider, Wolke, Schlagmüller, & Meyer, 2004). Effect sizes are larger for cohorts with more extreme low birthweight/low GA (Taylor et al., 2000a). Deficits in executive function, attention, memory, perceptual–motor abilities, and visual processing are especially prominent and cannot be attributed entirely to mental deficiency or to neurological or sensory disorders (Bohm, Smedler, & Forssberg, 2004; Foreman, Fielder, Minshell, Hurrion, & Sergienko, 1997; Goyen, Lui, & Woods, 1998; Harvey, O'Callaghan, & Mohay, 1999; Jakobson, Frisk, & Downie, 2006; Jakobson, Frisk, Knight, Downie, & Whyte, 2001; Kulseng et al., 2006; Marlow, Hennessy, Bracewell, & Wolke, 2007; Nosarti et al., 2007). Speech and language skills appear to be less consistently impaired during the school-age years than in early childhood (Luoma, Herrgard, Martikainen, & Ahonen, 1998). Aram, Hack, Hawkins, Weissman, and Borawski-Clark (1991) failed to find a higher rate of specific language impairment in 8-year-old children with VLBW than in controls with NBW; other studies reveal a relative sparing of verbal/semantic skills, articulation, and naming (Frisk & Whyte, 1994; Luoma et al., 1998; Taylor, Minich, Bangert, Filipek, & Hack, 2004a; Taylor, Klein, Drotar, Schluchter, & Hack, 2006).

The unevenness of the cognitive consequences of VLBW/VPTB is illustrated in Figure 2.2. This figure plots neuropsychological outcomes in three groups of children (48 with <750 g birthweight, 47 with 750–1,499 g birthweight, and 52 with NBW) followed in our research

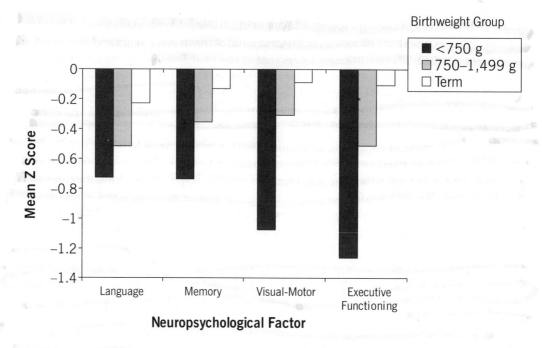

FIGURE 2.2. Differences among groups (<750 g birthweight, 750–1,499 g birthweight, and term) on four neuropsychological factor composites. The composites were means of the age-standardized scores for the measures loading on each factor. The *Language* factor consisted of the Boston Naming Test, the Synonyms and Pragmatic Language subtests of the Comprehensive Assessment of Spoken Language, and the Vocabulary subtest of either the Wechsler Intelligence Scale for Children—Third Edition (WISC-III) or the Wechsler Adult Intelligence Scale—Third Edition (WAIS-III). The *Memory* factor consisted of the California Verbal Learning Test—Children's Version Trials 1–5 Total score and a composite of the delayed-recall trials. The *Visual–Motor/Constructional* factor consisted of the Developmental Test of Visual–Motor Integration (VMI) and the organizational scores for the copy and delayed-recall trials of the Rey–Osterrieth Complex Figure (ROCF). The *Executive Functioning/Efficiency* factor consisted of Random A's, the Contingency Naming Test, the Purdue Pegboard Test, and the Spatial Span and Spatial Working Memory subtests of the Cambridge Neuropsychological Test Automated Battery. (See Taylor et al., 2004a, for more details about the composites.) Results of analyses of variance revealed significant group differences for Memory, $F (2, 144) = 3.32, p = .039$; Visual–Motor, $F (2, 144) = 19.89, p < .001$; and Executive Functioning, $F (2, 144) = 17.65, p < .001$; but not for Language, $F (2, 144) = 2.74, p = .07$. Simple effects tests indicated that the group with <750 g birthweight scored more poorly on the Memory, Visual–Motor, and Executive Functioning factors than the term group. The former group also scored significantly less well than the group with 750–1,499 g birthweight on the Visual–Motor and Executive Functioning composites. Differences between the group with 750–1,499 g birthweight and the controls, although consistently favoring the latter group, were not significant. The results show the differential sensitivity of different skill domains to the effects of VLBW/VPTB.

team's "School-Age Follow-Up Project" (Taylor et al., 2004a). Matched on age and sociode-mographic status, the three groups were first recruited at mean age 7 years and reassessed at mean ages 11, 12, 13, 14, and 16 years. Outcomes at the final assessment are summarized by four factor-derived age-adjusted composites: Language, Memory, Visual–Motor, and Executive Functioning. The figure shows group differences across the four composite scores, with analysis confirming a significantly larger group difference in Executive Functioning than in Language or Memory. The figure also illustrates the pervasive nature of cognitive sequelae and the more marked impairments in children with more extreme low birthweight. The tests of Memory and Executive Functioning at this and earlier assessments revealed that the group with <750 g birthweight was prone to specific types of cognitive impairments, including a slow rate of learning, impulsive responses, slowed processing times, and poorly organized approaches to multistep tasks (Taylor, Klein, Minich, & Hack, 2000c; Taylor, Minich, Klein, & Hack, 2004c).

Study findings further revealed both a downward shift in the cognitive skills across individual children, suggesting a continuum of sequelae, and a high rate of individual deficits in children without severe developmental handicaps. Figure 2.3 presents the frequencies of estimated IQs at the final follow-up visit for the three study groups for IQ bands from <70 to 130+. The figure shows a greater downward displacement of the IQ distribution with decreasing birthweight, as well as a bimodal distribution of scores most evident in the group with <750 g birthweight. The elevated rate of more severe IQ deficits suggests that a subset

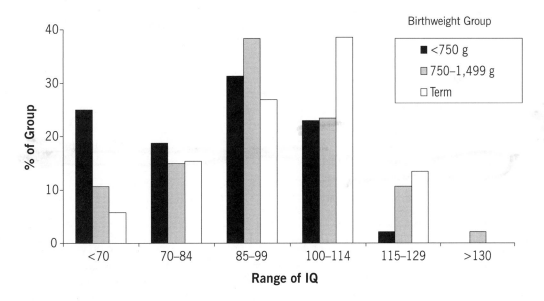

FIGURE 2.3. Distribution of IQ estimates for the three birthweight groups (<750 g birthweight, 750–1,499 g birthweight, and term). IQs were estimated from the Vocabulary and Block Design subtests of either the WISC-III or WAIS-III. Analysis of variance revealed a significant group difference in IQ, F (2, 144) = 8.92, p < .001. Tests of simple effects indicated significantly lower IQ for those with <750 g birthweight than for the controls, and a marginally significant difference between the groups with <750 g and 750–1,499 g birthweight. The results demonstrate both a downward shift in IQ scores and increased rate of cognitive deficiencies in the two groups with low birthweight.

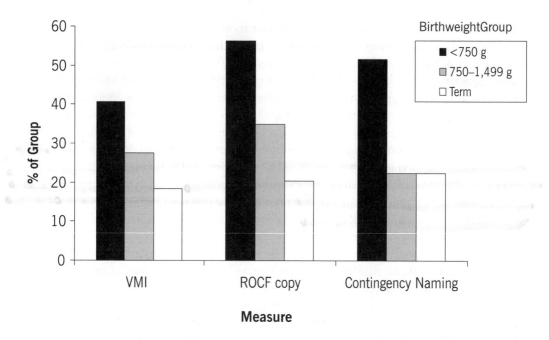

FIGURE 2.4. Rates of deficits on the VMI, ROCF copy, and Contingency Naming Test at mean age 16 years, excluding adolescents with IQs < 70 or with neurological or sensory disorders. According to results from logistic regression analysis, the odds of test deficits were significantly higher in the group with <750 g birthweight than in the term group. The results show deficits in tests of visual-perceptual skill and executive functioning for a substantial percentage of children with VLBW, especially those with more extreme low birthweight.

of the children sustained more severe brain insult. Figure 2.4 shows the rates of deficits on three of the tests administered as part of the neuropsychological battery at the final visit. Only the study participants with IQs ≥ 70 and without neurological or sensory impairments were considered in this analysis. The findings suggest that a large percentage of children with more extreme low birthweight have selective neuropsychological deficits that persist throughout the school-age years.

Behavior Outcomes

Behavioral consequences of VLBW/VPTB are evident shortly after birth. Wolf et al. (2002) administered the Neonatal Behavioral Assessment Scale (NBAS) and the Infant Behavioral Assessment (IBA) to infants with VLBW and NBW at term equivalent. The IBA and BSID-II Behavioral Rating Scale were also administered at 3 and 6 months corrected age. The group with VLBW scored more poorly than the group with NBW on NBAS measures of orientation, state control, motor function, autonomic stability, alertness, and irritability. The group with VLBW also showed more stress responses and fewer approach behaviors on the IBA at 3 and 6 months; lower attention/arousal and motor quality the BSID-II Behavioral Rating Scale at 3 months; and lower orientation, emotional regulation, and motor quality on the latter scale at 6 months. Research also documents differences between preterm and term infants in early temperament. Hughes, Shults, and Medoff-Cooper (2002) found that a preterm group was less regular and more distractible than a full-term stan-dardization sample at 6 weeks, less adaptable at 6 months, and less persistent at 12 months. Other studies suggest that young children with VLBW/VPTB are more insecurely attached to their parents and have lower social functioning and more behavior and mood prob-lems than controls with NBW (Eiser, Eiser, Mayhew, & Gibson, 2005; Mangelsdorf et al., 1996).

Later behavioral sequelae include deficits in adaptive behavior skills and social compe-tence, as well as more symptoms of inattention/hyperactivity, internalizing and external-izing problems, and atypical behaviors than in term-born children (Bhutta, Cleves, Casey, Cradock, & Anand, 2002; Klebanov, Brooks-Gunn, & McCormick, 1994; Taylor, Hack, & Klein, 1998a). These problems are documented by child behavior ratings from parents and teachers obtained at early school age (Hoff, Hansen, Munck, & Mortensen, 2004; Rose, Feldman, Rose, Wallace, & McCarton, 1992; Szatmari, Saigal, Rosenbaum, Campbell, & King, 1990), middle school age (Anderson et al., 2003; Breslau & Chilcoat, 2000; Hack et al., 1992; Hille et al., 2001; Taylor, Klein, Minich, & Hack, 2000b), adolescence (Gardner et al., 2004; Grunau, Whitfield, & Fay, 2004; Saigal, Pinelli, Hoult, Kim, & Boyle, 2003b), and young adulthood (Hack et al., 2004). Hille et al. (2001) reported parent ratings of social, thought, and attention problem scales for cohorts with ELBW that fell 0.5 to 1.2 standard deviations above those for controls. Findings from a study by Allin et al. (2006) of 18- and 19-year-olds with VPTB suggest that behavior consequences may also entail distinguishing personality traits. On the Eysenck Personality Questionnaire—Revised, the group with VPTB scored lower on extraversion (sociability), higher on neuroticism (anxi-ety, low mood, and low self-esteem), and higher on a "lie" scale than a full-term control group.

Formal psychiatric interviews reveal higher rates of attention-deficit/hyperactivity disorder (ADHD) and anxiety disorders, and more symptoms of depression, in children with VLBW/VPTB than in controls with NBW (Elgen, Sommerfelt, & Markestad, 2002; Indredavik et al., 2004). ADHD is especially prominent: Botting, Powls, and Cooke (1997) found that 23% of children with VLBW, but only 6% of a group, with NBW met criteria for this disorder. Some investigators have observed that ADHD is less often associated with conduct disorder in samples with VLBW/VPTB samples than in the broader population with ADHD, and that inattentiveness rather than hyperactivity better distinguishes them from their peers, suggesting a "purer" form of ADHD (Szatmari, Saigal, Rosenbaum, & Campbell, 1993).

Few studies have examined self-ratings or peer ratings of adjustment and social compe-tence. In the most comprehensive study on this topic, Hoy et al. (1992) compared children with VLBW and NBW on peer ratings of social competence and peer acceptance, and the children completed self-ratings of these same traits. The children with VLBW received higher peer ratings in social nonparticipation (e.g., "sad, plays by self, lonely") than the controls with NBW did; they also had higher self-ratings of sadness and social isolation, and lower self-ratings of cognitive and physical competence. Similarly, Saigal, Lambert, Russ, and Hoult (2002) found that children with ELBW rated themselves lower in athletic com-petence than those with NBW did. Other research, however, fails to document differences between groups with VLBW/VPTB and with NBW on self-ratings of behavior, emotional adjustment, or socialization (Gardner et al., 2004; Saigal, Pinelli, Hoult, Kim, & Boyle, 2003b; Taylor et al., 2000b).

Consequences for Academic Achievement and School Performance

Children with VLBW/VPTB score more poorly than controls with NBW on tests of reading, spelling, math, written expression, and handwriting (Anderson et al., 2003; Feder et al., 2005; Grunau, Whitfield, & Davis, 2002; Hack et al., 1992; Taylor et al., 2000b, 2006). Effect sizes for these comparisons range from slightly less than 0.5 to more than 1, with greater-magnitude effects associated with more extreme degrees of VLBW/VPTB (Anderson et al., 2003; Saigal et al., 2000b; Taylor et al., 2000b, 2006). These deficiencies persist through adolescence and are found even in analyses that exclude children with global intellectual deficits, neurological disorders, or sensory impairments (Breslau, Paneth, & Lucia, 2004; Grunau et al., 2004; Johnson & Breslau, 2000; Saigal et al., 2000b). Problems in math are especially prominent, with weaknesses in this area observed even when IQ is taken into account (Anderson et al., 2003; Botting, Powls, Cooke, & Marlow, 1998; Klebanov et al., 1994; Taylor et al., 2002).

Problems in school performance are further documented by teacher ratings and by high rates of grade repetition and special learning assistance (Botting et al., 1998; Buck, Msall, Schisterman, Lyon, & Rogers, 2000; Hille et al., 1994; Klebanov et al., 1994; Saigal et al., 1991). Saigal et al. (2000b) found that 58% of a regional cohort of children with ELBW ages 12–16 years either had repeated a grade or were receiving special educational assistance, compared with 13% of a matched control group. Similar rates of educational modifications are reported in other studies, as well as in four cross-national samples (Saigal et al., 2003a).

Several studies have found higher rates of learning disabilities in children with VLBW/VPTB than in children with NBW, whether such disabilities are defined in terms of low achievement by children of grossly normal IQ or in terms of achievement below expectation for IQ (Grunau et al., 2004; Litt, Taylor, Klein, & Hack, 2005; Saigal et al., 2000b). Children with VLBW/VPTB often have multiple learning disabilities, including math and written output in addition to reading (Grunau et al., 2002). Furthermore, low reading scores are more characteristic of these children than are reading scores that fall below predicted levels based on IQ (Litt et al., 2005; Samuelsson et al., 1999). Unfortunately, the educational needs of children with VLBW/VPTB and learning disabilities appear to be less well recognized than the needs of those with more severe developmental impairments. In a survey of kindergarten special education programs in Florida, Resnick et al. (1999) found that the degree of low birthweight was more closely related to placements in programs for mental, physical, or sensory disabilities than to placement in programs for learning disabilities. Litt et al. (2005) provide another reason to suspect that schools may be overlooking the needs of survivors with learning disabilities. Although children in this study with VLBW had higher rates of learning disabilities than controls with NBW, the groups did not differ in rates of special education placement in learning disabilities programs.

Developmental Changes and Later Outcomes

Hille et al. (1994) noted the possibility of increasing deficits with age as children with VLBW/VPTB face more complex cognitive and social demands. This expectation is further justified by evidence of emerging or more pronounced impairments with age in children with other forms of early brain insult (Taylor & Alden, 1997), as well as by the fact that children with VLBW/VPTB sustain damage to brain regions that continue to develop throughout childhood and adolescence (Huttenlocher & Dabholkar, 1997). Results from studies comparing outcomes in younger versus older school-age cohorts lend some support for this hypothesis (Zelkowitz, Papageorgiou, Zelazo, & Weiss, 1995). Several longitudinal studies also report slower development of cognitive abilities in children with VLBW/VPTB than in controls with NBW, or increasing deficits in groups with VLBW/VPTB at later ages (Botting et al., 1998; Breslau & Chilcoat, 2000; Koller, Lawson, Rose, Wallace, & McCarton, 1997; Landry et al., 1997; O'Brien et al., 2004; Rose et al., 1992; Saigal et al., 2000b). Evidence in this regard from the School-Age Follow-Up Project was obtained in analysis of changes across follow-up on tests of perceptual–motor skill and executive functioning (Taylor et al., 2004a). Figure 2.5 illustrates the increasing performance gap over time between the two groups with low birthweight and the controls on a test of executive functioning. The deficits that Nosarti et al. (2007) observed in young adults with VPTB are consistent with these findings.

However, there is no reason to suspect an overall decline in children's functioning over time. Many studies that have followed samples with VLBW/VPTB report stable cognitive and behavioral impairments (Breslau et al., 2001, 2004; Landry et al., 1993). Some investigations even document age-related improvements. Doyle et al. (2001) and Theunissen et al. (2000) observed fewer health problems over time in their samples. In following children with 600–1,250 g birthweight, Ment et al. (2003) found that standardized scores on a mea-

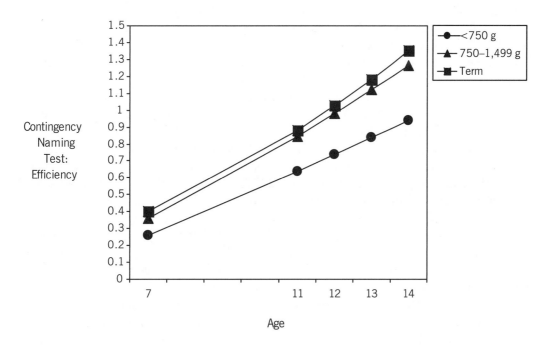

FIGURE 2.5. Changes over follow-up assessments on a measure of executive functioning, the Contingency Naming Test, for the three birthweight groups (<750 g, 750–1,499 g, and term) (Taylor et al., 2004a). The lines show estimated efficiency scores from mixed-model analysis. Mixed model analysis revealed a group × time interaction, $F (4, 363) = 4.28$, $p = .002$, with follow-up analysis indicating significantly greater gains with advancing age for the group with <750 g birthweight than for the controls.

sure of receptive vocabulary improved from ages 3 to 5 years for those with normal neonatal ultrasounds. Scores declined over this interval for the survivors with abnormal ultrasounds. Additional support for the possibility of a "catch-up" effect comes from our School-Age Follow-Up Project. In following children from early to middle school age, we observed faster gains in adaptive behavior skills for children with <750 g birthweight than for full-term controls, though this effect was evident only for children from more advantaged families (Taylor, Minich, Holding, Klein, & Hack, 2004b). Further support for the possibility of some catch-up growth is provided by Tideman (2000), who found attenuation of deficits in scholastic performance from ages 4 to 19 years in a lower-risk sample with <35 weeks GA; and by Samuelsson et al. (2006), who reported greater gains from 9 to 15 years in reading comprehension and orthographic reading for children with VLBW than for full-term controls. These different age trajectories may reflect differences in sample composition or in the types of outcomes assessed and their sensitivity to environmental influences.

Consistent with cross-age continuity of deficits, early outcomes of VLBW/VPTB are generally good predictors of later outcomes. Rose et al. (2005b) found that specific impairments in attention, speed of processing, and memory detected in infancy predict later cognitive outcomes; a number of other studies report associations of early childhood cognitive and motor abilities with later school-age outcomes (Dewey, Crawford, Creighton, & Sauve, 1999; Marlow, Roberts, & Cooke, 1993; Sullivan & McGrath, 2003). Normal scores on early tests of cognitive ability such as the BSID are reasonably accurate in predicting positive outcomes at later ages, as are severe early impairments in predicting later disability. But prediction is less accurate when early test scores indicate more mild degrees of impairment (Marlow, Wolke, Bracewell, Samara, & EPICure Study Group, 2005). Results from Hack et al. (2005b) suggest that even mild to moderate impairments on early cognitive tests may have poor predictive validity. In this study of children with ELBW, a score under 70 on the BSID-II Mental Development Index at 20 months corrected age was a poor predictor of a similar deficit on the Mental Processing Composite of the Kaufman Assessment Battery for Children (K-ABC) at mean age 8 years. The positive predictive value of an early deficit on the BSID-II in relation to a later deficit on the K-ABC was only .37. Although the predictive validity of an early impairment on the BSID-II was better for children with neurological or sensory abnormalities, 80% of children with early scores under 70 performed above this level in school-age testing. Hack et al. (2005b) speculated that the improved scores from early to later testing could reflect measurement problems or a change in children's functioning related to neural development or environmental influences.

The findings from studies of young adults with VLBW/VPTB suggest that outcomes are much the same as those measured in adolescence. In one of two major North American studies of young adult outcomes, Hack (2002, 2004) followed a large cohort with VLBW and controls with NBW to mean age 20 years. The group with VLBW had lower scores on tests of IQ and academic achievement than the controls, as well as higher systolic blood pressure, poorer respiratory function, and less involvement in physical activities. Males, but not females, with VLBW were smaller than the children with NBW in height, weight, and body mass index. In addition, fewer of the young adults with VLBW had graduated from high school or had obtained a General Education Diploma, and fewer of the men with VLBW than the men with NBW were in 4-year college or university programs. On parent behavior ratings of the young adults, men with VLBW were rated as having more thought and attention problems than men with NBW, and women with VLBW were rated as having more attention problems, anxious/depressed behaviors, and withdrawal than women with NBW. Self-reports also indicated more withdrawal in the women with VLBW. Outcomes for the cohort with VLBW were nevertheless positive in some respects. There were no group differences in rates of unemployment or in self-ratings of satisfaction with health; moreover, the group with VLBW reported less alcohol and drug use, fewer delinquent behaviors, and lower pregnancy rates than the controls. Studies in the United Kingdom and Sweden further document less drug and alcohol use, despite adverse effects on educational attainment (Cooke, 2004; Ericson & Kallen, 1998).

Similar results were obtained in a Canadian study of young adult survivors of ELBW by Saigal et al. (2007). Although these investigators did not find differences between this cohort and controls with NBW in educational attainment, the men with ELBW had higher rates of asthma than the control men, and the group with ELBW as a whole had higher rates of seizures, recurrent bronchitis, and placement on antidepressant medications than the controls. Functional limitations reported more frequently in the group with ELBW than in controls included vision difficulties, clumsiness and poor dexterity, and learning disabilities. This group also reported lower physical functioning and less participation in sports and strenuous activities.

Family Consequences

Research examining the family consequences of raising children with VLBW/VPTB is well justified, given the extensive stresses placed on parents and other family members at the time of such a child's birth and during the early neonatal period, as well as by the challenges families face in managing children at high risk for cognitive, school, and behavior problems (Deater-Deckard & Bulkley, 2000; Witt, Riley, & Coiro, 2003). The influences of the home environment on children's behavior and learning makes it even more imperative to examine family outcomes (Bradley, Caldwell, Rock, Casey, & Nelson, 1987; Landry, Miller-Loncar, Smith, & Swank, 2002). The family consequences of VLBW/VPTB during early childhood include increased parent stress and family burden and decreased parent well-being in the families of these children, compared to families of controls with NBW. Furthermore, the negative impact of VLBW/VPTB on families is greatest for children with longer neonatal hospitalizations or problems with health or development (Taylor et al., 2000a).

Although parent distress may diminish over time during early childhood, negative effects on families persist. A study by our research group used the Impact on Family scale (Drotar et al., 2006). This scale revealed that children with ELBW had a more negative impact on family finances and imposed more caretaker and familial burden than did children with NBW. Neurodevelopmental problems in the child, as defined by neurological or sensory disorders or impaired IQ or adaptive behavior skills, predicted a more negative family impact within the group with ELBW. Similarly, Saigal, Burrows, Stoskopf, Rosenbaum, and Streiner (2000a) found that the parents of the teens with ELBW, relative to parents of teens with NBW, reported that their children's health status had more negative effects on siblings and parental emotional health. Parents of teens with ELBW and neurological or sensory impairments also reported more limited time to attend to their personal needs than did parents of teens with ELBW but without these impairments, showing that the impact of ELBW varied with a teen's health status. On the positive side, the parents of the group with

ELBW indicated that their teens' health status brought them closer together. The investigators concluded that families adjusted fairly well in most respects, implying considerable resilience on the part of families.

Our research group's School-Age Follow-Up Project confirmed persisting effects of more extreme low birthweight on the family during middle childhood (Taylor, Klein, Minich, & Hack, 2001a). Based on data collected when the children were mean age 11 years, parents of the children in the group with <750 g birthweight reported less parenting competence, more problems with attachment, and a more negative impact of a child's health status on the family than parents of the group with NBW reported. Rates of adverse family outcomes in the group with 750–1,499 g birthweight fell between those of the other two groups but were not significantly higher than those for the control group, providing evidence for a gradient of family effects. The study also revealed that adverse family outcomes were related to SES and to problems in functional child health, as defined by a neurological or sensory impairment, a high behavior problem rating, or a low score on a measure of adaptive behavior. Associations between birthweight group and family outcomes were not significant in analyses that controlled for the latter child problems. The latter finding suggests that the adverse effects of <750 g birthweight on family outcomes may have been related in large part to the effects of VLBW/VPTB-related child morbidity.

To further examine the nature of family burdens, we administered a parent interview in which we asked parents to identify health, learning, or behavior problems in their children and to rate family concerns associated with these problems. Compared to the parents of controls with NBW, parents of children with <750 g birthweight reported greater burden related to disruptions in family routines and greater concerns about their children's future, need for supervision, self-esteem, and acceptance by peers. At the same time, many families seemed to fare well. Only about half of the families in the group with <750 g birthweight reported what we considered to be significant family concerns, compared with 36% of the group with 750–1,499 g and 27% of the group with NBW.

We (Moore, Taylor, Klein, Minich, & Hack, 2006) examined subsequent family assessments to investigate potential changes in family consequences from mean ages 11 to 14 years. A further aim was to explore associations of family characteristics with family outcomes. The family environment was assessed with measures of SES, family stressors, and family resources. Mixed-model analysis revealed that group differences in family burden changed over the follow-up period. In families with high resources, the parents of the group with <750 g birthweight reported significantly higher burden than the parents of the control group across all assessments, whereas this difference was evident only at ages 11 and 12 years for families with low resources. A possible explanation of this finding is that parents from low-resource families were more consumed with other concerns as their children became increasingly independent. The continued burden over time observed in parents with higher resources may be interpreted as a sign of greater sensitivity to the children's problems or of frustration that the supports provided were insufficient to meet the children's needs. A second finding was that parents of the children with <750 g birthweight reported significantly more psychological distress than the parents of the term group at ages 11 and 12 years, though not thereafter. The latter differences were only evident in families of lower SES, suggesting that other stressors or lack of supports may contribute to the difficulties these families have in effectively addressing their children's problems (McLoyd, 1998).

FACTORS RELATED TO CHILD OUTCOMES

Biological Risks

Chronic lung disease and intracranial ultrasound abnormalities (IVH, PVL, ventricular dilation) are especially robust and consistent predictors of poor outcomes of VLBW/ VPTB (Downie, Jakobson, Frisk, & Ushycky, 2003; Hack et al., 2000; Taylor et al., 2004a, 2006; Vohr et al., 2000; Whitaker et al., 1996, 1997; Wood et al., 2005). Other individual neonatal complications linked to poorer outcomes include NEC, postnatal steroid treatment, sepsis, meningitis, jaundice, hypothyroxinemia (reduced thyroid levels), hypocapnia (reduced carbon dioxide in the blood, often related to hyperventilation), hypotension, apnea, retinopathy of prematurity, seizures, and patent ductus arteriosus (Collins, Lorenz, Jetton, & Paneth, 2001; Cooke, 2005; Doctor et al., 2001; Hack et al., 2000; Hintz et al., 2005a; Ishaik, Mirabella, Asztalos, Perlma, & Rovet, 2000; Msall et al., 2000; Taylor, Klein, Schatschneider, & Hack, 1998b; Wood et al., 2005). The fact that complications co-occur in many infants makes it difficult to sort out their separate influences. Nevertheless, findings suggest that the degree of low birthweight/low GA, brain abnormalities on neonatal ultrasounds, chronic lung disease, retinopathy of prematurity, and postnatal steroids may predict different outcomes (Curtis, Lindeke, Georgieff, & Nelson, 2002; Laptook, O'Shea, Shankaran, Bhaskar, & the NICHD Neonatal Network, 2005; Schmidt et al., 2003; Short et al., 2003; Taylor et al., 2006). Existing research, for example, suggests that chronic lung disease predicts more global impairment than does the degree of low birthweight or brain abnormalities (Anderson, Doyle, & the Victorian Infant Collaborative Study Group, 2006; Taylor et al., 2004a), and that PVL and shunted hydrocephalus predict nonverbal abilities better than they do verbal skills (Jacobson, Ek, Fernell, Flodmark, & Broberger, 1996; Whitaker et al., 1996).

Because more severe neonatal illness is reflected in more of these complications and longer treatment, composites indices of neonatal risk are useful predictors of later outcomes. Such composites include the counts of neonatal complications, ratings of the severity of acute neonatal illness, time on ventilatory support, and length of neonatal hospitalization (Dorling, Field, & Manktelow, 2005; Laptook et al., 2005; Taylor et al., 2006). Associations of maternal chorioamnionitis and placental abnormalities with later neurological abnormalities and cognitive deficits suggest that outcomes are related to antenatal as well as neonatal risk factors (Redline, Minich, Taylor, & Hack, 2007; Wilson-Costello et al., 1998). Longer-term sequelae are additionally related to neurodevelopment impairments in early childhood (Wood et al., 2005).

More extreme degrees of low birthweight or GA also predict worse outcomes, even within the VLBW/VPTB range (Anderson et al., 2003; Horwood, Mogridge, & Darlow, 1998; Klebanov et al., 1994; Taylor et al., 2004a). These risk factors appear to be independent of the effects of neonatal complications (Short et al., 2003; Taylor et al., 1998b). Our research group found developmental impairment at early school age in 63% of a cohort with <750 g birthweight, 38% of the group with 750–1,499 g, and 18% of term-born controls (Taylor et al., 2000b). For this study, impairment was based on the presence of neurological or sensory disorder, low IQ, low score on achievement testing, behavior problems, ADHD, low adaptive behavior skills, or special education placement. Similarly, Wood, Marlow, Costeloe, Gibson, and Wilkinson (2000) found developmental or neuromotor disabilities in nearly half of a population-based cohort of children with GA ≤25 weeks examined at 30 months corrected age. Such sequelae are not limited to children with VLBW/VPTB, but extend across the broader continuum of low birthweight. Breslau, Chilcoat, DelDotto, Andreski, and Brown (1996) demonstrated "gradient" effects (i.e., higher birthweight associated with less marked consequences) on IQ and neuropsychological skills that extended to birthweights up to 3,000 g and Linnet et al. (2006) found an increased rate of hyperkinetic disorder in children with 34–36 weeks GA compared to term-born controls.

IUGR, small postnatal head circumference, and multiple births have also been examined as potential risk factors. Although IUGR is linked to poorer outcomes, the effects of this condition may be explained in large part by associated low birthweight, hypoxic ischemia, and subnormal fetal head growth (Gutbrod, Wolke, Soehne, Ohrt, & Riegel, 2000; Hack, 1997; Wallace & McCarton, 1997). Small head circumference after infancy has been more clearly associated with negative outcomes (Cooke, 2005; Peterson et al., 2006). Multiple births do not appear to confer a disadvantage relative to singleton births matched for birthweight, GA, brain lesions, and sex (Miyahara et al., 2003).

Abnormalities evident on MRI predict a number of outcomes. Predictors of cognitive ability include structural abnormalities in white and gray matter and increased ventricular size (Abernethy, Klafkowski, Foulder-Hughes, & Cooke, 2003; Edgin et al., 2008; Ment et al., 1999; Woodward, Anderson, Austin, Howard, & Inder, 2006); smaller cross-sectional area of the corpus callosum, and smaller volumes of white and gray matter and of individual structures such as the caudate, hippocampus, and cerebellum (Abernethy, Cooke, & Foulder-Hughes, 2004; Inder et al., 2005; Isaacs et al., 2000, 2004; Isaacs, Edmonds, Chong, Lucas, & Gadian, 2003; Nosarti et al., 2004; Peterson et al., 2000, 2003); and decreased FA (Skranes et al., 2007). With regard to academic achievement in children with VLBW/VPTB, Isaacs, Edmonds, Lucas, and Gadian (2001) found that smaller left parietal lobe volume predicted poorer calculation skills, and Allin et al. (2001) reported associations of smaller cerebellum volume with lower reading scores. Other studies report associations of parent ratings of inattention, hyperactivity, and problems in behavior adjustment with structural abnormalities on MRI, including white matter reduction and thinning of the corpus callosum (Indredavik et al., 2005), smaller caudate and hippocampal volumes (Abernethy, Palaniappan, & Cooke, 2002; Norsarti, Allin, Frangou, Rifkin, & Murray, 2005), and lower FA (Skranes et al., 2007). Evidence that MRI abnormalities and FA are related to developmental outcomes, even after neonatal risk factors are taken into account (Inder et al., 2006), indicates that prediction is enhanced by direct measurement of brain status.

Environmental Risks

Studies of predictors of outcomes of VLBW/VPTB show that environmental risks account for variability not explained by biological risks, thus confirming the additive effects of these two sets of risk factors (Hack et al., 1992; Taylor et al., 1998b, 2006; Vohr et al., 2003; Weisglas-Kuperus, Baerts, Smrkovsky, & Sauer, 1993). Distal measures of the family environment encompass ethnicity, parental education, occupation, and income; marital status; receipt of public assistance; and census-based descriptors of the neighborhood in which the family resides (e.g., percentage of poverty). Proximal measures encompass assessments of stimulation available to the child in the home environment, life stress, and parent social supports and psychological adjustment. Environmental factors also moderate the effects of biological risks on some outcomes of VLBW/VPTB. For example, Breslau and Chilcoat (2000) found that behavioral sequelae of VLBW were more pronounced in children from socially disadvantaged families; and Landry and her associates (Landry et al., 1997; Landry, Smith, Miller-Loncar, & Swank, 1998) reported that a high-risk VLBW group was more affected by the quality of the maternal–child interaction than a lower-risk group. In contrast, other studies have found that sequelae are attenuated by social disadvantage, indicating that the effects of VLBW may be overshadowed in some cases by environmental adversity (Taylor et al., 2000a, 2006).

Environmental and biological risks have "domain-specific" associations with outcomes of VLBW/VPTB. Performance on tests of executive function and perceptual–motor abilities are more closely related to biological risks than to environmental risks, whereas social risks are better predictors of verbal abilities, IQ, and behavioral outcomes (Dammann et al., 1996; Taylor et al., 1998b). To illustrate, Figure 2.6 shows the proportion of the variance in long-term neuropsychological outcomes of VLBW explained by sociodemographic factors (SES and race) versus neonatal risk in our School-Age Follow-Up Project sample (Taylor et

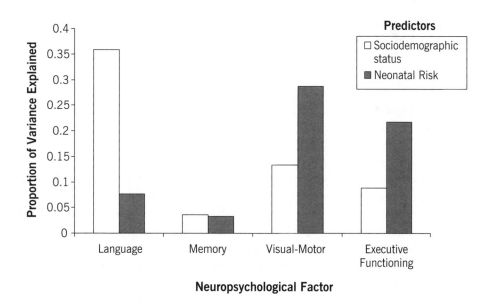

FIGURE 2.6. Proportions of variance in neuropsychological factor scores at mean age 16 years explained by sociodemographic status versus neonatal biological risk. Variance for sociodemographic status was determined by first entering neonatal biological risk as measured by birthweight and the Neonatal Risk Index (Taylor et al., 1998b) into a regression analysis, followed by SES and race. Variance for biological risk was determined by entering these variables in reverse order. Results indicated that both sets of factors accounted for significant variance in Memory, Visual–Motor, and Executive Functioning, but that neither set of factors accounted for variance in Memory. The findings suggest that sociodemographic factors are better predictors of Language, but that biological risk is a better predictor of Visual–Motor and Executive Functioning. Failure to predict Memory scores was unexpected but may relate to the fact that the memory test was administered in previous follow-up assessments, possibility reducing its utility as a measure of developmental outcome.

al., 2004a). Results showed that sociodemographic factors accounted for substantially more variance in language skills than neonatal risk, but that neonatal risk was a better predictor of visual–motor skill and executive functioning.

Sex Differences

Hintz, Kendrick, Vohr, Poole, and Higgins (2006) report that boys have a higher prevalence of neonatal complications and adverse early neurodevelopmental outcomes than girls. This study examined data from a large 1997–2000 birth cohort of children with <1,000 g birthweight and <28 weeks GA from the NICHD Neonatal Research Network. Boys had higher rates of multiple births, delivery room intubation, treatment with surfactant or postnatal steroids, grade III or IV IVH, and severe retinopathy of prematurity. Moreover, at 18–20 months corrected age the boys had higher rates of neurodevelopmental impairment as defined by CP, scores under 70 on the BSID-II Mental Development Index or Psychomotor Development Index, or deafness or blindness. Rates of neurodevelopmental impairment were likewise higher for boys in a large cohort of children born at ≤28 weeks GA (Wood et al., 2005). Other studies also report worse outcomes in boys (Hack et al., 2000; Johnson & Breslau, 2000), although these are not evident in all outcome studies (Saigal et al., 2000b; Taylor et al., 2004b). The reasons for a male disadvantage are not well understood, but may relate to a greater susceptibility of males to perinatal insults to the brain and lungs (Hintz et al., 2006; Lauterbach, Raz, & Sander, 2001).

Effects of Interventions

Treatments to improve outcomes for children with VLBW/VPTB range from neonatal medical management to environmental interventions in the neonatal nursery and programs to foster child development. Because these children are at high risk for complications, medical treatments are being continually evaluated as means to prevent or reduce adverse developmental consequences. For example, Ment et al. (2000) found that early postnatal administration of indomethacin reduced the rate of IVH in children with VLBW. Newer treatments include nutritional supplements (Ambalavanan et al., 2005; Clandinin et al., 2005), caffeine (Schmidt et al., 2006), and inhaled nitric oxide (Mestan, Marks, Hecox, Huo, & Schreiber, 2005). Postnatal steroids were given routinely to high-risk children for most of the 1990s, but are now only selectively employed because of evidence for deleterious effects (Wilson-Costello, 2007). To the extent that introduction or discontinuation of neonatal treatments alters survival or early medical morbidity, these interventions result in variations in long-term consequences according to birth year (i.e., cohort effects).

　　Researchers have also demonstrated positive effects of specialized care in the neonatal intensive care unit (NICU) and of early childhood interventions. Als's Neonatal Individualized Developmental Care and Assessment Program showed that environmental controls over exposures to light, loud noise, sleep interruptions, and other supportive developmental interventions resulted in decreased time on ventilators and tube feeding and in shorter hospitalizations, compared with routine neonatal care (Als, 1998; Als et al., 1994). Parent education and counseling during an infant's stay in the NICU and during the early postnatal period are additionally effective in improving short-term parent and infant outcomes (Browne & Talmi, 2005; Kaaresen, Ronning, Ulvund, & Dahl, 2006; Melnyk et al., 2001).

Other beneficial neonatal interventions include positioning and handling procedures, and efforts to encourage non-nutritive sucking and breastfeeding (Aucott, Donohue, Atkins, & Allen, 2002).

Early childhood interventions include center-based developmental programs and parent support and training. The best-known of these efforts, the Infant Health and Development Program (McCormick, McCarton, Brooks-Gunn, Belt, & Gross, 1998), compared the effects of an early childhood intervention program involving home visits, center-based developmental education, and parent support groups with pediatric follow-up only. The intervention was provided to children with low birthweight from term equivalent to 3 years corrected age. Children in both groups were stratified into heavier (2,001–2,500 g) and lighter (≤2000 g) subgroups. Assessments at 2 and 3 years corrected age revealed higher cognitive skills and reduced behavior problems in the intervention group than in the follow-up-only group. Group differences in cognitive performance were greater for children in the subgroup with heavier low birthweight, and were limited to mothers with a high school education or less. Although treatment effects diminished across subsequent posttreatment follow-ups at ages 5 and 8 years, a later follow-up at age 18 years indicated that the intervention participants with heavier low birthweight had higher scores on tests of math and receptive vocabulary and fewer high-risk behaviors than the controls (McCormick et al., 2006).

Other studies have demonstrated positive effects of early parenting programs on maternal adjustment and child development (Deater-Deckard & Bulkley, 2000). Achenbach, Howell, Aoki, and Rauh (1993) documented long-term benefits of a program to enhance mother–infant interactions in a sample of children with <2,250 g birthweight on the children's cognitive skills, academic achievement, and behavior. Landry, Smith, and Swank (2003) demonstrated that mothers of both preterm and full-term children could be taught to increase their use of contingent responsiveness to infants during the first year of life, and that these maternal changes were related to improvements in the infants' cognitive skills and social behaviors.

Some interventions have proved less successful. The Avon Premature Infant Project (1998) failed to document effects of interventions during the first two years of life for children born at ≤32 weeks GA. The infants in this project were randomly assigned to two early interventions: one emphasizing strategies to promote child development, and the other providing parent support. Both intervention groups obtained slightly higher scores on a developmental test than an untreated preterm group when social factors were controlled for. In addition, scores for higher-risk children, as defined by <1,251 g birthweight or evidence of brain insult on cerebral ultrasounds, were better for the developmental intervention group than for untreated controls. However, these initial benefits were not evident in a follow-up assessment conducted at 5 years (Johnson, Ring, Anderson, & Marlow, 2005). Similar findings were reported by Salokorpi, Rautio, Kajantie, and Von Wendt (2002). The investigators found immediate benefits of weekly occupational therapy provided to the children with ELBW from 6 to 12 months of age, but they did not find that these benefits persisted at later follow-ups after the therapy had ended. These studies suggest that early interventions may need to be sustained for substantial periods if they are to have lasting effects. Lack of parent participation in early interventions may also detract from the potential benefit of early intervention programs (Hill, Brooks-Gunn, & Waldfogel, 2003; Huber, Holditch-Davis, & Brandon, 1993).

METHODOLOGICAL CRITIQUE

The key methodological limitations of studies of the effects of VLBW/VPTB were clearly articulated 70 years ago in Benton's (1940) critique of early research on developmental outcomes. Prior to the advent of neonatal intensive care, only the "fittest" babies survived, and outcomes probably differed from those observed today. Nonetheless, Benton concluded from the evidence available at the time that low birthweight adversely affected early cognitive development and could result in behavior problems such as inattention and forgetfulness. Although he failed to find persuasive evidence for persisting cognitive deficits, he emphasized that research was limited by biases in sample recruitment, use of outcome measures that were narrow in scope or psychometrically inadequate, lack of comparison groups to control for background characteristics associated with high-risk birth, and failure to follow children over time or to take environmental influences into account.

According to Aylward (2002, 2005), these same problems continue to limit research in the modern era. Aylward additionally emphasizes the need to (1) take birthweight, GA, and neonatal complications into account as moderators of outcome; (2) control for both proximal and distal measures of the family environment; (3) correct for GA in computing age-adjusted performance, at least up to 2 years of age; (4) report rates of major neurodevelopmental disorders and examine the effect of including these children on group differences; (5) assess multiple facets of developmental outcome, including health status, distinct neuropsychological skills, school performance, adaptive behavior, behavioral problems, and quality of life; (6) document consequences in terms of both group means and impairment rates; (7) use outcome measures with adequate psychometric characteristics, including acceptable reliability, validity as potential markers of VLBW/VPTB-related consequences, and clinical utility (e.g., sensitivity and specificity) in identifying individual impairments; (8) assess children repeatedly over extended follow-up intervals, using the same test instruments as much as is feasible; and (9) consider possible changes in outcomes over successive birth cohorts related to advancements in neonatal care (cohort effects). Aylward further recommends that researchers use the most appropriate analytic tools, applying techniques such as structural equation models where appropriate to examine associations between latent constructs, or growth modeling to explore factors related to developmental change. In addition, he urges caution in interpreting group differences in outcomes solely in terms of the effects of low birthweight or preterm birth. Because the ultimate consequences of VLBW/VPTB may be moderated by genetic factors, early developmental interventions, and family circumstances, outcomes are not likely to be direct reflections of neonatal medical risk (Baron, Litman, Ahronovich, & Larson, 2007). Account also needs to be taken of potential variability between centers in medical treatment and outcomes (Vohr et al., 2004).

A sound practice when evaluating behavior outcomes is to obtain data from multiple informants, in part to reduce the potential for biased reporting. Research has documented low levels of agreement between parents and teachers (Kohen, Brooks-Bunn, McCormick, & Graber, 1997; Spiker, Kraemer, Constantine, & Bryant, 1992), suggesting that the children behave differently in different contexts and/or that parents and teachers use different criteria in evaluating child behavior. Behavioral researchers have thus advised obtaining ratings from both sources. Chilcoat and Breslau (1997) illustrate an elegant method for considering ratings from different informants in the same analysis, using general estimating equations. Self-impressions of behavior and adjustment also have a place, especially in evaluating subjective symptoms (Hack et al., 2005c). A limitation of self-reports is that they may be less revealing of negative outcomes (Hack et al., 2004; Saigal et al., 2003).

One especially thorny methodological problem not listed above is difficulty in identifying the presence and extent of prenatal exposures to drugs and alcohol. Because use of tobacco, alcohol, and cocaine during pregnancy is associated with decreased birthweight and may affect a child's development or signal problems in caregiving (Bada et al., 2005; Heffelfinger, Craft, White, & Shyken, 2002; Jacobson & Jacobson, 2001; Shankaran et al., 2007), control for such exposures would be useful in examining the effects of VLBW/VPTB. The challenge in this regard is that information on prenatal exposures obtained at the time of delivery through drug screens or interview with mothers may not be uniformly available and may be of variable quality. Interviews with mothers at follow-up about such exposures may be intrusive, and the validity of retrospective maternal reports is questionable (Jacobson, Chiodo, Sokol, & Jacobson, 2002).

Another unresolved issue is how long to continue correcting for low GA. Whereas Marlow (2004) recommends correcting for GA through 2 years of age, Rickards, Kitchen, Doyle, and Kelly (1989) advise that these corrections continue to be made up to 8½ years. Other researchers believe that such corrections provide an overly rosy picture of outcomes relative to real-life expectations, which are more typically based on chronological age. Further problems related to GA corrections include the imprecision of GA estimates and the artifactual drop in age-adjusted scores when corrections for prematurity are no longer applied (DiPietro & Allen, 1991; Landry et al., 1993).

RESEARCH DIRECTIONS

A Conceptual Framework

The conceptual framework presented in Figure 2.7 illustrates how the scope of future investigations might be broadened to better account for outcomes and to more accurately portray the influence of VLBW/VPTB on development. Several previous studies of outcomes of VLBW/VPTB have proposed similar causal networks (Taylor et al., 2002; Weisglas-Kuperus et al., 1993). The major assumption of this framework is that difficulties in learning and behavior in children with VLBW/VPTB can be best explained in terms of multiple influ-

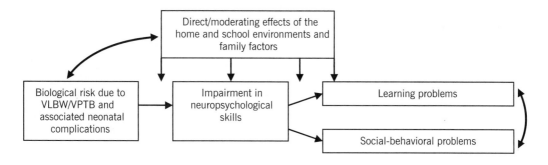

FIGURE 2.7. Conceptualization of the influences on learning and behavior in children with VLBW/VPTB.

ences on outcomes that include biological risks, impaired cognitive skills, and environ-mental influences. According to the model, biological risk results in neuropsychological impairment, which in turn leads to deficits in learning and behavior. The importance of examining mediation effects is their potential to enhance knowledge about the cogni-tive effects of VLBW/VPTB and the cognitive bases of children's academic and behavior problems (Martel, Lucia, Nigg, & Breslau, 2007). The curved arrow between biological and environmental factors represents potential covariation between these risks; the curved arrow on the right side of the figure represents the close association of academic achieve-ment with social competence and behavioral adjustment (McClelland, Morrison, & Hol-mes, 2000). A broader model of developmental outcomes would also consider changes with age in outcomes of VLBW/VPTB, although these are not shown in Figure 2.7. Rates of growth and changes in outcomes over time would then be examined in relation to the biological and environmental factors represented in the model.

Biological risk, shown on the left side of the figure, can be defined by comparing cohorts with VLBW/VPTB to term controls, or by examining low birthweight/GA or neo-natal complications as predictors of outcome within these cohorts. Brain insults related to VLBW/VPTB are conceived as varying in location and extent across children, and these variations are perceived as producing different cognitive outcomes. Tests of a broad range of ability domains are thus needed to fully assess cognitive outcomes. However, the model additionally acknowledges the special vulnerability of some brain structures to perinatal insult, including the basal ganglia, hippocampi, and frontostriatal white matter tracts. Because of the role of these structures in mediating executive functions and memory (Frisk & Whyte, 1994), tests of executive function and memory are of special importance in test-ing the model. We know little about genetic vulnerability to the adverse effects of preterm birth and perinatal neurological complications, but this is another relevant biological risk factor (Aylward, 2005).

The top part of the figure represents environmental influences on cognitive skills, learning, and behavior. These influences include sociodemographic status, parent psycho-logical distress, caretaker burden, family resources and stressors, and the support provided at home and at school for the child's development. The school and home environments are hypothesized to affect child outcomes more directly than biological risks (represented by downward-pointing arrows above these constructs). The model also incorporates poten-tial moderating influences of environmental factors on the causal linkages between the other model constructs (represented by downward-pointing arrows positioned above the left-to-right pathways in Figure 2.7). Environmental moderation of the effects of cognitive impairments on learning and behavior is of particular interest, as are protective factors. Environmental factors may affect children either directly or via their association with char-acteristics of the more proximal family environment, such as parenting support for achieve-ment, parent resources or stressors, and parent psychiatric symptoms or disorders (Klebanov, Brooks-Gunn, McCarton, & McCormick, 1998; Felner et al., 1995; McLoyd, 1998). Protec-tive factors, such as parental warmth and responsiveness, may help to account for favorable outcomes in children living in disadvantaged neighborhoods or those at high biological risk (Landry et al., 2003; McGrath, Sullivan, & Seifer, 1998; Tully, Arseneault, Caspi, Moffitt, & Morgan, 2004). Other contributing factors to consider are children's health status and experiential background, including histories of chronic illness, educational interventions, and opportunities for learning and socialization outside of school.

Important Research Initiatives

In addition to expanding the breadth of research, focused initiatives are needed to better understand VLBW/VPTB-related cognitive impairments, the biological basis of these deficits and their relevance to learning and behavior problems, and ways to optimize child outcomes. Examples of these initiatives are described below.

Differential Deficits and Their Association with Neuropathology

Attempts to specify the nature and neural basis of children's cognitive impairments will require more detailed studies of cognition, in combination with improved specification of the brain status of survivors. Areas of more pronounced cognitive impairment may be better determined by comparing levels of performance across a number of distinct skill areas than by examining performance relative to IQ. To the extent that a specific ability measure correlates with an omnibus measure of cognitive ability such as IQ, the latter procedure will undermine efforts to detect selective deficits. Assessment of relative strengths and weaknesses have been successful in clarifying the "core" deficiencies associated with other neurological disorders of childhood, such as hydrocephalus (Barnes & Dennis, 1998). Study of selective deficits in children with VLBW/VPTB is thus warranted. Research into differential deficits will involve using existing published measures and experimental tasks designed by neuropsychologists, cognitive scientists, and developmental psychologists to parse cognitive skills. Measures of both "crystallized" and "fluid" abilities will be useful in separating information storage from online mental processes and cognitive efficiency (Pennington, 1994; Isaacs et al., 2000). Assessments of discrete types of executive functioning, memory, and perceptual–motor skills also have potential to reveal dissociated deficits. To illustrate, existing evidence suggests that impairments may be greater in acquisition of verbal information than in retention (Taylor, Klein, Minich, & Hack, 2000c), that visual–motor skills are more vulnerable to PVL than nonmotor visual perception (Fazzi et al., 2004; Foreman et al., 1997), and that sustained attention is preserved relative to other executive functions in adolescents with VLBW (Kulseng et al., 2006). Additional study is required to identify the abilities most affected within the domains of executive functioning, memory, and perceptual–motor function, as well as specific cognitive deficits underlying weaknesses in math and social skills.

Hypotheses with regard to the types of brain insults incurred by these children may help guide the search for selective impairments. In view of evidence for localized brain insult, it would be fruitful to examine deficits consistent with specific forms of neuropathology, such as damage to the parieto-occipital pathway, or dorsal as opposed to ventral visual processing stream (Jakobson et al., 2001); frontal and subcortical regions (Curtis, Lindeke, Georgieff, & Nelson, 2002; Woodward et al., 2005); the white matter (Christ, White, Brunstrom, & Abrams, 2003; Edgin et al., 2008; Nagy, Westerberg, & Klingberg, 2004; Schatz, Craft, Koby, & Park, 1997); and the cerebellum (Allin et al., 2001). Because of substantial variability in how VLBW/VPTB affects brain substrate, these selective deficits are likely to be most evident in studies that examine cognitive outcomes in relation to variations in neuropathology, or that focus on children with specific types of brain insult. Measures of both localized and diffuse insult might be considered in attempting to account for cognitive outcomes.

Using fMRI to investigate differential patterns of brain activation in children with VLBW/VPTB versus controls with NBW is another brain-based approach to study of distinct neuropsychological outcomes of VLBW/VPTB. Group differences in patterns of brain activation during discrete tasks provide clues regarding neural reorganization of function following early insults. Differences in neural organization among children with VLBW/VPTB is suggested by hypoactivation of regions that would typically be engaged by a task, or by hyperactivation of regions less typically involved (Ment et al., 2006; Nosarti et al., 2006; Peterson et al., 2002; Rushe et al., 2004; Santhouse et al., 2002). A special advantage of fMRI studies is their potential to elucidate both brain dysfunction and compensatory mechanisms.

Effects on Early Learning Readiness

It would be useful to know more about the effects of VLBW/VPTB on children's readiness to learn when formal schooling begins and on how learning and behavior problems are manifested at this time. *Early learning readiness* refers to those cognitive and social skills needed to acquire beginning written language and math competencies (Blair, 2002). These skills include the abilities to pay attention to a task, to follow instructions, and to work collaboratively with teachers and peers. A focus on early childhood is justified by the fact that preacademic skills and social–behavioral competencies at the time of school entry predict later achievement and behavioral outcomes (Spira, Bracken, & Fischel, 2005). Early identification of special needs before or soon after school entry holds promise as a means to prevent or reduce adverse long-term educational and behavioral consequences of high-risk birth, at least if followed by appropriate interventions (Rimm-Kaufman, Pianta, & Cox, 2000). To identify children at risk and design effective early interventions, more information is needed about the ways in which these children fail to meet parent or teacher expectations. A clearer indication of the environmental demands and supports that exacerbate or buffer children's learning problems would also be useful.

Importance of Developmental Change

Additional longitudinal studies are needed for a fuller understanding of how outcomes of VLBW/VPTB change with age and what influences these changes. Longitudinal follow-up studies are critical for several reasons (Holmbeck, Bruno, & Jandasek, 2006). These studies provide greater precision in examining factors related to change and permit tests of mediators of the effects of early risks on later outcomes. Furthermore, the factors that affect change may differ from those that predict cross-sectional outcomes (Taylor et al., 2004c). Ideally, research on developmental change begins prior to school age (Baron et al., 2007; Breslau et al., 2004; Msall, 2006). Measures of early outcomes are important in determining the more immediate effects of neonatal complications or new neonatal treatments, and in identifying needs for early intervention. Continuing follow-up of children to later ages is then needed to establish the utility of shorter-term "surrogate" outcomes (Vohr, 2007). Further research to clarify the effects of VLBW/VPTB on specific cognitive skills during the preschool years may help to enhance the predictive validity of these early measures (Aylward, 2005; Espy et al., 2002). Early VLBW/VPTB-related deficits in specific information-processing skills may, in fact, help to account for the more generalized cognitive problems evident at later ages (Rose et al., 2005b). At the other end of the age continuum, we have much to learn about outcomes of VLBW/VPTB in middle and later adulthood. We know little about the implications of long-term weaknesses in executive function for adult educational and vocational functioning (Nosarti et al., 2007), and questions have been raised about risks for later-emerging cardiovascular, sleep, and mental health problems (Allin et al., 2006; Paavonen et al., 2007; Saigal et al., 2007).

Neonatal Complications as Predictors of Cognitive Outcomes

Data suggesting that lower GA, brain abnormalities, and chronic lung disease have different effects on cognition function (Curtis et al., 2002; Taylor et al., 2006) argue for additional study of neonatal factors as predictors of outcome. The rationale for such investigations is strengthened by recent findings relating neonatal brain abnormalities as assessed by MRI to childhood cognitive disabilities (Edgin et al., 2008; Woodward et al., 2005, 2006). MRI scans obtained during the neonatal or early postnatal periods reveal neuropathology not detected by ultrasounds and can illuminate neuropathological correlates of such risk factors as more extreme VLBW/VPTB, sepsis, and chronic lung disease (Gimenez et al., 2006; Inder et al., 2005; Kesler et al., 2004; Nosarti et al., 2004). Relating measures of early brain pathology to later brain status would also allow study of how early brain pathology effects subsequent brain development. Factors that could potentially mediate these changes, such as genetic risks, early interventions, or environmental supports, could then be examined to explore influences on neural reorganization. Outcomes of less extreme low birthweight/ prematurity also deserve further study as neonatal risk factors (Amiel-Tison, Allen, Lebrun, & Rogowski, 2002; Caravale, Tozzi, Albino, & Vicari, 2005; Linnet et al., 2006). Outcomes are generally more favorable for children with birthweights of 1,500–2,500 g and with 32–37 weeks GA than for those with VLBW/VPTB, and a smaller proportion of these "macropremies" may be adversely affected. Nevertheless, they are much more numerous, and we know relatively little about how they are affected or risks for poorer outcomes within this group.

Effects on Families and Mechanisms of Environmental Influence

Given the importance of environmental influences on outcomes, we need a better understanding of how families are affected by children with VLBW/VPTB, the ways in which families cope with children's problems and needs, and factors that facilitate or impede positive family adaptations. A related need is to increase our knowledge of how environments affect more positive child outcomes, whether by promoting neural plasticity, providing additional opportunities to develop compensatory skills, or employing child management techniques to encourage prosocial behaviors or enhance engagement in learning. The possibility that there are different environmental influences on different outcomes also deserves consideration. For example, Rose et al. (1992) reported different environmental influences on internalizing versus externalizing behaviors in young children with VLBW. Another issue worthy of investigation is whether VLBW or VPTB results in specific forms of psychopathology or confers a general vulnerability to psychopathology (Szatmari et al., 1993), possibly by limiting the individual's cognitive resources for dealing with environmental stress or negative life events. Although there is much to learn about the basis of environmental influences, efforts to promote family functioning and effective parenting methods may contribute to better child outcomes (Bradley et al., 1994; Landry et al., 2003).

Neuropsychological Basis of Learning and Behavior Problems

Several studies have demonstrated the utility of cognitive measures as predictors of academic achievement and behavior. Our research group has found that specific neuropsychological deficits predict poor academic achievement and attention problems in children with VLBW, even when general cognitive functioning is taken into account (Litt et al., 2005; Marlow et al., 2007; Taylor et al., 1998a). The relation of these skills to achievement differs according to the academic skills assessed. Other studies reveal associations of cognitive or motor skills to adaptive behavior and behavior problems (Breslau, Chilcoat, Johnson, Andreski, & Lucia, 2000; Rosenbaum, Saigal, Szatmari, & Hoult, 1995). Further research on the neuropsychological correlates of learning and behavior problems has the potential to clarify the specific skill deficits that contribute to these problems. Such research would identify children who are at high risk for learning and behavior disorders, and would guide efforts to facilitate learning and behavioral progress.

Interventions to Improve Outcomes

Finally, further studies of interventions to improve developmental outcomes are needed to determine what methods are most effective. Although preschool programs have failed to produce dramatic gains in outcomes, approaches that target parenting or specific developmental deficiencies may have more potential than more general efforts to facilitate child development (Landry et al., 2002). Few if any interventions have been directed at prevention or amelioration of academic or social–behavioral problems in school-age children with VLBW/VPTB. Appropriate interventions to consider would be those designed for children with executive deficits and with nonverbal learning disabilities, including direct instruction in organizational strategies, use of verbal mediation, and opportunities for extended time and practice (Litt et al., 2005; Taylor et al., 2004c). These programs could be either school- or home-based, but would probably require substantial individual programming to address the wide variability in deficits. It would also be relevant to determine whether some of the common sequelae of VLBW/VPTB, such as attention deficits, respond to medication and other interventions in a manner similar to such deficits in full-term children with ADHD.

SUMMARY AND CONCLUSIONS

Due in large part to recent advances in neonatal intensive care, survival of children with VLBW/VPTB has increased over the past few decades. This increase has been most dramatic among the children born at the lower end of the low-birthweight/low-GA spectrum. A large body of research indicates that these children are at risk for cognitive, learning, and behavior problems. Depending on the outcome measured and the degree of VLBW/

VPTB, comparisons between cohorts with VLBW/VPTB and controls with NBW yield moderate to large effect sizes. Global cognitive ability is mildly reduced in this population relative to the controls, but perceptual–motor skills, memory, and executive function are especially vulnerable. Academic deficits are evident in low scores on achievement tests; teacher ratings showing substandard school performance; and high rates of learning disabilities, special education placement, and grade repetition. Weaknesses in mathematics are especially pronounced. Behavior difficulties may include externalizing or internalizing symptoms, but most frequently entail attentional weaknesses. A better understanding of the effects of VLBW/VPTB on specific cognitive skills, along with efforts to link these skills to the specific forms of neuropathology, will clarify brain–behavior relationships and help account for children's learning and behavior problems.

Adverse effects of VLBW/VPTB on children's health and development persist throughout the school-age years and into adulthood. Health problems and early weaknesses in some language and adaptive behavior skills appear to attenuate somewhat with age. On the other hand, existing studies fail to suggest any general lessening with age of cognitive, learning, or behavior problems. In fact, a worsening of the degree of impairment relative to age expectations has been observed for a few tests of perceptual–motor skills and executive functioning. Research on developmental change across the school-age years is nevertheless scant. Additional investigation will be required to determine the domains in which improvement or worsening of outcomes may be possible, the factors associated with such changes, and the levels at which skills plateau as children approach adulthood.

The extent of children's deficits is related to the degree of low birthweight/low GA and to neonatal complications, such as IVH, PVL, and chronic lung disease. VLBW/VPTB-related reductions in brain volumes at birth and throughout childhood are other important markers of biological risk. Environmental disadvantage contributes to poor outcomes independently of biological risks, but may also moderate the effects of these risks. Study of multiple risk and protective factors has the potential to improve the accuracy of predictions of future outcomes, provide a clearer picture of the effects of birth-related neuropathology relative to other influences on development, and inform the design of interventions for children with VLBW/VPTB. Few studies have focused on high-risk survivors with good developmental outcomes, such as the minority of survivors at the extremes of low birthweight/low GA or with neonatal brain insults who appear to be faring well (Bassan et al., 2007; Shankaran et al., 2004). Investigations focused on these children may shed light on neural, genetic, or environmental factors that promote more positive outcomes.

Research has also confirmed adverse effects of VLBW/VPTB on children's families. Although negative effects on families are not universal in this population, the families of children with VLBW/VPTB are at greater risk for family burden, parenting stress, and parental psychological distress than are the families of children with NBW. These adverse consequences persist into adolescence for some families. Risks to families vary with a family's characteristics, a child's degree of low birthweight, and the child's neurodevelopmental outcome. Parent- and child-oriented interventions administered in early in childhood have been effective in lessening parent stress and improving child outcomes, but the needs of families of school-age children with VLBW/VPTB have been largely ignored. Evidence from other studies of bidirectional influences between child and family outcomes (Taylor et al., 2001b) implies that more positive family adaptations may benefit the child as well.

Future medical research is needed on the reasons for VLBW/VPTB, the antecedents to brain insult in survivors, and ways to reduce neurodevelopmental morbidities (Wilson-Costello, 2007). The Extremely Low Gestational Age Newborn Study is representative of such efforts (Laughon et al., 2007). Further neuropsychological studies of outcome will help to define the nature and neuropathological correlates of children's cognitive deficits, as well as the implications of these deficits for learning and behavior. Neuropsychological investigations will also be useful in selecting cognitive measures that are sensitive to variations in biological risk or neural reorganization; identifying early predictors of later outcomes and assessing longitudinal change; and recognizing genetic, environmental, and contextual factors that modulate the effects of biological risks on development.

ACKNOWLEDGMENTS

Work on this chapter was supported in part by Grant Nos. HD50309 and HD39756 from the National Institutes of Health (NIH). Past studies by our research team cited in the chapter were funded by NIH Grant Nos. HD39756, HD26554, and HD34177. I am indebted to Maureen Hack, MBChB, for her collaboration and leadership.

REFERENCES

Abernethy, L. J., Cooke, R. W. I., & Foulder-Hughes, L. (2004). Caudate and hippocampal volumes, intelligence, and motor impairment in 7-year-old children who were born preterm. *Pediatric Research*, 55, 884–893.

Abernethy, L. J., Klafkowski, G., Foulder-Hughes, L., & Cooke, R. W. I. (2003). Magnetic resonance imaging and T2 relaxometry of cerebral white matter and hippocampus in children born preterm. *Pediatric Research*, 54, 868–874.

Abernethy, L. J., Palaniappan, M., & Cooke, R. W. I. (2002). Quantitative magnetic resonance imaging of the brain in survivors of very low birth weight. *Archives of Disease in Childhood*, 87, 279–283.

Achenbach, T. M., Howell, C. T., Aoki, M., & Rauh, V. A. (1993). Nine-year outcome of the Vermont Intervention Program for Low Birth Weight Infants. *Pediatrics*, 91, 45–55.

Ajayi-Obe, M., Saeed, N., Cowan, F. M., Rutherford, M. A., & Edwards, A. D. (2000). Reduced development of cerebral cortex in extremely preterm infants. *Lancet*, 356, 1162–1163.

Alexander, G. R., & Slay, M. (2002). Prematurity at birth: Trends, racial disparities, and epidemiology. *Mental Retardation and Developmental Disabilities Research Reviews*, 8, 215–220.

Allin, M., Henderson M., Suckling, J., Nosarti, C., Rushe, T., Fearon, P., et al. (2004). Effects of very low birthweight on brain structure in adulthood. *Developmental Medicine and Child Neurology*, 46, 46–53.

Allin, M., Matsumoto, H., Santhouse, A. M., Nosarti, C., AlAsady, M. H. S., Stewart, A. L., et al. (2001). Cognitive and motor function and the size of the cerebellum in adolescents born very preterm. *Brain*, 124, 60–66.

Allin, M., Rooney, M., Cuddy, M., Wyatt, J., Walshe, M., Rifkin, L., et al. (2006). Personality in young adults who are born preterm. *Pediatrics*, 117, 309–316.

Als, H. (1998). Developmental care in the newborn intensive care unit. *Current Opinion in Pediatrics*, 10, 138–142.

Als, H., Lawhon, G., Duffy, F. H., McAnulty, G. B., Gibes-Grossman, R., & Blickman, J. G. (1994). Individualized developmental care for the very low-birth-weight preterm infant. *Journal of the American Medical Association*, 272, 853–858.

Ambalavanan, N., Tyson, J. E., Kennedy, K. A., Hansen, N. I., Vohr, B., Wright, L. L., et al. (2005). Vitamin A supplementation for extremely low birth weight infants: Outcome at 18 to 22 months. *Pediatrics, 115,* e249–e254.

Amiel-Tison, C., Allen, M. C., Lebrun, F., & Rogowski, J. (2002). Macropremies: Underpriviledged newborns. *Mental Retardation and Developmental Disabilities Research Reviews, 8,* 281–292.

Anderson, P., Doyle, L. W., & the Victorian Infant Collaborative Study Group. (2003). Neurobehavioral outcomes of school-age children born extremely low birth weight or very preterm in the 1990s. *Journal of the American Medical Association, 289,* 3264–3272.

Anderson, P., Doyle, L. W., & the Victorian Infant Collaborative Study Group (2006). Neurodevelopmental outcome of bronchopulmonary dysplasia. *Seminars in Perinatology, 30,* 227–232.

Aram, D. M., Hack, M., Hawkins, S. H., Weissman, B. M., & Borawski-Clark, E. (1991). Very-low-birthweight children and speech and language development. *Journal of Speech and Hearing Research, 34,* 1169–1179.

Aucott, S., Donohue, P. K., Atkins, E., & Allen, M. C. (2002). Neurodevelopmental care in the NICU. *Mental Retardation and Developmental Disabilities Research Reviews, 8,* 298–308.

Avon Premature Infant Project. (1998). Randomized trial of parental support for families with very preterm children. *Archives of Disease in Childhood: Fetal and Neonatal Edition, 79,* F4–F11.

Aylward, G. P. (2002). Methodological issues in outcome studies of at-risk infants. *Journal of Pediatric Psychology, 27,* 37–45.

Aylward, G. P. (2005). Neurodevelopmental outcomes of infants born prematurely. *Developmental and Behavioral Pediatrics, 26,* 427–440.

Bada, H. S., Das, A., Bauer, C. R., Shankaran, S., Lester, B. M., Gard, C. C., et al. (2005). Low birth weight and preterm births: Etiologic fraction attributable to prenatal drug exposure. *Journal of Perinatology, 25,* 631–637.

Barnes, M. A., & Dennis, M. (1998). Discourse after early-onset hydrocephalus: Core deficits in children of average intelligence. *Brain and Language, 61,* 309–334.

Baron, I. S., Litman, F. R., Ahronovich, M. D., & Larson, J. C. G. (2007). Neuropsychological outcomes of preterm triplets discordant for birthweight: A case report. *The Clinical Neuropsychologist, 21*(2), 338–362.

Bass, J. L., Corwin, M., Gozal, D., Moore, C., Nishida, H., Parker, S., et al. (2004). The effect of chronic or intermittent hypoxia on cognition in childhood: A review of the evidence. *Pediatrics, 114*(3), 805–816.

Bassan, J., Limperopoulos, C., Visconti, K., Mayer, D. L., Feldman, H. A., Avery, L., et al. (2007). Neurodevelopmental outcome in survivors of periventricular hemorrhagic infarction. *Pediatrics, 120,* 785–792.

Benton, A. L. (1940). Mental development of prematurely born children: A critical review of the literature. *American Journal of Orthopsychiatry, 10,* 719–746.

Bhutta, A. T., Cleves, M. A., Casey, P. H., Cradock, M. M., & Anand, K. J. S. (2002). Cognitive and behavioral outcomes of school-age children who were born preterm. *Journal of the American Medical Association, 288,* 728–737.

Blair, C. (2002). School readiness: Integrating cognition and emotion in a neurobiological conceptualization of children's functioning at school entry. *American Psychologist, 57,* 111–127.

Bohm, B., Smedler, A.-C., & Forssberg, H. (2004). Impulse control, working memory and other executive functions in preterm children when starting school. *Acta Paediatrica, 93,* 1363–1371.

Botting, N., Powls, A., & Cooke, R. W. I. (1997). Attention deficit hyperactivity disorders and other psychiatric outcomes in very low birthweight children at 12 years. *Journal of Child Psychology and Psychiatry, 8,* 931–941.

Botting, N., Powls, A., Cooke, R. W. I., & Marlow, N. (1998). Cognitive and educational outcome of very-low-birthweight children in early adolescence. *Developmental Medicine and Child Neurology, 40,* 652–660.

Bradley, R. H., Caldwell, B. M., Rock, S. L., Casey, P. M., & Nelson, J. (1987). The early development of low-birthweight infants: Relationship to health, family status, family context, family processes, and parenting. *International Journal of Behavioral Development, 10,* 301–318.

Bradley, R. H., Whiteside, L., Mundfrom, D. J., Casey, P. H., Kelleher, K. J., & Pope, S. K. (1994). Contribution of early intervention and early caregiving experiences to resilience in low-birthweight, premature children living in poverty. *Journal of Clinical Child Psychology, 23,* 425–434.

Breslau, N., & Chilcoat, H. D. (2000). Psychiatric sequelae of low birth weight at 11 years of age. *Biological Psychiatry, 47,* 1005–1011.

Breslau, N., Chilcoat, H. D., Johnson, E. O., Andreski, P., & Lucia, V. C. (2000). Neurologic soft signs and low birthweight: Their association and neuropsychiatric implications. *Biological Psychiatry, 47,* 71–79.

Breslau, N., Chilcoat, H. D., Susser, E. S., Matte, T., Liang, K., & Peterson, E. L. (2001). Stability and change in children's intelligence quotient scores: A comparison of two socioeconomically disparate communities. *American Journal of Epidemiology, 154,* 711–717.

Breslau, N., Chilcoat, J. D., DelDotto, J. E., Andreski, P., & Brown, G. G. (1996). Low birth weight and neurocognitive status at six years of age. *Biological Psychiatry, 40,* 389–397.

Breslau, N., Paneth, N. S., & Lucia, V. C. (2004). The lingering academic deficits of low birth weight children. *Pediatrics, 114,* 1035–1040.

Browne, J. V., & Talmi, A. (2005). Family-based intervention to enhance infant–parent relationships in the neonatal intensive care unit. *Journal of Pediatric Psychology, 30,* 667–677.

Buck, G. M., Msall, M. E., Schisterman, E. F., Lyon, N. R., & Rogers, B. T. (2000). Extreme prematurity and school outcomes, *Paediatric and Perinatal Epidemiology, 14,* 324–331.

Caravale, B., Tozzi, C., Albino, G., & Vicari, S. (2005). Cognitive development in low risk preterm infants at 3–4 years of life. *Archives of Disease in Childhood: Fetal and Neonatal Edition, 90,* F474–F479.

Chilcoat, H. D., & Breslau, N. (1997). Does psychiatry history bias mothers' reports?: An application of a new analytic approach. *Journal of the American Academy of Child and Adolescent Psychiatry, 36,* 971–979.

Christ, S. E., White, D. A., Brunstrom, J. E., & Abrams, R. A. (2003). Inhibitory control following perinatal brain injury. *Neuropsychology, 17,* 171–178.

Clandinin, M. T., Van Aerde, J. E., Merkel, K. L., Harris, C. L., Springer, M. A., Hansen, J. W., et al. (2005). Growth and development of preterm infants fed infant formulas containing docosahexaenoic acid and arachidonic acid. *Journal of Pediatrics, 146,* 461–468.

Cole, C., Hagadorn, J., & Kim, C. (2002, December). *Criteria for determining disability in infants and children: Low birth weight* (Evidence Report/Technology Assessment No. 70, Prepared by Tufts New England Medical Center Evidence-Based Practice Center under Contract No. 290-97-0019; AHRQ Publication No. 03-E010). Rockville, MD: Agency for Healthcare Research and Quality.

Collins, M. P., Lorenz, J. M., Jetton, J. R., & Paneth, N. (2001). Hypocapnia and other ventilation-related risk factors for cerebral palsy in low birth weight infants. *Pediatric Research, 50,* 712–719.

Cooke, R. W. I. (2004). Health, lifestyle, and quality of life for young adults born very preterm. *Archives of Disease in Childhood, 89,* 201–206.

Cooke, R. W. I. (2005). Perinatal and postnatal factors in very preterm infants and subsequent cognitive and motor abilities. *Archives of Disease in Childhood: Fetal and Neonatal Edition, 90,* F60–F63.

Costeloe, K., Hennessy, E., Gibson, A. T., Marlow, N., Wilkinson, A. R., & the EPICure Study Group. (2000). The EPICure study: Outcomes to discharge from hospital for babies born at the threshold of viability. *Pediatrics, 106,* 659–671.

Cunningham, C., Taylor, H. G., Klein, N., Minich, N., & Hack, M. (2001). Constipation in very-low-birth-weight children at 10 to 14 years of age. *Journal of Pediatric Gastroenterology and Nutrition, 33,* 23–27.

Curtis, W. J., Lindeke, L. L., Georgieff, M. K., & Nelson, C. A. (2002). Neurobehavioral functioning in neonatal intensive care unit graduates in late childhood and early adolescence. *Brain, 125,* 1646–1659.

Dammann, O., & Leviton, A. (1999). Brain damage in preterm newborns: Might enhancement of developmentally regulated endogenous protection open a door for prevention? *Pediatrics, 104,* 541–550.

Dammann, O., Walther, H., Allers, B., Schroder, M., Drescher, J., Lutz, D., et al. (1996). Developmental of a regional cohort of very-low-birthweight children at six years: Cognitive abilities are associated with neurological disability and social background. *Developmental Medicine and Child Neurology, 38,* 97–108.

Deater-Deckard, K., & Bulkley, J. (2000). Parent concerns in long-term follow-up. *Seminars in Neonatology, 5,* 171–178.

Dewey, D., Crawford, S. G., Creighton, D. E., & Sauve, R. S. (1999). Long-term neuropsychological outcomes in very low birth weight children free of sensorineural impairments. *Journal of Clinical and Experimental Neuropsychology, 21,* 851–865.

DiPietro, J. A., & Allen, M. C. (1991). Estimation of gestational age: Implications for developmental research. *Child Development, 62,* 1184–1199.

Doctor, B. A., Newman, N., Minich, N. M., Taylor, H. G., Fanaroff, A. A., & Hack, M. (2001). Clinical outcomes of neonatal meningitis in very-low-birth-weight infants. *Clinical Pediatrics, 40,* 473–480.

Dorling, J. S., Field, D. J., & Manktelow, B. (2005). Neonatal disease severity scoring systems. *Archives of Disease in Childhood: Fetal and Neonatal Edition, 90,* F11–F16.

Downie, A. L. S., Jakobson, L. S., Frisk, V., & Ushycky, I. (2003). Periventricular brain injury, visual motion processing, and reading and spelling abilities in children who were extremely low birthweight. *Journal of the International Neuropsychological Society, 9,* 440–449.

Doyle, L. W., Cheung, M. M. H., Ford, G. W., Olinsky, A., Davis, N. M., & Callanan, C. (2001). Birth weight <1501 g and respiratory health at age 14. *Archives of Disease in Childhood, 84,* 40–44.

Drotar, D., Hack, M., Taylor, H. G., Schluchter, M., Andreais, A., & Klein, N. (2006). The impact of extremely low birth weight on the families of school-aged children. *Pediatrics, 117,* 2006–2013.

Edgin, J. O., Inder, T. E., Anderson, P. J., Hood, K. M., Clark, C. A. C., & Woodward, L. J. (2008). Executive functioning in preschool children born very preterm: Relationship with early white matter pathology. *Journal of the International Neuropsychological Society, 14,* 90–101.

Eiser, C., Eiser, J. R., Mayhew, A. G., & Gibson, A. T. (2005). Parenting the premature infant: Balancing vulnerability and quality of life. *Journal of Child Psychology and Psychiatry, 46,* 1169–1177.

Elgen, I., Sommerfelt, K., & Markestad, T. (2002). Population based, controlled study of behavioural problems and psychiatric disorders in low birthweight children at 11 years of age. *Archives of Disease in Childhood: Fetal and Neonatal Edition, 87,* F128–F132.

Ericson, A., & Kallen, B. (1998). Very low birthweight boys at the age of 19. *Archives of Disease in Childhood: Fetal and Neonatal Edition, 78,* F171–F174.

Espy, K. A., Stalets, M. M., McDiarmid, M. M., Senn, T. E., Cwik, M. F., & Hamby, A. (2002). Executive functions in preschool children born preterm: Application of cognitive neuroscience paradigms. *Child Neuropsychology, 8,* 83–92.

Fanaroff, A. A., Hack, M., & Walsh, M. C. (2003). The NICHD Neonatal Research Network: Changes in practice and outcomes during the first 15 years. *Seminars in Perinatology, 27,* 281–287.

Fanaroff, A. A., Stoll, B. J., Wright, L. L., Carlo, W. A., Ehrenkranz, R. A., Stark, A. R., et al. (2007). Trends in neonatal morbidity and mortality for very low birthweight infants. *American Journal of Obstetrics and Gynecology, 196,* 147.e1–147.e8.

Fazzi, E., Bova, S. M., Uggetti, C., Signorini, S. G., Bianchi, P. E., Maraucci, I., et al. (2004). Visual-perceptual impairment in children with periventricular leukomalacia. *Brain and Development, 26,* 506–512.

Fearon, P., O'Connell, P., Frangou, S., Aquino, P., Nosarti, C., Allin, M., et al. (2004). Brain volumes in adult survivors of very low birth weight: A sibling-controlled study. *Pediatrics, 114,* 367–371.

Feder, K. P., Majnemer, A., Bourbonnais, D., Platt, R., Blayney, M., & Synnes, A. (2005). Handwriting performance in preterm children compared with term peers at age 6 to 7 years. *Developmental Medicine and Child Neurology, 47,* 163–170.

Felner, R. D., Brand, S., DuBois, D. L., Adan, A. M., Mulhall, P. F., & Evans, E. G. (1995). Socioeconomic disadvantage, proximal environmental experiences, and socioemotional and academic adjustment in early adolescence: Investigation of a mediated effects model. *Child Development, 66,* 774–792.

Fiscella, K. (2005). Race, genes and preterm birth. *Journal of the National Medical Association, 97,* 1516–1526.

Foreman, N., Fielder, A., Minshell, C., Hurrion, E., & Sergienko, E. (1997). Visual search, perception, and visual–motor skill in "healthy" children born at 27–32 weeks' gestation. *Journal of Experimental Child Psychology, 64,* 27–41.

Frisk, V., & Whyte, H. (1994). The long-term consequences of periventricular brain damage on language and verbal memory. *Developmental Neuropsychology, 10,* 313–333.

Gardner, F., Johnson, A., Yudkin, P., Bowler, U., Hockley, C., Mutch, L., et al. (2004). Behavioral and emotional adjustment of teenagers in mainstream school who were born before 29 weeks' gestation. *Pediatrics, 114,* 676–682.

Gimenez, M., Junque, C., Narberhaus, A., Bargallo, N., Botet, F., & Mercader, J. M. (2006). White matter volume and concentration reductions in adolescents with history of very preterm birth: A voxel-based morphometry study. *NeuroImage, 32,* 1485–1498.

Goldenberg, R. L., & Rouse, D. J. (1998). Prevention of premature birth. *New England Journal of Medicine, 229,* 313–320.

Goyen, T., Lui, K., & Woods, R. (1998). Visual–motor, visual-perceptual, and fine motor outcomes in very-low-birthweight children at 5 years. *Developmental Medicine and Child Neurology, 40,* 76–81.

Groenendaal, F., van der Grond, J., Eken, P., van Haastert, I. C., Rademaker, K. J., Toet, M. C., et al. (1997). Early cerebral proton MRS and neurodevelopmental outcome in infants with cystic leukomalacia. *Developmental Medicine and Child Neurology, 39,* 373–379.

Grunau, R. E., Kearney, S. M., & Whitfield, M. F. (1990). Language development at 3 years in pre-term children of birth weight below 1000 g. *British Journal of Disorders of Communication, 25,* 173–182.

Grunau, R. E., Whitfield, M. F., & Davis, C. (2002). Pattern of learning disabilities in children with extremely low birth weight and broadly average intelligence. *Archives of Pediatrics and Adolescent Medicine, 156,* 615–620.

Grunau, R. E., Whitfield, M. F., & Fay, T. B. (2004). Psychosocial and academic characteristics of extremely low birth weight (≤800 g) adolescents who are free of major impairment compared with term-born subjects. *Pediatrics, 114,* e725–e732.

Gutbrod, T., Wolke, D., Soehne, B., Ohrt, B., & Riegel, K. (2000). Effects of gestation and birth weight on the growth and development of very low birthweight small for gestational age infants: A matched group comparison. *Archives of Disease in Childhood: Fetal and Neonatal Edition, 82,* F208–F214.

Hack, M. (1997). Effects of intrauterine growth retardation on mental performance and behavior: Outcomes during adolescence and adulthood. *European Journal of Clinical Nutrition, 52*(Suppl. 1), 65–71.

Hack, M., Breslau, N., Aram, D., Weissman, B., Klein, N., & Borawski-Clark, E. (1992). The effect of very low birthweight and social risk on neurocognitive abilities at school age. *Journal of Developmental and Behavioral Pediatrics, 13,* 412–420.

Hack, M., & Fanaroff, A. A. (1999). Outcomes of children of extremely low birthweight and gestational age in the 1990s. *Early Human Development, 53,* 193–218.

Hack, M., Flannery, D. J., Schluchter, M., Carter, L., Borawski, E., & Klein, N. (2002). Outcomes in young adulthood for very-low-birthweight infants. *New England Journal of Medicine, 346,* 149–157.

Hack, M., Taylor, H. G., Drotar, D., Schluchter, M., Cartar, L., Andreias, L., et al. (2005a). Chronic conditions, functional limitations, and special health care needs of school-aged children born with extremely low-birth-weight in the 1990s. *Journal of the American Medical Association, 294,* 318–325.

Hack, M., Taylor, H. G., Drotar, D., Schluchter, M., Cartar, L., Wilson-Costello, D., et al. (2005b). Poor predictive validity of the Bayley Scales of Infant Development for cognitive function of extremely low birth weight children at school age. *Pediatrics, 10,* 333–341.

Hack, M., Weismann, B., Breslau, N., Klein, N., Borawski-Clark, E., & Fanaroff, A. (1993). Health status of VLBW children during their first 8 years. *Journal of Developmental and Behavioral Pediatrics, 122,* 887–892.

Hack, M., Wilson-Costello, D., Friedman, H., Taylor, H. G., Schluchter, M., & Fanaroff, A. A. (2000). Neurodevelopment and predictors of outcomes of children with birth weights of less than 1000g. *Archives of Pediatrics and Adolescent Medicine, 154,* 725–731.

Hack, M., Youngstrom, E., Cartar, L., Schluchter, M., Taylor, H. G., Flannery, D. J., et al. (2004). Behavioral outcomes and evidence of psychopatholgy among very low birth weight infants at age 20 years. *Pediatrics, 114,* 932–940.

Hack, M., Youngstrom, E., Cartar, L., Schluchter, M., Taylor, H. G., Flannery, D. J., et al. (2005c). Predictors of internalizing symptoms among very low birth weight young women. *Journal of Developmental and Behavioral Pediatrics, 26,* 93–104.

Hamilton, B. E., Martin, J. A., & Ventura, S. J. Births: Preliminary data for 2005. *Health E-Stats.* Retrieved November 21, 2006. *www.cdc.gov/nchs/products/pubd/hestats/prelimbirths05/prelimbirths05.htm.*

Hamilton, B. E., Martin, J. A., & Ventura, S. J. (2006). Births: Preliminary data for 2005. *National Vital Statistics Reports, 55.*

Harvey, J. M., O'Callaghan, M. J., & Mohay, H. (1999). Executive function of children with extremely low birthweight: A case study. *Developmental Medicine and Child Neurology, 41,* 292–297.

Heffelfinger, A. K., Craft, S., White, D. A., & Shyken, J. (2002). Visual attention in preschool children prenatally exposed to cocaine: Implications for behavioral regulation. *Journal of the International Neuropsychological Society, 8,* 12–21.

Hill, J. L., Brooks-Gunn, J., & Waldfogel, J. (2003). Sustained effects of high participation in an early intervention for low-birth-weight premature infants. *Developmental Psychology, 39,* 730–744.

Hille, E. T. M., den Ouden, A. L., Bauer, L., van de Oudenrijn, C., Brand, R., & Verloove-Vanhorick, S. P. (1994). School performance at nine years of age in very premature and very low birth weight infants: Perinatal risk factors and predictors at five years of age. *Pediatrics, 125,* 426–434.

Hille, E. T. M., den Ouden, A. L., Saigal, S., Wolke, D., Lambert, M., Whitaker, A., et al. (2001). Behavioural problems in children who weigh 1000 g at birth in four countries. *Lancet, 357,* 1641–1643.

Hintz, S. R., Kendrick, D. E., Stoll, B. J., Vohr, B. R., Fanaroff, A. A., Donovan, E. F., et al. (2005s). Neurodevelopmental and growth outcomes of extremely low birth weight infants after necrotizing enterocolitis. *Pediatrics, 115,* 696–703.

Hintz, S. R., Kendrick, D. E., Vohr, B. R., Poole, W. K., & Higgins, R. D. (2005b). Changes in neurodevelopmental outcomes at 18 and 22 months' corrected age among infants of less than 25 weeks' gestational age born in 1993–1999. *Pediatrics, 115,* 1645–1651.

Hintz, S. R., Kendrick, D. E., Vohr, B. R., Poole, W. K., & Higgins, R. D. (2006). Gender differences in neurodevelopmental outcomes among extremely preterm, extremely-low-birthweight infants. *Acta Paediatrica, 95,* 1239–1248.

Hoff, B., Hansen, B. M., Munck, H., & Mortensen, E. L. (2004). Behavioral and social development of children born extremely premature: 5-year follow-up. *Scandinavian Journal of Psychology, 45,* 285–292.

Holmbeck, G. N., Bruno, E. F., & Jandasek, B. (2006). Longitudinal research in pediatric psychology: An introduction to the special issue. *Journal of Pediatric Psychology, 31,* 995–1001.

Holzman, C., Lin, X., Senagore, P., & Chung, H. (2007). Histologic chorioamnionitis and preterm delivery. *American Journal of Epidemiology, 166,* 786–794.

Horbar, J. D., Badger, G. J., Carpenter, J. H. Fanaroff, A. A., Kilpartrick, S., LaCorte, M., et al. (2002). Trends in mortality and morbidity for very low birth weight infants, 1991–1999. *Pediatrics, 110,* 143–151.

Horwood, L. J., Mogridge, N., & Darlow, B. A. (1998). Cognitive, educational, and behavioural outcomes at 7 and 8 years in a national very low birthweight cohort. *Archives of Disease in Childhood, Fetal and Neonatal Edition, 79,* F12–F20.

Hoy, E. A., Sykes, D. H., Bill, J. M., Halliday, H. L., McClure, B. G., & Reid, M. M. (1992). The social competence of very-low-birthweight children: Teacher, peer, and self-perceptions. *Journal of Abnormal Child Psychology, 20,* 123–150.

Huber, C., Holditch-Davis, D., & Brandon, D. (1993). High-risk preterm infants at 3 years of age: Parental response to the presence of developmental problems. *Children's Health Care, 22,* 107–124.

Hughes, M., Shults, J., & Medoff-Cooper, B. (2002). Temperament characteristics of preterm infants during the first year of life. *Journal of Developmental and Behavioral Pediatrics, 23,* 430–435.

Huppi, P. S., & Inder, T. E. (2001). Magnetic resonance techniques in the evaluation of the perinatal brain: Recent advances and future directions. *Seminars in Neonatology, 6,* 195–210.

Huttenlocher, P. R., & Dabholkar, A. S. (1997). Regional differences in synaptogenesis in human cerebral cortex. *Journal of Comparative Neurology, 387,* 167–178.

Inder, T. E., Huppi, P. S., Warfield, S., Kikinis, R., Zientara, G. P., Barnes, P. D., et al. (1999a). Periventricular white matter injury in the premature infant is followed by reduced cerebral cortical gray matter volume at term. *Annals of Neurology, 46,* 755–760.

Inder, T. E., Huppi, P. S., Zientara, G. P., Maier, S. E., Jolesz, F. A., di Salvo, D., et al. (1999b). Early detection of periventricular leukomalacia by diffusion-weighted magnetic resonance imaging techniques. *Journal of Pediatrics, 134,* 631–634.

Inder, T. E., & Volpe, J. J. (2000). Mechanisms of perinatal brain injury. *Seminars in Neonatology, 5,* 3–16.

Inder, T. E., Warfield, S. K., Wang, H., Huppi, P. S., & Volpe, J. J. (2005). Abnormal cerebral structure is present at term in premature infants. *Pediatrics, 115,* 286–294.

Inder, T. E., Wells, S. J., Mogridge, N. B., Spencer, C., & Volpe, J. J. (2003). Defining the nature of the cerebral abnormalities in the premature infant: A qualitative magnetic resonance imaging study. *Journal of Pediatrics, 143,* 171–179.

Indredavik, M. S., Skranes, J. S., Vik, T., Heyerdahl, S., Romundstad, P., Myhr, G. E., et al. (2005). Low-birth-weight adolescents: Psychiatric symptoms and cerebral MRI abnormalities. *Pediatric Neurology, 33,* 259–266.

Indredavik, M. S., Vik, T., Heyerdahl, S., Kulseng, S., Fayers, P., & Brubakk, A. (2004). Psychiatric symptoms and disorders in adolescents with low birth weight. *Archives of Disease in Childhood: Fetal and Neonatal Edition, 89,* F445–F450.

Isaacs, E. B., Edmonds, C. J., Chong, W. K., Lucas, A., & Gadian, D. G. (2003). Cortical anomalies associated with visuospatial processing deficits. *Annals of Neurology, 53,* 768–773.

Isaacs, E. B., Edmonds, C. J., Chong, W. K., Lucas, A., Morley, R., & Gadian, D. G. (2004). Brain morphometry and IQ measurements in preterm children. *Brain, 127,* 2595–2607.

Isaacs, E. B., Edmonds, C. J., Lucas, A., & Gadian, D. G. (2001). Calculation difficulties in children of very low birthweight: A neural correlate. *Brain, 124,* 1701–1707.

Isaacs, E. B., Lucas, A., Chong, W. K., Wood, S. J., Johnson, C. L., Marshall, C., et al. (2000). Hippocampal volume and everyday memory in children of very low birth weight. *Pediatric Research, 47,* 713–720.

Ishaik, G., Mirabella, G., Asztalos, E., Perlma, K., & Rovet, J. (2000). Hypothyroxinemia of prematurity and the development of attention and memory in infants with low risk prematurity: A pilot study. *Journal of Developmental and Behavioral Pediatrics, 21,* 172–179.

Jacobson, L., Ek, U., Fernell, E., Flodmark, O., & Broberger, U. (1996). Visual impairment in preterm children with periventricular leukomalacia: Visual, cognitive, and neuropediatric characteristics relate to cerebral imaging. *Developmental Medicine and Child Neurology, 38,* 724–735.

Jacobson, S. W., Chiodo, L. M., Sokol, R. J., & Jacobson, R. J. (2002). Validity of maternal report of prenatal alcohol, cocaine, and smoking in relation to neurobehavioral outcome. *Pediatrics, 109,* 815–825.

Jacobson, S. W., & Jacobson, J. L. (2001). Alcohol and drug-related effects on development: A new emphasis on contextual factors. *Infant Mental Health Journal, 22,* 416–430.

Jakobson, L. S., Frisk, V., & Downie, A. L. (2006). Motion-defined form processing in extremely premature children. *Neuropsychologia, 44,* 1777–1786.

Jakobson, L. S., Frisk, V., Knight, R. M., Downie, A. L. S., & Whyte, H. (2001). The relationships between periventricular brain injury and deficits in visual processing among extremely-low-birth-weight (<1000 g) children. *Journal of Pediatric Psychology, 26(8),* 503–512.

Johnson, E. O., & Breslau, N. (2000). Increased risk of learning disabilities in low birthweight boys at age 11 years. *Biological Psychiatry, 47,* 490–500.

Johnson, S. (2007). Cognitive and behavioural outcomes following very preterm birth. *Seminars in Fetal and Neonatal Medicine, 12,* 363–373.

Johnson, S., Ring, W., Anderson, P., & Marlow, P. (2005). Randomized trial of parental support for families with very preterm children: Outcome at 5 years. *Archives of Disease in Childhood, 90,* 909–915.

Kaaresen, P. I., Ronning, J. A., Ulvund, S. E., & Dahl, L. B. (2006). A randomized, controlled trial of the effectiveness of an early-intervention program in reducing parenting stress after preterm birth. *Pediatrics, 118,* e9–e19.

Kesler, S. R., Ment, L. R., Vohr, B., Pajot, S. K., Schneider, K. C., Katz, K. H., et al. (2004). Volumetric analysis of regional cerebral development in preterm children. *Pediatric Neurology, 31,* 318–325.

Klebanov, P. K., Brooks-Gunn, J., McCarton, C., & McCormick, M. C. (1998). The contribution of neighborhood and family income to developmental test scores over the first three years of life. *Child Development, 69,* 1420–1436.

Klebanov, P. K., Brooks-Gunn, J., & McCormick, M. C. (1994). School achievement and failure in very low birthweight children. *Journal of Developmental and Behavioral Pediatrics, 15,* 248–256.

Kohen, D. E., Brooks-Gunn, J., McCormick, M., & Graber, J. A. (1997). Concordance of maternal and teacher ratings of school and behavior problems in children of varying birth weights. *Journal of Developmental and Behavioral Pediatrics, 18,* 295–303.

Koller, H., Lawson, K., Rose, S. A., Wallace, I., & McCarton, C. (1997). Patterns of cognitive development in very low birth weight children during the first six years of life. *Pediatrics, 99,* 383–389.

Kulseng, S., Jennekens-Schinkel, A., Naess, P., Romundstad, P., Indredavik, M., Vik, T., et al. (2006). Very-low-birthweight and term small-for-gestational-age adolescents: Attention revisited. *Acta Paediatrica, 95,* 224–230.

Landry, S. H., Fletcher, J. M., Denson, S. E., & Chapieski, M. L. (1993). Longitudinal outcome for low birth weight infants: Effects of intraventricular hemorrhage and bronchopulmonary dysplasia. *Journal of Clinical and Experimental Neuropsychology, 15,* 205–218.

Landry, S. H., Miller-Loncar, C. L., Smith, K. E., & Swank, P. R. (2002). The role of early parenting in children's development of executive processes. *Developmental Neuropsychology, 21,* 15–41.

Landry, S. H., Smith, K. E., Miller-Loncar, C. L., & Swank, P. R. (1997). Predicting cognitive–language and social growth curves from early maternal behaviors in children at varying degrees of biological risk. *Developmental Psychology, 33,* 1040–1053.

Landry, S. H., Smith, K. E., Miller-Loncar, C. L., & Swank, P. R. (1998). The relation of change in maternal interactive styles to the developing social competence of full-term and preterm children. *Child Development, 69,* 105–123.

Landry, S. H., Smith, K. E., & Swank, P. R. (2003). The importance of parenting during early childhood for school-age development. *Developmental Neuropsychology, 24,* 559–591.

Laptook, A. R., O'Shea, M., Shankaran, S., Bhaskar, B., & the NICHD Neonatal Network. (2005). Adverse neurodevelopmental outcomes among extremely low birth weight infants with a normal head ultrasound: Prevalence and antecedents. *Pediatrics, 115,* 673–680.

Laughon, M., Bose, C., Allred, E., O'Shea, T. M., Van Marter, L. J., Bednarek, F., et al. (2007). Factors associated with treatment for hypotension in extremely low gestational age newborns during the first postnatal week. *Pediatrics, 119,* 273–280.

Lauterbach, M. D., Raz, S., & Sander, C. J. (2001). Neonatal hypoxic risk in preterm birth infants: The influence of sex and severity of respiratory distress on cognitive recovery. *Neuropsychology, 15,* 411–420.

Limperopoulos, C., Soul, J. S., Gauvreau, K., Huppi, P. S., Warfield, S. K., Bassan, J., et al. (2005). Late gestation cerebellar growth is rapid and impeded by premature birth. *Pediatrics, 115,* 688–695.

Linnet, K. M., Wisborg, K., Agerbo, E., Secher, N. J., Thomsen, P. H., & Henriksen, T. B. (2006). Gestational age, birth weight, and the risk of hyperkinetic disorder. *Archives of Disease in Childhood, 91,* 655–660.

Litt, J., Taylor, H. G., Klein, N., & Hack, M. (2005). Learning disabilities in children with very low birth weight: Prevalence, neuropsychological correlates, and educational interventions. *Journal of Learning Disabilities, 38*, 130–141.

Lorenz, J. M., Paneth, N., Jetton, J. R., Den Ouden, L., & Tyson, J. E. (2001). Comparison of management strategies for extreme prematurity in New Jersey and the Netherlands: Outcomes and resource expenditure. *Pediatrics, 108*, 1269–1274.

Lou, H. C. (1996). Etiology and pathogenesis of attention-deficit hyperactivity disorder (ADHD): Significance of prematurity and perinatal hypoxic–haemodynamic encephalopathology. *Acta Paediatrica, 85*, 1266–1271.

Luoma, L., Herrgard, E., Martikainen, A., & Ahonen, T. (1998). Speech and language development of children born at <32 weeks gestation: A 5-year prospective follow-up study. *Developmental Medicine and Child Neurology, 40*, 380–387.

Mangelsdorf, S. C., Plunkett, J. W., Dedrick, C. F., Berlin, M., Meisels, S. J., McHale, J. L., et al. (1996). Attachment security in very low birth weight infants. *Developmental Psychology, 32*, 914–920.

Marlow, N. (2004). Neurocognitive outcome after preterm birth. *Archives of Disease in Childhood: Fetal and Neonatal Edition, 89*, F224–F228.

Marlow, N., Hennessy, E. M., Bracewell, M. A., & Wolke, D. (2007). Motor and executive function at 6 years of age after extremely preterm birth. *Pediatrics, 120*, 793–804.

Marlow, N., Roberts, L., & Cooke, R. (1993). Outcome at 8 years for children with birth weights of 1250 g or less. *Archives of Disease in Childhood, 68*, 286–290.

Marlow, N., Wolke, D., Bracewell, M. A., Samara, M., & EPICure Study Group (2005). Neurologic and developmental disabilities at six years of age after extremely preterm birth. *New England Journal of Medicine, 352*, 9–19.

Martel, M. M., Lucia, V. C., Nigg, J. T., & Breslau, N. (2007). Sex differences in the pathway from low birth weight ton inattention/hyperactivity. *Journal of Abnormal Child Psychology, 35*, 87–96.

Martin, J. A., Hamilton, B. E., Ventura, S. J., Menacker, F., & Park, M. M. (2002). Births: Final data from 2000. *National Vital Statistics Reports, 50*, 1–104.

McClelland, M. M., Morrison, F. J., & Holmes, D .L. (2000). Children at risk for early academic problems: The role of learning-related social skills. *Early Childhood Research Quarterly, 15*, 307–329.

McCormick, M., Brooks-Gunn, J., Buka, S. L., Goldman, J., Yu, J., Mikhail, S., et al. (2006). Early intervention in low birth weight premature infants: Results at 18 years of age for the Infant Health and Development Program. *Pediatrics, 117*, 771–780.

McCormick, M., McCarton, C., Brooks-Gunn, J., Belt, P., & Gross, R. T. (1998). The Infant Health and Development Program: Interim summary. *Journal of Developmental and Behavioral Pediatrics, 19*, 359–370.

McGrath, M. M., Sullivan, M. C., & Seifer, R. (1998). Maternal interaction patterns and preschool competence in high-risk children. *Nursing Research, 47*, 309–317.

McLoyd, V. C. (1998). Socioeconomic disadvantage and child development. *American Psychologist, 53*, 185–204.

Melnyk, B. M., Alpert-Gillis, L., Feinstein, N. F., Fairbanks, E., Schultz-Czarniak, J., Hust, D., et al. (2001). Improving cognitive development of low-birth-weight premature infants with the COPE Program: A pilot study of the benefit of early NICU intervention with mothers. *Research in Nursing and Health, 24*, 373–389.

Ment, L. R., Peterson, B. S., Vohr, B., Allan, W., Schneider, K. C., Lacadie, C., et al. (2006). Cortical recruitment patterns in children born prematurely compared with control subjects during a passive listening functional magnetic resonance imaging task. *Journal of Pediatrics, 149*, 490–498.

Ment, L. R., Vohr, B., Allan, W., Katz, K. H., Schneider, K. C., Westerveld, M., et al. (2003). Change in cognitive function over time in very low-birth-weight infants. *Journal of the American Medical Association, 289*, 705–711.

Ment, L. R., Vohr, B., Allan, W., Westerveld, M., Katz, K. H., Schneider, K. C., et al. (1999). The etiology and outcome of cerebral ventriculomegaly at term in very low birth weight preterm infants. *Pediatrics, 104*, 243–248.

Ment, L. R., Vohr, B., Allan, W., Westerveld, M., Sparrow, S. S., Schneider, K. C., et al. (2000). Outcome of children in the indomethacin intraventricular hemorrhage prevention trial. *Pediatrics, 105,* 485–491.

Mestan, K. K., Marks, J. D., Hecox, K., Huo, D., & Schreiber, M. D. (2005). Neurodevelopmental outcomes of premature infants treated with inhaled nitric oxide. *New England Journal of Medicine, 353,* 23–32.

Miller, C. L., Landry, S. H., Smith, K. E., Wildin, S. R., Anderson, A. E., & Swank, P. R. (1995). Developmental change in the neuropsychological functioning of very low birth weight infants. *Child Neuropsychology, 1,* 224–236.

Miyahara, M., Jongmans, M. J., Mercuri, E., deVries, L. S., Henderson, L., & Henderson, S. E. (2003). Multiple birth versus neonatal brain lesions in children born prematurely as predictors of perceptuo-motor impairment at age 6. *Developmental Neuropsychology, 24,* 435–459.

Moore, M., Taylor, H. G., Klein, N., Minich, N., & Hack, M. (2006). Longitudinal changes in family outcomes of very low birth weight. *Journal of Pediatric Psychology, 31,* 1024–1035.

Msall, M. E. (2006). Neurodevelopmental surveillance in the first 2 years after extremely preterm birth: Evidence, challenges, and guidelines. *Early Human Development, 82,* 157–166.

Msall, M. E., Buck, G. M., Rogers, B. J., & Catanzaro, N. L. (1992). Kindergarten readiness after extreme prematurity. *American Journal of Diseases of Children, 146,* 1371–1378.

Msall, M. E., Phelps, D. L., DiGaudio, K. M., Dobson, V., Tung, B., McClead, R. E., et al. (2000). Severity of neonatal retinopathy of prematurity is predictive of neurodevelopmental functional outcome at age 5.5 years. *Pediatrics, 106,* 998–1005.

Nagy, Z., Westerberg, H., & Klingberg, T. (2004). Maturation of white matter is associated with the development of cognitive functions during childhood. *Journal of Cognitive Neuroscience, 16,* 1227–1233.

Nagy, Z., Westerberg, H., Skare, S., Andersson, J. L., Lilja, A., Flodmark, O., et al. (2003). Preterm children have disturbances of white matter at 11 years of age as shown by diffusion tensor imaging. *Pediatric Research, 54,* 672–679.

Nosarti, C., AlAsady, M. H. S., Frangou, S., Stewart, A. L., Rifkin, L., & Murray, R. M. (2002). Adolescents who were born very preterm have decreased brain volumes. *Brain, 125,* 1616–1623.

Nosarti, C., Allin, M. P., Frangou, S., Rifkin, L., & Murray, R. M. (2005). Hyperactivity in adolescents born very preterm is associated with decreased caudate volume. *Biological Psychiatry, 57,* 662–666.

Nosarti, C., Giouroukou, E., Micali, N., Rifkin, L., Morris, R. G., & Murray, R. M. (2007). Impaired executive functioning in young adults born very preterm. *Journal of the International Neuropsychological Society, 13,* 571–581.

Nosarti, C., Rubia, K., Smith, A. B., Frearson, S., Williams, S. C., Rifkin, L., et al. (2006). Altered functional neuroanatomy of response inhibition in adolescent males who were born very preterm. *Developmental Medicine & Child Neurology, 48,* 265–271.

Nosarti, C., Rushe, T. M., Woodruff, P. W. R., Stewart, A. L., Rifkin, L., & Murray, R. M. (2004). Corpus callosum size and very preterm birth: Relationship to neuropsychological outcome. *Brain, 127,* 2080–2089.

O'Brien, F., Roth, S., Stewart, A., Rifkin, L., Rushe, T., & Wyatt, J. (2004). The neurodevelopmental progress of infants less than 33 weeks into adolescence. *Archives of Disease in Childhood, 89,* 207–211.

Paavonen, E. J., Strang-Karlsson, S., Raikkonen, K., Heinonen, K., Pesonen, A., Hovi, P., et al. (2007). Very low birth weight increase risk for sleep-disordered breathing in young adulthood: The Helsinki Study of Very Low Birth Weight Adults. *Pediatrics, 120,* 778–784.

Paneth, N. (1995). The problem of low birth weight. *The Future of Children, 5,* 19–34.

Pennington, B. F. (1994). The working memory function of the prefrontal cortices: Implications for developmental and individual differences in cognition. In M. M. Haith, J. Benson, R. Roberts, & B. F. Pennington (Eds.), *The development of future oriented processes* (pp. 243–289). Chicago: University of Chicago Press.

Peterson, B. S., Anderson, A. W., Ehrenkranz, R., Staib, L. H., Tageldin, M., Colson, E., et al. (2003). Regional brain volumes and their later neurodevelopmental correlates in term and preterm infants. *Pediatrics, 111,* 939–948.

Peterson, B. S., Vohr, B., Kane, M. J., Whalen, D. J., Schneider, K. C., Katz, K. J., et al. (2002). A functional magnetic resonance imaging study of language processing and its cognitive correlates in prematurely born children. *Pediatrics, 110,* 1153–1162.

Peterson, B. S., Vohr, B., Staib, L. H., Cannistraci, C. J., Dolberg, A., Schneider, K. C., et al. (2000). Regional brain volume abnormalities and long-term cognitive outcome in preterm infants. *Journal of the American Medical Association, 284,* 1939–1947.

Peterson, J., Taylor, H. G., Minich, N., Klein, N., & Hack, M. (2006). Subnormal head circumference in very low birth weight children: Neonatal correlates and school-age consequences. *Early Human Development, 82,* 325–334.

Petrou, S. (2003). Economic consequences of preterm birth and low birthweight. *International Journal of Obstetrics and Gynaecology, 110,* 17–23.

Redline, R. W., Minich, N., Taylor, H. G., & Hack, M. (2007). Placental lesions as predictors of cerebral palsy and abnormal neurocognitive function at 8 years of age in extremely low birth weight infants (<1 kg). *Pediatric and Developmental Pathology, 10*(4), 282–292.

Reiss, A. L., Kesler, S. R., Vohr, B., Duncan C. C., Katz, K. H., Pajot, S., et al. (2004). Sex differences in cerebral volumes of 8-year-olds born preterm. *Journal of Pediatrics, 145,* 242–249.

Resnick, M. B., Gueorguieva, R. V., Carter, R. L., Ariet, M., Sun, Y., Roth, J., et al. (1999). The impact of low birth weight, prenatal conditions, and sociodemographic factors on educational outcome in kindergarten. *Pediatrics, 104,* e74.

Rickards, A. L., Kitchen, W. H., Doyle, L. W., & Kelly, E. A. (1989). Correction of developmental and intelligence test scores for premature birth. *Australian Journal of Paediatrics, 25,* 127–129.

Rimm-Kaufman, S. E., Pianta, R. C., & Cox, M. J. (2000). Teachers' judgments of problems in the transition to kindergarten. *Early Childhood Research Quarterly, 15,* 147–166.

Rose, S. A., Feldman, J. F., & Jankowski, J. J. (2005a). Recall memory in the first three years of life: A longitudinal study of preterm and term children. *Developmental Medicine and Child Neurology, 47,* 653–659.

Rose, S. A., Feldman, J. F., Jankowski, J. J., & Van Rossem, R. (2005b). Pathways from prematurity and infant abilities to later cognition. *Child Development, 76,* 1172–1184.

Rose, S. A., Feldman, J. F., Rose, S. L., Wallace, I. F., & McCarton, C. (1992). Behavior problems at 3 and 6 years: Prevalence and continuity in full-terms and preterms. *Development and Psychopathology, 4,* 361–374.

Rosenbaum, P., Saigal, S., Szatmari, P., & Hoult, L. (1995). Vineland Adaptive Behavior Scales as a summary of functional outcome of extremely low-birthweight children. *Developmental Medicine and Child Neurology, 37,* 577–586.

Roth, J., Figlio, D. N., Chen, Y., Ariet, M., Carter, R. L., Resnick, M. B., et al. (2004). Maternal and infant factors associated with excess kindergarten costs. *Pediatrics, 114,* 720–728.

Rushe, T. M., Temple, C. M., Rifkin, L., Woodruff, P. W. R., Bullmore, E. T., Stewart, A. L., et al. (2004). Lateralisation of language function in young adults born very preterm. *Archives of Disease in Childhood: Fetal and Neonatal Edition, 89,* F112–F118.

Saigal, S. (2000). Follow-up of very low birthweight babies to adolescence. *Seminars in Neonatology, 5,* 107–118.

Saigal, S., Burrows, E., Stoskopf, B. L., Rosenbaum, P. L., & Streiner, D. (2000a). Impact of extreme prematurity on families of adolescent children. *Journal of Pediatrics, 137,* 701–706.

Saigal, S., den Ouden, L., Wolke, D., Hoult, L., Paneth, N., Streiner, D. L., et al. (2003a). School-age outcomes in children who were extremely low birth weight from four international population-based cohorts. *Pediatrics, 112,* 943–950.

Saigal, S., Hoult, L. A., Streiner, D. L., Stoskopf, B. L., & Rosenbaum, P. L. (2000b). School difficulties at adolescence in a regional cohort of children who were extremely low birthweight. *Pediatrics, 105,* 325–331.

Saigal, S., Lambert, M., Russ, C., & Hoult, L. (2002). Self-esteem of adolescents who were born prematurely. *Pediatrics, 109*, 429–433.

Saigal, S., Pinelli, J., Hoult, L., Kim, M. M., & Boyle, M. (2003b). Psychopathology and social competencies of adolescents who were extremely low birth weight. *Pediatrics, 111*, 969–975.

Saigal, S., Rosenbaum, P., Szatmari, P., & Campbell, D. (1991). Learning disabilities and school problems in a regional cohort of extremely low birthweight (< 1000 grams) children: A comparison with term controls. *Journal of Developmental and Behavioral Pediatrics, 12*, 294–300.

Saigal, S., Stoskopf, B., Boyle, M., Paneth, N., Pinelli, J., Streiner, D., et al. (2007). Comparison of current health, functional limitations, and health care of young adults who were born with extremely low birth weight and normal birth weight. *Pediatrics, 119*, e562–e573.

Saigal, S., Szatmari, P., & Rosenbaum, P. (1992). Can learning disabilities in children who were extremely low birth weight be identified at school entry? *Journal of Developmental and Behavioral Pediatrics, 13*, 356–362.

Salokorpi, T., Rautio, T., Kajantie, E., & Von Wendt, L. (2002). Is early occupational therapy in extremely pre-term infants of benefit in the long run? *Pediatric Rehabilitation, 5*, 91–98.

Samuelsson, S., Bylund, B., Cervin, T., Finnstrom, O., Gaddlin, P., Leijon, I., et al. (1999). The prevalence of reading disabilities among very-low-birth-weight children at 9 years of age: Dyslexics or poor readers? *Dyslexia, 5*, 94–112.

Samuelsson, S., Finnstrom, O., Flodmark, O., Gaddline, P., Leijon, I., & Wadsby, M. (2006). A longitudinal study of reading skills among very-low-birthweight children: Is there a catch-up? *Journal of Pediatric Psychology, 31*, 967–977.

Santhouse, A. M., Fytche, D. H., Howard, R. J., Williams, S. C. R., Stewart, A. L., Rooney, M., et al. (2002). The functional significance of perinatal corpus callosum damage: An fMRI study in young adults. *Brain, 125*, 1782–1792.

Schatz, J., Craft, S., Koby M., & Park, T. S. (1997). Associative learning in children with prenatal brain injury. *Journal of the International Neuropsychological Society, 3*, 521–527.

Schmidt, B., Asztalos, E. V., Roberts, R. S., Robertson, C. M. T., Sauve, R. S., & Whitfield for the Trial of Indomethacin Prophylasix in Preterms (TIPP) Investigators. (2003). Impact of bronchopulmonary dysplasia, brain injury, and severe retinopathy on the outcome of extremely low-birth-weight infants at 18 months. *Journal of the American Medical Association, 289*, 1124–1129.

Schmidt, B., Roberts, R. S., Davis, P., Doyle, L. W., Barrington, K. J., Ohlsson, A., et al. (2006). Caffeine therapy for apnea of prematurity. *New England Journal of Medicine, 354*, 2112–2121.

Schneider, W., Wolke, D., Schlagmüller, M., & Meyer, R. (2004). Pathways to school achievement in very preterm and full term children. *European Journal of Psychology of Education, 19*, 385–406.

Shankaran, S., Johnson, Y., Langer, J. C., Vohr, B. R., Fanaroff, A. A., Wright, L. L., et al. (2004). Outcome of extremely-low-birth-weight infants at highest risk: Gestational age ≤24 weeks, birth weight ≤750 g, and 1-minute Apgar ≤3. *American Journal of Obstetrics and Gynecology, 191*, 1084–1091.

Shankaran, S., Lester, B. M., Das, A., Bauer, C. R., Bada, H. S., Lagasse, L., et al. (2007). Impact of maternal substance use during pregnancy on childhood outcome. *Seminars in Fetal and Neonatal Medicine, 12*, 143–150.

Short, E. J., Klein, N. K., Lewis, B. A., Fulton, S., Eisengart, S., Kercsmar, C., et al. (2003). Cognitive and academic consequences of bronchopulmonary dysplasia and very low birth weight: 8-year-old outcomes. *Pediatrics, 112*, e359–e366.

Skranes, J., Vangberg, T. R., Kulseng, S., Indredavik, M. S., Evensen, K. A. I., Martinussen, M., et al. (2007). Clinical findings and white matter abnormalities seen on diffusion tensor imaging in adolescents with very low birth weight. *Brain, 130*, 654–666.

Spiker, D., Kraemer, H. C., Constantine, N. A., & Bryant, D. (1992). Reliability and validity of behavior problem checklists as measures of stable traits in low birth weight, premature preschoolers. *Child Development, 63*, 1481–1496.

Spira, E. G., Bracken, S. S., & Fischel, J. E. (2005). Predicting improvement after first-grade reading difficulties: The effects of oral language, emergent literacy, and behavior skills. *Developmental Psychology, 41*, 225–234.

Srinivasan, L., Dutta, R., Counsell, S. J., Allsop, J. M., Boardman, J. P., Rutherford, M. A., et al. (2007). Quantification of deep gray matter in preterm infants at term-equivalent age using manual volumetry of 3-Tesla magnetic resonance images. *Pediatrics, 119,* 759–765.

St. John, E. B., Nelson, K. G., Cliver, S. P., Bishnoi, R. R., & Goldenberg, R. L. (2000). Cost of neonatal care according to gestational age at birth and survival status. *American Journal of Obstetrics and Gynecology, 182,* 170–175.

Sullivan, M. C., & McGrath, M. M. (2003). Perinatal morbidity, mild motor delay, and later school outcomes. *Developmental Medicine and Child Neurology, 45,* 104–112.

Szatmari, P., Saigal, S., Rosenbaum, P., & Campbell, D. (1993). Psychopathology and adaptive functioning among extremely low birthweight children at eight years of age. *Development and Psychopathology, 5,* 345–357.

Szatmari, P., Saigal, S., Rosenbaum, P., Campbell, D., & King, S. (1990). Psychiatric disorders at five years among children with birthweights <1000 gram: A regional perspective. *Developmental Medicine and Child Neurology, 32,* 954–962.

Taylor, H. G., & Alden, J. (1997). Age-related differences in outcomes following childhood brain insults: An introduction and overview. *Journal of the International Neuropsychological Society, 3,* 555–567.

Taylor, H. G., Burant, C., Holding, P. A., Klein, N., & Hack, M. (2002). Sources of variability in sequelae of very low birth weight. *Child Neuropsychology, 8,* 164–178.

Taylor, H. G., Hack, M., & Klein, N. (1998a). Attention deficits in children with <750 gm birth weight. *Child Neuropsychology, 4,* 21–34.

Taylor, H. G., Klein, N., Drotar, D., Schluchter, M., & Hack, M. (2006). Consequences and risks for <1000-g birth weight for neuropsychological skills, achievement, and adaptive functioning. *Journal of Developmental and Behavioral Pediatrics, 27,* 459–469.

Taylor, H. G., Klein, N., & Hack, M. (2000a). School-age consequences of <750 g birth weight: A review and update. *Developmental Neuropsychology, 17,* 289–321.

Taylor, H. G., Klein, N., Minich, N., & Hack, M. (2000b). Middle school-age outcomes in children with very low birthweight. *Child Development, 71,* 1495–1511.

Taylor, H. G., Klein, N., Minich, N., & Hack, M. (2000c). Verbal memory deficits in children with less than 50 g birth weight. *Child Neuropsychology, 6,* 49–63.

Taylor, H. G., Klein, N., Minich, N. M., & Hack, M. (2001a). Long-term family outcomes for children with very low birth weights. *Archives of Pediatrics and Adolescent Medicine, 155,* 155–161.

Taylor, H. G., Klein, N., Schatschneider, C., & Hack, M. (1998b). Predictors of early school age outcomes in very low birthweight children. *Journal of Developmental and Behavioral Pediatrics, 19,* 235–243.

Taylor, H. G., Minich, N., Bangert, B., Filipek, P. A., & Hack, M. (2004a). Long-term neuropsychological outcomes of very low birth weight: Associations with early risks for periventricular brain insults. *Journal of the International Neuropsychological Society, 10,* 987–1004.

Taylor, H. G., Minich, N., Holding, P., Klein, N., & Hack, M. (2004b). *Longitudinal changes in behavior and achievement in children with VLBW.* Paper presented at the meeting of the American Academy of Clinical Neuropsychology, Minneapolis, MN.

Taylor, H. G., Minich, N. M., Klein, N., & Hack, M. (2004c). Longitudinal outcomes of very low birth weight: Neuropsychological findings. *Journal of the International Neuropsychological Society, 10,* 149–163.

Taylor, H. G., Yeates, K. O., Wade, S. L., Drotar, D., Stancin, T., & Burant, C. (2001b). Bidirectional child–family influences on outcomes of traumatic brain injury in children. *Journal of the International Neuropsychological Society, 7,* 755–767.

Theunissen, N. C. M., den-Ouden, L., Meulman, J. J., Koopman, H. M., Verloove-Vanhorick, S. P., & Wit, J. (2000). Health status development in a cohort of preterm children. *Journal of Pediatrics, 137,* 534–539.

Tideman, E. (2000). Longitudinal follow-up of children born preterm: Cognitive development at age 19. *Early Human Development, 58,* 81–90.

Tully, L. A., Arseneault, L., Caspi, A., Moffitt, T. E., & Morgan, J. (2004). Does maternal warmth moderate the effects of birth weight on twins' attention-deficit/hyperactivity disorder (ADHD) symptoms and low IQ? *Journal of Consulting and Clinical Psychology, 72*, 218–226.

Vicari, S., Caravale, B., Carlesimo, G. A., Casadei, A. M., & Allemand, F. (2004). Spatial working memory deficits in children at ages 3–4 who were low birth weight, preterm infants. *Neuropsychology, 18*, 673–678.

Vohr, B., Allan, W. C., Westerveld, M., Schneider, K. C., Katz, K. H., Makuch, R. W., et al. (2003). School-age outcomes of very low birth weight infants in the Indomethacin Intraventricular Hemorrhage Prevention Trial. *Pediatrics, 111*, e340–e346.

Vohr, B. R. (2007). How should we report early childhood outcomes of very low birth weight infants? *Seminars in Fetal and Neonatal Medicine, 12*, 355–362.

Vohr, B. R., Wright, L. L., Dusick, A. M., Mele, L., Verter, J., Steichen, J. J., et al. (2000). Neurodevelopmental and functional outcomes of extremely low birth weight infants in the National Institute of Child Health and Human Development Neonatal Research Network, 1993–1994. *Pediatrics, 105*, 1216–1226.

Vohr, B. R., Wright, L. L., Dusick, A. M., Perritt, R., Poole, W. K., Tyson, J. E., et al. (2004). Center differences and outcomes of extremely low birth weight infants. *Pediatrics, 113*, 781–789.

Wallace, I. F., & McCarton, C. M. (1997). Neurodevelopmental outcomes of the premature, small-for-gestational-age infant through age 6. *Clinical Obstetrics and Gynecology, 40*, 843–852.

Weisglas-Kuperus, N., Baerts, W., Smrkovsky, M., & Sauer, P. J. J. (1993). Effects of biological and social factors on the cognitive development of very low birth weight children. *Pediatrics, 92*, 658–665.

Whitaker, A. H., Feldman, J. F., Van Rossem, R., Schonfeld, I. S., Pinto-Martin, J. A., Torre, C., et al. (1996). Neonatal cranial ultrasound abnormalities in low birth weight infants: Relation to cognitive outcomes at six years of age. *Pediatrics, 98*, 719–729.

Whitaker, A. H., Van Rossem, R., Feldman, J. F., Schonfeld, I. S., Pinto-Martin, J. A., Torre, C., et al. (1997). Psychiatric outcomes in low-birth-weight children at age 6 years: Relation to neonatal cranial ultrasound abnormalities. *Archives of General Psychiatry, 54*, 847–856.

Wilson-Costello, D. (2007). Is there evidence that long-term outcomes have improved with intensive care? *Seminars in Fetal and Neonatal Medicine, 12*, 344–354.

Wilson-Costello, D., Borawski, W., Friedman, H., Redline, R., Fanaroff, A. A., & Hack, M. (1998). Perinatal correlates of cerebral palsy and other neurologic impairment among very low birth weight children. *Pediatrics, 102*, 315–322.

Wilson-Costello, D., Friedman, H., Minich, N., Fanaroff, A. A., & Hack, M. (2005). Improved survival rates with increased neurodevelopmental disability for extremely low birth weight infants in the 1990s. *Pediatrics, 115*, 997–1003.

Wilson-Costello, D., Friedman, H., Minich, N., Siner, B., Taylor, G., Schluchter, M., et al. (2007). Improved neurodevelopmental outcomes for extremely low birth weight infants in 2000–2002. *Pediatrics, 110*, 37–45.

Witt, W. P., Riley, A. W., & Coiro, M. J. (2003). Childhood functional status, family stressors, and psychosocial adjustment among school-aged children with disabilities in the United States. *Archives of Pediatrics and Adolescent Medicine, 157*, 687–695.

Wolf, M., Koldewijn, K., Beelen, A., Smit, B., Hedlund, R., & de Groot, I. J. M. (2002). Neurobehavioral and developmental profile of very low birthweight preterm infants in early infancy. *Acta Paediatrica, 91*, 930–938.

Wolke, D., & Meyer, R. (1999). Cognitive status, language attainment, and prereading skills of 6-year-old very preterm children and their peers: The Bavarian Longitudinal Study. *Developmental Medicine and Child Neurology, 41*, 94–109.

Wood, N. S., Costeloe, K., Gibson, A. T., Hennessy, E. M., Marlow, N., & Wilkinson, A. R. (2003). The EPICure study: Growth and associated problems in children born at 25 weeks or less gestational age. *Archives of Disease in Childhood: Fetal and Neonatal Edition, 88*, F492–F500.

Wood, N. S., Costeloe, K., Gibson, A. T., Hennessy, E. M., Marlow, N., & Wilkinson, A. R. (2005). The EPICure study: Associations and antecedents of neurological and developmental disability at 30 months of age following extremely preterm birth. *Archives of Disease in Childhood: Fetal and Neonatal Edition, 90*, F134–F140.

Wood, N. S., Marlow, N., Costeloe, K., Gibson, A. T., & Wilkinson, A. R. (2000). Neurologic and developmental disability after extremely preterm birth. *New England Journal of Medicine, 343*, 378–384.

Woodward, L. J., Anderson, P. J., Austin, N. C., Howard, K., & Inder, T. E. (2006). Neonatal MRI to predict neurodevelopmental outcomes in preterm infants. *New England Journal of Medicine, 355*, 685–694.

Woodward, L. J., Edgin, J. O., Thompson, D., & Inder, T. E. (2005). Object working memory deficits predicted by early brain injury and development in the preterm infant. *Brain, 128*, 2578–2587.

Zelkowitz, P., Papageorgiou, A., Zelazo, P. R., & Weiss, M. J. S. (1995). Behavioral adjustment in very low and normal birth weight children. *Journal of Clinical Child Psychology, 24*, 21–30.

CHAPTER 3

Childhood Epilepsy

MICHAEL WESTERVELD

Because epilepsy is a common childhood neurological condition with diverse etiologies and phenotypes, neuropsychological comorbidity in epilepsy is an important but challenging topic. Numerous factors interact to produce a unique clinical picture in each individual with seizures. First, the primary symptomatic expression of the disorder (clinical seizures) is paroxysmal and, with the exception of a few known triggers, unpredictable. During the interictal period, many patients may or may not have cognitive issues related to their disorder; however, the unpredictability of the disorder combined with the stigma can produce psychological and psychosocial consequences even in the absence of cognitive impairments. Second, similar clinical expression (e.g., complex partial seizures) may be due to one of many different underlying neurological conditions (e.g., hippocampal sclerosis, neoplasm, focal disorders of neuroblast migration). As a result, the neuropsychological comorbidities vary widely and depend on numerous factors (many of which remain unknown) that produce a virtually infinite number of possible cognitive outcomes. Finally, the manner in which the same underlying neuroanatomical cause of epilepsy is manifested with respect to cognitive function can also vary widely from person to person. As a result, attempts to characterize a neuropsychological "syndrome" associated with epilepsy are often inadequate, particularly when such models are applied to children with diverse individual backgrounds whose development is ongoing and in whom neuroplasticity still exists. The manner in which endogenous biological factors interact with environmental factors can be difficult to predict and understand. The purpose of this chapter is to provide a summary of known factors that can affect cognitive function in children with epilepsy.

EPIDEMIOLOGY OF SEIZURES AND DEFINITIONS OF EPILEPSY

Epilepsy is among the most common neurological disorders of childhood. According to the World Health Organization (2008), approximately 5% of the population will have at least one seizure during their lifetime. The estimated worldwide prevalence of epilepsy, defined as recurrent unprovoked seizures, is upwards of 50 million individuals at any given point in time. Thus epilepsy constitutes a major public health issue for children. More important, since epilepsy and related treatments can have a significant impact on cognition, epilepsy also represents a developmental challenge that neuropsychologists are uniquely qualified to address by virtue of their combined knowledge of neuropathology and development of cognitive and psychological function.

It is important to note that a single seizure occurrence is not sufficient for a diagnosis of epilepsy, and that not all epilepsy is intractable or resistant to treatment. It is estimated that approximately 40–50% of children with a first unprovoked seizure will have a second unprovoked seizure, with the majority of recurrences occurring within 2 years of the initial event (Berg, 2008b). An *unprovoked* seizure is defined as a seizure that occurs outside the context of an acute event, such as a fever or traumatic brain injury. Unprovoked seizures may be either *symptomatic* or *cryptogenic*, with symptomatic seizures being the result of a known underlying cause (e.g., neoplasm, stroke), whereas cryptogenic seizures are without a known neuropathological cause. It is estimated that 60–80% of new cases in children are without a known cause; that approximately 20% are associated with causes present from birth; and that the remaining cases are associated with a variety of acquired etiologies, such as trauma, central nervous system (CNS) infection, or stroke (Hauser, 2001). When seizures do recur, they may be associated with varying degrees of cognitive morbidity.

The degree of cognitive impairment that may be associated with epilepsy is closely related to factors that determine the likelihood of recurrence, as well as to the frequency of seizures and other factors, such as age at seizure onset, the underlying cause of seizures, and localization of seizure onset. Risk factors for recurrence can be categorized broadly, with the most commonly cited factors including whether a first seizure is treated, the presence of an electroencephalographic (EEG) abnormality, or an abnormal neurological examination (Berg, 2008b). These factors are interrelated, in that the decision whether to treat a first seizure is likely to be based on EEG findings and presence of neurological abnormality. However, not all first seizures are treated, since a single febrile seizure with no further recurrence is common among children, and unnecessary treatment may itself be associated with adverse side effects. Prospective studies aimed at identifying risk of recurrence and cognitive outcomes are rare. In one study that randomly assigned children to a deferred-treatment or immediate-treatment arm, the immediate-treatment group had an approximately 60% reduction of risk for recurrence (First Seizure Trial Group, 1993), regardless of other factors (e.g., presence or absence of neurological abnormality). Thus the decision to treat a first seizure or not may have a significant impact on whether seizures recur, and also on related cognitive morbidities.

Risk factors for seizure recurrence can also be identified with greater specificity. These include prolonged febrile convulsions that may induce neurological injury (Sagar & Oxbury, 1987); neoplasm (Spencer, Spencer, Mattson, & Williamson, 1984); disorders of neuroblast migration, such as cortical dysplasia and heterotopias (Sarnat & Flores-Sarnat, 2006); and traumatic brain injury (Annegers et al., 1980). Genetic factors also play a role in recurrent seizures. There have been several studies demonstrating increased concordance for epilepsy in monozygotic compared with dizygotic twins, and there are also several well-defined epileptic syndromes with identified genetic linkages (Ottman, 2001).

CLASSIFICATION OF SEIZURES

There are several ways that recurrent seizures, or epilepsy, may be classified. The International League Against Epilepsy (ILAE) has endorsed a classification scheme for epileptic seizures (Commission on Classification and Terminology of the ILAE, 1981) and a classification for epilepsy syndromes (Commission on Classification and Terminology of the ILAE, 1989). The epileptic seizures themselves are classified on the basis of the EEG and behavioral characteristics of the event, with the nature of the recurrent seizures defining the syndrome. For example, seizures are classified based on whether they are *partial* or *generalized* in origin—that is, whether the first clinical and EEG signs originate in part of one cerebral hemisphere (partial seizures, also known as *focal* or *localized*), or simultaneously throughout both cerebral hemispheres (generalized seizures). Partial seizures (also sometimes referred to as focal seizures, or localization-related seizures) that do not involve an alteration in consciousness are classified as *simple partial* seizures. Partial seizures that involve alteration of awareness or consciousness are classified as *complex partial seizures*. Epileptiform activity in partial seizures may also spread, producing a secondarily generalized seizure, although the onset is localized.

Primary generalized seizures typically involve both hemispheres at seizure onset, with impairment in consciousness often being the first clinical sign. Those that do not involve any significant motor symptoms are classified as *absence* seizures. Generalized seizures that involve motor activity are classified as *myoclonic, tonic, atonic, clonic,* or *tonic–clonic* seizures. Myoclonic seizures involve a brief spasmodic event, often involving multiple muscle groups simultaneously. Tonic seizures involve sudden, usually brief increase in muscle tone. Atonic seizures, also known as *akinetic* seizures or (colloquially) as "drop attacks," involve a sudden brief loss of muscle tone throughout the body. Clonic seizures involve rhythmic jerking movements of the limbs, and can vary in duration. Clonic seizures are relatively uncommon alone, and clonus (rhythmic jerking) is more often preceded by a tonic event, referred to as a tonic–clonic seizure. The tonic–clonic seizures are also commonly referred to as *grand mal* seizures.

The type of seizure event often defines part of a syndrome. Epilepsy syndromes are classified according to several characteristics of the individual seizures as described above, including whether the seizures are localization-related (also referred to as *partial* or *focal* epilepsies) or generalized; what behaviors that occur during the seizure (also referred to as *ictal semiology*); and whether the seizures are idiopathic or symptomatic. Localization-related epilepsies may have characteristic behaviors that are related to the site of origin in the brain. For example, occipital lobe epilepsies are often characterized by visual phenomena that may include perceptive illusions, positive visual phenomena (e.g., flashes of light, sparks), or negative visual effects (e.g., transient scotoma or hemianopsia). The more common temporal lobe epilepsy (TLE) may include psychic phenomena such as an aura of déjà vu, followed by alteration of awareness with behavioral automatisms (repetitive, purposeless behaviors) for which the patient is typically amnestic. Ictal speech (speech that occurs during a seizure) may be aphasic in dominant-hemisphere TLE, or confused in nondominant-hemisphere TLE. Transient postictal aphasia may occur, and can provide important information about lateralization of temporal lobe seizures. Generalized epilepsy syndromes may be classified according to whether the seizures are symptomatic (e.g., Lennox–Gastaut syndrome [LGS]) or idiopathic (e.g., childhood absence epilepsy). Some epilepsy syndromes are not clearly defined as having focal or generalized origins, but may still have a clearly defined set of symptoms (e.g., Landau–Kleffner syndrome [LKS]) or course (e.g., Rasmussen syndrome).

As any "syndrome" is, epileptic syndromes are defined by characteristic clusterings of symptoms that occur uniquely together. There are several epilepsy syndromes that are associated with neuropsychological impairments; some of these syndromes are progressive, but others are self-limiting and spontaneously remit. Collectively referred to as *epileptic encephalopathies*, these include infantile-onset syndromes such as West syndrome, and later-onset syndromes such as LGS and LKS. West syndrome is characterized by seizures manifesting as infantile spasms, an EEG pattern referred to as hypsarrhythmia (near-continuous, random high-voltage spike-and-wave discharges), and global cognitive impairments with low IQ. Onset of seizures in West syndrome occurs in the first few months of life, and West syndrome is typically self-limiting in terms of seizure events and EEG abnormality, with most children experiencing spontaneous remission by 4 years of age (Ohtahara & Yamatogi, 2001). However, cognitive impairments usually persist after seizure remission. Although the cognitive prognosis is typically poor, recent studies have shown that early treatment with adrenocorticotropic hormone (ACTH) may improve cognitive outcome (Hattori et al., 2006), particularly if treatment is initiated early (Kivity et al., 2004).

LGS is defined by an EEG pattern consisting of diffuse slow spike–wave discharges, less than 3 Hz. Children with LGS typically have several different seizure types, with the most common being tonic or absence seizures, although many different seizure types are often present in an individual child with LGS. Seizure onset may occur any time in childhood, but typically occurs in preschool aged children; some children may have a prior history of diagnosis with West syndrome. LGS is typically associated with global cognitive deficits, and cognitive impairment is considered a defining feature, although some children may have normal development prior to the onset of seizures in LGS. The typical cognitive profile is one of global cognitive impairment with low IQ, and prognosis is worse with early seizure onset and symptomatic (vs. idiopathic) origins.

LKS is a rare syndrome that is associated with progressive aphasia in children after a period of relatively normal language development. Because the primary cognitive symptom is language regression, LKS is also referred to as *acquired epileptic aphasia*. Although LKS is considered an "epilepsy" syndrome, the occurrence of seizures is not a prerequisite for the diagnosis. Instead, the diagnosis is based primarily on the appearance of language impairment in association with EEG abnormalities. Clinical seizure events may not occur in as many as 20–30% of patients with LKS (Neville & Cross, 2006). During wakefulness, the EEG may show normal background activity, with occasional high-amplitude focal discharges in the temporoparietal region. However, during sleep the EEG will show more significant abnormality, with bilateral spike–wave activity in the temporal regions, particularly in primary auditory cortex (Deonna & Roulet-Perez, 2005). Although there are no specific neuroanatomical findings on imaging in LKS, recent work has observed reduced volume in the superior temporal regions bilaterally (Takeoka et al., 2004). The language disturbance begins with predominantly receptive language disturbance, specifically auditory agnosia, and progresses to include reduced expressive language. Although studies using a variety of methods have indicated that abnormalities are primarily limited to perisylvian receptive language areas (Boyd, Rivera-Gaxiola, Towell, Harkness, & Neville, 1996; da Silva, Chugani, Muzik, & Chugani, 1997; Neville & Cross, 2006), continued development and maintenance of expressive speech are dependent upon auditory feedback (Deonna & Roulet-Perez, 2005). In addition to language regression, LKS is associated with behavior problems, particularly attention and disruptive behavior disorders (Neville & Cross, 2006). LKS is also of particular interest due to similarities between the regression in some autism spectrum disorders and LKS, prompting some to consider the possibility of a pathophysiological similarity between the two disorders (Mantovani, 2000).

IMAGING IN PEDIATRIC EPILEPSY

Epilepsy is predominantly a functional disturbance, defined by electrophysiological characteristics. Individual brain imaging results are often interpreted as normal, with no gross structural abnormalities identified. However, there are some types of seizures that do have specific imaging signatures, such as mesial temporal sclerosis associated with TLE (Jack, 2001). Moreover, the increasing sensitivity and resolution of imaging techniques have led to increased identification of pathologies on imaging that might previously have been missed (Sawaishi et al., 2005).

Although many cases of new-onset seizures in children are associated with normal structural imaging, magnetic resonance imaging (MRI) is the most widely used technique to investigate structural changes associated with epilepsy, due to the sensitivity to the most common underlying substrates. Consequently, MRI should be considered a primary diagnostic tool for new-onset cases in children (Peretti, Raybaud, Dravet, Mancini, & Pinsard, 1989). In cases with known pathology, the most common underlying features are developmental abnormalities, such as focal cortical dysplasia, or more significant abnormalities, such as hemimegancephaly or schizencephaly (Kuzniecky, 2001). Focal cortical dysplasia may be more difficult to detect; it may be manifested as thickened cortex or abnormal gray–white matter architecture (Kuzniecky, 2001), such as blurring of the gray–white matter junction on MRI. In children with partial complex seizures, temporal lobe abnormalities, including hippocampal sclerosis, may be identified on imaging. When present, the MRI characteristics of hippocampal sclerosis in children are similar to those of adults and include volumetric atrophy and increased signal on T2-weighted images (Kuzniecky, 2001). MRI indications of mesial temporal sclerosis in children are more likely to be observed when there is a history of early seizure onset and complex febrile convulsions (Kodama et al., 1995).

As noted above, many children with new-onset seizures do not present with MRI-detected pathology. However, even among patients in whom imaging does not show a pathological structural abnormality, MRI may be useful in understanding how seizures affect brain development and cognitive function. For example, Hermann et al. (2002) found significant reductions in white matter tissue volume throughout the brain in patients with childhood-onset epilepsy, compared with patients with later-onset epilepsy. This finding suggests an adverse neurodevelopmental impact of childhood epilepsy that is correlated with clinically significant alterations in cognitive function.

Functional neuroimaging techniques are also increasingly applied in pediatric epilepsy. Techniques that are designed to measure functional activation or base rate metabolism may be sensitive to pathologies in epilepsy, as well as being related to cognitive impairments. Positron emission tomography is useful for detecting regional metabolic abnormalities that may be indicative of underlying pathology. However, because of the poor temporal resolution due to slow uptake of commonly used tracer delivery (e.g., fluorodeoxyglucose), more direct assessment of changes in regional metabolism associated with seizure onset, or performance on cognitive tasks, is not possible. Single-photon emission computed tomography (SPECT), which measures blood flow, may be useful in identifying regional metabolic abnormalities in the interictal state. The increased temporal resolution also makes SPECT useful for studying transient changes associated with seizure onset and propagation, although interpretive caution is needed, depending on the time elapsed between seizure onset and injection of the tracer (Kuzniecky, 2001; Lee et al., 2006).

In children who may be candidates for surgical treatment, assessment of language lateralization and memory function is needed. Results of intracarotid Amytal procedures (so-called "Wada testing") have been shown to be quite successful in lateralizing language and predicting surgical outcome (Lee, Westerveld, Blackburn, Park, & Loring, 2005; Westerveld et al., 1994), but such procedures are invasive, and it is not always possible to perform them. Recent studies have demonstrated the utility of functional MRI (fMRI) in evaluating language lateralization in children (Anderson et al., 2006). However, concordance with other methods of language lateralization (e.g., cortical stimulation) is not 100%, and individual results may not be as reliable as correlations at the group level. Furthermore, to date there are no studies evaluating fMRI assessment of memory with respect to postsurgical memory outcome in children.

NEUROPSYCHOLOGICAL COMORBIDITIES IN EPILEPSY

Although the preceding discussion of some selected syndromes indicates that there may be characteristic features of some disorders, most epilepsies do not have signature cognitive impairments. Cognitive function in children with epilepsy can vary widely—from completely normal function with minimal or no impairments, to catastrophic cognitive impairments. One of the primary determinants of cognitive impairments is the underlying pathology or risk factor for epilepsy. The underlying pathology will produce different cognitive profiles, depending on other factors (such as the degree to which pathology is localized, where it is localized, and the developmental stage during which the pathology emerges). Depending on the nature of the underlying pathology, there may also be comorbidities and iatrogenic factors that contribute to cognitive and/or psychological disturbance. Owing to the vast number of potential underlying causes of epilepsy and the large number of distinctly different epilepsy syndromes, it is difficult if not impossible to identify a single cognitive phenotype of epilepsy. However, there are some aspects of cognitive function that tend to be disrupted more commonly among children with different forms of epilepsy.

Intellectual Function

Studies of intelligence in children with epilepsy have obtained mixed results, probably because of differences in the populations included in studies, as well as differences in methodology (e.g., cross-sectional vs. longitudinal studies, comparison group differences) (Vingerhoets, 2006). For example, while some studies have found that children with epilepsy tend to have lower IQs than comparison groups, others have found that more specific relationships between IQ and seizures exist (Jokeit & Ebner, 2002). In one of the first studies to prospectively examine changes in cognitive function in children with epilepsy, Bourgeois, Prensky, Palkes, Talent, and Busch (1983) found that intelligence in most such children was normal, with an average IQ (99.7) that did not differ significantly from that of sibling controls. Follow-up assessments of the children in their study also found that in most children with epilepsy, IQ remained stable over time. However, there were risk factors associated with intellectual deterioration, including medication usage. Children with a history of more difficult-to-control seizures and toxic levels of medication had a greater risk of decline in IQ of 10 points or more. This study also implicated age at seizure onset as a factor in worse cognitive outcome, with younger age of onset associated with greater cognitive impairment.

Other researchers have also identified age at seizure onset as one of the most important factors determining cognitive outcome. Berg et al. (2008) studied 613 children with epilepsy enrolled in a community-based longitudinal study. In this study, more than 25% of these children had borderline IQ scores or lower (i.e., 26.4% had IQs less than 80). Several risk factors were identified as independently contributing to cognitive dysfunction, with the most significant being seizure onset before 5 years of age. The association of age at onset with general intellectual function appears to be independent of other factors thought to be related to cognitive decline, such as seizure frequency or location of seizure onset (Kramer et al., 2006; Strauss, Hunter, & Wada, 1995).

The effects of epilepsy on IQ have also been thought to be related to the site of seizure origin. In particular, there is a widely held belief that seizures originating in the left hemisphere are more likely to affect Verbal IQ, whereas seizures originating in the right hemisphere are more likely to affect Performance IQ. However, this has proven to be an inaccurate assumption in both adult and pediatric populations. Early onset of cerebral injury related to development of epilepsy may also affect the cortical representation of language, resulting in mixed or right-hemisphere dominance. The related effect on IQ is in part dependent on the lateralization of language (Loring et al., 1999), with many patients who have left-hemisphere seizure onset demonstrating lower Performance IQ scores and relatively well-preserved Verbal IQ. However, the failure to identify lateralized effects on IQ in adults may be the result of the cumulative learning that takes place after the initial injury, rather than a lack of relationship between lateralization of injury and material-specific cognitive function, and assessment of IQ in childhood may produce different results. In fact, other authors have failed to find a lateralizing effect on IQ in children. Blackburn et al. (2007) reviewed the IQ scores of 130 children undergoing evaluation for epilepsy surgery. They found that even large discrepancies (greater than 15 points) between Verbal and Performance IQ were not necessarily lateralizing indicators, and that Verbal–Performance discrepancies lacked sensitivity and specificity as indicators of hemispheric seizure onset.

Although lowered IQ is an important consequence of epilepsy in some cases, many children with epilepsy have normal general intellectual function. However, even children with normal IQ may have impairments in more specific cognitive abilities. Children with epilepsy and normal IQ scores still have a higher prevalence of academic difficulties, characterized by increased utilization of educational support services and lower academic achievement scores (Bailet & Turk, 2000). It is likely that global measures like IQ mask more specific cognitive deficits in children with epilepsy, including difficulties with memory, disorders of attention and other executive functions, and specific language and learning disabilities.

Memory

Memory is one of the most widely studied cognitive functions in patients with epilepsy, due to the involvement of the hippocampal complex in many seizure disorders and the importance of this system for memory. TLE, characterized by complex partial seizures and often associated with hippocampal sclerosis, is associated with specific learning disabilities and impaired learning and memory. Moreover, there are numerous studies that characterize the memory impairments in adult patients with epilepsy. These studies report that epilepsy originating in the dominant hemisphere, particularly the temporal lobes, is associated with impaired learning and memory for verbal information, and that memory impairment can be directly attributed to damage in the hippocampus (Sass et al., 1990). Seizures originating in the nondominant hemisphere are often associated with impaired learning and recall for visual information, although the relationship is less robust than for verbal information and dominant-hemisphere seizures (Barr et al., 1997). Although lateralized seizure onset and material-specific memory impairments are among the most widely reported findings in adults with epilepsy, there are fewer studies in children. More important, while some authors have reported findings similar to those in adults, others have not.

In a study that compared 24 children with lateralized TLE (12 left, 12 right), Cohen (1992) found that when these children were administered a battery of memory tasks, those with right TLE performed more poorly on visual memory tasks than those with left TLE. Conversely, left TLE was associated with worse performance on verbal memory measures. This pattern appears to be more prevalent in studies in which children are evaluated for surgery, particularly temporal lobectomy (e.g., Jambaque, Dellatolas, Dulac, Ponsot, & Signoret, 1993), which may account for some of the differences in findings. Even though hippocampal sclerosis as a primary pathology in TLE is less common among children than among adults, candidates for surgery may be more likely to have localized damage associated with more specific cognitive patterns.

Other authors investigating material-specific memory impairments in children have not found lateralized effects, even for children with temporal lobe seizures. Mabbott and Smith (2003) studied 44 children undergoing surgery for epilepsy; they found that with the exception of face recognition, material-specific memory impairments were not present before or after surgery and were not associated with lateralization or temporal lobe surgery. Specific memory impairment may be more difficult to detect in children, for many reasons. Cognitive skills tend to be less differentiated in younger children, and the development of declarative memory is dependent upon these emerging skills. Also, in children whose language is less well developed, there may naturally be less dependence on the material-specific encoding tapped by measures of verbal or nonverbal memory. This may account for the observations of Lespinet, Bresson, N'Kaoua, Rougier, and Claverie (2002), who studied 56 children with lateralized TLE and found that children with earlier seizure onset (before age 5) had global, nonspecific memory deficits, while children with later seizure onset (over 10 years of age) had more specific deficits in material-dependent memory associated with side of seizure onset.

Others have investigated whether the failure to identify patterns of memory impairment similar to those observed in adults is related to the laterality of the lesion in TLE. Gonzalez, Anderson, Wood, Mitchell, and Harvey (2007) studied a sample of 43 children with right (n = 22) or left (n = 21) TLE, using a battery of verbal and visual memory measures. Like Mabbott and Smith (2003), Gonzalez et al. found that with the exception of face recognition, there was not a material-specific pattern of memory impairment associated with right versus left temporal lobe seizure onset. Gonzalez et al. also investigated the role of the location of the lesion within the temporal lobe (e.g., mesial vs. lateral temporal lobe), to determine whether this was a factor in whether material-specific memory impairment was present. They found that lesions involving the mesial temporal lobe structures were associated with verbal and visual memory impairments regardless of side, while children with lesions in the lateral temporal neocortex did not have memory impairments. The authors concluded that their findings supported a general associative learning model of hippocampal function in children that could not be extrapolated from adult material-specific models of memory.

Despite differences between adults and children in the nature of the memory impairment, there is clear evidence that TLE is associated with learning and memory deficits in children, and in many cases this may be due to the same underlying pathology as in adults—damage to the medial temporal lobe structures (including the hippocampus and perirhinal cortex) that are associated with temporal lobe seizures. It appears that early-onset seizures exert a more global deleterious effect on learning and memory, while later seizure onset is associated with patterns of performance more similar to those reported in adults. This makes sense, because studies of memory impairments in adults with TLE tend to focus on patients with hippocampal sclerosis. Although early febrile seizure is a risk factor for hippocampal sclerosis, onset of refractory seizures with hippocampal sclerosis as the primary pathology is more likely to occur in adolescence and adulthood than in early childhood (Berg, 2008a).

Executive Functions and Attention

Selected executive functions may be disrupted by seizures originating virtually anywhere, but particularly in the frontal lobes. Frontal lobe seizures differ from temporal lobe or other seizures in a variety of ways, including the clinical manifestations of the seizures themselves. The ictal behaviors observed in frontal lobe seizures vary greatly, owing to the complexity and diversity of behaviors mediated by the frontal lobes. Clinical manifestations will vary according to the region of seizure onset within the frontal lobe. Frontal lobe seizures tend to be brief, with rapid recovery and return to baseline, and tend to be more frequently nocturnal (Fogarasi, Janszky, Faveret, Pieper, & Tuxhorn, 2001). Seizure types can involve simple motor seizures, such as tonic posturing or forced head turning (Janszky, Fogarasi, Jokeit, & Ebner, 2001). However, more complex motor and other behavior changes may be observed, some of which appear bizarre and may lead to misinterpretation of ictal behaviors as behavior problems or psychiatric disturbance. For example, repeated walking in circles/rotating may be observed (Leung et al., 2008). Also, ictal vocalizations such as sudden screaming or moaning are common (Fogarasi et al., 2001; Rego, Arnold, & Noachtar, 2006). Gelastic seizures (pathological laughing), which are most often associated with hypothalamic hamartomas, also occur in frontal lobe epilepsy (Cheung, Parrent, & Burneo, 2007; Garcia, Gutierrez, Barrasa, & Herranz, 2000). Rarely, more severe behavioral or psychiatric disturbance, such as aggressive outbursts (Sumer, Atik, Unal, Emre, & Atasoy, 2007), or psychosis with violent hallucinations (Fornazzari, Farcnik, Smith, Heasman, & Ichise, 1992), may occur. Although a complete review of clinical manifestations in frontal lobe epilepsy is beyond the scope of this chapter, it is clear that the spectrum of behaviors is broad, and seizures should be ruled out in cases in which repeated episodes of similar atypical or bizarre behaviors occur.

With respect to the more general issue of executive functions in epilepsy, clinical studies suggest that 30–40% of children with all types of epilepsy have difficulties with attention, and that the predominantly inattentive type of attention-deficit/hyperactivity disorder (ADHD) is more common than the hyperactive–impulsive or combined types (Dunn & Kronenberger, 2005; Hermann et al., 2007). Attention problems among children with epilepsy differ from those in the general population not only in the general prevalence, but also in the fact that boys and girls with epilepsy are equally affected (Dunn, Austin, Harezlak, & Ambrosius, 2003). Although the combined subtype of ADHD is less commonly observed in children with seizures, it may be related to severity of epilepsy when it is present. Like others, Sherman, Slick, Connolly, and Eyrl (2007) found that the inattentive subtype of ADHD was more common, but that the combined subtype was associated with earlier age of onset, a higher degree of intractability, and lower quality of life. Although treatment with some antiepileptic drugs (AEDs) may produce attention difficulties as a side effect (see below), in most cases attention problems are not accounted for by medication effects alone. Problems with attention often precede development of seizures (Hesdorffer et al., 2004), suggesting that there may be an antecedent neurobiological insult or developmental abnormality (Hermann et al., 2006; Hesdorffer et al., 2004). In a subsequent study, Hermann et al. (2007) found an association between ADHD in epilepsy and quantitative MRI volumetrics in the frontal lobes and brainstem, suggesting that attention problems and later development of seizures may be different manifestations of the same underlying processes affecting development of brain structures that are important for attention.

Aside from attention, other dimensions of executive function in children with focal epilepsy have been very little studied. Although memory deficits may be more commonly observed among children with epilepsy originating in the temporal lobes, developmental emergence of executive function is more likely to be suppressed by frontal lobe seizures. Interictal effects in frontal lobe epilepsy may be more subtle, and may be manifested as deficient development in aspects of executive function. In a comparison of children with frontal or temporal lobe seizures, Culhane-Shelburne, Chapieski, Hiscock, and Glaze (2002) found an association between impaired executive function and frontal lobe epilepsy, whereas children with TLE did not show the same pattern of deficits. In this study, children with frontal lobe epilepsy showed impairments in planning and problem solving but not memory, while children with TLE showed the opposite pattern. Interestingly, both groups demonstrated impairment on a continuous-performance measure of attention. Similarly,

Hernandez et al. (2003) found that children with frontal lobe epilepsy demonstrated a variety of cognitive impairments associated with frontal lobe dysfunction, compared to children with TLE or absence seizures. In their study, frontal lobe epilepsy was associated with lower performance on a continuous-performance attention measure, slower processing speed, greater susceptibility to interference and intrusion errors in memory testing, and more frequent parent-reported attention problems on behavior rating forms.

Although primary localized effects on executive function may be more likely with frontal lobe seizures, temporal lobe seizures may result in secondary impairment in executive function through a diaschisis effect (Guimaraes et al., 2007; Rzezak et al., 2007). Rzezak et al. found that children with TLE also had impaired executive functions, and that age of onset was a factor in the severity of observed impairments. In addition, medication effects may contribute to attention and executive function deficits in children with focal epilepsy (Loring & Meador, 2004). The severity of epilepsy may also be a factor in whether executive function deficits are present. In a study of children with intractable epilepsy, Slick, Lautzenhiser, Sherman, & Eyrl (2006) found that 36% had four or more clinically significant elevations on the Behavior Rating Inventory of Executive Function, a parent report form for executive function in children. Sixty-nine percent had at least one clinically significant scale elevation, with the most commonly reported problems cited in the areas of working memory and planning/organization.

In sum, children with epilepsy appear to be more prone to problems with executive functions, particularly deficits in attention. Developmental abnormalities in brain structures associated with attention have been noted, and may be responsible for symptomatic expression as both attention problems and seizures.

Learning Disabilities

Children with epilepsy have a much higher rate of special education classification, and receive more educational support services, than children who do not have epilepsy (Berg et al., 2005). This overrepresentation of children with epilepsy in special needs programs is not attributable to the general effects of having a chronic medical condition. In one study comparing children with epilepsy to children with chronic asthma, the children with epilepsy were found to have significantly lower academic achievement scores (Austin, Huberty, Huster, & Dunn, 1998). There have been several studies investigating the factors that may be responsible for the impaired academic skills of children with epilepsy, particularly seizure-related variables (Holdsworth & Whitmore, 1974; Stores & Hart, 1976; Suurmeijer, 1991; Zelnik, Sa'adi, Silman-Stolar, & Goikhman, 2001). However, the relationship between educational achievement and epilepsy is complex and may be affected by multiple factors, not just seizures. Although such factors as seizure frequency, treatment (Zelnik et al., 2001), and type and severity of epilepsy (Aldenkamp, Weber, Overweg-Plandsoen, Reijs, & vanMil, 2005) are important, educational achievement continues to lag behind even when seizures remit or are well controlled (Suurmeijer, 1991). Furthermore, the influence of these variables is not uniform across different areas of academic achievement. Seidenberg et al. (1986) found that a high frequency of children with epilepsy had lower academic achievement scores than expected for their general intellectual ability. The worst performance was found on measures of mathematical achievement, but performance was also poor in spelling, reading comprehension, and word reading. The influence of seizure-related variables was greater for math and spelling than for reading achievement. Finally, while overall level of intellectual function is also an important factor, children with epilepsy may have lower academic achievement scores even when overall IQ is normal (Bailet & Turk, 2000). When achievement is considered against a child's potential as measured by IQ testing, a discrepancy is still likely.

Surprisingly, there is little information about specific patterns of academic under-achievement in children with epilepsy, or about how these patterns fit into models of learning disability. Many studies simply report the percentage of children who have received special education services, without specifying the nature or intensity of the services (Berg et al., 2005). Other investigators have tried to link epilepsy-related variables to specific aspects of learning disability, but have found no clear evidence of specific learning disability types in children with epilepsy (Vermeulen, Kortstee, Alpherts, & Aldenkamp, 1994). However, some research has found specific patterns of dysfunction among children with epilepsy that are related to the underlying pathology. In a comparison of children with three different seizure types (TLE, benign rolandic epilepsy, and idiopathic generalized epilepsy), the children with TLE performed significantly worse on reading tasks than the other two groups did (Chaix et al., 2006). Lower academic achievement in the TLE group was related to phonological, semantic, and verbal working memory impairments, reflecting the role of the temporal lobe in these abilities. Children with idiopathic generalized epilepsy had more general cognitive impairments, but to a lesser degree, suggesting a more general effect than that associated with temporal lobe seizures. Others have also noted specific deficits that are related to the region of epileptic discharge, in that there appears to be some specificity in the relationship between the occurrence of discharges and the types of impairments observed. For example, left-sided interictal discharges are more likely to be associated with reading errors or errors on verbal tasks, while right-sided discharges are more likely to produce errors on nonverbal tasks (Binnie, Channon, & Marston, 1990).

The association of localized pathology with learning disabilities may go beyond the electrophysiological abnormalities found in localization-related epilepsies. There is increasing evidence that there are neuroanatomical differences in children with otherwise "normal" imaging (i.e., nonlesional epilepsy). Hermann et al. (2006) found that children with epilepsy who had the most abnormal cognitive function and associated learning disabilities also had significantly lower gray matter volumes in the left parietal and occipital lobes. Children with epilepsy overall lacked the developmental association between cognitive function and cerebral tissue volumes demonstrated in normal children. This indicates that there may indeed be a direct relationship between specific neurodevelopmental abnormalities and learning impairments in children with epilepsy.

There is a justifiable focus on biological variables in learning disability and other impairments in children with epilepsy; however, nonbiological factors also need to be considered. Stigma associated with epilepsy is an important variable that is associated with adjustment and quality of life in children with epilepsy. However, there is also evidence that stigma may be a factor in educational achievement. Teachers tend to rate children with epilepsy as having lower ability when they are aware of the children's history of epilepsy, even when there is no difference in their actual level of academic achievement (Katzenstein, Fastenau, Dunn, & Austin, 2007). Educators' perceptions of the intellectual potential of children with seizures may affect the services or attention that these children receive, and may thus further contribute to the psychological adjustment issues that are increasingly observed among children with epilepsy.

PSYCHOLOGICAL AND PSYCHOSOCIAL ASPECTS OF EPILEPSY

There is increased recognition that the well-described psychological and psychosocial problems associated with epilepsy in adults begin during childhood and adolescence. Epidemiological studies have identified higher rates of psychological disturbance in children with epilepsy than in the general population (Davies, Heyman, & Goodman, 2003). Children with epilepsy also have a higher prevalence of psychological problems and worse quality of life than children with other chronic diseases, such as diabetes (Davies et al., 2003). Psychological manifestations of mood disturbance, such as depression and anxiety, are among the most commonly reported. Even among children who have not been formally diagnosed with a mood disorder, increased symptoms of depression and anxiety are present (Ettinger et al., 1998). However, although mood disorders and internalizing behaviors are more common, externalizing behaviors also occur with greater frequency among children with epilepsy than among children with other disorders (Plioplys, Dunn, & Caplan, 2007).

Psychological distress among children with epilepsy, like cognitive impairment, is complex in its genesis. Most models recognize this, and several studies have helped to delineate psychosocial factors that contribute to psychological disturbance. There is some contribution of factors that are inherent to chronic diseases in general, such as family burden (Rodenburg, Stams, Meijer, Aldenkamp, & Dekovic, 2005). These factors may interact with new-onset epilepsy to increase vulnerability to depression, since it has been noted that family problems in children with epilepsy who are depressed predate the diagnosis of epilepsy (Oostrom, Schouten, Olthof, Peters, & Jennekens-Schinkel, 2000), and that low family mastery increases the risk of behavior problems in children with new-onset epilepsy (Baum et al., 2007). Although psychosocial factors do play an important role, the increased prevalence of psychopathology in epilepsy also implicates epilepsy-specific variables. However, the specific nature of the relationship of epilepsy variables to psychological disturbance has been difficult to pin down. Factors such as laterality of seizure onset have proved inconsistent, with some authors finding higher rates of depression among patients with right-hemisphere seizure onset (Quigg, Broshek, Heidal-Schiltz, Maedgen, & Bertram, 2003), while others have found the opposite (Altshuler, Devinsky, Post, & Theodore, 1990). Although it is possible that there are different mechanisms underlying depression in patients with differently lateralized onset, it is difficult to predict depression from laterality of seizures. Other seizure-related variables that have proven to be important for cognitive development, such as age at seizure onset, have not been shown to be risk factors for development of psychological or behavioral problems—although an indirect relationship exists, in that greater cognitive impairment is associated with increased behavior problems such as hyperactivity and impulse control disorders (Plioplys et al., 2007). Similarly, seizure frequency does not appear to be a risk factor, once cognition is controlled for. Although age of onset and frequency of seizures do not appear to be significant in the development of psychological and behavioral problems, the nature of the epileptic syndrome does. Children with idiopathic seizures have more frequent behavior problems than those with symptomatic epilepsy (Berg et al., 2007). Children with symptomatic epilepsy also report lower quality of life than those with idiopathic epilepsy, although children with different symptomatic partial epilepsies (frontal lobe, TLE) do not seem to differ from one another (Sabaz et al., 2003).

Although psychosocial factors clearly play an important role, these factors act on a disturbed neurobiological substrate that may predispose an individual to development of mood disorders. Some have even suggested a bidirectional relationship between epilepsy and mood disorders, specifically depression, that suggests a shared common pathology involving multiple neuroanatomical and neurotransmitter systems (Kanner, 2008). A common underlying substrate would explain the recent findings of several authors that behavioral and affective disturbance is present before the onset of seizures (Kanner, 2008), and that it persists into adulthood even in patients with seizure remission who are no longer taking seizure medications (Berg et al., 2007; Jalava, Sillanpaa, Camfield, & Camfield, 1997; Kokkonen, Kokkonen, Saukkonen, & Pennanen, 1997).

IATROGENIC COGNITIVE AND BEHAVIORAL CONSEQUENCES

Most cases of epilepsy are treated adequately with medication. However, AEDs used to treat seizures may be associated with some adverse cognitive symptoms. Unfortunately, the majority of studies investigating cognitive morbidity associated with AED treatment have been conducted in adults, due to methodological and ethical difficulties in conducting such studies with children. As a result, studies in children tend to be observational and are fraught with methodological problems that limit direct attribution of observed problems to a specific AED. Nonetheless, there is some evidence that commonly used AEDs may affect cognitive function. One of the oldest AEDs still in common use, phenobarbital, has been shown to have a lasting effect on IQ scores in children (Sulzbacher, Farwell, Temkin, Lu, & Hirtz, 1999). However, IQ is generally not considered a sensitive indicator, since AED effects may be present in more limited domains (such as attention, memory, or language), but are not necessarily associated with a global decline in IQ. It appears from studies with adult patients that AED effects are nonspecific, in that attention and processing speed are more vulnerable, regardless of the mechanism of action for a particular AED. Effects on attention and reaction time have been noted for carbamezapine (Hessen, Lossius, Reinvang, & Gjerstad, 2006) and phenytoin (Aldenkamp et al., 1994).

Newer AEDs appear to be associated with fewer cognitive side effects (Loring & Meador, 2004), with a few notable exceptions. Topiramate, whose antiepileptic properties appear to derive from multiple mechanisms of action (including enhancing the action of the inhibitory neurotransmitter gamma-aminobutyric acid and inhibiting the excitatory neurotransmitter glutamate), has been associated with adverse cognitive side effects. Studies have reported impairments on measures of language functions, including Verbal IQ (Thompson, Baxendale, Duncan, & Sander, 2000) and word-finding tasks (Coppola et al., 2008). Impairments have also been found in other general cognitive abilities, such as memory, attention, and processing speed (Lee et al., 2003). Aside from topiramate, however, the newer AEDs appear to have fewer adverse cognitive side effects, and some may even have beneficial effects on aspects of cognitive function through improved seizure control (Loring & Meador, 2004).

DEVELOPMENTAL CONSIDERATIONS

Epilepsy is predominantly a disorder with childhood onset, owing to several developmental factors. For one, genetic predispositions to develop epilepsy are more likely to be manifested in childhood. In addition, children have a higher chance of exposure to, and are also more vulnerable to, risk factors for development of epilepsy. For example, children are more vulnerable to CNS infection because of the immature blood–brain barrier. Also, exposure to risk factors in childhood is more likely to result in seizures, due to a developmental imbalance between excitatory and inhibitory processes in the brain (Velisek & Moshe, 2001).

The increased risk of seizure onset during childhood also increases the risk that seizures will disrupt normal developmental processes. Although there is a belief that early injury may be associated with better long-term outcome, due to plasticity of the maturing nervous system, recent studies implicating earlier age of seizure onset as an important factor for various negative cognitive and neurobehavioral outcomes have indicated that this is not necessarily the case (Berg et al., 2008). The finding that earlier age of onset is associated with worse cognitive outcome may seem counterintuitive when such factors as presumed greater plasticity of the younger brain are considered. However, it appears that seizures may adversely affect important neurodevelopmental processes resulting in structural as well as functional impairments (Hermann et al., 2006).

The importance of developmental aspects in epilepsy, including the cumulative long-term effects on cognitive and psychosocial function, have resulted in advocates for more aggressive early intervention—including surgical resection when single focal onset sites are clearly identifiable. However intuitive the appeal of early surgery may seem, the evidence to support assumptions that aggressive early treatment has better long-term outcome is lacking. Although some authors have found favorable outcomes for surgery in children, others have obtained equivocal results. Gleissner, Sassen, Schramm, Elger, and Helmstaedter (2005) compared the memory outcome in a sample of children who underwent temporal lobectomy with that of an adult surgery group. Groups were matched for pathology and surgery type, and studied at postoperative intervals of 3 months and 1 year. Both groups experienced memory decline after surgery, but only the pediatric group showed recovery to baseline at 1 year after surgery. In addition to better memory outcome, Gleissner et al. reported better seizure control and improved attention. Others have also reported better outcome with surgery in childhood (e.g., Jambaque et al., 1993) However, not all studies have found significant improvement in cognition or quality of life in children after epilepsy surgery (Smith, Elliott, & Lach, 2004). Whether the promise of reduced psychosocial and cognitive problems with early surgery as a treatment for medically refractory seizures is realized has yet to be determined (Westerveld, 2006).

CONCLUSIONS AND DIRECTIONS FOR FUTURE STUDY

Emerging technologies provide a clearer window into the association of various neurobiological factors and cognitive dysfunction in epilepsy. It is becoming more evident that the symptomatic expression of seizures and the associated cognitive and behavioral impairments share a common substrate that varies greatly, depending on individual factors (including age of seizure onset and the nature of the underlying pathology). Imaging studies have identified global and local structural changes in the developing brains of children with epilepsy. Electrophysiological studies have been helpful in differentiating transient cognitive deficits due to interictal epileptiform activity from the more basic cognitive impairments associated with underlying structural abnormalities. Finally, increased understanding of early emergence of specific cognitive skills and earlier assessment of diverse cognitive functions have also led to a greater appreciation for the subtle cognitive effects of various forms of epilepsy and the sensitivity of the developing brain to the effects of seizures.

Despite these advances, our ability to predict from a detailed understanding of these factors which individual child is at risk for cognitive impairments is lacking, and our understanding of the evolution of cognitive function and processes that guide development is minimal. We need to increase the scope of neuropsychological methods in collaborative interdisciplinary and translational research that combines detailed neurobiological studies with longitudinal assessment of cognitive development, in order to clarify our understanding of the processes leading to development of neuropsychological impairments. Specifically, controlled studies designed to elucidate the complex nature of the interaction between iatrogenic factors (e.g., AED side effects) and disease-specific factors are needed; in such studies, neuropsychological evaluations must be conducted at the time of diagnosis, prior to initiation of AED treatment. Although the nature of epilepsy precludes a true randomized controlled study due to practical and ethical concerns, observational studies that begin with the very first seizure event can provide useful information regarding the effects of seizures and AEDs on development of function. In addition, serial imaging studies that utilize comparisons to typically developing children without epilepsy are needed, to better define both the impact of epilepsy on brain development and its relationship to cognitive function. Structure–function correlational studies, like that of Hermann et al. (2006), provide a model for accomplishing this type of research. Follow-up imaging studies can track changes in brain development that are correlated with seizure remission, treatment variables, and cognitive outcome. Better utilization of emerging technologies such as fMRI can also add to the understanding of mechanisms of epilepsy and plasticity in cognitive development. This type of research has already begun to emerge in studies of children born preterm (Ment & Constable, 2007) and is ideally suited to understanding the mechanisms of epilepsy and cognitive development in children with seizures.

Finally, epilepsy has a rich history of contributing to basic knowledge of brain–behavior relationships. Extending this tradition to include basic science efforts to understand the role of specific neurotransmitters and cellular pathologies in epilepsy can contribute to better understanding of mechanisms of cognitive function. Epilepsy research programs include analysis of cellular excitability and long-term potentiation, as well as the role of neurotransmitters in altering neuronal function in epilepsy. Studies of cognitive development in relation to these more basic mechanisms of neuronal function can provide insights into how cognition is mediated at the most basic level. For example, examining the relationship of in vivo changes in neurotransmitter release during seizures and cognitive tasks through microdialysis can provide insight into how epileptic alterations of neurotransmitters (e.g., glutamate) affect cognitive function. There is a virtually infinite landscape for the interaction of cognitive neuroscience and basic science in studying cognitive development. Neuropsychologists are uniquely qualified to contribute to this type of research, through designing assessment paradigms that incorporate appreciation for the developmental changes in cognitive function over time (e.g., emergence of executive functions from childhood through adolescence and adulthood) with technologies for assessing neuroanatomical function.

REFERENCES

Aldenkamp, A. P., Alpherts, W. C., Diepman, L., van't Slot, B., Overweg, J., & Vermeulen, J. (1994). Cognitive side-effects of phenytoin compared with carbamazepine in patients with localization-related epilepsy. *Epilepsy Research, 19*(1), 37–43.

Aldenkamp, A. P., Weber, B., Overweg-Plandsoen, W. C., Reijs, R., & vanMil, S. (2005). Educational underachievement in children with epilepsy: A model to predict the effects of epilepsy on educational achievement. *Journal of Child Neurology, 20*(3), 175–180.

Altshuler, L. L., Devinsky, O., Post, R.M., Theodore, W. (1990). Depression, anxiety, and temporal lobe epilepsy. Laterality of focus and symptoms. *Archives of Neurology, 47*(3), 284–288.

Anderson, D. P., Harvey, A. S., Saling, M. M., Anderson, V., Kean, M., Abbott, D. F., et al. (2006). FMRI lateralization of expressive language in children with cerebral lesions. *Epilepsia, 47*(6), 998–1008.

Annegers, J. F., Grabow, J. D., Groover, R. V., Laws, E. R., Jr., Elveback, L. R., & Kurland, L. T. (1980). Seizures after head trauma: A population study. *Neurology, 34*, 746–758.

Austin, J. K., Huberty, T. J., Huster, G. A., & Dunn, D. W. (1998). Academic achievement in children with epilepsy or asthma. *Developmental Medicine and Child Neurology, 40*(4), 248–255.

Bailet, L. L., & Turk, W. R. (2000). The impact of childhood epilepsy on neurocognitive and behavioral performance: A prospective longitudinal study. *Epilepsia, 41*(4), 426–431.

Barr, W., Chelune, G. J., Hermann, B. P., Loring, D. W., Perrine, K. R., Strauss, E., et al. (1997). The use of figural reproduction tests as measures of nonverbal memory in epilepsy surgery candidates. *Journal of the International Neuropsychological Society, 3*(5), 35–43.

Baum, K. T., Byars, A. W., deGrauw, T. J., Johnson, C. S., Perkins, S. M., Dunn, D. W., et al. (2007). Temperament, family environment, and behavior problems in children with new-onset seizures. *Epilepsy and Behavior, 10*(2), 319–327.

Berg, A. T. (2008a). The natural history of mesial temporal lobe epilepsy. *Current Opinion in Neurology, 21*(2), 173–178.

Berg, A. T. (2008b). Risk of recurrence after a first unprovoked seizure. *Epilepsia, 49*(Suppl. 1), 13–18.

Berg, A. T., Langfitt, J. T., Testa, F. M., Levy, S. R., Dimario, F., Westerveld, M., et al. (2008). Global cognitive function in children with epilepsy: A community-based study. *Epilepsia, 49*(4), 608–614.

Berg, A. T., Smith, S. N., Frobish, D., Levy, S. R., Testa, F. M., Beckerman, B., et al. (2005). Special education needs of children with newly diagnosed epilepsy. *Developmental Medicine and Child Neurology, 47*, 749–753.

Berg, A. T., Vickrey, B. G., Testa, F. M., Levy, S. R., Shinnar, S., & DiMario, F. (2007). Behavior and social competency in idiopathic and cryptogenic childhood epilepsy. *Neurology, 49*(7), 487–492.

Binnie, C. D., Channon, S., & Marston, D. (1990). Learning disabilities in epilepsy: Neurophysiological aspects. *Epilepsia, 31*(Suppl. 4), S2–S8.

Blackburn, L. B., Lee, G. P., Westerveld, M., Hempel, A., Park, Y. D., & Loring, D. W. (2007). The Verbal IQ/Performance IQ discrepancy as a sign of seizure focus laterality in pediatric patients with epilepsy. *Epilepsy and Behavior, 10*(1), 84–88.

Bourgeois, B., Prensky, A. L., Palkes, H. S., Talent, B. K., Busch, & S. G. (1983). Intelligence in epilepsy: A prospective study in children. *Annals of Neurology, 14*(4), 438–444.

Boyd, S. G., Rivera-Gaxiola, M., Towell, A. D., Harkness, W., & Neville, B. G. (1996). Discrimination of speech sounds in a boy with Landau–Kleffner syndrome: An intraoperative event-related potential study. *Neuropediatrics, 27*(4), 211–215.

Chaix, Y., Laguitton, V., Lauwers-Cances, V., Daquin, G., Cances, C., Demonet, J. F., et al. (2006). Reading abilities and cognitive functions of children with epilepsy: Influence of epileptic syndrome. *Brain and Development, 28*(2), 122–130.

Cheung, C. S., Parrent, A. G., & Burneo, J. G. (2007). Gelastic seizures: Not always hypothalamic hamartoma. *Epileptic Disorders*, 9(4), 453–458.

Cohen, M. (1992). Auditory/verbal and visual/spatial memory in children with complex partial epilepsy of temporal lobe origin. *Brain and Cognition*, 20(2), 315–326.

Commission on Classification and Terminology of the International League Against Epilepsy (ILAE). (1981). Proposal for revised clinical and electroencephalographic classification of epileptic seizures. *Epilepsia*, 22, 489–501.

Commission on Classification and Terminology of the International League Against Epilepsy (ILAE). (1989). Proposal for revised classification of epilepsies and epileptic syndromes. *Epilepsia*, 26, 268–278.

Coppola, F., Rossi, C., Mancini, M., Corbelli, I., Nardi, K., Sarchielli, P., et al. (2008). Language disturbances as a side effect of prophylactic treatment of migraine. *Headache*, 48(1), 86–94.

Culhane-Shelburne, K., Chapieski, L., Hiscock, M., & Glaze, D. (2002). Executive functions in children with frontal and temporal lobe epilepsy. *Journal of the International Neuropsychological Society*, 8(5), 623–632.

da Silva, E. A., Chugani, D. C., Muzik, O., & Chugani, H. T. (1997). Landau–Kleffner syndrome: Metabolic abnormalities in temporal lobe are a common feature. *Neurology*, 12(8), 489–495.

Davies, S., Heyman, I., & Goodman, R. (2003). A population survey of mental health problems in children with epilepsy. *Developmental Medicine and Child Neurology*, 45, 292–295.

Deonna, T., & Roulet-Perez, E. (2005). *Cognitive and behavioural disorders of epileptic origin in children*. London: Mac Keith Press.

Dunn, D. W., Austin, J. K., Harezlak, J., & Ambrosius, W. T. (2003). (2003). ADHD and epilepsy in childhood. *Developmental Medicine and Child Neurology*, 45(1), 50–54.

Dunn, D. W., & Kronenberger, W. G. (2005). Childhood epilepsy, attention problems, and ADHD: Review and practical considerations. *Seminars in Pediatric Neurology*, 12(4), 222–228.

Ettinger, A. B., Weisbrot, D. M., Nolan, E. E., Gadow, K. D., Vitale, S. A., Andriola, M. R., et al. (1998). Symptoms of depression and anxiety in pediatric epilepsy patients. *Epilepsia*, 39(6), 595–599.

First Seizure Trial Group. (1993). Randomized clinical trial of the efficacy of antiepileptic drugs in reducing the risk of relapse after a first unprovoked tonic–clonic seizure.. *Neurology*, 43, 478–483.

Fogarasi, A., Janszky, J., Faveret, E., Pieper, T., & Tuxhorn, I. (2001). A detailed analysis of frontal lobe seizure semiology in children younger than 7 years. *Epilepsia*, 42(1), 80–85.

Fornazzari, L., Farcnik, K., Smith, I., Heasman, G. A., & Ichise, M. (1992). Violent visual hallucinations and aggression in frontal lobe dysfunction: Clinical manifestations of deep orbitofrontal foci. *Journal of Neuropsychiatry and Clinical Neurosciences*, 4(1), 42–44.

Garcia, A., Gutierrez, M. A., Barrasa, J., & Herranz, J. L. (2000). Cryptogenic gelastic epilepsy of frontal lobe origin: A paediatric case report. *Seizure*, 9(4), 297–300.

Gleissner, U., Sassen, R., Schramm, J., Elger, C. E., & Helmstaedter, C. (2005). Greater functional recovery after temporal lobe epilepsy surgery in children. *Brain*, 128(12), 2822–2829.

Gonzalez, L. M., Anderson, V. A., Wood, S. J., Mitchell, L. A., & Harvey, A. S. (2007). The localization and lateralization of memory deficits in children with temporal lobe epilepsy. *Epilepsia*, 48(1), 124–132.

Guimaraes, C. A., Li, L. M., Rzezak, P., Fuentes, D., Franzon, R. C., Augusta-Montenegro, M., et al. (2007). Temporal lobe epilepsy in childhood: Comprehensive neuropsychological assessment. *Journal of Child Neurology*, 22(7), 836–840.

Hattori, A., Ando, N., Hamaguchi, K., Hussein, M. H., Fujimoto, S., Ishikawa, T., et al. (2006). Short-duration ACTH therapy for cryptogenic West syndrome with better outcome. *Pediatric Neurology*, 35(6), 415–418.

Hauser, W. A. (2001). Epidemiology of epilepsy in children. In J. M. Pellock, W. E. Dodson, & B. F. D. Bourgeois (Eds.), *Pediatric epilepsy: Diagnosis and therapy* (2nd ed., pp. 81–96). New York: DEMOS.

Hermann, B., Jones, J., Dabbs, K., Allen, C. A., Sheth, R., Fine, J., et al. (2007). The frequency, complications and aetiology of ADHD in new onset paediatric epilepsy. *Brain*, 130(12), 3135–3148.

Hermann, B., Jones, J., Sheth, R., Dow, C., Koehn, M., & Seidenberg, M. (2006). Children with new-onset epilepsy: Neuropsychological status and brain structure. *Brain, 129,* 2609–2619.

Hermann, B., Seidenberg, M., Bell, B., Rutecki, P., Sheth, R., Ruggles, K., et al. (2002). The neurodevelopmental impact of childhood-onset temporal lobe epilepsy on brain structure and function. *Epilepsia, 43*(9), 1062–1071.

Hernandez, M. T., Sauerwein, H. C., Jambaque, I., deGuise, E., Lussier, F., Lortie, A., et al. (2003). Attention, memory, and behavioral adjustment in children with frontal lobe epilepsy. *Epilepsy and Behavior, 4*(5), 522–536.

Hesdorffer, D. C., Ludvigsson, P., Olafsson, E., Gudmundsson, G., Kjartansson, O., & Hauser, W. A. (2004). ADHD as a risk factor for incident unprovoked seizures and epilepsy in children. *Archives of General Psychiatry, 61*(7), 731–736.

Hessen, E., Lossius, M. I., Reinvang, I., & Gjerstad, L. (2006). Influence of major antiepileptic drugs on attention, reaction time, and speed of information processing: Results from a randomized, double-blind, placebo-controlled withdrawal study of seizure-free epilepsy patients receiving monotherapy. *Epilepsia, 47*(12), 2038–2045.

Holdsworth, L., & Whitmore, K. (1974). A study of children with epilepsy attending ordinary school. *Developmental Medicine and Child Neurology, 16,* 746–758.

Jack, C. R. (2001). Neuroimaging of the temporal lobe. In H. O. Luders & Y. G. Comair (Eds.), *Epilepsy surgery* (2nd ed., pp. 227–238). Philadelphia: Lippincott Williams & Wilkins.

Jalava, M., Sillanpaa, M., Camfield, C., & Camfield P. (1997). Social adjustment and competence 35 years after onset of childhood epilepsy: A prospective controlled study. *Epilepsia, 38,* 708–715.

Jambaque, I., Dellatolas, G., Dulac, O., Ponsot, G., & Signoret, J. L. (1993). Verbal and visual memory impairment in children with epilepsy. *Neuropsychologia, 31*(12), 1321–1337.

Janszky, J., Fogarasi, A., Jokeit, H., & Ebner, A. (2001). Lateralizing value of unilateral motor and somatosensory manifestations in frontal lobe seizures. *Epilepsy Research, 43*(2), 125–133.

Jokeit, H., & Ebner, A. (2002). Effects of chronic epilepsy on intellectual functions. *Progress in Brain Research, 135,* 455–463.

Kanner, A. M. (2008). Depression in epilepsy: A complex relation with unexpected consequences. *Current Opinion in Neurology, 21,* 190–194.

Katzenstein, J. M., Fastenau, P. S., Dunn, D. W.,& Austin, J. K. (2007). Teachers' ratings of the academic performance of children with epilepsy. *Epilepsy and Behavior, 10*(3), 426–431.

Kivity, S., Lerman, P., Ariel, R., Danziger, Y., Mimouni, M., & Shinnar, S. (2004). Long-term cognitive outcomes of a cohort of children with cryptogenic infantile spasms treated with high-dose adrenocorticotropic hormone. *Epilepsia, 45*(3), 255–262.

Kodama, K., Murakami, A., Yamanouchi, N., Koseki, K., Iwasa, H., Okada, S., et al. (1995). MR in temporal lobe epilepsy: Early childhood onset versus later onset. *American Journal of Neuroradiology, 16*(3), 523–529.

Kokkonen, J., Kokkonen, E. R., Saukkonen, A. L., & Pennanen, P. (1997). Psychosocial outcome of young adults with epilepsy in childhood. *Journal of Neurology, Neurosurgery, and Psychiatry, 62,* 265–268.

Kramer, U., Kipervasser, S., Neufeld, M. Y., Fried, I., Nagar, S., & Andelman, F. (2006). Is there any correlation between severity of epilepsy and cognitive abilities in patients with temporal lobe epilepsy? *European Journal of Neurology, 13*(2), 130–134.

Kuzniecky, R. I. (2001). Neuroimaging in pediatric epilepsy. In J. M. Pellock, W. E. Dodson, & B. F. D. Bourgeois (Eds.), *Pediatric epilepsy: Diagnosis and therapy* (2nd ed., pp. 133–143). New York: DEMOS.

Lee, G. P., Westerveld, M., Blackburn, L. B., Park, Y. D., & Loring, D. W. (2005). Prediction of verbal memory decline after epilepsy surgery in children: Effectiveness of Wada memory asymmetries. *Epilepsia, 46*(1), 97–103.

Lee, S., Sziklas, V., Andermann, F., Farnham, S., Risse, G., Gustafson, M., et al. (2003). The effects of adjunctive topiramate on cognitive function in patients with epilepsy. *Epilepsia, 44*(3), 339–347.

Lee, S. K., Lee, S. Y., Yun, C. H., Lee, H. Y., Lee, J. S., & Lee, D. S. (2006). Ictal SPECT in neocortical epilepsies: Clinical usefulness and factors affecting the pattern of hyperperfusion. *Neuroradiology, 48*(9), 678–684.

Lespinet, V., Bresson, C., N'Kaoua, B., Rougier, A., & Claverie, B. (2002). Effect of age of onset of temporal lobe epilepsy on the severity and the nature of preoperative memory deficits. *Neuropsychologia, 40*(9), 1591–1600.

Leung, H., Schindler, K., Clusmann, H., Bien, C. G., Popel, A., Schramm, J., et al. (2008). Mesial frontal epilepsy and ictal body turning along the horizontal body axis. *Archives of Neurology, 65*(1), 71–77.

Loring, D. W., & Meador, K. J. (2004). Cognitive side effects of antiepileptic drugs in children. *Neurology, 62*(6), 872–877.

Loring, D. W., Strauss, E., Hermann, B. P., Perrine, K. R., Trenerry, M. R., Barr, W. B., et al. (1999). Effects of anomalous language representation on neuropsychological performance in temporal lobe epilepsy. *Neurology, 53,* 260–264.

Mabbott, D. J., & Smith, M. L. (2003). Memory in children with temporal or extra-temporal excisions. *Neuropsychologia, 41*(8), 995–1007.

Mantovani, J. F. (2000). Autistic regression and Landau–Kleffner syndrome: progress or confusion? *Developmental Medicine and Child Neurology, 42*(5), 349–353.

Ment, L. R., & Constable, R. T. (2007). Injury and recovery in the developing brain: Evidence from functional MRI studies of prematurely born children. *Nature Clinical Practice: Neurology, 3*(10), 558–571.

Neville, B., & Cross, H. (2006). Continuous spike wave of slow sleep and Landau Kleffner syndrome. In E. Wyllie (Ed.), *The treatment of epilepsy: Principles and practice* (4th ed., pp. 455–462). Philadelphia: Lippincott Williams & Wilkins.

Ohtahara, S., & Yamatogi, Y. (2001). Severe encephalopathic epilepsy in infants: West syndrome. In J. M. Pellock, W. E. Dodson, & B. F. D. Bourgeois (Eds.), *Pediatric epilepsy: Diagnosis and therapy* (2nd ed., pp. 177–192). New York: DEMOS.

Oostrom, K. J., Schouten, A., Olthof, T., Peters, A. C., & Jennekens-Schinkel, A. (2000). Negative emotions in children with newly diagnosed epilepsy. *Epilepsia, 41,* 326–331.

Ottman, R. (2001). Genetic influence on risk for epilepsy. In J. M. Pellock, W. E. Dodson, & B. F. D. Bourgeois (Eds.), *Pediatric epilepsy: Diagnosis and therapy* (2nd ed., pp. 61–68). New York: DEMOS.

Peretti, P., Raybaud, C., Dravet, C., Mancini, J., & Pinsard, N. (1989). Magnetic resonance imaging in partial epilepsy of childhood: Seventy-nine cases. *Journal of Neuroradiology, 16*(4), 308–316.

Plioplys, S., Dunn, D. W., & Caplan, R. (2007). 10-year research update review: Psychiatric problems in children with epilepsy. *Journal of the American Academy of Child and Adolescent Psychiatry, 46*(11), 1389–1402.

Quigg, M., Broshek, D. K., Heidal-Schiltz, S., Maedgen, J. W., & Bertram, E. H. (2003). Depression in intractable partial epilepsy varies by laterality of focus and surgery. *Epilepsia, 44*(3), 419–424.

Rego, R., Arnold, S., & Noachtar, S. (2006). Frontal lobe epilepsy manifesting with seizures consisting of isolated vocalization. *Epileptic Disorders, 8*(4), 274–276.

Rodenburg, R., Stams, G. J., Meijer, A. M., Aldenkamp, A. P., & Dekovic, M. (2005). Psychopathology in children with epilepsy: A meta-analysis. *Journal of Pediatric Psychology, 30*(6), 453–468.

Rzezak, P., Fuentes, D., Guimaraes, C. A., Thome-Souza, S., Kuczynski, E., Li, L. M., et al. (2007). Frontal lobe dysfunction in children with temporal lobe epilepsy. *Pediatric Neurology, 37*(3), 176–185.

Sabaz, M., Cairns, D. R., Bleasel, A. F., Lawson, J. A., Grinton, B., Scheffer, I. E., et al. (2003). The health-related quality of life of childhood epilepsy syndromes. *Journal of Paediatrics and Child Health, 39*(9), 690–696.

Sagar, H. J., & Oxbury, J. M. (1987). Hippocampal neuron loss in temporal lobe epilepsy: Correlation with early childhood convulsions. *Annals of Neurology, 22,* 334–340.

Sarnat, H., & Flores-Sarnat, L. (2006). Human nervous system development and malformations. In E. Wyllie (Ed.), *The treatment of epilepsy: Principles and practice* (4th ed., pp. 13–36). Philadelphia: Lippincott Williams & Wilkins.

Sass, K., Spencer, D. D., Kim, J. H., Westerveld, M., Novelly, R. A., & Lencz, T. (1990). Verbal memory impairment correlates with hippocampal pyramidal cell density. *Neurology, 40,* 1694–1697.

Sawaishi, Y., Sasaki, M., Yano, T., Hirayama, A., Akabane, J., & Takada, G. (2005). A hippocampal lesion detected by high-field 3 Tesla magnetic resonance imaging in a patient with temporal lobe epilepsy. *Tohoku Journal of Experimental Medicine, 205*(3), 287–291.

Seidenberg, M., Beck, N., Geisser, M., Giordani, B., Sackellares, J. C., Berent, S., et al. (1986). Academic achievement of children with epilepsy. *Epilepsia, 27*(6), 753–759.

Sherman, E. M., Slick, D. J., Connolly, M. B., & Eyrl, K. L. (2007). ADHD, neurological correlates and health-related quality of life in severe pediatric epilepsy. *Epilepsia, 48*(6), 1083–1091.

Slick, D. J., Lautzenhiser, A., Sherman, E. M., & Eyrl, K. (2006). Frequency of scale elevations and factor structure of the Behavior Rating Inventory of Executive Function (BRIEF) in children and adolescents with intractable epilepsy. *Child Neuropsychology, 12*(3), 181–189.

Smith, M. L., Elliott, I. M., & Lach, L. (2004). Cognitive, psychosocial, and family function one year after pediatric epilepsy surgery. *Epilepsia, 45*(6), 650–660.

Spencer, D. D., Spencer, S. S., Mattson, R. H., & Williamson, P. D. (1984). Intracerebral masses in patients with intractable partial epilepsy. *Neurology, 34,* 432–436.

Stores, G., & Hart, J. (1976). Reading skills of children with generalized or focal epilepsy attending ordinary school. *Developmental Medicine and Child Neurology, 18,* 705–716.

Strauss, E., Hunter, M., & Wada, J. (1995). Risk factors for cognitive impairment in epilepsy. *Neuropsychology, 9*(4), 457–463.

Sulzbacher, S., Farwell, J. R., Temkin, N., Lu, A. S., & Hirtz, D. G. (1999). Late cognitive effects of early treatment with phenobarbital. *Clinical Pediatrics, 38*(7), 387–394.

Sumer, M. M., Atik, L., Unal, A., Emre, U., & Atasoy, H. T. (2007). Frontal lobe epilepsy presented as ictal aggression. *Neurological Sciences, 28*(1), 48–51.

Suurmeijer, T. (1991). Treatment, seizure-free periods, and educational achievements: A follow-up study among children with epilepsy and healthy children. *Family Practice, 8*(4), 320–328.

Takeoka, M., Riviello, J. J., Duffy, F. H., Kim, F., Kennedy, D. N., Makris, N., et al. (2004). Bilateral volume reduction of the superior temporal areas in Landau–Kleffner syndrome. *Neurology, 63*(7), 1289–1292.

Thompson, P. J., Baxendale, S. A., Duncan, J. S., & Sander, J. W. (2000). Effects of topiramate on cognitive function. *Journal of Neurology, Neurosurgery, and Psychiatry, 69*(5), 636–641.

Velisek, L., & Moshe, S. L. (2001). Pathophysiology of seizures and epilepsy in the immature brain: Cells, Synapses, and Circuits. In J. M. Pellock, W. E. Dodson, & B. F. D. Bourgeois (Eds.), *Pediatric epilepsy: Diagnosis and therapy* (2nd ed., pp. 1–24). New York: DEMOS.

Vermeulen, J., Kortstee, S. W., Alpherts, W. C., & Aldenkamp, A. P. (1994). Cognitive performance in learning disabled children with and without epilepsy. *Seizure, 3*(1), 13–21.

Vingerhoets, G. (2006). Cognitive effects of seizures. *Seizure, 15*(4), 221–226.

Westerveld, M. (2006). Cognitive and psychosocial benefits of early surgical intervention: What do we know? In J. Miller & D. Silbergeld (Eds.), *Epilepsy surgery: Principles and controversies* (pp. 148–153). New York: Taylor & Francis.

Westerveld, M., Zawacki, T., Sass, K. J., Spencer, S. S., Novelly, R. A., & Spencer, D. D. (1994). Intracarotid amytal procedure evaluation of hemispheric speech and memory function in children and adolescents. *Journal of Epilepsy, 7*(4), 295–302.

World Health Organization. (2008). Epilepsy: Aetiology, epidemiology and prognosis. Retrieved from *www.who.int/mediacentre/factsheets/fs165/en/*

Zelnik, N., Sa'adi, L., Silman-Stolar, Z., & Goikhman, I. (2001). Seizure control and educational outcome in childhood-onset epilepsy. *Journal of Child Neurology, 16*(11), 820–824.

CHAPTER 4

Pediatric Brain Tumors

M. DOUGLAS RIS
RICHARD ABBEY

Cancer in childhood is much less common than it is in adults (Ries et al., 2006). Yet when we consider the consequences in terms of net years of disability and years of life lost, pediatric cancer's impact on public health is disproportionate to its incidence. Brain tumors, or intracranial neoplasms, are the most common solid tumors in childhood (Ries et al., 2006). Whereas great strides have been made in the last several decades in the treatment of some other childhood cancers (such as acute lymphoblastic leukemia), no "silver bullets" have been found for brain tumors, where progress has been incremental. Advances have come from improved treatments, but also from improved characterization of tumors in terms of histology, imaging, and disease staging. Essentially, more is being discovered about the innumerable ways in which brain tumors vary and which of these are most relevant for treatment and survival.

Fundamental to an understanding of pediatric brain tumors is that they are actually a collection of diseases common in the sense that they affect the brain, but highly diverse in their histology, location, response to various treatments, and survival. A thorough treatment of pediatric brain tumors is difficult to accomplish in a book, much less a chapter; thus, out of necessity, we neglect some matters and give only cursory treatment to others while attempting to focus on issues of most importance to neuropsychologists and other behavioral scientists and practitioners. Neuropsychology's impact, scientifically and clinically, has been greatest in the area of *late effects* (i.e., long-term or remote sequelae of cancer and its treatments), and so we focus on these effects in this chapter. A review of official taxonomies of brain tumors is one matter that must be left to other authoritative sources (Rorke, Gilles, Davis, & Becker, 1985). For our purposes, we utilize a simplified classification system based on tumor location borrowed from Strother et al. (2002) (Table 4.1). This scheme assigns tumors to three major categories: (1) *infratentorial* (sometimes designated as

TABLE 4.1. Simple Typology of Pediatric Brain Tumors

Infratentorial tumors	Midline tumors	Supratentorial tumors
• Medulloblastoma (MB)/primitive neuroectodermal tumor (PNET) • Cerebellar glioma • Diffuse (malignant) brainstem glioma • Benign (focal) brainstem glioma • Ependymoma	• Optic pathway glioma/ chiasmatic–hypothalamic glioma • Craniopharyngioma • Germinoma • Malignant germ cell tumor • Pineal parenchymal tumor	• Low-grade glioma • High-grade glioma • Ganglioglioma • Ependymoma • Choroid plexus tumor • PNET

Note. Based on Strother et al. (2002).

posterior fossa or *fourth ventricle*), (2) *midline* (sometimes referred to as *third ventricle* or *dien-cephalic*), and (3) *supratentorial* (sometimes designated as *lateral ventricle* or *hemispheric*).

Since the neuropsychological literature is organized not only by the tumor type/location but also by the toxicity of treatments, we can classify pediatric brain tumors according to both dimensions, resulting in a 3 × 3 matrix (Table 4.2). The five tumor types in Table 4.2 have been selected to be presented in more detail because they represent the spectrum of toxicity in treatments, the diversity of tumor locations, and the highest-incidence tumors in pediatric populations. Together, they account for approximately two-thirds of the population with pediatric brain tumors and for the majority of the neurobehavioral literature, which has tended to focus on those conditions posing the most risk for long-term neurobehavioral morbidity. The toxicity classifications in Table 4.2 also reflect the empirically justifiable assertion that in regard to long-term neurobehavioral effects, extensive-field radiotherapy (RT) protocols (i.e., whole-brain/cranial and craniospinal RT) are generally more toxic; local-field RT protocols are less toxic; and surgery alone or in conjunction with chemotherapy is least toxic. We hasten to add, though, that "low toxicity" does not imply that these treatments have no effect on neuropsychological functioning. Indeed, Carpentieri et al. (2003) have documented neuropsychological impairment in patients shortly after surgery and before any other treatments, although their study could not determine the persistence of these deficits.

We acknowledge that this organizational scheme simplifies reality along both dimensions. For example, there are midline/diencephalic low-grade gliomas that receive low-

TABLE 4.2. Major Pediatric Brain Tumors by Location and Treatment Toxicity

Tumor type	High toxicity	Intermediate toxicity	Low toxicity
Infratentorial	MB/PNET		Cerebellar low-grade (LGA) astrocytoma
Midline		Optic pathway glioma/ chiasmatic–hypothalamic glioma Craniopharyngioma	
Supratentorial			Low-grade glioma (including LGA and oligodendroglioma)

toxicity treatments, as well as supratentorial PNETs that receive high-toxicity treatments. Assignments to toxicity categories in Table 4.2 are based upon the *modal* treatment, and do not represent such situations as treatment with local RT for residual disease in supratentorial low-grade gliomas.

Within this structure, we further delineate conditions that are most prevalent; those for which there is a substantial neurobehavioral literature; and, relatedly, those for which the rate of survival is sufficient to warrant an interest in neurobehavioral outcome. For each of the types of pediatric brain tumors addressed in greater detail below, we summarize the incidence, pathophysiology, treatments, and neuropsychological effects. This is followed by a brief discussion of the neurobehavioral toxicity of chemotherapy; a few examples of studies that pose specific neuropsychological hypotheses; clinical interventions for neurobehavioral morbidities; an overall scientific critique of the literature on pediatric brain tumors; and projections on where the field is, or should be, headed. It is apparent through this review that the field of neuropsychology is an important contributor to both the scientific investigation and clinical care of children with brain tumors.

MEDULLOBLASTOMA

Incidence and Pathophysiology

MB is among the most common of the pediatric tumors (approximately 20%) but rare in adults, making it the quintessential childhood brain tumor (Blaney et al., 2006). The peak age of diagnosis is 5–7 years, with 1.5–2 times higher risk for boys than for girls. These tumors typically arise from the fourth ventricle, invading the cerebellar vermis and fourth ventricle, and consist of poorly differentiated epithelial cells. Controversy about the nomenclature of MB and PNET dates back many years and continues to this day. MB is maintained in the current World Health Organization (Kleihues & Sobin, 2000) nosology, and so it is the term used here. Desmoplastic MB is a histological variant with a more favorable prognosis, occurring mostly in the cerebellar hemispheres of adolescents and adults. Large-cell MB and large-cell anaplastic MB are a particularly aggressive variants. For treatment and prognostic purposes, the Chang staging system is often used. This system classifies tumors by size and local infiltration (T1–T4), as well as degree of cerebrospinal fluid (CSF) dissemination (M0–M4). M stage has been found to be consistently predictive of outcome, while T stage has not. Age is also related to survival, with younger age associated with a poorer prognosis. Presenting symptoms are most often those associated with increased intracranial pressure (e.g., headache and vomiting), due to mass effect of the tumor and resultant hydrocephalus secondary to obstruction at the fourth ventricle and cerebral aquaduct.

Treatments

Multimodal therapy is common for MB, with surgery and RT being most common. These lesions are typically approached through an incision in the cerebellar vermis. Gross total resection of the tumor is often achieved, and is associated with increased progression-free survival (PFS) compared with subtotal resection. The treatment of MB is risk-adapted, in that patients with "standard-risk" MB (age greater than 3 years, little residual tumor, and no evidence of dissemination) typically receive less toxic treatment than those with "high-risk" MB (3 years old or less, residual tumor greater than 1.5 cm², evidence of dissemination).

MB is a highly radiosensitive tumor, and so RT remains the mainstay of treatment. Depending upon the M stage, treatment may be limited to the tumor and surrounding tissue; however, because of this tumor's propensity to disseminate through the CSF, it most often encompasses the entire neuroaxis with a boost to the tumor site. Modern conformal RT, in which radiation is delivered in multiple planes, allows improved precision in maximizing the dose to the tumor while sparing healthy brain tissue. Basically, with three-dimensional conformal RT, ionizing radiation is delivered in small doses through multiple planes, resulting in steeper radiation gradients with a high aggregate dose to the clinical target volume and much lower doses to surrounding (ostensibly healthy) tissue. Intensity-modulated radiation therapy, stereotactic radiosurgery, and proton radiation therapy are additional modern approaches used to concentrate high doses to the tumor while limiting exposure to healthy neural tissues. Much of the existing literature on late effects is based upon samples receiving conventional two-dimensional parallel-opposed lateral-field RT, in which larger volumes are exposed to higher doses than in the modern techniques noted above.

MBs also tend to be chemosensitive, and so chemotherapy is most often used as *adjuvant* therapy (meaning that it is applied after the primary treatment). For the most part, chemotherapy is intended to provide further local control, as well as limit disease dissemination in the subarachnoid space. For standard-risk MB, 5-year PFS rates in the range of 81–86% have been reported (Packer et al., 2006); for high-risk MB, the corresponding survival rate is in the range of 40–57% (Zeltzer et al., 1999).

Neuropsychological Effects

Most of the literature on neuropsychological effects in pediatric brain tumors has focused on the long-term outcomes of survivors as measured by intelligence tests. A smaller literature is available on acute effects, but certainly the late effects are most pertinent to neuropsychologists engaged in the management of disease and treatment sequelae. Some of the most serious effects are either late-developing or late-emerging, and one of the most challenging aspects of this research is the multitude of factors that can potentially affect the brain and its subsequent development in these children. Acutely, there are the direct physiological and mechanical effects of the tumor at the site, local and remote compression effects (e.g., herniation), and disruption in the flow of CSF. There is also the impact of treatments, the effects of which may not emerge until years later. All this being said, there is convincing evidence that RT is the single disease or treatment factor accounting for the most variance in neurobehavioral outcome in diseases like MB. The pathophysiology of these RT late effects is itself complicated and incompletely understood (Wong & Van der Kogel, 2004). It probably involves apoptotic cell death and secondary cell death mediated by hypoxic–ischemic and inflammatory responses, culminating in damage to the intimal lining of the cerebral vasculature, disruption of the blood–brain barrier, and direct damage to (particularly developing) cerebral white matter. RT-related vascular damage not only may account for some of the documented late effects, but also places patients at significantly increased risk for stroke 10 or more years after treatment (Bowers et al., 2006).

Effects on intellectual development are associated with radiation dose and age, with younger children treated with higher doses being most at risk for eventual declines in IQ of up to 25–30 points (Packer et al., 1987). Until fairly recently, "standard" therapy for MB was 5,400 cGy to the posterior fossa and 3,600 cGy to the neuroaxis. Several clinical trials over the past decade have demonstrated comparable disease control with reduced-dose craniospinal RT (2,400 cGy). Adverse effects appear to be mitigated by reduced-dose RT protocols (Kieffer-Renaux et al., 2000); however, declines in functioning can still be substantial, especially for young children (Ris, Packer, Goldwein, Jones-Wallace, & Boyett, 2001; Mulhern et al., 1998). Recent studies at St. Jude Children's Research Hospital have shown an association between decreases in normal cerebral white matter and long-term effect on IQ in children treated for MB (Mulhern et al., 1999, 2001). A recent study from the Toronto Hospital for Sick Children of a sample composed mostly of patients treated for MB demonstrated continued declines in intellectual functioning for up to 4 years posttreatment, with an average decline in IQ of 2–4 points per year (Spiegler, Bouffet, Greenburg, Rutka, & Mabbot, 2004). Palmer et al. (2003) found different trajectories for older and younger patients. Older patients (mean age at diagnosis = 11 years) showed early preservation followed by later, gradual decline. Younger patients (mean age at diagnosis = almost 6 years) showed early decline followed by later stabilization of IQ.

Investigation of specific neuropsychological effects has been the trend in recent years. For example, Nagel et al. (2006) reported both retrieval and recognition deficits on the Children's Version of the California Verbal Learning Test (Delis, Kramer, Kaplan, & Ober, 1994). And Reeves et al. (2006) found attention deficits in patients with MB, whose omission errors on a continuous-performance task predicted lower math and reading scores. Specific effects based on conventional neuropsychological typologies (e.g., memory, language, visuospatial, etc.) may be less relevant in the context of these diseases than in others, because (1) the insult to the brain is often widespread, (2) the brain is often in an early stage of development, and (3) RT effects on white matter pathways are likely to disrupt multiple neurobehavioral systems/networks. Consequently, measurement of *supramodal capacities* (e.g., processing speed and attention) may ultimately provide us with the best insights into the adverse effects suffered by these children (Ris, 2007), since these functions may mediate the acquisition of higher cognitive functions, as asserted by Shatz, Kramer, Ablin, and Matthay (2000) and Fry and Hale (1996).

Research on *cerebellar mutism* (Pollack, Polinko, Albright, Towbin, & Fitz, 1995; Robertson et al., 2006) indicates that this may be a heretofore underappreciated factor in accounting for late effects. Cerebellar mutism is characterized by onset of mutism 1–2 days after surgery, emotional lability, and high-pitched cry. In some cases, recovery is slow and incomplete. The etiology is not well understood, but may be related to surgical trauma or vasospasm. The most recent report by Robertson et al. (2006) suggests that as many as 24% of patients with MB are so affected, which means that a significant amount of variance in long-term outcome may be accounted for by this syndrome. Indeed, Grill et al. (2004) reported lower Verbal IQ, Performance IQ, and fine motor deficits in patients with posterior fossa tumors who had mutism than in those who did not.

SUPRATENTORIAL AND INFRATENTORIAL LOW-GRADE GLIOMA

Incidence and Pathophysiology

Most supratentorial low-grade gliomas in childhood are LGAs, oligodendrogliomas, or mixtures of these. They are histologically benign and generally nonaggressive clinically, and they are the most prevalent supratentorial tumor in childhood with very favorable long-term survival. Some 80–85% of cerebellar gliomas are pilocytic astrocytomas, with approximately half of these having cystic components. Infrequently, these tumors may also involve the brainstem. Unlike the other major tumor of the posterior fossa, MB, cerebellar LGAs rarely seed through the neuraxis. As it is for supratentorial gliomas, long-term survival for low-grade cerebellar tumors is high, estimated at about 90% (Pollock, 1999).

Treatment

Gross total resection is associated with greater than 75% 5-year PFS in LGA of the supratentorium. Such radical resections are more frequent in hemispheric than in diencephalic tumors. Tumors that subsequently progress are usually amenable to second surgery. Although most would agree that additional treatment after a gross total resection is not necessary, treatment following subtotal resection is controversial. In such cases, focal RT may improve PFS, if not overall survival rate. Chemotherapy has no proven role in the treatment of these tumors.

For cerebellar LGA, aggressive resection is the most effective treatment and is usually achieved unless there is significant involvement of the cerebellar peduncles and brainstem. As with supratentorial LGAs, RT may further control the disease in incomplete resections, while chemotherapy does not appear to make a significant contribution to the treatment of these tumors.

Neuropsychological Effects

As a group, little is known about the neurobehavioral morbidity associated with supratentorial LGAs. Some of these patients are included in samples of third-ventricle/diencephalic tumors. As we will see, the limited research available indicates that such patients are at increased risk for neurobehavioral sequelae. For those with tumors situated in the cerebral hemispheres, there are few empirical data. We recently reported on a large sample (N = 94) of patients with midline and hemispheric LGA receiving only surgical treatment (Ris et al., 2008). There was evidence of mild cognitive dysfunction, particularly for those with left-hemisphere lesions (mean Verbal IQ = 88, Performance IQ = 93, and Full Scale IQ = 89).

Somewhat more is known about the neuropsychological outcome in patients with cerebellar gliomas, partly because such patients offer a conceptually attractive and convenient comparison group for investigations of MB. One study by Chadderton et al. (1995) recalled 50 patients several years after treatment for LGAs. Thirty-two of these patients had tumors in the cerebellum. Of these, patients who received surgery only had a mean Full Scale IQ of 105, while those treated with surgery and radiation to the posterior fossa (4,250 cGy) had a mean Full Scale IQ of 83. Levisohn, Cronin-Golomb, and Schmahmann (2000) evaluated 19 patients with cerebellar tumors treated surgically, and found executive, visuospatial, expressive language, verbal memory, and affect regulation problems.

In the largest study to date, Beebe et al. (2005) found lower than expected IQs (Verbal = 97, Performance = 95, Full Scale = 96) compared to test norms, as well as deficits in adaptive functioning on the Vineland Adaptive Behavior Scale and Child Behavior Checklist, in a sample of 103 surgery-only patients. There was no association found between the location of the lesion and cognitive or adaptive/behavioral results. In this study, pre-, peri-, and postsurgical complications did not predict outcomes. However, Roncadin, Dennis,

Greenberg, and Spiegler (2008) reported that adverse medical events in the perioperative and especially the short-term survival period (5 years posthospitalization) accounted for 15–32% of the variance in intelligence, perhaps reflecting the predictive value of persisting sensory and motor disturbances. An Israeli group (Berger et al., 2005a, 2005b) reported evidence of behavioral rigidity on switching and serial reaction time tasks despite normal learning in a small but well-controlled study of patients with posterior fossa tumors receiving surgery only. Finally, on a quality-of-life measure, there was evidence that patients with LGAs of the posterior fossa were at increased risk for social adjustment problems and withdrawal years after treatment (Aarsen et al., 2005).

It is difficult to draw firm conclusions from this limited number of studies so diverse in methodology. However, they do raise concerns about possible subtle cognitive and behavioral effects associated with these tumors, particularly when radiation is added to the treatment. In the case of supratentorial LGA, such effects would be consistent with site-specific compromise of neural systems subserving various neuropsychological functions. In the case of infratentorial LGA, the growing literature identifying the cerebellum in circuits subserving several cognitive and emotional regulatory functions provides some biological plausibility to these early findings (Karatekin, Lazareff, & Asarnow, 2000; Levisohn et al., 2000). Such concerns are compounded when we consider that these children have not been studied as thoroughly as those with other types of tumors. Because neurobehavioral morbidity is less salient in these children than in children with some other tumors (e.g., MB), they have not received as much attention and their clinical outcomes are not as closely followed. Yet they constitute about a quarter of those diagnosed with pediatric brain tumors, and presumably an even greater proportion of long-term survivors. From the perspective of net social burden, then, this group of children may be one of the most at-risk groups treated for brain tumors.

OPTIC PATHWAY/CHIASMATIC–HYPOTHALAMIC GLIOMA

Incidence and Pathophysiology

Approximately 5% of pediatric intracranial tumors are gliomas that arise from the optic nerves, chiasm, and hypothalamus (Blaney et al., 2006). A majority of these tumors are diagnosed before the age of 5 years. Optic nerve involvement is common in patients with neurofibromatosis type 1 (NF-1), while involvement of the optic chiasm is more common in patients without NF-1. Histologically, these are usually low-grade gliomas that tend to spread slowly along the visual pathways. Tumors involving the chiasm and hypothalamus tend to have a higher recurrence rate. As one would expect from the location of these tumors, visual disturbances are frequent presenting symptoms.

Treatment

Surgery to remove the exophytic portion of chiasmatic–hypothalamic gliomas is common, although because of the infiltration of eloquent structures (e.g., the optic chiasm), a complete resection is often not possible. Focal RT has been used to stabilize residual disease, while chemotherapy has been used to forestall the use of radiation in younger patients and avert radiation-related developmental sequelae. Survival rates for these low-grade tumors tend to be quite high (e.g., 86% for a series of patients with chiasmatic–hypothalamic tumors reported by Fouladi et al., 2003), although recurrence is common, and so PFS rates are more modest (36% in the Fouladi et al. series).

Neuropsychological Effects

Intellectual impairment can occur in patients with these anterior midline lesions. Fouladi et al. (2003) reported initial impairment at diagnosis (IQ = 86), but no further decline following local irradiation, and there was no difference in IQ between those irradiated and those not irradiated. In contrast, Lacaze et al. (2003) reported that those children treated with chemotherapy alone had well-preserved intelligence (IQ = 107), whereas those who received local RT showed evidence of IQ decline (IQ = 88). Complicating the interpretation of these studies are patients with NF-1 who present with other intracranial abnormalities and neuropsychological deficits (Moore, Ater, Needle, Slopis, & Copeland, 1994). Overall, though, these patients are at increased risk for neurobehavioral morbidity because of their younger age at diagnosis and the risk to critical diencephalic structures.

CRANIOPHARYNGIOMA

Incidence and Pathophysiology

Craniopharyngiomas arise in the sella and suprasellar region and account for 6–9% of brain tumors in children, with a peak incidence at 8–10 years of age (Blaney et al., 2006). They tend to be lobulated masses with calcifications and cystic components. Though histologically benign, they have a propensity to infiltrate surrounding tissue. Presenting symptoms include short stature and other endocrine-related problems, symptoms of increased intracranial pressure, visual field disturbance, and behavioral symptoms. Hydrocephalus secondary to obstruction of the third ventricle and foramen of Monro occurs in about 50% of these patients.

Treatment

In those patients who receive gross total resection of their lesion, tumor recurrence is uncommon. However, craniopharyngiomas tend to attach themselves to the pituitary stalk, optic chiasm, hypothalamus, and vessels of the circle of Willis. Aggressive surgery therefore can result in significant postsurgical morbidity, particularly panhypopituitarism. For this reason, some argue for less aggressive surgery followed by focal RT (Merchant et al., 2002). Chemotherapy has no established role in the treatment of these tumors.

Neuropsychological Effects

Because of the diverse neural structures implicated in this disease and its treatments (pituitary, optic chiasm, frontal lobe, diencephalon), craniopharyngiomas are among the most interesting pediatric tumors from a neurobehavioral standpoint. In a paper from the Boston group (Waber et al., 2006), everyday memory problems were found in 10 patients with craniopharyngiomas, but except for processing speed, neuropsychological test scores were within normal limits. From St. Jude (Merchant et al., 2006), there is a recent report on a larger sample (N = 28) of children treated with conformal RT, in which long-term effects on IQ were found to be related to multiple surgical factors (e.g., extent of surgery, shunt), subject age, and volume of brain irradiated. In an earlier report from this group, it was concluded that there was less cognitive and endocrine morbidity in patients treated with limited surgery followed by RT than in those patients treated with more aggressive surgery (Merchant et al., 2002). It would appear that limited surgery followed by RT may produce a better outcome, despite the risk of radiation-related long-term effects. It should also be noted that some of these tumors are prechiasmatic and extraventricular, and so can be excised *in toto* without the need for RT; patients with such tumors have perhaps the best all-around outcome of all, although this conclusion is based on limited data (Pierre-Kahn et al., 2005).

TUMORS OF INFANCY AND EARLY CHILDHOOD

A small but expanding neurobehavioral outcome literature has developed around children diagnosed with tumors before the age of 3 years who constitute approximately 20–25% of the population with pediatric brain tumors (Rickert & Paulus, 2001). As they are for adolescents and adults, supratentorial tumors are more common for children below age 2 years, whereas infratentorial tumors predominate during midchildhood. Infants and preschoolers are particularly vulnerable, not only because of their age, but because their tumors often require aggressive management with chemotherapy and/or RT. In the largest series of such patients reported to date (Fouladi et al., 2005), at a median follow-up of 7.6 years, 126 children diagnosed at an average age of 1.8 years were found to have a mean IQ decline of −0.29 points per year. This decline was significantly associated with RT: Those receiving craniospinal RT had a mean decline of −1.34 points per year; those receiving local RT had a mean decline of −0.51 points per year; and those who received no RT had a mean *increase* of 0.91 points per year. This confirms the findings of an earlier report by Copeland, deMoor, Moore, and Ater (1999). The marked neurodevelopmental toxicity of craniospinal RT is also driven home by the finding that 71.4% of children receiving such therapy had IQs less than 70 5+ years after diagnosis. To address this unfortunate situation, treatment protocols have been proposed that use either reduced doses of craniospinal RT, or chemotherapy alone as a means of delaying RT until a child is older (Kalifa & Grill, 2005).

OTHER TUMORS

As stated from the outset, some tumors of childhood are not covered in this chapter. This may merely reflect variations in terminology/specificity (e.g., fibrillary astrocytoma is a type of cerebellar low-grade glioma) or the relative rarity of the tumor and so the absence of a significant neuropsychological literature (e.g., germ cell tumors, choroid plexus tumors), although such tumors may be included in large, diagnostically heterogeneous samples. Historically, neurobehavioral outcome research in oncology increases in direct relation to improved survival rates. For some tumors, therefore, survival rates remain so poor as to preclude the study of neurobehavioral outcomes. Such is the case for diffuse intrinsic brainstem glioma, glioblastoma multiforme, and highly anaplastic astrocytomas.

Ependymomas constitute approximately 7% of pediatric tumors (Central Brain Tumor Registry of the United States, 2002) and so are common enough to deserve mention. Two-thirds of ependymomas arise in the posterior fossa, and, like MB, they are more common in males than females. These tumors are radiosensitive and so are often studied along with other tumors of the posterior fossa receiving multimodal therapy. Surgery for these tumors can be more complicated than for MB because of their propensity to attach themselves to the brainstem and cranial nerves. Contemporary protocols have achieved good disease control with local irradiation. Encouraging results for this disease were recently reported from St. Jude, where they were able to achieve a high rate of gross total or near-total resection (91%) followed by 5,400–5,940 cGy to the posterior fossa, with reduced clinical target volume producing a 3-year PFS, rate of 74.5%. Moreover, the IQs of these children were maintained over a 4-year follow-up (Merchant et al., 2004). This finding is particularly encouraging, because this tumor tends to occur at younger ages than MB.

CHEMOTHERAPY AND NEUROBEHAVIORAL LATE EFFECTS

As noted above, some pediatric brain tumors have been found to be chemoresponsive, and so various agents are increasingly being used. It is because chemotherapy has been found to be much less neurotoxic than RT that it is of less concern to neuropsychologists interested in late effects. For example, in the Palmer et al. (2003) longitudinal study of patients with MB, chemotherapy did not predict late effects on estimated IQ. Reddick et al. (1998) found no chemotherapy-related reductions in white or gray matter volumes in 56 patients with pediatric brain tumors. Leukoencephalopathy, though, was found in a majority of children treated with a chemotherapy-only regimen consisting of intravenous methotrexate, cyclophosphamide, carboplatin, etoposide, and vincristine as well as intraventricular methotrexate for MB, although these magnetic resonance imaging (MRI) abnormalities were described as asymptomatic and resolved spontaneously in two-thirds of these patients (Rutkowski et al., 2005). Still, the research on delayed neurotoxicity of methotrexate in particular (summarized by Cole & Kamen, 2006) and of high-dose steroids (Waber et al., 2000) from the literature on acute lymphoblastic leukemia cautions against a total dismissal of chemotherapy-related neurobehavioral effects. Furthermore, the evaluation of patients receiving chemotherapy can be complicated by ototoxic (from platinum analogs) and peripheral neuropathy (from vincristine) effects that can be confused with central nervous system effects.

NEUROPSYCHOLOGY-DIRECTED INVESTIGATIONS

In a 1994 review of the literature, Ris and Noll encouraged more research guided by neuropsychological/neurodevelopmental theory and constructs. Although the foregoing discussion attests to the significant recent advances in the quality and volume of neurobehavioral research on pediatric brain tumors (see Ris, 2007, for the historical progression), much of this research could be described as "toxicity ascertainment" in which greater sophistication has been applied to generate a better understanding of these children's outcomes. Encouragingly, increasing numbers of studies have also been oriented toward investigating neurobehavioral constructs in greater detail.

For example, Buono et al. (1998) investigated a particular neurobehavioral phenotype (nonverbal learning disability) in children treated for brain tumors, finding partial support for its relevance to this population. In another example, King et al. (2004) compared patients with third-ventricle tumors to those with cerebellar tumors, demonstrating a double dissociation on measures of verbal memory and immediate memory span; that is, those with third-ventricle tumors were more impaired in verbal memory, while patients with cerebellar tumors were more impaired in immediate memory span. The aforementioned studies by the Israeli group (Berger et al., 2005a, 2005b) could also be considered recent examples of this promising trend toward research that goes beyond just documenting neurobehavioral toxicity and makes neuropsychological constructs the subjects of investigation.

CLINICAL APPLICATIONS AND INTERVENTIONS

What are the clinical implications of this research for those who care for these patients? First of all, this research allows us to better direct limited resources to those patients at highest risk for adverse neurobehavioral outcomes. For example, young children receiving radiation to large brain volumes are clearly in need of close, protracted neuropsychological surveillance coupled with early, comprehensive educational and psychosocial support/intervention. On the other hand, patients at "low" risk (such as those treated with surgery only for cerebellar LGAs) are not necessarily at "no" risk and should be monitored, albeit less intensively, for the emergence of posttreatment neurobehavioral complications.

Surveillance should be tailored to the degree and temporal nature of risks these patients face. Evidence indicating "declines" in functioning for several years after treatment with cranial RT would argue for repeated evaluations for 4–5 years posttreatment. Those patients not treated with RT may be followed less intensively over a shorter period of time. Nevertheless, for young children in particular, late effects may emerge as a developmental phenomenon (see Dennis, 1988) even in the absence of late pathological changes in the brain associated with RT, and this must be considered when a surveillance plan is formulated. This is consistent with the usual interpretation of declining IQ scores as reflecting failure to keep pace with normally developing peers, rather than an absolute loss of abilities.

The research cited above cautions us neither to overfocus our neurobehavioral inquiries nor to rely upon abbreviated or screening measures, since the effects in many of these patients can be highly diverse. This also means that psychoeducational evaluations geared toward common developmental disabilities (e.g., reading disability, mental retardation) are inadequate when it comes to pediatric brain tumors and should not be relied upon to direct educational interventions. Above all, patients with these tumors require deficit-adapted intervention plans that draw upon a range of neurobehavioral tools, as well as skill in coordinating care over time with many others (including parents, educators, occupational therapists, physical therapists, speech therapists, and physicians of various specialties). Indeed, once these patients are stabilized and their tumors are in remission, medical professionals and their various methods typically recede into the background, while neuropsychologists and their methods assume an increasingly central role in the care of these patients—often for many years to come. The hybrid training of neuropsychologists in brain–behavior relationships makes them uniquely suited for this.

A comprehensive neuropsychological evaluation is an important first step in providing efficacious interventions for children with pediatric brain tumors and is recommended in the Children's Oncology Group Long-Term Follow-Up Guidelines for Survivors of Childhood, Adolescent, and Young Adult Cancers (Landier et al., 2004). Reevaluation at 12- to 18-month intervals is important to detect neuropsychological late effects of treatment, and these findings can be used to update intervention recommendations (Armstrong, Blumberg, & Toledano, 1999).

Educational interventions are crucial parts of a comprehensive program for children with pediatric brain tumors. A formal plan for school reentry and interventions for educational needs should be implemented both during and after treatment (Mitby et al., 2003). Specialized cancer centers typically have protocols that include peer, parent and teacher education about a child's educational and physical needs. School personnel workshops increase understanding about the child's medical condition (see Prevatt, Heffer, & Lowe, 2000; Rynard, Chambers, Klinck, & Gray, 1998), and peer education programs increase other children's interest in interacting with a peer who has cancer and helps decrease concerns about the ill peer (Benner & Marlow, 1991; Treiber, Schramm, & Mabe, 1986).

Psychopharmacological research has demonstrated the efficacy of stimulant medication for improving attentional deficits in children with pediatric brain tumors. Thompson et al. (2001) found that methylphenidate (MPH; 0.6 mg/kg) significantly improved sustained attention in children with childhood cancer. Mulhern et al. (2004) extended these results by demonstrating that significant improvements were evident in the areas of attention and cognition on standardized parent and teacher rating inventories, and that the teacher ratings also indicated significant improvement in social skills and academic competence. There were no differences between low-dose (0.3 mg/kg) and moderate-dose (0.6 mg/kg) MPH in these findings. However, teachers reported significant improvement in problem behaviors with moderate-dose but not low-dose MPH.

Preliminary research supports the effectiveness of social skills training for pediatric brain tumors. Barakat et al. (2003) provided six social skills group sessions for children treated for brain tumors and their parents. Target skills included nonverbal communication, maintaining conversation, cooperation, empathy, and conflict resolution. Significant improvement was found in social competence and internalizing behavior problems. This research, though, is still in its infancy, and so it is not clear whether larger and better-designed studies will replicate these provisional results.

Although few research studies have investigated the effectiveness of cognitive remediation, its potential to improve cognitive functioning is promising. The Cognitive Remediation Program (Butler, 1998; Butler & Copeland, 2002) has demonstrated consistent improvements in the area of attention in children with childhood cancer, and preliminary results of a randomized controlled intervention trial support academic generalization (Butler & Mulhern, 2005).

CRITIQUE

Although contemporary neuro-oncology research reflects increasing differentiation of (and somewhat shifting terminology for) pediatric brain tumors along histological, clinical, and molecular genetic lines, much of the neuropsychological literature lags behind these developments. Samples of children with brain tumors are often heterogeneous, reflecting practical concerns (e.g., small samples available for study at any single site) as well as the focus of a particular study (e.g., the long-term effects of RT, regardless of tumor type). The brain tumor nomenclature used in this chapter may serve to facilitate discussion of these diseases, but the neuropsychological literature does not easily map onto these divisions. In appraising the neuropsychological literature, it is also important to keep in mind that, particularly for retrospective studies, patients in these samples may not have been treated uniformly as a consequence of improvements in therapies over the time span sampled (e.g., decreased dose of RT or volume of brain irradiated).

Most of the weaknesses in this literature (small heterogeneous samples, overrepresentation of cross-sectional designs, overreliance on global outcome measures, need for comparison groups) that have been pointed out in early reviews (e.g., Mulhern, Crisco, & Kun, 1983; Ris & Noll, 1994) still apply, but to a lesser degree (Ris, 2007). Given the statistical rarity of pediatric brain tumors (only about 3.3 cases per 100,000 children in the United States; Ries et al., 2006), larger sample sizes are often assembled at the expense of diagnostic homogeneity and/or contemporaneousness. Few single institutions see enough of these patients to overcome these obstacles. Studies coming from cooperative groups can acquire large homogeneous samples, but poor adherence to psychological/neuropsychological requirements in these protocols is common. Also, with these large research platforms come tradeoffs in data quality and neurobehavioral sophistication. The growth in this literature over the past 20 years, though, is impressive and has provided not only a large *volume* of research on the neurobehavioral outcomes in pediatric brain tumors, but also substantial methodological *variety* as grist for quantitative and qualitative analyses of converging evidence. There is every reason to believe that these methodological and conceptual improvements will continue.

One particular challenge is for research on neurobehavioral outcomes to move in synchrony with improved treatments of pediatric brain tumors. This is made even more difficult by the fact that we are dealing with constantly changing organisms in which adverse effects may not emerge until long after the precipitating event(s). Changes in developmental trajectory are not easily discerned with little to no premorbid history to speak of. Yet if we do not closely coordinate our efforts with those of professionals in other disciplines (neurosurgeons, oncologists, radiation oncologists) as they continue to "push the envelope" with their innovative treatments, our findings risk being obsolete by the time they are published.

FUTURE DIRECTIONS

Measurement is a fundamental scientific enterprise, and so models of neurobehavioral outcome in pediatric brain tumors are only as good as our precision in measuring the multitude of variables comprising these models. One limiting factor has been the crude means by which the "radiation lesion" is characterized. Groups formed on the basis of prescribed dose (e.g., 2,400 cGy vs. 3,600 cGy) or presence versus absence of craniospinal RT fail to capture the substantial diversity in contemporary RT protocols. More recently, investigators have incorporated detailed dose–volume information produced by modern RT software to improve the precision of this measurement (Merchant, Kiehna, Li, Xiong, & Mulhern,

2005; Ris et al., 2005). Small- and intermediate-scale prospective studies, in particular, are well positioned to make use of dosimetry data in their longitudinal modeling of late effects. Better models can then drive further refinements in treatment and more accurate prediction of sequelae.

Improved precision of *in vivo* brain "assays" through modern imaging are also being incorporated into studies of neurobehavioral late effects. Volumetrics (Nagel et al., 2004), diffusion tensor imaging (Khong et al., 2006), and functional MRI (Zou et al., 2005) have all been recently introduced into this literature and present exciting opportunities for neuropsychologists to relate their distal measures of brain function to the more proximal measures offered by these techniques.

These advances in radiation oncology and brain imaging, however, must be matched by developments in "behavioral" measurement. By this we mean not only the application of more sophisticated neuropsychological metrics in place of omnibus measures like IQ, but also the use of paradigms drawn from cognitive neuroscience (e.g., Akshoomoff & Courchesne, 1992; Posner & Peterson, 1990). Furthermore, we should not assume that all of the meaningful neurobehavioral morbidity in these patients can be captured by laboratory-based measures. Some of the most meaningful effects in these children elude such contrived procedures, and so a comprehensive assessment strategy must make use of *proxy reports* of educational performance/adjustment, life course/adaptive behavior, psychological/behavioral adjustment, and neuropsychological constructs such as functional executive skills (Gioia, Isquith, Retzlaff, & Espy, 2002) and everyday memory (Waber et al., 2006). More comprehensive and innovative outcome measurement will lead to interventions that are not just focused on the neurocognitive dimension. For example, the few studies available indicate that children with brain tumors are at increased risk for social isolation (Vannatta, Garstein, Short, & Noll, 1998), and a better understanding of these risks within a broader social neuroscience framework (Yeates et al., 2007) will be important.

Any future outcome research making claims to be comprehensive must also take into account "contextual" factors that mediate and moderate outcomes. In this respect, the study by Carlson-Green, Morris, and Krawiecki (1995) continues to be instructive after well over 10 years. As one would predict from the literature on other neurobehavioral conditions of childhood (e.g., Taylor et al., 2001), family factors account for a significant amount of variance in behavioral and intellectual outcome in pediatric brain tumor patients. As we progressively home-in on the biophysical processes related to neurobehavioral outcome, it is easy to overlook the simple fact that even the most powerful predictors of outcome, such as RT, account for far less than half of the variance in intellectual outcome (e.g., 12% in the Silber et al., 1992, study). Those of us who have worked with longitudinal data sets from samples of children with brain tumors cannot help being impressed by the heterogeneity in individual outcomes, which serves as a constant reminder of the limitations of measures of central tendency (e.g., mean IQ decline) and our tenuous grasp of the complex matter under investigation.

Attempts to develop comprehensive models of outcome will help define realistic expectations for the benefits of improved therapies, and will also inform educational, family, and behavioral interventions designed to mitigate neurobehavioral sequelae. As we have seen, such intervention research specifically tailored to neuro-oncology populations is just now emerging. These early results are promising and should be enthusiastically pursued with more, larger-scale efforts. Researchers should draw not only from research on other neurobehavioral conditions, but also from research on other oncology populations, where important investigations of maternal problem solving (Sahler et al., 2002), social skills training (Varni & Katz, 1989), and posttraumatic stress (Kazak et al., 2004) are underway.

Investigations into genetic polymorphisms relevant to neuropsychological development (Blackman, Worley, & Strittmatter, 2005) and treatment toxicity (Krull et al., 2008) may provide us with a better explanation for the highly diverse outcomes that we see in these children. Animal models are also being developed with direct implications for human outcome research. For example, a recent series of papers reports on how cognitive effects in mice exposed to radiation may be related to depletion of neural precursor cells (Otsuka et al., 2006). One of these studies found increased numbers of immature neurons only in mice undergoing cognitive training, suggesting that environmental enrichment may provide protection from such effects (Rola et al., 2004). Neurobehavioral researchers' collaboration with basic scientists in translational research of this type would surely accelerate the process by which discoveries move from "bench" to "bedside."

CONCLUSIONS

The last 20 years in particular have witnessed a significant expansion and maturing of the empirical literature on the neurobehavioral effects associated with pediatric brain tumors. In this chapter, we have attempted to direct our readers' attention to some of the most salient issues in this research, as well as some of the more durable and recent findings in this literature. The challenge before us is one of establishing and sustaining multidisciplinary relationships that will "feed" the increasingly sophisticated outcome models required for this disease complex. Our studies must be increasingly prospective, in the sense of keeping current with and even anticipating new methods of treatment for these children, as retrospective samples will insufficiently enlighten us about the needs of children who are currently undergoing treatment for intracranial neoplasms. The recursive influence of neurobehavioral toxicity research on treatment protocol development has been of genuine benefit to recent generations of neuro-oncology patients, and this should certainly continue. We are also on the cusp, though, of being able to offer proven treatments to lessen the long-term ill effects of these diseases and their treatments, and this may be the most exciting possibility of all.

REFERENCES

Aarsen, F. K., Paquier, P. F., Reddingius, R. E., Streng, I. C., Arts, W. F. M., Evera-Preesman, M., et al. (2005). Functional outcome after low-grade astrocytomas treatment in childhood. *Cancer, 106,* 396–402.

Armstrong, F. D., Blumberg, M. J., & Toledano, S. R. (1999). Neurobehavioral issues in childhood cancer. *School Psychology Review, 28,* 194–204.

Akshoomoff, N. A., & Courchesne, E. (1992). A new role for the cerebellum in cognitive operations. *Behavioral Neuroscience, 106,* 731–738.

Barakat, L. P., Hetzke, J. D., Foley, B., Carey, M. E., Gyato, K., & Phillips, P. D. (2003). Evaluation of social skills training group intervention with children treated for brain tumors: A pilot study. *Journal of Pediatric Psychology, 28,* 299–307.

Beebe, D. W., Ris, M. D., Armstrong, F. D., Fontanesi, J., Mulhern, R., Homes, E., et al. (2005). Cognitive and adaptive outcome in low grade pediatric cerebellar astrocytomas: Evidence of increased risk in national collaborative research studies (CCG9891/POG9130). *Journal of Clinical Oncology, 23,* 5198–5204.

Benner, A. E., & Marlow, L. S. (1991). The effect of a workshop on childhood cancer on students' knowledge, concerns, and desire to interact with a classmate with cancer. *Children's Health Care, 20,* 101–108.

Berger, A., Sadeh, S., Tzur, G., Shuper, A., Kornreich, L., Inbar, D., et al. (2005a). Task switching after cerebellar damage. *Neuropsychology, 19,* 362–370.

Berger, A., Sadeh, S., Tzur, G., Shuper, A., Kornreich, L., Inbar, D., et al. (2005b). Motor and non-motor sequence learning in children and adolescents with cerebellar damage. *Journal of the International Neuropsychological Society, 11,* 482–487.

Blackman, J. A., Worley, G., & Strittmatter, W. J. (2005). Apolipoprotein E and brain injury: Implications for children. *Developmental Medicine and Child Neurology, 47,* 64–70.

Blaney, S. M., Kun, L. E., Hunter, J., Rorke-Adams, L. B., Lau, C., Strother, D., et al. (2006). Tumors of the central nervous system. In P. A. Pizzo & D. G. Pollack (Eds.), *Principles and practices of pediatric oncology* (5th ed., pp. 786–864). Philadelphia: Lippincott Williams & Wilkins.

Bowers, D. C., Liu, Y., Leisenring, W., McNeil, E., Stovall, M., Gurney, J. G., et al. (2006). Late-occurring stroke among long- term survivors of childhood leukemia and brain tumors: A report from the Childhood Cancer Survivor Study. *Journal of Clinical Oncology, 24,* 5277–5282.

Buono, L. A., Morris, M. K., Morris, R. D., Krawiecki, N., Norris, F. H., Foster, M. A., et al. (1998). Evidence for the syndrome of nonverbal learning disabilities in children with brain tumors. *Child Neuropsychology, 4,* 144–157.

Butler, R. W. (1998). Attentional processes and their remediation in childhood cancer. *Medical and Pediatric Oncology, 30(Suppl. 1),* 75–78.

Butler, R. W., & Copeland, D. R. (2002). Attentional processes and their remediation in children treated for cancer: A literature review and the development of a therapeutic approach. *Journal of the International Neuropsychological Society, 8,* 115–124.

Butler, R. W., & Mulhern, R. K. (2005). Neurocognitive interventions for children and adolescents surviving cancer. *Journal of Pediatric Psychology, 30,* 65–78.

Carlson-Green, B., Morris, R. D., & Krawiecki, N. (1995). Family and illness predictors of outcome in pediatric brain tumors. *Journal of Pediatric Psychology, 20,* 769–784.

Carpentieri, S. C., Waber, D. P., Pomeroy, S. L., Scott, R. M., Goumnerova, L. C., Kieran, M. W., et al. (2003). Neuropsychological functioning after surgery in children treated for brain tumor. *Neurosurgery, 52,* 1348–1357.

Central Brain Tumor Registry of the United States. (2002). *Statistical report: Primary brain tumors in the United States, 1995–1999.* Hinsdale, IL: Author.

Chadderton, R. D., West, C. G. H., Schulz, S., Quirke, D. C., Gattamaneni, R., & Taylor, R. (1995). Radiotherapy in the treatment of low-grade astrocytomas: The physical and cognitive sequelae. *Child's Nervous System, 11,* 443–448.

Cole, P. D., & Kamen, B. A. (2006). Delayed neurotoxicity associated with therapy for children with acute lymphoblastic leukemia. *Mental Retardation and Developmental Research Reviews, 12,* 174–183.

Copeland, D. R., deMoor, C., Moore, B. D., III, & Ater, J. L. (1999). Neurocognitive development of children after a cerebellar tumor in infancy: A longitudinal study. *Journal of Clinical Oncology, 17,* 3476–3486.

Delis, D. C., Kramer, J. H., Kaplan, E., & Ober, B. A. (1994). *California Verbal Learning Test—Children's Version: Manual.* San Antonio, TX: Psychological Corporation.

Dennis, M. (1988). Language and the young damaged brain. In T. Boll & B. K. Bryant (Eds.), *Clinical neuropsychology and brain function: Research measurement and practice* (pp. 89–123). Washington, DC: American Psychological Association.

Fouladi, M., Gilger, E., Kocak, M., Wallace, D., Buchanan, G., Reeves, G., et al. (2005). Intellectual and functional outcome of children three years old or younger who have CNS malignancies. *Journal of Clinical Oncology, 23*, 7152–7160.

Fouladi, M., Wallace, D., Langston, J. W., Mulhern, R., Rose, S. R., Gajjar, A., et al. (2003). Survival and functional outcome of children with hypothalamic/chiasmatic tumors. *Cancer, 97*, 1084–1092.

Fry, A. F., & Hale, S. (1996). Processing speed, working memory, and fluid intelligence: Evidence for a developmental cascade. *Psychological Science, 7*, 237–241.

Gioia, G. A., Isquith, P. K., Retzlaff, P. D., & Espy, K. A. (2002). Confirmatory factor analysis of the Behavior Rating Inventory of Executive Function (BRIEF) in a clinical sample. *Child Neuropsychology, 8*, 249–257.

Grill, J., Viguier, D., Kieffer, V., Bulteau, C., Sainte-Rose, C., Hartmann, O., et al. (2004). Critical risk factors for intellectual impairment in children with posterior fossa tumors: The role of cerebellar damage. *Journal of Neurosurgery: Pediatrics, 101*, 152–158.

Kalifa, C., & Grill, J. (2005). The therapy of infantile malignant brain tumors: Current status? *Childhood Brain Tumors, 75*, 279–285.

Karatekin, C., Lazareff, J. A., & Asarnow, R. F. (2000). Relevance of the cerebellar hemispheres for executive functions. *Pediatric Neurology, 22*, 106–112.

Kazak, A., Alderfer, M., Streisand, R., Simms, S., Rourke, M., Barakat, L. P., et al. (2004). Treatment of posttraumatic stress symptoms in adolescent survivors of childhood cancer and their families: A randomized trial. *Journal of Family Psychology, 18*, 493–504.

Khong, P. L., Leung, L. H. T., Fung, D. Y. T., Qui, D., Kwong, D. L. W., Ooi, G. C., et al. (2006). White matter anisotropy in post-treatment childhood cancer survivors: Preliminary evidence of association with neurocognitive function. *Journal of Clinical Oncology, 24*, 884–890.

Kieffer-Renaux, V., Bulteau, C., Grill, J., Kalifa, C., Viguier, D., & Jambaque, I. (2000). Patterns of neuropsychological deficits in children with medulloblastoma according to craniospatial irradiation doses. *Developmental Medicine and Child Neurology, 42*, 741–745.

King, T. Z., Fennell, E. B., Williams, L., Algina, J., Boggs, S., Crosson, B., et al. (2004). Verbal memory abilities of children with brain tumors. *Child Neuropsychology, 10*, 76–88.

Kleihues, P., & Sobin, L. H. (2000). World Health Organization classification of tumors. *Cancer, 88*, 2887.

Krull, K. R., Brouwers, P., Jain, N., Zhang, L., Bomgaars, L., Dreyer, Z., et al. (2008). Folate pathway genetic polymorphisms are related to attention disorders in childhood leukemia survivors. *Journal of Pediatrics, 152*, 101–105.

Lacaze, E., Keiffer, V., Streri, A., Lorenzi, C., Gentaz, E., Habrand, J. L., et al. (2003). Neuropsychological outcome in children with optic pathway tumours when first-line treatment is chemotherapy. *British Journal of Cancer, 89*, 2038–2044.

Landier, W., Bhatia, S., Eshelman, D. A., Forte, K. J., Sweeney, T., Hester, A. L., et al. (2004). Development of risk-based guidelines for pediatric cancer survivors: The Children's Oncology Group Long-Term Follow-Up Guidelines from the Children's Oncology Group Late Effects Committee and Nursing Discipline. *Journal of Clinical Oncology, 22*, 4979–4990.

Levisohn, L., Cronin-Golomb, A., & Schmahmann, J. D. (2000). Neuropsychological consequences of cerebellar tumor resection in children: Cerebellar cognitive affective syndrome in a pediatric population. *Brain, 123*, 1041–1050.

Merchant, T. E., Kiehna, E. N., Kun, L. E., Mulhern, R. K., Li, C., Xiong, X., et al. (2006). Phase II trial of conformal radiation therapy for pediatric patients with craniopharyngioma and correlation of surgical factors and radiation dosimetry with change in cognitive function. *Journal of Neurosurgery: Pediatrics, 104*, 94–102.

Merchant, T. E., Kiehna, E. N., Li, C., Xiong, X., & Mulhern, R. K. (2005). Radiation dosimetry predicts IQ after conformal radiation therapy in pediatric patients with localized ependymoma. *International Journal of Radiation Oncology, Biology, Physics, 63*, 1546–1554.

Merchant, T. E., Kiehna, E. N., Sanford, R. A., Mulhern, R. K., Thompson, S. J., Wilson, M. W., et al. (2002). Craniopharyngioma: The St. Jude Children's Research Hospital experience 1984–2001. *International Journal of Radiation Oncology, Biology, Physics, 53*, 533–542.

Mitby, P. A., Robison, L. L., Whitton, J. A., Zevon, M. A., Gibbs, I. C., Tersak, J. M., et al. (2003). Utilization of special education services and educational attainment among long-term survivors of childhood cancer: A report from the Childhood Cancer Survivor Study. *Cancer, 97,* 115–126.

Moore, B. D., Ater, S. L., Needle, M. N., Slopis, J. S., & Copeland, D. R. (1994). Neuropsychological profile of children with neurofibromatosis, brain tumor, or both. *Journal of Child Neurology, 9,* 368–377.

Mulhern, R. K., Crisco, J. J., & Kun, L. (1983). Neuropsychological sequelae of childhood brain tumors: A review. *Journal of Clinical Child Psychology, 12,* 66–73.

Mulhern, R. K., Kepner, J. L., Thomas, P. R., Armstrong, F. D., Friedman, H. S., & Kun, L. E. (1998). Neuropsychologic functioning of survivors of childhood medulloblastoma randomized to receive conventional or reduced-dose craniospinal irradiation: A pediatric oncology group study. *Journal of Clinical Oncology, 16*(5), 1–7.

Mulhern, R. K., Khan, R. B., Kaplan, S., Helton, S., Christensen, R., Bonner, M., et al. (2004). Short-term efficacy of methylphenidate: A randomized, double-blind, placebo-controlled trial among survivors of childhood cancer. *Journal of Clinical Oncology, 22,* 4743–4751.

Mulhern, R. K., Palmer, S. L., Reddick, W. E., Glass, J. O., Kun, L. E., Taylor, J., et al. (2001). Risks of young age for selected neurocognitive deficits in medulloblastoma are associated with white matter loss. *Journal of Clinical Oncology, 19,* 472–479.

Mulhern, R. K., Reddick, W. E., Palmer, S. L., Glass, J. O., Elkin, T. D., Kun, L. E., et al. (1999). Neurocognitive deficits in medulloblastoma survivors and white matter loss. *Annals of Neurology, 46,* 834–841.

Nagel, B. J., Delis, D. C., Palmer, S. L., Reeves, C., Gajjar, A., & Mulhern, R. K. (2006). Early patterns of verbal memory impairment in children treated for medulloblastoma. *Neuropsychology, 20,* 105–112.

Nagel, B. J., Palmer, S. L., Reddick, W. E., Glass, J. O., Helton, K. J., Wu, S., et al. (2004). Abnormal hippocampal development in children with medulloblastoma treated with risk-adapted irradiation. *American Journal of Neuroradiology, 25,* 1575–1582.

Otsuka, S., Coderre, J. A., Micca, P. L., Morris, G. M., Hopewell, J. W., Rola, R., et al. (2006). Depletion of neural precursor cells after local brain irradiation is due to radiation dose to the parenchyma, not the vasculature. *Radiation Research, 165,* 582–591.

Packer, R. J., Gajjar, A., Vezina, G., Rorke-Adams, L., Burger, P. C., Robertson, P. L., et al. (2006). Phase III study of craniospinal radiation therapy followed by adjuvant chemotherapy for newly diagnosed average-risk medulloblastoma. *Journal of Clinical Oncology, 24,* 4202–4208.

Packer, R. J., Sposto, R., Atkins, T. E., Sutton, L. N., Bruce, D. A., Seigle, K. R., et al. (1987). Quality of life in children with primitive neuroectodermal tumors (medulloblastoma) of posterior fossa. *Pediatric Neuroscience, 13,* 169–175.

Palmer, S. L., Gajjar, A., Reddick, W. E., Glass, J. O., Kun, L. E., Wu, S., et al. (2003). Predicting intellectual outcome among children treated with 35–40 Gy craniospinal irradiation for medulloblastoma. *Neuropsychology, 17,* 548–555.

Pierre-Kahn, A., Recassens, C., Pinto, G., Thalassinos, C., Chokron, S., Soubervielle, J. C., et al. (2005). Social and psycho-intellectual outcome following radical removal of craniopharyngioma in childhood: A prospective series. *Child's Nervous System, 21,* 817–824.

Pollack, I. F. (1999). Pediatric brain tumors. *Seminars in Surgical Oncology, 16,* 73–90.

Pollack, I. F., Polinko, P., Albright, L., Towbin, R., & Fitz, C. (1995). Mutism and pseudobullar symptoms after resection of posterior fossa tumors in children: Incidence and pathophysiology. *Neurosurgery, 37,* 885–893.

Posner, M. I., & Petersen, S. E. (1990). The attention system of the human brain. *Annual Review of Neuroscience, 13,* 25–42.

Prevatt, F. F., Heffer, R. W., & Low, P. A. (2000). A review of school reintegration programs for children with cancer. *Journal of School Psychology, 38,* 447–467.

Reddick, W. E., Mulhern, R. K., Elkin, D., Glass, J. O., Merchant, T. E., & Langston, J. W. (1998). A hybrid neural network analysis of subtle brain volume differences in children surviving brain tumors. *Magnetic Resonance Imaging, 16,* 413–421.

Reeves, C. B., Palmer, S. L., Reddick, W. E., Merchant, T. E., Buchanan, G. M., Gajjar, A., et al. (2006). Attention and memory functioning among pediatric patients with medulloblastoma. *Journal of Pediatric Psychology, 31,* 272–280.

Rickert, C. H., & Paulus, W. (2001). Epidemiology of central nervous system tumors in childhood and adolescence based on new WHO classification. *Child's Nervous System, 17,* 503–511.

Ries, L. A. G., Harkins, D., Krapcho, M., Mariotto, A., Miller, B. A., Feuer, E. J., et al. (Eds.). (2006). *SEER cancer statistics review, 1975–2003.* Retrieved from *seer.cancer.gov/csr/1975_2003/*

Ris, M. D. (2007). Lessons in pediatric neuropsycho-oncology: What we've learned since Johnny Gunther. *Journal of Pediatric Psychology, 32,* 1029–1037.

Ris, M. D., Beebe, D. W., Armstrong, F. D., Fontanesi, J., Holmes, E., Sanford, R. A., et al. (2008). Cognitive and adaptive outcome in extracerebellar low-grade brain tumors in children: A report from the Children's Oncology Group. *Journal of Clinical Oncology, 26,* 4765–4770.

Ris, M. D., & Noll, R. B. (1994). Long-term neurobehavioral outcome in pediatric brain-tumor patients: Review and methodological critique. *Journal of Clinical and Experimental Neuropsychology, 16,* 21–42.

Ris, M. D., Packer, R., Goldwein, J., Jones-Wallace, D., & Boyett, J. M. (2001). Intellectual outcome after reduced-dose radiation therapy plus adjuvant chemotherapy for medulloblastoma: A Children's Cancer Group study. *Journal of Clinical Oncology, 19,* 3470–3476.

Ris, M. D., Ryan, P. M., Lamba, M., Brenemen, J., Cecil, K., Succop, P., et al. (2005). An improved methodology for modeling neurobehavioral late-effects of radiotherapy in pediatric brain tumors. *Pediatric Blood and Cancer, 44*(5), 487–493.

Robertson, P. L., Muraszko, K. M., Holmes, E. J., Spasto, R., Packer, R. J., Gajjar, A., et al. (2006). Incidence and severity of postoperative cerebellar mutism syndrome in children with medulloblastoma: A prospective study by the Children's Oncology Group. *Journal of Neurosurgery, 105,* 444–451.

Rola, R., Raber, J., Rizk, A., Otsuka, S., VandenBerg, S. R., Morhardt, D. R., et al. (2004). Radiation-induced impairment of hippocampal neurogenesis is associated with cognitive deficits in young mice. *Experimental Neurology, 188,* 316–330.

Roncadin, C., Dennis, M., Greenberg, M. L., & Spiegler, B. J. (2008). Adverse medical events associated with cerebellar astrocytomas and medulloblastomas: Natural history and relation to very long-term neurobehavioral outcomes. *Child's Nervous System, 24,* 995–1002.

Rorke, L. B., Gilles, F. H., Davis, R. L., & Becker, L. E. (1985). Revision of the World Health Organization classification of brain tumors for childhood brain tumors. *Cancer, 56,* 1869–1886.

Rutkowski, S., Bode, U., Deinlein, F., Ottensmeier, H., Warmuth-Metz, M., Soerensen, N., et al. (2005). Treatment of early childhood medulloblastoma by postoperative chemotherapy alone. *New England Journal of Medicine, 352,* 978–986.

Rynard, D. W., Chambers, A., Klinck, A. M., & Gray, J. D. (1998). School support programs for chronically ill children: Evaluating the adjustment of children with cancer at school. *Children's Health Care, 27,* 31–46.

Sahler, O. J., Varni, J., Fairclough, D., Butler, R., Dolgin, M., & Phipps, S. (2002). Problem-solving skills training for mothers of children with newly diagnosed cancer: A randomized trial. *Developmental and Behavioral Pediatrics, 23,* 77–86.

Shatz, J., Kramer, J. H., Ablin, A., & Matthay, K. K. (2000). Processing speed, working memory, and IQ: A developmental model of cognitive deficits following cranial radiation therapy. *Neuropsychology, 14,* 189–200.

Silber, J. H., Radcliffe, J., Peckham, V., Perilongo, G., Kishnavi, P., Fridman, M., et al. (1992). Whole-brain irradiation and decline in intelligence: The influence of dose and age on IQ scores. *Journal of Clinical Oncology, 10,* 1390–1396.

Spiegler, B. J., Bouffet, E., Greenburg, M. L., Rutka, J. T., & Mabbot, D. J. (2004). Change in neurocognitive functioning after treatment with cranial radiation in childhood. *Journal of Clinical Oncology, 22,* 208–212.

Strother, D. R., Pollack, I. F., Fisher, P. G., Hunter, J. V., Woo, S. Y., Pomeroy, S. L., et al. (2002). Tumors of the central nervous system. In P. A. Pizzo & D. G. Poplack (Eds.), *Principles and practice of pediatric oncology* (4th ed., pp. 751–824). Philadelphia: Lippincott Williams & Wilkins.

Taylor, H. G., Yeates, K. O., Wade, S. L., Drotar, D., Stancin, T., & Burant, C. (2001). Bidirectional child–family influences on outcomes of traumatic brain injury in children. *Journal of the International Neuropsychological Society, 7,* 755–67.

Thompson, S. J., Leigh, L., Christensen, R., Xiong, X., Kun, L. E., Heideman, R. L., et al. (2001). Immediate neurocognitive effects of methylphenidate on learning-impaired survivors of childhood cancer. *Journal of Clinical Oncology, 19,* 1802–1808.

Treiber, F. A., Schramm, L., & Mabe, P. A. (1986). Children's knowledge and concerns towards a peer with cancer: A workshop intervention approach. *Child Psychiatry and Human Development, 16,* 249–260.

Vannatta, K., Garstein, M. S., Short, A., & Noll, R. B. (1998). A controlled study of peer relationships of children surviving brain tumors: Teacher, peer, and self-rating. *Journal of Pediatric Psychology, 23,* 279–287.

Varni, J. W., & Katz, E. R. (1989). *Social skills training manual for children with cancer.* Unpublished manuscript.

Waber, D. P., Carpentieri, S. C., Klar, N., Silverman, L. B., Schwenn, M., Hurwitz, C. A., et al. (2000). Cognitive sequelae in children treated for acute lymphoblastic leukemia with dexamethasone or prednisone. *Journal of Pediatric Hematology/Oncology, 22,* 206–213.

Waber, D. P., Pomeroy, S. L., Chiverton, A. M., Kieran, M. W., Scott, R. M., Goumnerova, L. C., et al. (2006). Everyday cognitive function after craniopharyngioma in childhood. *Pediatric Neurology, 34,* 13–19.

Wong, C. S., & Van der Kogel, A. J. (2004). Mechanisms of radiation injury to the central nervous system: Implications for neuroprotection. *Molecular Interventions, 4,* 273–284.

Yeates, K. O., Dennis, M., Rubin, K. H., Taylor, A. G., Bigler, E. D., Gethardt, C. A., et al. (2007). Social outcomes in childhood brain disorder: A heuristic integration of social neuroscience and developmental psychology. *Psychological Bulletin, 132,* 535–556.

Zeltzer, P. M., Boyett, J. M., Finlay, J. L., Albright, A. L., Rorke, L. B., Milstein, J. M., et al. (1999). Metastasis stage, adjuvant treatment, and residual tumor are prognostic factors for medulloblastoma in children: Conclusions from the Children's Cancer Group 921 randomized phase III study. *Journal of Clinical Oncology, 17,* 832–845.

Zou, P., Mulhern, R. K., Butler, R. W., Li, C. S., Langston, J. W., & Ogg, R. J. (2005). BOLD responses to visual stimulation in survivors of childhood cancer. *NeuroImage, 24,* 61–69.

CHAPTER 5

Traumatic Brain Injury

KEITH OWEN YEATES

Traumatic brain injury (TBI) resulting from closed-head trauma in children is a major public health problem, resulting in total annual health care costs exceeding $1 billion (Schneier, Shields, Hostetler, Xiang, & Smith, 2006). TBI is a leading cause of death and disability among youth, and represents the most common source of acquired brain injury among children and adolescents. Hence it is a major source of referrals for pediatric neuropsychologists in clinical practice (Yeates, Ris, & Taylor, 1995b), and also has been of long-standing interest to researchers in pediatric neuropsychology.

The research literature pertaining to the neuropsychological consequences of TBI in children is extensive and has been the subject of several recent reviews (Bodin & Yeates, in press; Kirkwood, Yeates, & Bernstein, in press; Taylor, 2004, in press). Compared to the state of the field when the first edition of this book appeared (Yeates, 2000), substantial advances have been made in understanding the neurobehavioral outcomes of pediatric TBI. Nevertheless, much remains to be learned (Anderson & Yeates, in press; Kochanek, 2006). The goals of the present chapter are to provide an overview of the current state of knowledge regarding pediatric TBI; to critique the existing research and recommend conceptual and methodological improvements; and to suggest potentially fruitful directions for future investigation.

EPIDEMIOLOGY

Incidence and Prevalence

Accurate statistics regarding the incidence and prevalence of TBI in the United States are difficult to obtain. Few registries for TBI have been established at a local, regional, or national level, and existing registries are often concerned only with injuries that involve hospital care, thereby omitting many cases of mild TBI. Moreover, as Kraus (1995) has noted, epidemiological studies have varied widely in terms of definition of injury, sources of data, data collection techniques, description of cases, and ages of the target populations. The most recent and complete data on incidence and prevalence come from the Centers for Disease Control and Prevention (CDC; Langlois, Rutland-Brown, & Thomas, 2006), which estimated a total of 475,000 TBI cases annually for children ages 0–14, with an overall annual incidence of 799 per 100,000 population (based on deaths, hospitalizations, and emergency department visits).

Incidence and prevalence vary as a function of injury severity. The most common measure of injury severity is the Glasgow Coma Scale (Teasdale & Jennett, 1974), on which scores range from 3 to 15 (see Table 5.1). By convention, scores from 13 to 15 represent mild injuries, scores from 9 to 12 represent moderate injuries, and scores of 8 and less represent severe injuries. Studies using the Glasgow Coma Scale as the measure of severity have found that the majority of children with TBI have mild TBI. For instance, the National Pediatric Trauma Registry (Lescohier & DiScala, 1993) reported that 76% of TBI cases in the registry were mild, 10% moderate, and 13% severe. Similarly, using data from a 14-state

TABLE 5.1. Glasgow Coma Scale

Category	Score	Description
Eye Opening		
None	1	Not attributable to ocular swelling.
To pain	2	Pain stimulus is applied to chest or limbs.
To speech	3	Nonspecific response to speech or shout; does not imply patient obeys command to open eyes.
Spontaneous	4	Eyes are open, but this does not imply intact awareness.
Motor Response		
No response	1	Flaccid.
Extension	2	Decerebrate posturing: Adduction, internal rotation of shoulder, and pronation of forearm.
Abnormal flexion	3	Decorticate posturing: Abnormal flexion, adduction of the shoulder.
Withdrawal	4	Normal flexor response; withdraws from pain stimulus with abduction of the shoulder.
Localizes pain	5	Pain stimulus applied to supraocular region or fingertip causes limb to remove it.
Obeys commands	6	Follows simple commands.
Verbal Response		
No response	1	No vocalization.
Incomprehensible	2	Vocalizes, but no recognizable words.
Inappropriate	3	Intelligible speech (e.g., shouting or swearing), but no sustained or coherent conversation.
Confused	4	Responds to questions in a conversational manner, but the responses indicate disorientation.
Oriented	5	Normal orientation to time, person, and place.

Note. Glasgow Coma Scale score = Eye Opening score + Motor Response score + Verbal Response score (range 3 to 15). Based on Teasdale and Jennett (1974).

surveillance system, the CDC estimated that 71–77% of hospital discharges for TBI across youth ages 0–19 years were classified as mild, 7–11% as moderate, and 8–12% as severe (Langlois et al., 2003). These estimates almost certainly underestimate the proportion of mild TBI cases, many of which go unreported entirely or are treated in outpatient settings and do not result in hospital visits.

Cause of Injury

Data regarding the external cause of TBI can provide important information about the mechanism of brain injuries. The categorization of external causes is often inconsistent from one study to another, and the coding of external cause of injury in emergency departments and hospitals is often incomplete or inaccurate. Nonetheless, the most common causes of TBI involve transportation and falls. Together, those two causes account for more than 50% of all pediatric TBI cases (Langlois et al., 2006). The distribution of causes varies significantly as a function of age (Keenan & Bratton, 2006). Infants are especially likely to sustain TBI through falls, as well as via inflicted injuries secondary to child abuse. Young children are most likely to be injured through falls and motor vehicle collisions (as either occupants or pedestrians). In older children, sports and recreational accidents and pedestrian or bicycle collisions with motor vehicles account for an increasing proportion of TBI. Adolescents are especially likely to be injured in motor vehicle collisions.

Demographic Variation

The incidence and prevalence of TBI also vary significantly according to demographic factors, such as sex and age. Boys are about twice as likely to sustain TBI as girls, although the ratio varies somewhat with age (Langlois et al., 2006). Children ages 0–4 are most likely to visit emergency departments for evaluation of TBI, with an annual incidence of about 1,100 per 100,000, suggesting that milder injuries may be especially common among younger children. In contrast, older adolescents ages 15–19 show the highest rate of hospitalizations and deaths, with a combined annual incidence of about 150 per 100,000, probably reflecting the increasing severity of TBI in that age group as a function of motor vehicle collisions.

Incidence/prevalence rates also may vary as a function of race and socioeconomic status. Among children 0–9 years of age, blacks demonstrate higher rates of hospitalization and death than whites for motor-vehicle-related TBI (Langlois, Rutland-Brown, & Thomas, 2005). In the United Kingdom, epidemiological data showed that social disadvantage was a risk factor for more severe TBI (Parslow, Morris, Tasker, Forsyth, & Hawley, 2005).

Mortality and Morbidity

Traumatic injuries constitute the leading cause of death among children and adolescents, and about 40–50% of the deaths resulting from trauma are associated with TBI (Kraus, 1995). Overall, mortality rates are lower among children than among adolescents and adults. The CDC estimates an annual mortality rate of about 4.5 per 100,000 for children 0–14 years of age, but a rate of about 24 per 100,000 for 15- to 19-year-olds (Langlois et al., 2006). The mortality rate is highest among children with severe injuries, and is virtually nil among those with mild injuries. Kraus (1995) found case fatality rates among hospital admissions to range from 12% to 62% for severe injuries, but to be less than 4% for moderate injuries and less than 1% for mild injuries.

Survivors of TBI frequently experience adverse consequences. One gross measure of outcome that has been employed in epidemiological studies is the Glasgow Outcome Scale (Jennett & Bond, 1975). The Glasgow Outcome Scale differentiates five outcome categories: death, persistent vegetative state, severe disability; moderate disability, and so-called "good recovery." In his review, Kraus (1995) found that between 75% and 95% of children with TBI displayed a "good recovery," about 10% showed a moderate disability, 1–3% showed a severe disability, and fewer than 1% were in a persistent vegetative state. However, a "good recovery" according to the Glasgow Outcome Scale does not preclude neurobehavioral impairment or associated functional disabilities (Koelfen et al., 1997).

NEUROPATHOLOGY AND PATHOPHYSIOLOGY

TBI is associated with multiple forms of neuropathology (see Table 5.2). These include overt damage to brain tissue, including both focal and diffuse lesions, as well as disruptions in brain function at a cellular level. The pathophysiology of TBI begins at the time of impact, but continues over a period of days or weeks and perhaps even longer. Indeed, recent research indicates that the brain damage resulting from TBI involves more complex, prolonged, and interwoven processes than investigators previously recognized (Farkas & Povlishock, 2007; Giza & Hovda, 2001; Povlishock & Katz, 2005).

Although pathophysiological commonalities exist among all types of TBI, the immature brain responds differently to trauma than does the mature brain of the adult (Giza, Mink, & Madikians, 2007). For example, children are more likely to display posttraumatic brain swelling, hypoxic–ischemic insult, and diffuse rather than focal injuries. The biomechanical properties of the young brain may explain at least some of these differences. Com-

TABLE 5.2. Neuropathology of TBI

Type of insult	Neuropathology
Primary	• Skull fracture • Intracranial contusions and hemorrhage • Shear–strain injury
Secondary	• Brain swelling • Cerebral edema • Elevated intracranial pressure • Hypoxia–ischemia • Mass lesions (hematoma)
Neurochemical	• Excessive production of free radicals • Excessive release of excitatory neurotransmitters • Alterations in glucose metabolism • Decreased cerebral blood flow
Late/delayed	• White matter degeneration and cerebral atrophy • Posttraumatic hydrocephalus • Posttraumatic seizures

pared to adults, children have a greater head-to-body ratio, less myelination, and greater relative proportion of water content and cerebral blood volume. Once children reach adolescence, TBI-related pathology begins to more closely resemble that seen in adults.

Primary and Secondary Injuries

Observable injuries resulting from closed-head trauma can be classified into two broad categories: *primary* and *secondary*. Primary injuries result directly from the trauma itself. They include skull fractures, contusions/lacerations, and mechanical injuries to nerve fibers and blood vessels. Secondary injuries arise indirectly from the trauma, and in children include brain swelling/edema, hypoxia/hypotension, increased intracranial pressure, and mass lesions.

The primary injuries that arise from closed-head trauma reflect biomechanical forces that are not fully understood in children (Margulies & Coats, in press). Most of the common causes of TBI in children, including falls and motor vehicle collisions, give rise to acceleration–deceleration injuries. Acceleration injuries can involve both *translational* and *rotational* trauma. Translational trauma involves linear acceleration along an axis that passes through the center of the head. The acceleration can result in deformation of the skull or skull fractures, as well as contusions at the site of impact. Isolated translational trauma is rare, however, and is usually combined with rotational trauma. Rotational trauma occurs when the axis of impact does not pass directly through the center of the head, and hence results in a combination of both linear and angular acceleration. Rotational trauma arises when the skull is stopped by the impact, but the brain continues to move in the skull because of its angular acceleration. The movement results in the tearing or bruising of blood vessels that gives rise to focal contusions or hemorrhage, as well as in shearing or straining of nerve fibers that can give rise to diffuse axonal injury.

Focal contusions are especially likely to occur in the frontal and temporal cortex, because of its proximity to the bony prominences in the anterior and middle fossa of the skull (Bigler, 2007). Thus neuroimaging consistently reveals an anterior–posterior gradient in the focal lesions associated with TBI. Focal lesions are generally larger and occur more frequently in frontal and anterior temporal regions than in posterior temporal, parietal, or occipital regions (Wilde et al., 2005). In contrast, diffuse axonal injury appears to be most common at the boundaries between gray and white matter, and tends to occur most often around the basal ganglia, periventricular regions, superior cerebellar peduncles, fornices, corpus callosum, and fiber tracts of the brainstem.

In most cases, medical management of TBI focuses not on primary injuries, but instead on the secondary injuries that arise indirectly following the initial trauma. Brain swelling and cerebral edema are two major secondary complications of TBI, and are especially common in children (Bruce, 1995; Kochanek, 2006). Brain swelling and cerebral edema are thought to result from a disruption of the normal relationships among blood, brain tissue, and cerebrospinal fluid. A disruption of these relationships can result in decreased cerebral blood flow, increased cerebral blood volume, and increased intracranial pressure, which together can give rise to ischemic and hypoxic injury, as well as to brain herniation and death (Bruce, 1995). Decreases in cerebral blood flow are often exacerbated by hypotension, or low blood pressure, which is a common symptom of shock. Pulmonary insufficiency can also contribute to hypoxia.

In contrast to brain swelling and cerebral edema, mass lesions are less common in children than in adults (Bruce, 1995). Mass lesions involve the accumulation of fluid, usually blood associated with contusion and hemorrhage. *Hematomas* are blood clots that occur in various locations in and around the brain. Epidural hematomas result from bleeding into the space between the dura and the skull, often in association with a skull fracture that disrupts the middle meningeal artery. Epidural hematomas occasionally become clinically apparent only after several days. Subdural hematomas result from bleeding into the space between the dura and the arachnoid membranes, frequently because of a tear in the bridging veins of the sagittal sinus, and are more often acute in nature. Intracerebral hematomas occur within the brain parenchyma, and often follow the same spatial distribution as contusions. They may result from shear injuries to brain tissue. Subarachnoid or intraventricular hemorrhages are also common in TBI.

Neurochemical and Neurometabolic Mechanisms

The mechanical forces involved in head trauma are no longer thought to account for the majority of diffuse axonal injury. Instead, reactive axonal changes occur following the trauma and lead only gradually to brain damage. These reactive changes are mediated by a cascade of biochemical and metabolic reactions following a TBI (Farkas & Povlishock, 2007; Novack, Dillon, & Jackson, 1996). TBI can result in a variety of neurochemical events, including the production of free radicals and excitatory amino acids, the disruption of normal calcium homeostasis, and changes in glucose metabolism and cerebral blood flow (Giza & Hovda, 2001). These events act in concert to exacerbate the hypoxic–ischemic insult that commonly occurs following TBI.

Free radicals are normal by-products of metabolism. Excessive production of free radicals, however, can affect cell membrane integrity and cause lipid peroxidation or attack cell organelles, such as the mitochondria. Brain tissue may be especially vulnerable to free radicals, because it is rich in cholesterol and polyunsaturated fatty acid. Experimental research with animals has shown that treatment with radical scavengers can reduce brain injury (Novack et al., 1996).

Excitatory amino acids normally function as neurotransmitters. They can be harmful in excessive amounts, however, disrupting cell function and eventually resulting in cell death. Glutamate and aspartate are two common excitatory amino acids. These compounds have an affinity for receptors that are especially prevalent in such regions as the hippocampus and thalamus. Experimental studies of animals indicate that the release of glutamate and aspartate is especially sensitive to hypoxic–ischemic events and increases dramatically after TBI. Thus excitotoxicity may help to account for the severe effects of hypoxia–ischemia on the hippocampus, which has many glutamate receptors, and also may explain the vulnerability of the hippocampus in TBI (Wilde et al., 2007). Experimental research indicates that substances that block glutamate receptors can reduce the brain damage associated with hypoxia–ischemia. Other neurotransmitters, including acetylcholine, also are thought to contribute to brain injury.

The disruption of cellular calcium homeostasis by hypoxia–ischemia is another indirect source of brain injury. Hypoxic–ischemic insults interrupt normal ion-pumping mechanisms and induce the release of intracellular calcium. The influx of calcium exacerbates the effects of hypoxia–ischemia on the normal metabolic process of oxidative phosphorylation and further reduces adenosine triphosphate, which is the major energy source for cell function. In addition, the calcium influx triggers other chemical events, including the release of free radicals, excitatory neurotransmitters, and cystein proteases. The disruption of calcium homeostasis also can result in vasoconstriction, leading to further hypoxic–ischemic insult.

Late Effects

TBI can be associated with a variety of late effects. Neuroimaging studies have indicated that severe TBI often results in a gradual and prolonged process of white matter degeneration and cortical thinning, with associated cerebral atrophy and ventricular enlargement (Ghosh et al., 2009; Merkley et al., 2008). In some cases, ventricular dilation results from an actual disturbance in the circulation of cerebrospinal fluid and is associated with hydrocephalus. Posttraumatic hydrocephalus, as opposed to cerebral atrophy and associated ventricular enlargement, is relatively uncommon; it typically develops only after severe injuries associated with certain predisposing factors, such as subarachnoid hemorrhage (McLean et al., 1995).

Early posttraumatic seizures, defined as occurring within the first week after TBI, occur in many children and can involve focal status epilepticus (Statler, 2006). Younger children seem especially vulnerable to early posttraumatic seizures. The occurrence of seizures soon after injury does not clearly place children at risk for later epilepsy, which occurs in about 10–20% of children with severe TBI. Posttraumatic epilepsy is more common in children with penetrating injuries, inflicted injuries, or depressed skull fracture. Most posttraumatic seizures occur within the first 2 postinjury years, although the occurrence of posttraumatic seizures increases with longer follow-up duration.

NEUROBEHAVIORAL CONSEQUENCES

The literature on the neuropsychological consequences of pediatric TBI is extensive, and a detailed review of all individual studies is beyond the scope of this chapter. In general, research indicates that TBI, especially when severe, can produce deficits in a variety of domains: alertness and orientation; intellectual functioning; language and communication skills; nonverbal skills; attention, memory, and executive functions; corticosensory and motor skills; academic achievement; social functioning; behavioral adjustment; psychiatric disorder; and adaptive functioning. The following sections provide a selective overview of the existing literature and highlight recent research findings.

Alertness and Orientation

Orientation and alertness are often disturbed following TBI, particularly during the initial phase of recovery. Most children with TBI, especially those that are moderate or severe, experience a period of fluctuations in arousal, as well as disorientation, confusion, and memory loss after the injury. These changes in mental status occur during what is usually referred to as the period of *posttraumatic amnesia* (PTA), which is a common measure of injury severity. Various standardized measures are available to assess the presence and duration of PTA in children, such as the Children's Orientation and Amnesia Test (COAT; Ewing-Cobbs, Levin, Fletcher, Miner, & Eisenberg, 1990) and the Westmead PTA Scale (Marosszeky, Batchelor, Shores, Marosszelcy, & Boonschate, 1993).

Intellectual Functioning

The seminal Isle of Wight studies by Rutter and colleagues were among the first to document deficits in intellectual functioning following TBI in children (Chadwick, Rutter, Brown, Shaffer, & Traub, 1981). Intellectual deficits have since been shown to occur whether children with TBI are compared to healthy controls or to children with orthopedic injuries not involving the head, and the magnitude of the deficits is related to injury severity. Early research suggested that IQ scores reflecting nonverbal skills are particularly likely to be depressed, presumably because those measures require fluid problem-solving skills and involve speeded motor output. In contrast, verbal intelligence was thought to be less vulnerable, because its assessment depends more on previously acquired knowledge and makes few demands for speeded responses or motor control. However, more recent studies have found deficits in both nonverbal and verbal intellectual functioning (Anderson, Morse, Catroppa, Haritou, & Rosenfeld, 2004; Anderson, Catroppa, Morse, Haritou, & Rosenfeld, 2005b; Taylor et al., 1999).

Prospective longitudinal studies indicate that children demonstrate significant recovery in intellectual functioning following TBI. Thus IQ scores tend to increase over time following TBI, with the largest increases occurring among children with more severe injuries (Yeates et al., 2002). The increases in IQ scores occur most rapidly immediately after injury; thus IQ scores tend to plateau after 1–2 years. Despite substantial recovery, IQ scores often continue to be depressed relative to premorbid levels. Persistent deficits in IQ appear to be especially likely among children with severe TBI and those injured early in life (Anderson et al., 2004; Anderson, Catroppa, Morse, Haritou, & Rosenfeld, 2005a).

Traditional omnibus IQ measures do not provide much insight into the specific cognitive deficits that characterize children with TBI (Taylor, 2004, in press). However, studies using more recent versions of IQ tests have suggested more specific deficits in processing speed, as opposed to either verbal or nonverbal skills per se (Donders & Janke, 2008). Nevertheless, current neuropsychological research on childhood TBI now tends to focus on more specific cognitive domains, rather than on global measures of intellectual functioning.

Language and Communication Skills

Spontaneous mutism and expressive language deficits are common immediately after TBI (Levin et al., 1983), but overt aphasic disorders rarely persist following acute recovery. However, subtle language difficulties often persist, again most often following moderate to severe injuries. Long-term deficits have been identified on tests measuring a variety of basic linguistic skills, including syntactical comprehension, sentence repetition, confrontation naming, object description, and verbal fluency (Ewing-Cobbs & Barnes, 2002). Language deficits typically improve over time, with the most improvement seen following severe TBI (Catroppa & Anderson, 2004).

Children with TBI also display more pronounced difficulties with the pragmatic aspects of language (Chapman, 1995; Dennis & Barnes, 1990). Deficits have been demonstrated in a variety of skills, such as interpreting ambiguous sentences, making inferences, formulating sentences from individual words, and explaining figurative expressions. Deficits in such skills are construed as reflecting a general impairment in *discourse*, which can be defined as the ability to convey a message by communicating a series of ideas, usually in sentences. Studies of narrative discourse, using story recall as the dependent measure, indicate that children with severe TBI use fewer words and sentences in their stories (Chapman, 1995; Chapman et al., 2004). Moreover, their stories contain less information, are not as well organized, and are less complete than those produced by children with milder injuries or by normal controls. The differences remain significant even after word knowledge and verbal memory are controlled. Because of the importance of communication skills for success in school, discourse deficits may account for some of the academic difficulties that children with TBI often experience.

Nonverbal Skills

Long-term deficits in nonverbal skills are relatively frequent consequences of pediatric TBI, and encompass both perceptual/spatial and constructional abilities. Deficits following head injuries have been reported on a variety of constructional tasks, including block and puzzle tasks such as the Block Design subtest on the Wechsler Intelligence Scale for Children—Fourth Edition, and drawing tasks such as the Developmental Test of Visual—Motor Integration (Thompson et al., 1994; Yeates et al., 2002) and the Rey–Osterrieth Complex Figure (Yeates, Patterson, Waber, & Bernstein, 2003). Less research has focused on examining perceptual or spatial skills with measures that do not involve motor output, but children with TBI have shown deficits on such tasks in a variety of studies (Lehnung et al., 2001; Verger et al., 2000).

Attention

Complaints about attention problems are very common following childhood TBI (Yeates et al., 2005). However, studies using standardized measures of attention were relatively infrequent until the past decade. In recent years, a substantial literature has documented deficits in many different aspects of attention. Early studies generally focused on continuous-performance tests (e.g., Dennis, Wilkinson, Koski, & Humphreys, 1995). On such measures, children with TBI display poorer response modulation, especially in the presence of distraction, as well as slower reaction times. More recent studies have shown deficits in sustained, selective, shifting, and divided attention, particularly on more complex and timed measures (Anderson, Fenwick, Manly, & Robertson, 1998; Catroppa & Anderson, 2005; Catroppa, Anderson, Morse, Haritou, & Rosenfeld, 2007; Ewing-Cobbs et al., 1998b). The deficits show some recovery, but can persist across time, especially in more severely injured children.

Memory

Childhood TBI frequently results in complaints of memory deficits (Ward, Shum, Dick, McKinlay, & Baker-Tweney, 2004). Deficits have been reported on a wide variety of tasks assessing explicit memory; the magnitude of these impairments depends on injury severity

(Catroppa & Anderson, 2002, 2007; Levin et al., 1988; Yeates, Blumenstein, Patterson, & Delis, 1995a; Yeates et al., 2003). Research has attempted to delineate more precisely the specific components of memory that are impaired. For instance, research using the California Verbal Learning Test suggests that deficits occur in a variety of memory components, including storage, retention, and retrieval (Roman et al., 1998; Yeates et al., 1995a).

Guided by advances in the developmental neuroscience of memory (Nelson, 1995), research has recently begun to examine types of memory other than those measured solely by traditional standardized tasks requiring explicit recall. For instance, an important distinction has been drawn between *explicit* and *implicit* memory. Explicit memory involves the conscious recollection of past events or experiences and is typically measured through recall or recognition, whereas implicit memory involves demonstrations of learning or facilitation of performance in the absence of conscious recollection. Several studies, using measures of both procedural learning and perceptual and conceptual priming, have indicated that children with TBI are less likely to show deficits in implicit memory than in explicit memory (Shum, Jamieson, Bahr, & Wallace, 1999; Ward, Shum, Wallace, & Boon, 2002; Yeates & Enrile, 2005).

Prospective memory is another type of recall that has received recent attention. Prospective memory essentially involves remembering to perform an intended action at some time in the future. Children and adolescents with moderate to severe TBI display deficits in prospective memory when compared to children with orthopedic injuries (McCauley & Levin, 2004; McCauley, McDaniel, Pedroza, Chapman, & Levin, 2009) or to typically developing children (Ward, Shum, McKinlay, Baker, & Wallace, 2007).

Executive Functions

Deficits in executive functions occur frequently after childhood TBI. Over the past decade, research on executive functions in TBI has begun to examine not only performance on standardized cognitive tests, but also various aspects of emotional and behavioral regulation. Levin and his colleagues have studied executive functions extensively, and have found that children with TBI display deficits on a variety of tasks meant to assess such executive functions as working memory, inhibitory control, and planning (Levin et al., 1996; Levin & Hanten, 2005). The magnitude of deficits on executive function tasks has been shown to correlate with the volume of lesions in the frontal lobes, but not with extrafrontal lesion volume (Levin et al., 1994, 1997). Young children and those with severe injuries are particularly vulnerable to executive deficits following TBI (Anderson & Catroppa, 2005; Ewing-Cobbs, Prasad, Landry, Kramer, & DeLeon, 2004b), and the deficits can persist for years after injury (Nadebaum, Anderson, & Catroppa, 2007).

Because of concerns about the ecological validity of performance-based tests of executive functions, research has also begun to focus on executive problems that children with TBI display in everyday settings (Mangeot, Armstrong, Colvin, Yeates, & Taylor, 2002; Sesma, Slomine, Ding, & McCarthy, 2008). Children with TBI, particularly those with more severe TBI, are consistently reported to demonstrate executive deficits that extend to their emotional and behavioral regulation, as well as to their working memory, cognitive flexibility, and planning skills. Moreover, these deficits have been linked to broader difficulties with social and behavioral adjustment (Ganesalingam, Sanson, Anderson, & Yeates, 2006, 2007).

Corticosensory and Motor Skills

Children with TBI often demonstrate deficits in corticosensory and complex motor skills. Levin and Eisenberg (1979) found that approximately 25% of children with severe injuries displayed deficits on tests of stereognosis, finger localization, and graphesthesia. Similarly, Bawden and his colleagues (Bawden, Knights, & Winogron, 1985; Winogron, Knights, & Bawden, 1984) showed deficits on various measures of fine motor skills, especially those that were timed, among children with severe TBI. More recent studies have demonstrated sustained deficits in gait and gross motor skills as well (Katz-Leurer, Rotem, Lewitus, Keren, & Meyer, 2008; Kuhtz-Buschbeck et al., 2003).

Academic Performance

As might be anticipated from the litany of neurocognitive deficits described above, pediatric TBI is frequently associated with reports of declines in academic performance (Ewing-Cobbs et al., 2004a; Taylor et al., 2002) and with an increased risk of grade retention, placement in special education, and other indicators of academic difficulties (Ewing-Cobbs, Fletcher, Levin, Iovino, & Meyer, 1998a; Taylor et al., 2003). However, the reported academic difficulties do not necessarily translate into deficits on formal achievement testing. Deficits in academic achievement following TBI are most likely to be apparent in children injured at a young age (Ewing-Cobbs et al., 2004a, 2006). Children injured at a later age do not necessarily display deficits on standardized achievement tests (Kinsella et al., 1995; Taylor et al., 2002).

The academic difficulties that children with TBI face are predicted by a variety of different factors, including a child's premorbid academic functioning (Catroppa & Anderson, 2007) and postinjury neuropsychological functioning (Kinsella et al., 1997; Miller & Donders, 2003; Stallings, Ewing-Cobbs, Francis, & Fletcher, 1996), as well as the child's postinjury behavioral adjustment (Yeates & Taylor, 2006). Interestingly, the family environment also moderates academic performance, such that more supportive and functional homes lessen the impact of TBI (Taylor et al., 2002). In contrast, standardized achievement testing is not always a strong predictor of academic outcomes after TBI (Yeates & Taylor, 2006).

Social Functioning

Childhood TBI often results in problems with social functioning. A growing literature indicates that children with severe TBI are rated as less socially competent and lonelier than healthy children or children with injuries not involving the brain, and that their poor social outcomes persist over time (Andrews, Rose, & Johnson, 1998; Bohnert, Parker, & Warschausky, 1997; Dennis, Guger, Roncadin, Barnes, & Schachar, 2001a; Yeates et al., 2004). The relationship between TBI and social outcomes appears to be moderated by environmental variables (Yeates et al. 2004). More specifically, poor social outcomes following TBI can be exacerbated by poor family functioning, lower socioeconomic status, and lack of family resources.

The poor social outcomes displayed by children with TBI may be mediated by deficits in social information processing. Following TBI, children display deficits in the understanding of emotion (Dennis, Barnes, Wilkinson, & Humphreys, 1998) and mental states (Dennis, Purvis, Barnes, Wilkinson, & Winner, 2001b), as well as in social problem solving (Hanten et al., 2008; Janusz, Kirkwood, Yeates, & Taylor, 2002; Warschausky, Cohen, Parker, Levendosky, & Okun, 1997). Collectively, deficits in executive functions, language pragmatics, and social problem solving account for significant variance in social outcomes among children with TBI (Yeates et al., 2004).

The social deficits shown by children with TBI may be linked specifically to damage to anterior brain regions. Children with frontal lobe injury in association with TBI are more likely to have problems with social discourse (Dennis et al., 2001a) and social problem solving (Hanten et al., 2008), as well as more generally with social functioning (Levin et al., 2004). In the future, the integration of models and methods from social-cognitive neuroscience and developmental psychology is likely to result in a better understanding of social outcomes following childhood TBI (Yeates et al., 2007).

Behavioral Adjustment

Numerous studies have documented that moderate to severe TBI in children increases the risk for a wide range of emotional and behavioral problems (Fletcher, Ewing-Cobbs, Miner, Levin, & Eisenberg, 1990; Schwartz et al., 2003; Taylor et al., 2002). For example, Schwartz et al. (2003) found that at 4 years after injury, 36% of a group with severe TBI displayed significant behavioral problems, compared with 22% of a group with moderate TBI and 10% of a comparison group with orthopedic injury. In contrast to cognitive difficulties, which often show recovery in the initial months after injury, behavioral problems are more likely to show a stable or even worsening pattern over time (Fay et al., 2009).

Most previous research has relied on generic rating scales, such as the Child Behavior Checklist (Achenbach & Rescorla, 2001), to assess behavioral adjustment. Such scales were not designed to be sensitive to the effects of TBI (Drotar, Stein, & Perrin, 1995; Perrin, Stein, & Drotar, 1991). Research focusing on specific symptoms that arise following TBI may be more informative. For instance, we (Yeates et al., 2001) found high rates of neurobehavioral symptoms in the first year following TBI. However, cognitive and somatic symptoms (e.g., fatigue, headache, inattention) tended to decline in the first year, whereas emotional and behavioral symptoms (e.g., aggression, impulsivity) tended to increase over time, especially in children with severe TBI and in those with poor family functioning.

Research on behavioral adjustment can be confounded by the high prevalence of preinjury behavior problems in children with TBI. Asarnow and colleagues (Asarnow et al., 1995; Light et al., 1998) found that children with mild TBI displayed higher rates of preinjury behavior problems than did children with no injury. In contrast, their preinjury behavioral functioning did not differ from that of children with injuries not involving the head. The latter findings suggest that the presence of premorbid behavior problems increases the likelihood of traumatic injuries. Indeed, Bloom et al. (2001) found that children with preinjury psychiatric disorders, such as attention-deficit/hyperactivity disorder (ADHD) and anxiety disorders, were more likely to experience a head injury than were children without such preinjury disorders.

Behavioral functioning following childhood TBI does not appear to be closely related to cognitive outcomes. For instance, Fletcher et al. (1990) found small and generally nonsignificant correlations between five neuropsychological measures and measures of adaptive functioning and behavioral adjustment. Thus cognitive and behavioral outcomes may be somewhat independent following TBI, and their determinants may differ considerably. For instance, cognitive outcomes are related more strongly to injury-related variables, whereas behavioral outcomes are related more strongly to measures of preinjury family functioning (Yeates et al., 1997).

Psychiatric Disorder

Pediatric TBI is associated with a variety of specific psychiatric symptoms and disorders. Several studies have reported a risk of new psychiatric disorders following pediatric TBI. For instance, Bloom et al. (2001) found that 58% of their sample developed a novel psychiatric disorder following a TBI. Max et al. (1997a, 1997b, 1997c, 1998d) conducted a series of studies following the development of new psychiatric disorders in a cohort of children with TBI at 3, 6, 12, and 24 months after injury. They found that 46% of the participants met criteria for a new psychiatric disorder at 3 months, 24% at 6 months, 37% at 12 months, and 35% at 24 months.

The most common psychiatric diagnoses that are identified following childhood TBI are oppositional defiant disorder (Max et al., 1998a), ADHD (Gerring et al., 1998; Levin et al., 2007; Massagli et al., 2004; Max et al., 2005b; Yeates et al., 2005), and organic personality syndrome (now termed personality change due to TBI; Max et al., 2000; Max, Robertson, & Lansing, 2001; Max et al., 2005a). Internalizing disorders have also been documented following pediatric TBI, including obsessive–compulsive symptoms, generalized anxiety, separation anxiety, and depression (Grados et al., 2008; Luis & Mittenberg, 2002; Vasa et al., 2002). Symptoms of posttraumatic stress disorder (PTSD) are also elevated following childhood TBI, although relatively few children meet full diagnostic criteria for PTSD (Gerring et al., 2002; Levi, Drotar, Yeates, & Taylor, 1999; Max et al., 1998b).

Following mild TBI, various somatic, cognitive, and behavioral complaints commonly referred to as *postconcussive symptoms* are often reported by children and parents. Postconcussion syndrome is a controversial diagnosis for which research criteria have been included in the most recent version (fourth edition, text revision) of the *Diagnostic and Statistical Manual of Mental Disorders* (DSM-IV; American Psychiatric Association, 2000). Several studies have shown that children with mild TBI show more postconcussive symptoms than children with injuries not involving the brain (Mittenberg, Wittner, & Miller, 1997; Ponsford et al., 1999; Yeates et al., 1999). We (Yeates et al., 2009) recently examined longitudinal trajectories of such symptoms in children with mild TBI as compared to children with orthopedic injuries. We found that children with mild TBI, particularly those with more severe injury, were more likely to demonstrate trajectories showing high acute levels of postconcussive symptoms, as well as persistent increases in these symptoms, in the first postinjury year.

Adaptive Functioning and Quality of Life

Moderate or severe TBI is also associated with persistent adaptive behavior deficits (e.g., poorer communication, socialization, and daily living skills) and functional limitations (Fay et al., 2009; Max et al., 1998c; Taylor et al., 1999). Deficits in adaptive behavior appear to be especially likely in the presence of family dysfunction (Taylor et al., 1999). More generally, children with TBI demonstrate significant declines in their overall quality of life, although the differences are more pronounced in parental reports than in children's self-reports (McCarthy et al., 2006; Stancin et al., 2002).

PREDICTION OF OUTCOMES

The preceding summary of the neurobehavioral outcomes of pediatric TBI is based largely on the results of group comparisons (e.g., children with severe TBI vs. children with orthopedic injuries). Although the generalizations are valid, they must be tempered by the realization that children with TBI display substantial variation in outcomes, even when they are grouped according to injury severity. These individual differences in outcomes reflect a complex interplay among injury characteristics, non-injury-related influences, and developmental factors.

Injury Characteristics

Injury severity has consistently proven to be a major determinant of the consequences of TBI. Generally speaking, a dose–response relationship has been established between injury severity and neuropsychological outcome, such that more severe injuries are associated with poorer outcomes. Injury severity has been assessed by using a variety of clinical metrics, including level of consciousness, duration of impaired consciousness, and length of PTA. Injury severity has also been assessed by using a variety of specific medical indicators, including brainstem abnormalities (e.g., pupillary reactivity), seizures, and elevated intracranial pressure.

The Glasgow Coma Scale (see Table 5.1; Teasdale & Jennett, 1974) is most often used to assess level of consciousness; it not only predicts cognitive recovery and functional outcome, but is also correlated with later cerebral atrophy (Ghosh et al., 2009). The Motor Response scale on the Glasgow Coma Scale can be used to assess duration of impaired consciousness, which is usually defined as the amount of time that elapses from an injury until a child is able to follow commands consistently (i.e., the number of days during which the Motor Response scale on the Glasgow Coma Scale falls below 6). An injury is usually considered severe when the duration of impaired consciousness lasts more than 24 hours. Unlike the Glasgow Coma Scale, which is a measure of a child's neurological status at a given point in time, the duration of impaired consciousness is an indirect indicator of rate of recovery, because it reflects the speed with which a child's mental status improves acutely after injury. The length of PTA, or the time that elapses from the injury until a child is oriented and displays intact memory for daily events, also indirectly reflects the child's rate of recovery. As noted earlier, standardized measures have been developed to assess PTA in children.

The relationship between various clinical measures of injury severity and neuropsychological outcomes has been explored in several studies (Ewing-Cobbs, Fletcher, Levin, Hastings, & Francis, 1996; McDonald et al., 1994). Across studies, the durations of coma, impaired consciousness, and PTA were generally better predictors of outcome than was any static measure, such as the lowest postresuscitation Glasgow Coma Scale score. The predictive utility of the duration measures may be related to their utility as markers of recovery, rather than as measures of neurological status immediately after injury.

However severity is designated, moderate to severe TBI is widely agreed to result in substantial neurobehavioral morbidity. In contrast, the outcomes of mild TBI are a matter of controversy. Both parents and children frequently report somatic, cognitive, and emotional symptoms following mild TBI (Yeates et al., 2009); yet these postconcussive symptoms often occur in the absence of objective evidence of brain injury, such as abnormal neuroimaging findings or deficits on standardized cognitive testing (Asarnow et al., 1995; Satz, 2001; Satz, Zaucha, McCleary, Light, & Asarnow, 1997). However, methodological shortcomings hamper definitive conclusions. Differences in findings across studies are probably related to lack of a common definition of mild TBI, differences in recruitment strategies, and variations in research designs and outcome measures (Yeates & Taylor, 2005). Overall, the literature suggests that at least some cases of mild TBI are associated with demonstrable brain insults and with persistent cognitive deficits and postconcussive symptoms (Bigler, 2008; Kirkwood et al., 2008; Yeates et al., 2009).

The classification of severity has begun to move beyond simple clinical metrics, such as the Glasgow Coma Scale, to more sophisticated indices that are linked more closely to the pathophysiology of TBI (Saatman et al., 2008). One of the major advances in assessing severity involves neuroimaging. Computed tomography (CT) is the preferred method of neuroimaging during the acute phase of TBI, because it is rapidly and widely available and relatively inexpensive, and is also sensitive to lesions such as epidural hematomas that may necessitate neurosurgical intervention (Bigler, 1999, 2003; Poussaint & Moeller, 2002). However, magnetic resonance imaging (MRI) is superior to CT in documenting most pathology associated with TBI, because of its sensitivity to both focal lesions and diffuse axonal injury, and particularly the subacute and chronic changes that can occur across time following TBI (Bigler, 2003; Sigmund et al., 2007).

Numerous advanced imaging procedures have been developed to assess both structural and functional brain abnormalities in childhood TBI. An extensive review of these methods is beyond the scope of this chapter, but such reviews can be found in the literature (see Ashwal, in press; Ashwal, Holshouser, & Tong, 2006b; Munson, Schroth, & Ernst, 2006). Newer MRI technologies that show increased sensitivity to the structural effects of pediatric TBI include susceptibility-weighted MRI (Ashwal et al., 2006a; Babikian et al., 2005) and diffusion tensor imaging (Wilde et al., 2006; Yuan et al., 2007). Imaging techniques such as functional MRI (Kramer et al., 2008), proton magnetic resonance spectroscopy (Ashwal et al., 2006a; Babikian et al., 2006), positron emission tomography, and single-photon emission CT are able to assess brain function directly (Munson et al., 2006).

Neuroimaging studies in children with TBI generally indicate that the more prevalent the structural or functional abnormalities, the greater the morbidity (Brenner, Freier, Holshouser, Burley, & Ashwal, 2003). Moreover, studies have also shown predictable brain–behavior relationships in children with TBI. For instance, frontal lesions have been associated with poorer social outcomes (Levin et al., 2004), and brain activation on working memory tasks is altered in frontal regions following TBI (Newsome et al., 2008). However, research also suggests that brain–behavior relationships based on adult models are not necessarily applicable after childhood TBI. For instance, frontal lesion volume is not a consistent predictor of attention or executive function (Power, Catroppa, Coleman, Ditchfield, & Anderson, 2007; Slomine et al., 2002), and lesions within the frontotemporal regions are not stronger predictors of memory performance than lesions outside those regions (Salorio et al., 2005). Taken together, these studies suggest that brain–behavior relationships in children may differ from those in adults.

In addition to neuroimaging, other potential indices of injury severity include serum biomarkers, such as S100B and neuron-specific enolase, that may be tied to the neuro-chemical cascade occurring in TBI (Berger, Adelson, Richichi, & Kochanek, 2006; Shore et al., 2007). The use of biomarkers may be particularly important for diagnosing TBI in young children, for whom conventional indices such as the Glasgow Coma Scale are often invalid, and for children with inflicted TBI, who may suffer head trauma that is not disclosed (Berger, Hayes, Wang, & Kochanek, in press; Berger, Ta'Asan, Rand, Lokshin, & Kochanek, 2009).

Non-Injury-Related Influences

Most previous studies of the prediction of recovery following childhood TBI have emphasized injury-related variables, even though injury severity fails to account for most of the variance in postinjury outcomes (Fletcher et al., 1995). Recently, however, research has begun to focus on non-injury-related influences on recovery. For instance, children's premorbid functioning may be an important determinant of the outcomes of childhood TBI. We (Yeates et al., 2005) showed that premorbid attention problems increased the risk of an increase in postinjury attention problems among children with moderate to severe TBI. Findings such as this are consistent with theories of cognitive and brain reserve capacity, which suggest that children's vulnerability to neurological insults varies as a function of their preinjury cognitive abilities and brain integrity (Dennis, 2000; Dennis, Yeates, Taylor, & Fletcher, 2007).

Environmental influences are another potential source of non-injury-related variance in outcomes. Research suggests that a child's environment is a significant predictor of the outcomes following TBI. General measures of socioeconomic status and family demographics are consistent predictors of outcomes, as are more specific measures of family status and the social environment (Taylor et al., 1999, 2002; Yeates et al., 1997, 2004). One critical issue addressed by studies of environmental factors as determinants of recovery is whether the environment affects the functioning of children with TBI in the same way that it does the functioning of children without such injuries, or whether it moderates the impact of TBI by buffering or exacerbating its direct, neurologically based consequences. In a prospective, longitudinal study designed to examine the role of the family and social environment as determinants of children's recovery from TBI, measures of both pre- and postinjury family status were shown to moderate outcomes (Taylor et al., 1999, 2002; Yeates et al., 1997, 2004). Specifically, the effects of severe TBI relative to orthopedic injuries were more pronounced for children from dysfunctional families than for children from more functional families. Interestingly, this pattern was observed for both cognitive and behavioral measures—although the relative importance of injury severity and family environment varied across the two outcome domains, with injury severity playing a larger role for cognitive outcomes, and the family environment assuming more importance for behavioral and functional outcomes.

Another potentially critical influence on children's recovery from TBI is the treatment they receive, ranging from acute medical care to ongoing rehabilitation and education. Guidelines exist for the acute medical management of childhood TBI, but are by and large not based on rigorous evaluation through randomized controlled trials (Adelson et al., 2003; Jankowitz & Adelson, 2006; McLean et al., 1995). Thus we do not know whether or how acute medical care affects long-term outcomes. Comprehensive reviews of the inpatient and outpatient rehabilitation of children with TBI have been published, but again these highlight the relative paucity of empirical evidence (Anderson & Catroppa, 2006; Beaulieu, 2002; Ylvisaker et al., 2005a). Even less is known regarding the effectiveness of educational interventions for children with TBI (Ylvisaker et al., 2001). The inclusion of family members in the rehabilitation of children with TBI has been supported by many studies (Braga, Da Paz Júnior, & Ylvisaker, 2005; Wade, in press), as has the integration of home and school services following discharge from inpatient rehabilitation (Ylvisaker et al., 2005a).

Research regarding treatments for the psychosocial and cognitive sequelae of pediatric TBI is also relatively limited (Donders, 2007). Surprisingly little is known regarding the effectiveness of psychotropic medications for managing behavioral or cognitive difficulties, and most of the existing literature pertains to adults rather than children (Deb & Crownshaw, 2004; Tenovuo, 2006). Studies of the effectiveness of psychological and behavioral treatments following pediatric TBI are also rare. Empirical support exists for treatments of behavioral and social problems following pediatric TBI (Ylvisaker, Turkstra, & Coelho, 2005b; Ylvisaker et al., 2007). More specifically, operant conditioning has been found to be effective in decreasing aggressive behaviors following TBI in children and adolescents, and school-based social interventions have received empirical support as well (Warschausky, Kewman, & Kay, 1999). In contrast, few studies have focused on treatments for internalizing problems (i.e., depression and anxiety) following TBI.

Cognitive remediation programs have been developed for pediatric TBI, but few have been the focus of empirical validation (Butler, 2007; Van't Hooft, in press). Laatsch et al. (2007) conducted an evidence-based review of cognitive and behavioral treatment studies of pediatric TBI and determined that cognitive remediation for attention skills is supported by the literature, as is the involvement of family members as active members of the treatment team. Catroppa and Anderson (2006) conducted a review of intervention studies of executive deficits following childhood TBI and concluded that few methodologically sound outcome studies had been conducted in this area, although they found limited support for specific interventions.

Developmental Variation

The outcomes associated with childhood TBI depend not only on injury characteristics and various non-injury-related influences, but also on developmental factors. Research suggests that outcomes can vary along three distinct but interrelated age-related dimensions: the age of the child at the time of injury, the amount of time that has passed since the injury, and the child's age at the time of outcome assessment (Taylor & Alden, 1997).

Most studies of childhood TBI have focused on school-age children and adolescents. Across this age range, age at injury has not been found to be strongly related to outcomes. In contrast, studies of preschool children suggest that injuries sustained during infancy or early childhood are associated with more persistent deficits than are injuries occurring during later childhood and adolescence (Anderson et al., 2005a; Ewing-Cobbs et al.,

1997, 2006). Even mild TBI may have particularly deleterious effects for preschool children (Gronwall, Wrightson, & McGinn, 1997).

Longitudinal research on the relationship of time since injury to the outcomes of TBI suggests that children generally display a gradual recovery over the first few years after injury, with the most rapid improvement occurring soon after the injury (Yeates et al., 2002). The initial rate of recovery is often more rapid among children with severe TBI than among those with mild TBI, although severe injuries are also more likely to be associated with persistent deficits after the rate of recovery slows (Fay et al., 2009). Recent studies of long-term outcomes 5 or more years after injury suggest that children with severe TBI rarely show any progressive deterioration in neuropsychological functioning relative to noninjured peers after their initial recovery, despite clinical lore to the contrary (Cattelani, Lombardi, Brianti, & Mazzucchi, 1998; Jonsson, Horneman, & Emanuelson, 2004; Klonoff, Clark, & Klonoff, 1995). On the other hand, the rate of recovery varies as a function of factors other than injury severity, including age at injury. More specifically, younger children appear to demonstrate a slower rate of change over time and more significant residual deficits after their recovery plateaus than do older children with injuries of equivalent severity (Catroppa, Anderson, Morse, Haritou, & Rosenfeld, 2008; Koskiniemi, Kyykka, Nybo, & Jarho, 1995).

Of the three age-related dimensions potentially related to outcomes, the influence of age at testing has been the focus of the least research. The effects of age at testing would be reflected in latent or delayed sequelae resulting from children's failure to meet new developmental demands following a head injury. The demonstration of such effects will be difficult, because it requires evidence that differences in the consequences of pediatric TBI are due specifically to age at testing, as opposed to age at injury or time since injury—and it is difficult to disentangle these dimensions, even in the context of longitudinal research (Taylor & Alden, 1997).

METHODOLOGICAL CRITIQUE OF EXISTING RESEARCH

Sample Selection, Recruitment, and Attrition

Many previous studies on TBI suffer from shortcomings in the selection and recruitment of research participants. Children with TBI have sometimes been selected retrospectively, based on admission to a rehabilitation facility or referral for neuropsychological evaluation (e.g., Yeates et al., 1995a). Samples selected on this basis are likely to differ in important ways from samples that are recruited prospectively from consecutive admissions to a large hospital or trauma center. The latter method of recruitment is more likely to yield representative groups of children with TBI.

Even when samples are recruited prospectively from consecutive cases, they may not be representative of the larger population from which they are drawn, or they may become unrepresentative because of selective attrition over time. The agreement to participate in scientific research is not a random decision, nor is the decision to discontinue participation. However, relatively few studies report participation rates, much less compare participants and nonparticipants in terms of family demographics or child injury characteristics, to determine whether study participation introduces bias into sample selection. Similarly, few studies have compared children who are available for follow-up to those who drop out, to determine whether attrition affects the outcomes studied (Francis, Copeland, & Moore, 1994). Statistical procedures such as pattern-mixture analysis can be used to determine whether attrition is likely to have biased study results (Hedeker & Gibbons, 1997).

The selection of comparison groups in research on TBI has also been problematic. In some cases, children with mild TBI have been used as a comparison group, despite ongoing controversy regarding the outcomes associated with mild TBI (Satz et al., 1997; Yeates et al., 2009). In other cases, noninjured children matched for age, gender, and other demographic variables have been used as a comparison group (Jaffe, Polissar, Fay, & Liao, 1995). Noninjured children may not constitute the best comparison group, however, because they are not equated to children with TBI in terms of the experience of a traumatic injury or ensuing medical treatment. To the extent that traumatic injuries do not occur at random, moreover, noninjured children may also differ from children with TBI in various premorbid characteristics that are not controlled for by matching on demographic factors alone. Several studies suggest that children who sustain injuries are more likely to display preexisting behavioral, developmental, and learning problems than children who are not injured (Asarnow et al., 1995; Bijur & Haslum, 1995); they are also more likely to come from families that are more socially disadvantaged, as well as more stressed and less cohesive (Christoffel, Donovan, Schofer, Wills, & Lavigne, 1996; Howard, Joseph, & Natale, 2005; Parslow et al., 2005). Background differences between children with TBI and noninjured controls or between children with TBI of varying severities are not reported in all studies (Anderson et al., 1997). Nevertheless, a comparison group of children who have sustained injuries not involving the head and who have undergone comparable medical treatment is often regarded as desirable.

Measurement

Injury Characteristics

A substantial amount of the variability in the literature on TBI is attributable to differences in the characterization of injury severity. Although measures of injury severity are usually correlated, differences in how and when severity is assessed have increased the variability in results across studies. Greater uniformity in the assessment of severity would allow more meaningful cross-study comparisons (Saatman et al., 2008). Future studies are likely to need to incorporate multidimensional approaches to classifying severity that incorporate clinical indicators, neuroimaging, and possibly biomarkers.

Specific criticisms can be raised about each of the clinical indices of injury severity described earlier. The Glasgow Coma Scale (see Table 5.1) is problematic when used with infants and young children, despite attempts to make suitable modifications (Durham et al., 2000). The timing of assessment is also of concern when the Glasgow Coma Scale is used, because scores vary over time, and are not always lowest at the scene of an accident or upon arrival at a hospital.

The duration of impaired consciousness can be difficult to assess reliably, because it is often measured retrospectively, based on clinical assessments by nursing staff or physicians. Similarly, in many studies PTA has been assessed based on retrospective reports from caretakers, such as health care providers or parents. Prospective administration of standardized instruments such as the COAT (Ewing-Cobbs et al., 1990) can provide a more reliable and objective measure of PTA.

As noted earlier, advances in neuroimaging have now begun to permit the characterization of injury severity based on underlying neuropathology, as opposed to clinical indicators. The advent of more advanced structural imaging techniques, such as susceptibility-weighted imaging and diffusion tensor imaging, as well as functional imaging techniques, such as functional MRI and proton magnetic resonance spectroscopy, should provide a much more precise measures of both the diffuse and focal neuropathology associated with TBI. These measurements can in turn be used to predict neurobehavioral outcomes (Levin et al., 1993, 2004; Newsome et al., 2008).

Non-Injury-Related Influences

The literature on TBI in children has paid increasing attention to the influence of non-injury-related factors on morbidity. Outcomes such as behavioral adjustment and adaptive functioning are not as strongly related to injury severity as cognitive functioning is; they appear to be more dependent on such factors as children's premorbid status and family functioning (Fletcher et al., 1990; Taylor et al., 1999, 2002; Yeates et al., 2005). Future research should increasingly incorporate measures of children's premorbid status, including genetic differences (Moran et al., in press), that are likely to moderate the effects of TBI. Research will also need to incorporate more detailed measures of children's environments to determine the mechanisms by which these environments affect the outcomes of childhood TBI. Recent research on parenting skills in preschool children with TBI provides an example of such an approach (Wade et al., 2008).

The existing literature can be further criticized for failing to assess the effectiveness of the interventions used to manage TBI. The conduct of clinical trials in children with TBI is challenging (Adelson, in press; Natale, Joseph, Pretzlaff, Silber, & Guerguerian, 2005), but trials are badly needed to evaluate the efficacy and effectiveness of potential medical treatments, such as hypothermia (Adelson, 2009). Research is also required to test the benefits of postacute medical interventions, such as psychotropic or anticonvulsant medications, rehabilitative and educational programs, and psychological and behavioral interventions targeted to children and their families (Wade, in press). Indeed, the need for intervention research focusing on childhood TBI is glaring.

Outcomes

The outcome measures used in studies of pediatric TBI often suffer from limitations. Most outcome measures can be classified into one of three categories: clinical judgments, psychometric tests, and rating scales and interviews (Fletcher, Ewing-Cobbs, Francis, & Levin, 1995). Clinical judgments, such as those reflected in the Glasgow Outcome Scale (Jennett & Bond, 1975), often lack sensitivity to more subtle differences in outcomes. Compared to clinical judgments, psychometric tests generally provide more reliable and sensitive outcome measures. The interpretation of psychometric results is complicated, however, by the multifactorial nature of test performance. Tests that are designed to assess specific aspects of skill deficits, or that employ experimental manipulations of task demands, may yield more precise information about the nature and brain basis of cognitive sequelae of TBI (Taylor, in press).

Psychometric testing often cannot be used to assess some of the most important outcomes following TBI, including social competence, behavioral adjustment, and adaptive functioning. The latter outcomes are generally assessed with rating scales and interviews. As noted earlier, however, many commonly used rating scales, such as the Child Behavior Checklist (Achenbach & Rescorla, 2001), were not developed for use with children with TBI and may prove misleading or insensitive when used in this population (Drotar et al., 1995; Perrin et al., 1991). The use of rating scales that are more specifically targeted to children with TBI may be more informative (Yeates et al., 2001).

Another shortcoming is the restricted range of outcomes assessed in studies of childhood TBI. Outcomes that have been assessed include cognitive functioning, behavioral adjustment, and adaptive functioning. Less attention has been paid to other important outcomes, such as emotional and social functioning (Yeates et al., 2007), family functioning (Taylor et al., 1995; Wade et al., 2006), school performance (Taylor et al., 2003), or quality of life (McCarthy et al., 2006). These outcomes are not strongly related to children's cognitive abilities and are more likely to be moderated by contextual demands and supports.

Mechanisms of Effects

Most of the previous research on childhood TBI has been descriptive (Fletcher, 1995). Few studies have attempted to explain the mechanisms that underlie the sequelae of TBI in children (Taylor, in press). For instance, we do not know why younger children display less recovery from TBI than older children, although research on nonhuman animals suggests that important differences in neural plasticity may play a role (Bittigau et al., 1999; Giza & Prins, 2006). Future studies that investigate causal mechanisms will need to draw on theoretical models of brain–behavior relationships, developmental approaches to the outcomes of childhood brain disorders (Taylor & Alden, 1997), and experimental paradigms based on research on brain injury in nonhuman animals (Kolb, Gibb, & Robinson, 2003). The models and methods used to study causal mechanisms will also need to incorporate broader frameworks that acknowledge the role of non-injury-related influences in development (e.g., Dennis, 2000; Yeates et al., 2007).

Assessment of Recovery and Analysis of Change

Most previous studies of childhood TBI have employed cross-sectional designs. The use of cross-sectional designs precludes investigation of the process of postinjury recovery of function. Longitudinal studies are needed to examine recovery over time and to determine the relative importance of age at injury and time since injury as predictors of outcomes (Taylor & Alden, 1997). Previous longitudinal studies, moreover, have followed children for relatively brief periods. Prospective longitudinal investigations that are of much longer duration are needed to document the long-term outcomes of childhood TBI, not only in later childhood and adolescence, but also into adulthood (Klonoff et al., 1995).

Existing longitudinal studies also can be criticized for failing to adopt a developmental approach in modeling the process of recovery. Traditional approaches to data analysis in longitudinal designs, which rely on repeated-measures analyses of variance, view outcomes as static endpoints. These approaches model change as a group phenomenon that is incremental in nature, with individual differences in change treated as error variance. They reflect a variable-centered approach to data analysis, which focuses on the significance of group differences in means. Because development and recovery in children inherently involve change that is continuous and heterogeneous in nature, individual differences in developmental change should represent a major focus in studies of childhood TBI. Research should begin to incorporate alternative statistical methods that reflect a person-centered approach (Laursen & Hoff, 2006).

Growth curve modeling and related statistical approaches permits the investigation of change at an individual level (Francis, Fletcher, Stuebing, Davidson, & Thompson, 1991). In this approach, intraindividual change is conceptualized in terms of growth curves that quantify the rate of development, changes in that rate over time, and the eventual level of outcome. The role of injury-related and other factors as determinants of recovery from TBI can be studied by analyzing rates of change and levels of outcomes separately for individual children and collectively for groups of children (Thompson et al., 1994; Yeates et al., 1997).

Mixture modeling is another approach that can be used to examine intraindividual change. It can be used to empirically identify latent classes of individuals based on different developmental trajectories (Nagin, 1999). Figure 5.1 provides an example of this approach; it shows distinct developmental trajectories of postconcussive symptoms in children with mild TBI (Yeates et al., 2009). In this study, children with mild TBI were more likely than

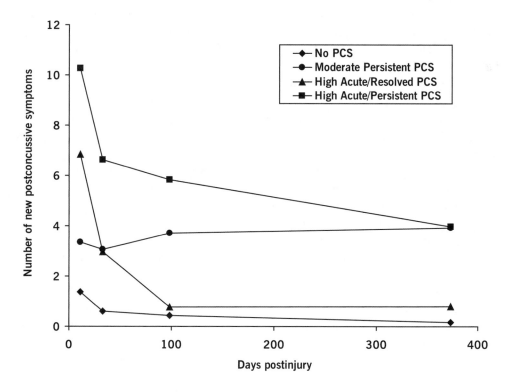

FIGURE 5.1. Postconcussive symptom trajectory groups in children with mild TBI and orthopedic injuries. From Yeates et al., 2009. Copyright 2009 by the American Academy of Pediatrics. Reprinted by permission.

those with orthopedic injuries to demonstrate the two trajectories involving high acute levels of symptoms, and the differences were particularly pronounced for children with mild TBI whose acute clinical presentation reflected more severe injury.

FUTURE DIRECTIONS

The preceding critique indicates a number of potential avenues for future research on childhood TBI. For instance, additional studies are needed of outcomes in domains other than cognitive and behavioral functioning. Of particular importance will be studies examining children's general adaptation to their environment. At this time, we know relatively little about the implications of TBI for school placement, friendships and peer relationships, health care utilization, or overall quality of life. Studies are also needed that examine the links between neuropsychological abilities and these more functional outcomes, to determine the ecological validity of neuropsychological assessment in childhood TBI (Farmer & Eakman, 1995).

Research regarding the neural substrates of the neuropsychological deficits that occur in childhood TBI is needed as well. Studies that capitalize on advances in neuroimaging to measure underlying neuropathology, and that correlate these measures with assessments of neuropsychological functioning, will enhance our understanding of the predictors and outcomes of TBI. Such research also will provide more general insights into the nature of brain–behavior relationships in children.

Studies of the brain–behavior relationships following TBI should not be conducted without also considering a child's broader environment as a predictor of outcomes. A growing literature has clearly demonstrated that measures of the family and social environment are related to the outcomes of TBI, and that these environmental factors often act in concert with injury-related factors to determine eventual outcomes (Taylor et al., 2002; Yeates et al., 2002, 2004). Future research is needed to clarify which aspects of the environment influence which outcomes, and to delineate the mechanisms by which the environment affects children's functioning.

In addition, research efforts must incorporate a developmental perspective reflecting the complex interplay of age-related factors in neurobehavioral outcomes. Studies are needed that follow children for extended periods of time after injury, and preferably into adulthood. Prospective, longitudinal studies that follow children over a period of years will allow us to move beyond the characterization of group differences in outcomes toward a better understanding of individual recovery and the influences on this process. In so doing, research will provide a more thorough understanding of the variability in outcomes that characterize children with TBI.

Finally, future research on pediatric TBI will need to occur outside traditional academic silos. Research is needed that is integrative, cutting across domains or disciplines, as well as translational, promoting the application of knowledge to clinical care. The scientific advances that have occurred within domains are not likely to result in significant progress in the clinical management of children with TBI until they become the topics of collaborative research that cuts across multiple levels of analysis. Thus the time appears to be ripe for interdisciplinary efforts that promote integrative and translational research (Anderson & Yeates, in press).

REFERENCES

Achenbach, T. M., & Rescorla, L. A. (2001). *Integrative guide for the 1991 CBCL/6–18, YSR, and TRF profiles*. Burlington: University of Vermont, Department of Psychiatry.

Adelson, P. D. (2009). Hypothermia following pediatric traumatic brain injury. *Journal of Neurotrauma*, 26, 429–436.

Adelson, P. D. (in press). Clinical trials and pediatric traumatic brain injury. In V. A. Anderson & K. O. Yeates (Eds.), *Pediatric traumatic brain injury: New directions in clinical and translational research*. New York: Oxford University Press.

Adelson, P. D., Bratton, S. L., Carney, N. A., Chesnut, R. M., du Coudray, H. E., Goldstein, B., et al. (2003). Guidelines for the acute medical management of severe traumatic brain injury in infants, children, and adolescents. Chapter 1: Introduction. *Pediatric Critical Care Medicine*, 4(Suppl. 3), S2–S4.

American Psychiatric Association. (2000). *Diagnostic and statistical manual of mental disorders* (4th ed., text rev.). Washington, DC: Author.

Anderson, V., & Catroppa, C. (2005). Recovery of executive skills following paediatric traumatic brain injury (TBI): A 2 year follow-up. *Brain Injury*, 19, 459–470.

Anderson, V., & Catroppa, C. (2006). Advances in postacute rehabilitation after childhood acquired brain injury: A focus on cognitive, behavioral, and social domains. *American Journal of Physical Medicine and Rehabilitation*, 85, 767–778.

Anderson, V. A., Catroppa, C., Morse, S., Haritou, F., & Rosenfeld, J. (2005a). Functional plasticity or vulnerability after early brain injury? *Pediatrics*, 116, 1374–1382.

Anderson, V., Catroppa, C., Morse, S., Haritou, F., & Rosenfeld, J. (2005b). Identifying factors contributing to child and family outcome at 30 months following traumatic brain injury in children. *Journal of Neurology, Neurosurgery and Psychiatry*, 76, 401–408.

Anderson, V., Fenwick, T., Manly, T., & Robertson, I. (1998). Attentional skills following traumatic brain injury in childhood: A componential analysis. *Brain Injury*, 12, 937–949.

Anderson, V. A., Morse, S., Catroppa, C., Haritou, F., & Rosenfeld, J. (2004). Thirty month outcome from early childhood head injury: A prospective analysis of neurobehavioural recovery. *Brain*, 127, 2608–2620.

Anderson, V. A., Morse, S. A., Klug, G., Catroppa, C., Haritou, F., Rosenfeld, J. V., et al. (1997). Predicting recovery from head injury in young children: A prospective analysis. *Journal of the International Neuropsychological Society*, 3, 568–580.

Anderson, V. A., & Yeates, K. O. (Eds.). (in press). *Pediatric traumatic brain injury: New directions in clinical and translational research*. New York: Oxford University Press.

Andrews, T. K., Rose, F. D., & Johnson, D. A. (1998). Social and behavioural effects of traumatic brain injury in children. *Brain Injury*, 12, 133–138.

Asarnow, R. F., Satz, P., Light, R., Zaucha, K., Lewis, R., & McCleary, C. (1995). The UCLA study of mild closed head injuries in children and adolescents. In S. H. Broman & M. E. Michel (Eds.), *Traumatic head injury in children* (pp. 117–146). New York: Oxford University Press.

Ashwal, S. (in press). Neuroimaging in pediatric traumatic brain injury. In V. A. Anderson & K. O. Yeates (Eds.), *Pediatric traumatic brain injury: New directions in clinical and translational research*. New York: Oxford University Press.

Ashwal, S., Babikian, T., Gardner-Nichols, J., Freier, M. C., Tong, K. A., & Holshouser, B. A. (2006a). Susceptibility-weighted imaging and proton magnetic resonance spectroscopy in assessment of outcome after pediatric traumatic brain injury. *Archives of Physical Medicine and Rehabilitation*, 87, 50–58.

Ashwal, S., Holshouser, B. A., & Tong, K. A. (2006b). Use of advanced neuroimaging techniques in the evaluation of pediatric traumatic brain injury. *Developmental Neuroscience*, 28, 309–326.

Babikian, T., Freier, M. C., Ashwal, S., Riggs, M. L., Burley, T., & Holshouser, B. A. (2006). MR spectroscopy: Predicting long-term neuropsychological outcome following pediatric TBI. *Journal of Magnetic Resonance Imaging*, 24, 801–811.

Babikian, T., Freier, M. C., Tong, K. A., Nickerson, J. P., Wall, C. J., Holshouser, B. A., et al. (2005). Susceptibility weighted imaging: Neuropsychologic outcome and pediatric head injury. *Pediatric Neurology, 33,* 184–94.

Bawden, H. N., Knights, R. M., & Winogron, H. W. (1985). Speeded performance following head injury in children. *Journal of Clinical Neuropsychology, 7,* 39–54.

Beaulieu, C. L. (2002). Rehabilitation and outcome following pediatric traumatic brain injury. *Surgical Clinics of North America, 82,* 393–408.

Berger, R. P., Adelson, P. D., Richichi, R., & Kochanek, P. M. (2006). Serum biomarkers after traumatic and hypoxemic brain injuries: Insights into the biochemical response of the pediatric brain to inflicted brain injury. *Developmental Neuroscience, 28,* 327–335.

Berger, R. P., Hayes, R. L., Wang, K. K. W., & Kochanek, P. (in press). Using serum biomarkers to diagnose, assess, treat and predict outcome after pediatric TBI. In V. A. Anderson & K. O. Yeates (Eds.), *Pediatric traumatic brain injury: New directions in clinical and translational research.* New York: Oxford University Press.

Berger, R. P., Ta'Asan, S., Rand, R., Lokshin, A., & Kochanek, P. (2009). Multiplex assessment of serum biomarker concentrations in well-appearing children with inflicted brain injury. *Pediatric Research, 65,* 97–102.

Bigler, E. D. (1999). Neuroimaging in pediatric traumatic head injury: Diagnostic considerations and relationships to neurobehavioral outcome. *Journal of Head Trauma Rehabilitation, 14,* 406–423.

Bigler, E. D. (2003). Neurobiology and neuropathology underlie the neuropsychological deficits associated with traumatic brain injury. *Archives of Clinical Neuropsychology, 18,* 595–621.

Bigler, E. D. (2007). Anterior and middle cranial fossa in traumatic brain injury: Relevant neuroanatomy and neuropathology in the study of neuropsychological outcome. *Neuropsychology, 21,* 515–531.

Bigler, E. D. (2008). Neuropsychology and clinical neuroscience of persistent post-concussive syndrome. *Journal of the International Neuropsychological Society, 14,* 1–22.

Bijur, P. E., & Haslum, M. (1995). Cognitive, behavioral, and motoric sequelae of mild head injury in a national birth cohort. In S. H. Broman & M. E. Michel (Eds.), *Traumatic head injury in children* (pp. 147–164). New York: Oxford University Press.

Bittigau, P., Sifringer, M., Pohl, D., Stadrhaus, D., Ishimaru, M., Shimizu, H., et al. (1999). Apoptotic neurodegeneration following trauma is markedly enhanced in the immature brain. *Annals of Neurology, 45,* 724–735.

Bloom, D. R., Levin, H. S., Ewing-Cobbs, L., Saunders, A. E., Song, J., Fletcher, J. M., et al. (2001). Lifetime and novel psychiatric disorders after pediatric traumatic brain injury. *Journal of the American Academy of Child and Adolescent Psychiatry, 40,* 572–579.

Bodin, S. D., & Yeates, K. O. (in press). Traumatic brain injury. In R. J. Shaw & D. R. DeMaso (Eds.), *Textbook of pediatric psychosomatic medicine: Consultation on physically ill children.* Washington, DC: American Psychiatric Publishing.

Bohnert, A. M., Parker, J. G., & Warschausky, S. A. (1997). Friendship and social adjustment of children following a traumatic brain injury: An exploratory investigation. *Developmental Neuropsychology, 13,* 477–486.

Braga, L. W., Da Paz Júnior, A. C., & Ylvisaker, M. (2005). Direct clinician-delivered versus indirect family-supported rehabilitation of children with traumatic brain injury: A randomized controlled trial. *Brain Injury, 19,* 819–831.

Brenner, T., Freier, M. C., Holshouser, B. A., Burley, T., & Ashwal, S. (2003). Predicting neuropsychologic outcome after traumatic brain injury in children. *Pediatric Neurology, 28,* 104–114.

Bruce, D. A. (1995). Pathophysiological responses of the child's brain. In S. H. Broman & M. E. Michel (Eds.), *Traumatic head injury in children* (pp. 40–51). New York: Oxford University Press.

Butler, R. W. (2007). Cognitive rehabilitation. In S. J. Hunter & J. Donders (Eds.), *Pediatric neuropsychological intervention* (pp. 444–464). New York: Cambridge University Press.

Catroppa, C., & Anderson, V. (2002). Recovery in memory function in the first year following TBI in children. *Brain Injury, 16,* 369–384.

Catroppa, C., & Anderson, V. (2004). Recovery and predictors of language skills two years following pediatric traumatic brain injury. *Brain and Language, 88*, 68–78.

Catroppa, C., & Anderson, V. (2005). A prospective study of the recovery of attention from acute to 2 years post pediatric traumatic brain injury. *Journal of the International Neuropsychological Society, 11*, 84–98.

Catroppa, C., & Anderson, V. (2006). Planning, problem-solving, and organizational abilities in children following traumatic brain injury: Intervention techniques. *Pediatric Rehabilitation, 9*, 89–97.

Catroppa, C., & Anderson, V. (2007). Recovery in memory function, and its relationship to academic success, at 24 months following pediatric TBI. *Child Neuropsychology, 13*, 240–261.

Catroppa, C., Anderson, V. A., Morse, S. A., Haritou, F., & Rosenfeld, J. V. (2007). Children's attentional skills 5 years post-TBI. *Journal of Pediatric Psychology, 32*, 354–369.

Catroppa, C., Anderson, V. A., Morse, S. A., Haritou, F., & Rosenfeld, J. V. (2008). Outcome and predictors of functional recovery 5 years following pediatric traumatic brain injury. *Journal of Pediatric Psychology, 33*, 707–718.

Cattelani, R., Lombardi, F., Brianti, R., & Mazzucchi, A. (1998). Traumatic brain injury in childhood: Intellectual, behavioural and social outcome into adulthood. *Brain Injury, 12*, 283–296.

Chadwick, O., Rutter, M., Brown, G., Shaffer, D., & Traub, M. (1981). A prospective study of children with head injuries: II. Cognitive sequelae. *Psychological Medicine, 11*, 49–61.

Chapman, S. B. (1995). Discourse as an outcome measure in pediatric head-injured populations. In S. H. Broman & M. E. Michel (Eds.), *Traumatic head injury in children* (pp. 95–116). New York: Oxford University Press.

Chapman, S. B., Sparks, G., Levin, H. S., Dennis, M., Roncadin, C., Zhang, L., et al. (2004). Discourse macrolevel processing after severe pediatric traumatic brain injury. *Developmental Neuropsychology, 25*, 37–60.

Christoffel, K., Donovan, M., Schofer, J., Wills, K., & Lavigne, J. (1996). Psychosocial factors in childhood pedestrian injury: A matched case–control study. *Pediatrics, 97*, 33–42.

Deb, S., & Crownshaw, T. (2004). The role of pharmacotherapy in the management of behaviour disorders in traumatic brain injury patients. *Brain Injury, 18*, 1–31.

Dennis, M. (2000). Childhood medical disorders and cognitive impairment: Biological risk, time, development, and reserve. In K. O. Yeates, M. D. Ris, & H. G. Taylor (Eds.), *Pediatric neuropsychology: Research, theory, and practice* (pp. 3–22). New York: Guilford Press.

Dennis, M., & Barnes, M. A. (1990). Knowing the meaning, getting the point, bridging the gap, and carrying the message: Aspects of discourse following closed head injury in childhood and adolescence. *Brain and Language, 39*, 428–446.

Dennis, M., Barnes, M. A., Wilkinson, M., & Humphreys, R. P. (1998). How children with head injury represent real and deceptive emotion in short narratives. *Brain and Language, 61*, 450–483.

Dennis, M., Guger, S., Roncadin, C., Barnes, M., & Schachar, R. (2001a). Attentional–inhibitory control and social-behavioral regulation after childhood closed head injury: Do biological, developmental, and recovery variables predict outcome? *Journal of the International Neuropsychological Society, 7*, 683–692.

Dennis, M., Purvis, K., Barnes, M. A., Wilkinson, M., & Winner, E. (2001b). Understanding of literal truth, ironic criticism, and deceptive praise following childhood head injury. *Brain and Language, 78*, 1–16.

Dennis, M., Wilkinson, M., Koski, L., & Humphreys, R. P. (1995). Attention deficits in the long term after childhood head injury. In S. H. Broman & M. E. Michel (Eds.), *Traumatic head injury in children* (pp. 165–187). New York: Oxford University Press.

Dennis, M., Yeates, K. O., Taylor, H. G., & Fletcher, J. M. (2007). Brain reserve capacity, cognitive reserve capacity, and age-based functional plasticity after congenital and acquired brain injury in children. In Y. Stern (Ed.), *Cognitive reserve* (pp. 53–83). New York: Taylor & Francis.

Donders, J. (2007). Traumatic brain injury. In S. J. Hunter & J. Donders (Eds.), *Pediatric neuropsychological intervention* (pp. 91–111). New York: Cambridge University Press.

Donders, J., & Janke, K. (2008). Criterion validity of the Wechsler Intelligence Scale for Children—Fourth Edition after pediatric traumatic brain injury. *Journal of the International Neuropsychological Society, 14*, 651–655.

Drotar, D., Stein, R. E. K., & Perrin, E. C. (1995). Methodological issues in using the Child Behavior Checklist and its related instruments in clinical child psychology research. *Journal of Clinical Child Psychology, 24*, 184–192.

Durham, S. R., Clancy, R. R., Leuthardt, E., Sun, P., Kamerling, S., Dominquez, T., et al. (2000). CHOP Infant Coma Scale ('Infant Face Scale'): A novel coma scale for children less than two years of age. *Journal of Neurotrauma, 17*, 729–737.

Ewing-Cobbs, L., & Barnes, M. (2002). Linguistic outcomes following traumatic brain injury in children. *Seminars in Pediatric Neurology, 9*, 209–217.

Ewing-Cobbs, L., Barnes, M., Fletcher, J. M., Levin, H. S., Swank, P. R., & Song, J. (2004a). Modeling of longitudinal academic achievement scores after pediatric traumatic brain injury. *Developmental Neuropsychology, 25*, 107–133.

Ewing-Cobbs, L., Fletcher, J. M., Levin, H. S., Francis, D. J., Davidson, K., & Miner, M. E. (1997). Longitudinal neuropsychological outcome in infants and preschoolers with TBI. *Journal of the International Neuropsychological Society, 3*, 581–591.

Ewing-Cobbs, L., Fletcher, J. M., Levin, H. S., Hastings, P. Z., & Francis, D. J. (1996). Assessment of injury severity following closed head injury in children: Methodological issues. *Journal of the International Neuropsychological Society, 2*, 39.

Ewing-Cobbs, L., Fletcher, J. M., Levin, H. S., Iovino, I., & Miner, M. E. (1998a). Academic achievement and academic placement following traumatic brain injury in children and adolescents: A two-year longitudinal study. *Journal of Clinical and Experimental Neuropsychology, 20*, 769–781.

Ewing-Cobbs, L., Levin, H. S., Fletcher, J. M., Miner, M. E., & Eisenberg, H. M. (1990). The Children's Orientation and Amnesia Test: Relationship to severity of acute head injury and to recovery of memory. *Neurosurgery, 27*, 683–691.

Ewing-Cobbs, L., Prasad, M. R., Fletcher, J. M., Levin, H. S., Miner, M. E., & Eisenberg, H. M. (1998b). Attention after pediatric traumatic brain injury: A multidimensional assessment. *Child Neuropsychology, 4*, 35–48.

Ewing-Cobbs, L., Prasad, M. R., Kramer, L., Cox, C. S., Jr., Baumgartner, J., Fletcher, S., et al. (2006). Late intellectual and academic outcomes following traumatic brain injury sustained during early childhood. *Journal of Neurosurgery, 105*, 2887–2896.

Ewing-Cobbs, L., Prasad, M. R., Landry, S. H., Kramer, L., & DeLeon, R. (2004b). Executive functions following traumatic brain injury in young children: A preliminary analysis. *Developmental Neuropsychology, 26*, 487–512.

Farkas, O., & Povlishock, J. T. (2007). Cellular and subcellular change evoked by diffuse traumatic brain injury: A complex web of change extending far beyond focal damage. *Progress in Brain Research, 161*, 43–59.

Farmer, J. E., & Eakman, A. M. (1995). The relationship between neuropsychological functioning and instrumental activities of daily living following acquired brain injury. *Applied Neuropsychology, 2*, 107–115.

Fay, T. B., Yeates, K. O., Wade, S. L., Drotar, D., Stancin, T., & Taylor, H. G. (2009). Predicting longitudinal patterns of functional deficits in children with traumatic brain injury. *Neuropsychology, 23*, 271–282.

Fletcher, J. M., Ewing-Cobbs, L., Francis, D. J., & Levin, H. S. (1995). Variability in outcomes after traumatic brain injury in children: A developmental perspective. In S. H. Broman & M. E. Michel (Eds.), *Traumatic head injury in children* (pp. 3–21). New York: Oxford University Press.

Fletcher, J. M., Ewing-Cobbs, L., Miner, M. E., Levin, H. S., & Eisenberg, H. M. (1990). Behavioral changes after closed head injury in children. *Journal of Consulting and Clinical Psychology, 58*, 93–98.

Francis, D. J., Copeland, D. R., & Moore, B. D. (1994). Neuropsychological changes in children with cancer: The treatment of missing data in longitudinal studies. *Neuropsychology Review, 4*, 199–222.

Francis, D. J., Fletcher, J. M., Stuebing, K. K., Davidson, K. C., & Thompson, N. M. (1991). Analysis of change: Modeling individual growth. *Journal of Consulting and Clinical Psychology, 59*, 27–37.

Ganesalingam, K., Sanson, A., Anderson, V., & Yeates, K. O. (2006). Self-regulation and social and behavioral functioning following childhood traumatic brain injury. *Journal of the International Neuropsychological Society, 12*, 609–621.

Ganesalingam, K., Sanson, A., Anderson, V., & Yeates, K. O. (2007). Self-regulation as a mediator of the effects of childhood traumatic brain injury on social and behavioral functioning. *Journal of the International Neuropsychological Society, 13*, 298–311.

Gerring, J. P., Brady, K. D., Chen, A., Vasa, R., Grados, M., Bandeen-Roche, K., et al. (1998). Premorbid prevalence of ADHD and development of secondary ADHD after closed head injury. *Journal of the American Academy of Child and Adolescent Psychiatry, 37*, 647–654.

Gerring, J. P., Slomine, B., Vasa, R. A., Grados, M., Chen, A., Rising, W., et al. (2002). Clinical predictors of posttraumatic stress disorder after closed head injury in children. *Journal of the American Academy of Child and Adolescent Psychiatry, 41*, 157–165.

Ghosh, A., Wilde, E. A., Hunter, J. V., Bigler, E. D., Chu, Z., Li, X., et al. (2009). The relation between Glasgow Coma Scale score and later cerebral atrophy in pediatric traumatic brain injury. *Brain Injury, 23*, 228–233.

Giza, C. C., & Hovda, D. (2001). The neurometabolic cascade of concussion. *Journal of Athletic Training, 36*, 228–235.

Giza, C. C., Mink, R. B., & Madikians, A. (2007) Pediatric traumatic brain injury: Not just little adults. *Current Opinions in Critical Care, 13*, 143–152.

Giza, C. C., & Prins, M. L. (2006). Is being plastic fantastic?: Mechanisms of altered plasticity after developmental traumatic brain injury. *Developmental Neuroscience, 28*, 364–379.

Grados, M. A., Vasa, R. A., Riddle, M. A., Slomine, B. S., Salorio, C., Christensen, J., et al. (2008). New onset obsessive–compulsive symptoms in children and adolescents with severe traumatic brain injury. *Depression and Anxiety, 25*, 398–407.

Gronwall, D., Wrightson, P., & McGinn, V. (1997). Effect of mild head injury during the preschool years. *Journal of the International Neuropsychological Society, 3*, 592–597.

Hanten, G., Wilde, E. A., Menefee, D. S., Li, X., Lane, S., Vasquez, C., et al. (2008). Correlates of social problem solving during the first year after traumatic brain injury in children. *Neuropsychology, 22*, 357–370.

Hedeker, D., & Gibbons, R. D. (1997). Application of random-effects pattern-mixture models for missing data in longitudinal studies. *Psychological Methods, 2*, 64–78.

Howard, I., Joseph, J. G., & Natale, J. E. (2005). Pediatric traumatic brain injury: Do racial/ethnic disparities exist in brain injury severity, mortality, or medical disposition? *Ethnicity and Disease, 15*, S551–S556.

Jaffe, K. M., Polissar, N. L., Fay, G. C., & Liao, S. (1995). Recovery trends over three years following pediatric traumatic brain injury. *Archives of Physical Medicine and Rehabilitation, 76*, 17–26.

Jankowitz, B. T., & Adelson, P. D. (2006). Pediatric traumatic brain injury: Past, present, and future. *Developmental Neuroscience, 28*, 264–275.

Janusz, J. A., Kirkwood, M. W., Yeates, K. O., & Taylor, H. G. (2002). Social problem-solving skills in children with traumatic brain injury: Long-term outcomes and prediction of social competence. *Child Neuropsychology, 8*, 179–194.

Jennett, B., & Bond, M. (1975). Assessment of outcome after severe brain damage: A practical scale. *Lancet, i*, 480–484.

Jonsson, C. A., Horneman, G., & Emanuelson, I. (2004). Neuropsychological progress during 14 years after severe traumatic brain injury in childhood and adolescence. *Brain Injury, 18*, 921–934.

Katz-Leurer, M., Rotem, H., Lewitus, H., Keren, O., & Meyer, S. (2008). Relationship between balance abilities and gait characteristics in children with post-traumatic brain injury. *Brain Injury, 22*, 153–159.

Keenan, H. T., & Bratton, S. L. (2006). Epidemiology and outcomes of pediatric traumatic brain injury. *Developmental Neuroscience, 28*, 256–263.

Kinsella, G., Prior, M., Sawyer, M., Murtagh, D., Eisenmajer, R., Anderson, V., et al. (1995). Neuropsychological deficit and academic performance in children and adolescents following TBI. *Journal of Pediatric Psychology, 20,* 753–767.

Kinsella, G., Prior, M., Sawyer, M., Ong, B., Murtagh, D., Eisenmajer, R., et al. (1997). Predictors and indicators of academic outcome in children 2 years following traumatic brain injury. *Journal of the International Neuropsychological Society, 3,* 608–616.

Kirkwood, M. W., Yeates, K. O., & Bernstein, J. H. (in press). Traumatic brain injury in childhood. In J. Donders & S. Hunter (Eds.), *Principles and practice of lifespan developmental neuropsychology.* New York: Cambridge University Press.

Kirkwood, M. W., Yeates, K. O., Taylor, H. G., Randolph, C., McCrea, M., & Anderson, V. A. (2008). Management of pediatric mild traumatic brain injury: A neuropsychological review from injury through recovery. *The Clinical Neuropsychologist, 22,* 769–800.

Klonoff, H., Clark, C., & Klonoff, P. S. (1995). Outcomes of head injuries from childhood to adulthood: A twenty-three year follow-up study. In S. H. Broman & M. E. Michel (Eds.), *Traumatic head injury in children* (pp. 219–234). New York: Oxford University Press.

Kochanek, P. M. (2006). Pediatric traumatic brain injury: Quo vadis? *Developmental Neuroscience, 28,* 244–255.

Koelfen, W., Freund, M., Dinter, D., Schmidt, B., Koenig, S., & Schultze, C. (1997). Long-term follow up of children with head injuries classified as "good recovery" using the Glasgow Outcome Scale: Neurological, neuropsychological, and magnetic resonance imaging results. *European Journal of Pediatrics, 156,* 230–235.

Kolb, B., Gibb, R., & Robinson, T. E. (2003). Brain plasticity and behavior. *Current Directions in Psychological Science, 12,* 1–5.

Koskiniemi, M., Kyykka, T., Nybo, T., & Jarho, L. (1995). Long-term outcome after severe brain injury in preschoolers is worse than expected. *Archives of Pediatrics and Adolescent Medicine, 149,* 249–254.

Kramer, M. E., Chiu, C. Y. P., Walz, N. C., Holland, S. K., Yuan, W., Karunanayaka, P., et al. (2008). Long-term neural processing of attention following early childhood traumatic brain injury: fMRI and neurobehavioral outcomes. *Journal of the International Neuropsychological Society, 14,* 424–235.

Kraus, J. F. (1995). Epidemiological features of brain injury in children: Occurrence, children at risk, causes and manner of injury, severity, and outcomes. In S. H. Broman & M. E. Michel (Eds.), *Traumatic head injury in children* (pp. 22–39). New York: Oxford University Press.

Kuhtz-Buschbeck, J. P., Hoppe, B., Golge, M., Dreesmann, M., Damm-Stunitz, U., & Ritz, A. (2003). Sensorimotor recovery in children after traumatic brain injury: Analyses of gait, gross motor, and fine motor skills. *Developmental Medicine and Child Neurology, 12,* 821–828.

Laatsch, L., Harrington, D., Hotz, G., Marcantuono, J., Mozzoni, M. P., Walsh, V., et al. (2007). An evidence-based review of cognitive and behavioral rehabilitation treatment studies in children with acquired brain injury. *Journal of Head Trauma Rehabilitation, 22,* 248–256.

Langlois, J. A., Kegler, S. R., Butler, J. A., Gotsch, K. E., Johnson, R. L., Reichard, A. A., et al. (2003). Traumatic brain injury-related hospital discharges: Results from a 14-state surveillance system, 1997. *Morbidity and Mortality Weekly Report, 52,* 1–18.

Langlois, J. A., Rutland-Brown, W., & Thomas, K. E. (2005). The incidence of traumatic brain injury among children in the United States: Differences by race. *Journal of Head Trauma Rehabilitation, 20,* 229–238.

Langlois, J. A., Rutland-Brown, W., & Thomas, K. E. (2006). *Traumatic brain injury in the United States: Emergency department visits, hospitalizations, and deaths.* Atlanta, GA: Centers for Disease Control and Prevention, National Center for Injury Prevention and Control.

Laursen, B., & Hoff, E. (2006). Person-centered and variable-centered approaches to longitudinal data. *Merrill–Palmer Quarterly, 52,* 377–389.

Lehnung, M., Leplow, B., Herzog, A., Benz, B., Ritz, A., Stolze, H., et al. (2001). Children's spatial behavior is differentially affected after traumatic brain injury. *Child Neuropsychology, 7,* 59–71.

Lescohier, I., & DiScala, C. (1993). Blunt trauma in children: Causes and outcomes of head versus extracranial injury. *Pediatrics, 91,* 721–725.

Levi, R. B., Drotar, D., Yeates, K. O., & Taylor, H. G. (1999). Posttraumatic stress symptoms in children following orthopedic or traumatic brain injury. *Journal of Clinical Child Psychology, 28,* 232–243.

Levin, H. S., Culhane, K. A., Mendelsohn, D., Lilly, M. A., Bruce, D., Fletcher, J. M., et al. (1993). Cognition in relation to magnetic resonance imaging in head-injured children and adolescents. *Archives of Neurology, 50,* 897–905.

Levin, H. S., & Eisenberg, H. M. (1979). Neuropsychological impairment after closed head injury in children and adolescents. *Journal of Pediatric Psychology, 4,* 389–402.

Levin, H. S., Fletcher, J. M., Kufera, J. A., Howard, H., Lilly, M. A., Mendelsohn, D., et al. (1996). Dimensions of cognition measured by the Tower of London and other cognitive tasks in head-injured children and adolescents. *Developmental Neuropsychology, 12,* 17–34.

Levin, H. S., & Hanten, G. (2005). Executive functions after traumatic brain injury in children. *Pediatric Neurology, 33,* 79–93.

Levin, H. S., Hanten, G., Max, J., Li, X., Swank, P., Ewing-Cobbs, L., et al. (2007). Symptoms of attention-deficit/hyperactivity disorder following traumatic brain injury in children. *Journal of Developmental and Behavioral Pediatrics, 28,* 108–118.

Levin, H. S., High, W. M., Ewing-Cobbs, L., Fletcher, J. M., Eisenberg, H. M., Miner, M. E., et al. (1988). Memory functioning during the first year after closed head injury in children and adolescents. *Neurosurgery, 22,* 1043–1052.

Levin, H. S., Madison, C. F., Bailey, C. B., Meyers, C. A., Eisenberg, H. M., & Guinto, F. C. (1983). Mutism after closed head injury. *Archives of Neurology, 40,* 601–606.

Levin, H. S., Mendelsohn, D., Lilly, M. A., Fletcher, J. M., Culhane, K. A., Chapman, S. B., et al. (1994). Tower of London performance in relation to magnetic resonance imaging following closed head injury in children. *Neuropsychology, 8,* 171–179.

Levin, H. S., Song, J., Scheibel, R. S., Fletcher, J. M., Harward, H., Lilly, M., et al. (1997). Concept formation and problem solving following closed head injury in children. *Journal of the International Neuropsychological Society, 3,* 598–607.

Levin, H. S., Zhang, L., Dennis, M., Ewing-Cobbs, L., Schachar, R., Max, J., et al. (2004). Psychosocial outcome of TBI in children with unilateral frontal lesions. *Journal of the International Neuropsychological Society, 10,* 305–316.

Light, R., Asarnow, R., Satz, P., Zaucha, K., McCleary, C., & Lewis, R. (1998). Mild TBI in children and adolescents: Behavior problems and academic outcomes. *Journal of Consulting and Clinical Psychology, 66,* 1023–1029.

Luis, C. A., & Mittenberg, W. (2002). Mood and anxiety disorders following pediatric traumatic brain injury: A prospective study. *Journal of Clinical and Experimental Neuropsychology, 24,* 270–279.

Mangeot, S., Armstrong, K., Colvin, A. N., Yeates, K. O., & Taylor, H. G. (2002). Long-term executive function deficits in children with traumatic brain injuries: Assessment using the Behavior Rating Inventory of Executive Function (BRIEF). *Child Neuropsychology, 8,* 271–284.

Margulies, S., & Coats, B. (in press). Biomechanics of pediatric traumatic brain injury. In V. A. Anderson & K. O. Yeates (Eds.), *Pediatric traumatic brain injury: New directions in clinical and translational research.* New York: Oxford University Press.

Marosszeky, N. E., Batchelor, J., Shores, E. A., Marosszeky, J. E., & Boonschate, M. (1993). The performance of hospitalised, non-head injured children on the Westmead PTA Scale. *The Clinical Neuropsychologist, 7,* 85–95.

Massagli, T. L., Fann, J. R., Burington, B. E., Jaffe, K. M., Katon, W. J., & Thompson, R. S. (2004). Psychiatric illness after mild traumatic brain injury in children. *Archives of Physical Medicine and Rehabilitation, 85,* 1428–1434.

Max, J. E., Castillo, C. S., Bokura, H., Robin, D. A., Lindgren, S. D., Smith, W. L., et al. (1998a). Oppositional defiant disorder symptomatology after traumatic brain injury: A prospective study. *Journal of Nervous and Mental Disease, 186,* 325–332.

Max, J. E., Castillo, C. S., Robin, D. A., Lindgren, S. D., Smith, W. L., Jr., Sato, Y., et al. (1998b). Posttraumatic stress symptomatology after childhood traumatic brain injury. *Journal of Nervous and Mental Disease, 186,* 589–596.

Max, J. E., Koele, S. L., Castillo, C. C., Lindgren, S. D., Arndt, S., Bokura, H., et al. (2000). Personality change disorder in children and adolescents following traumatic brain injury. *Journal of the International Neuropsychological Society, 6,* 279–289.

Max, J. E., Koele, S. L., Lindgren, S. D., Robin, D. A., Smith, W. L., Jr., Sato, Y., et al. (1998c). Adaptive functioning following traumatic brain injury and orthopedic injury: A controlled study. *Archives of Physical Medicine and Rehabilitation, 79,* 893–899.

Max, J. E., Levin, H. S., Landis, J., Schachar, R., Saunders, A., Ewing-Cobbs, L., et al. (2005a). Predictors of personality change due to traumatic brain injury in children and adolescents in the first six months after injury. *Journal of the American Academy of Child and Adolescent Psychiatry, 44,* 434–442.

Max, J. E., Lindgren, S. D., Robin, D. A., Smith, W. L., Sato, Y., Mattheis, P. J., et al. (1997a). TBI in children and adolescents: Psychiatric disorders in the second three months. *Journal of Nervous and Mental Disease, 185,* 394–401.

Max, J. E., Robertson, B. A., & Lansing, A. E. (2001). The phenomenology of personality change due to traumatic brain injury in children and adolescents. *Journal of Neuropsychiatry and Clinical Neuroscience, 13,* 161–170.

Max, J. E., Robin, D. A., Lindgren, S. D., Smith, W. L., Sato, Y., Mattheis, P. J., et al. (1997b). TBI in children and adolescents: Psychiatric disorders at two years. *Journal of the American Academy of Child and Adolescent Psychiatry, 36,* 1278–1285.

Max, J. E., Robin, D. A., Lindgren, S. D., Smith, W. L., Sato, Y., Mattheis, P. J., et al. (1998d). Traumatic brain injury in children and adolescents: Psychiatric disorders at one year. *Journal of Neuropsychiatry and Clinical Neuroscience, 10,* 290–297.

Max, J. E., Robin, D. A., Lindgren, S. D., Smith, W. L., Jr., Sato, Y., Mattheis, P. J., et al. (1997c). Traumatic brain injury in children and adolescents: Psychiatric disorders at two years. *Journal of the American Academy of Child and Adolescent Psychiatry, 36,* 1278–1285.

Max, J. E., Schachar, R. J., Levin, H. S., Ewing-Cobbs, L., Chapman, S. B., Dennis, M., et al. (2005b). Predictors of secondary attention-deficit/hyperactivity disorder in children and adolescents 6 to 24 months after traumatic brain injury. *Journal of the American Academy of Child and Adolescent Psychiatry, 44,* 1041–1049.

McCarthy, M. L., MacKenzie, E. J., Durbin, D. R., Aitken, M. E., Jaffe, K. M., Paidas, C. N., et al. (2006). Health-related quality of life during the first year after traumatic brain injury. *Archives of Pediatric and Adolescent Medicine, 160,* 252–260.

McCauley, S. R., & Levin, H. S. (2004). Prospective memory in pediatric traumatic brain injury: A preliminary study. *Developmental Neuropsychology, 25,* 5–20.

McCauley, S. R., McDaniel, M. A., Pedroza, C., Chapman, S. B., & Levin, H. S. (2009). Incentive effects on event-based prospective memory performance in children and adolescents with traumatic brain injury. *Neuropsychology, 23,* 201–209.

McDonald, C. M., Jaffe, K. M., Fay, G. C., Polissar, N. L., Martin, K. M., Liao, S., et al. (1994). Comparison of indices of TBI severity as predictors of neurobehavioral outcomes in children. *Archives of Physical Medicine and Rehabilitation, 75,* 328–337.

McLean, D. E., Kaitz, E. S., Kennan, C. J., Dabney, K., Cawley, M. F., & Alexander, M. A. (1995). Medical and surgical complications of pediatric brain injury. *Journal of Head Trauma Rehabilitation, 10,* 1–12.

Merkley, T. L., Bigler, E. D., Wilde, E. A., McCauley, S. R., Hunter, J. V., & Levin, H. S. (2008). Diffuse changes in cortical thickness in pediatric moderate-to-severe traumatic brain injury. *Journal of Neurotrauma, 25,* 1343–1345.

Miller, L. M., & Donders, J. (2003). Prediction of educational outcome after pediatric traumatic brain injury. *Rehabilitation Psychology, 48,* 237–241.

Mittenberg, W., Wittner, M. S., & Miller, L. J. (1997). Postconcussion syndrome occurs in children. *Neuropsychology, 11,* 447–452.

Moran, L. M., Taylor, H. G., Ganesalingam, K., Gastier-Foster, J. M., Frick, J., Bangert, B., et al. (in press).

Apolipoprotein E4 as a predictor of outcomes in pediatric mild traumatic brain injury. *Journal of Neurotrauma.*

Munson, S., Schroth, E., & Ernst, M. (2006). The role of functional neuroimaging in pediatric brain injury. *Pediatrics, 117,* 1372–1381.

Nadebaum, C., Anderson, V., & Catroppa, C. (2007). Executive function outcomes following traumatic brain injury in young children: A five year follow-up. *Developmental Neuropsychology, 32,* 703–728.

Nagin, D. S. (1999). Analyzing developmental trajectories: A semi-parametric, group-based approach. *Psychological Methods, 4,* 129–177.

Natale, J. E., Joseph, J. G., Pretzlaff, R. K., Silber, T. J., & Guerguerian, A.-M. (2005). Clinical trials in pediatric traumatic brain injury: Unique challenges and potential responses. *Developmental Neuroscience, 28,* 276–290.

Nelson, C. A. (1995). The ontogeny of human memory: A cognitive neuroscience perspective. *Developmental Psychology, 31,* 723–738.

Newsome, M. R., Steinberg, J. L., Scheibel, R. S., Troyanskaya, M., Chu, Z., Hanten, G., et al. (2008). Effects of traumatic brain injury on working memory-related brain activation in adolescents. *Neuropsychology, 22,* 419–425.

Novack, T. A., Dillon, M. C., & Jackson, W. T. (1996). Neurochemical mechanisms in brain injury and treatment: A review. *Journal of Clinical and Experimental Neuropsychology, 18,* 685–706.

Parslow, R. C., Morris, K. P., Tasker, R. C., Forsyth, R. J., & Hawley, C. A. (2005). Epidemiology of traumatic brain injury in children receiving intensive care in the UK. *Archives of Disease in Childhood, 90,* 1182–1187.

Perrin, E. C., Stein, R. E., & Drotar, D. (1991). Cautions in using the Child Behavior Checklist: Observations based on research about children with a chronic illness. *Journal of Pediatric Psychology, 16,* 411–421.

Ponsford, J., Willmott, C., Rothwell, A., Cameron, P., Ayton, G., Nelms, R., et al. (1999). Cognitive and behavioral outcomes following mild traumatic head injury in children. *Journal of Head Trauma Rehabilitation, 14,* 360–372.

Poussaint, T. Y., & Moeller, M. D. (2002). Imaging of pediatric head trauma. *Neuroimaging Clinics of North America, 12,* 271–294.

Povlishock, J. T., & Katz, D. I. (2005). Update of neuropathology and neurological recovery after traumatic brain injury. *Journal of Head Trauma Rehabilitation, 20,* 76–94.

Power, T., Catroppa, C., Coleman, L., Ditchfield, M., & Anderson, V. (2007). Do lesion site and severity predict deficits in attentional control after preschool traumatic brain injury (TBI)? *Brain Injury, 21,* 279–292.

Roman, M. J., Delis, D. C., Willerman, L., Magulac, M., Demadura, T. L., de la Peña, J. L., et al. (1998). Impact of pediatric TBI on components of verbal memory. *Journal of Clinical and Experimental Neuropsychology, 20,* 245–258.

Saatman, K. E., Duhaime, A.-C., Bullock, R., Mass, A. I. R., Valadka, A., Manley, G. T., et al. (2008). Classification of traumatic brain injury for targeted therapies. *Journal of Neurotrauma, 25,* 719–738.

Salorio, C. F., Slomine, B. S., Grados, M. A., Vasa, R. A., Christensen, J. R., & Gerring, J. P. (2005). Neuroanatomic correlates of CVLT-C performance following pediatric traumatic brain injury. *Journal of the International Neuropsychological Society, 11,* 686–696.

Satz, P. (2001). Mild head injury in children and adolescents. *Current Directions in Psychological Science, 10,* 106–109.

Satz, P., Zaucha, K., McCleary, C., Light, R., & Asarnow, R. (1997). Mild head injury in children and adolescents: A review of studies (1970–1995). *Psychological Bulletin, 122,* 107–131.

Schneier, A. J., Shields, B. J., Hostetler, S. G., Xiang, H., & Smith, G. A. (2006). Incidence of pediatric traumatic brain injury and associated hospital resource utilization in the United States. *Pediatrics, 118,* 483–492.

Schwartz, L., Taylor, H. G., Drotar, D., Yeates, K. O., Wade, S. L., & Stancin, T. (2003). Long-term

behavior problems following pediatric traumatic brain injury: Prevalence, predictors, and correlates. *Journal of Pediatric Psychology, 28*, 251–263.

Sesma, H. W., Slomine, B. S., Ding, R., & McCarthy, M. L. (2008). Executive functioning in the first
year after pediatric traumatic brain injury. *Pediatrics, 121*, e1686–e1695.

Shore, P. M., Berger, R. P., Varma, S., Janesko, K. L., Wisniewski, S. R., Clark, R. S., et al. (2007). Cerebrospinal fluid biomarkers versus Glasgow Coma Scale and Glasgow Outcome Scale in pediatric
traumatic brain injury: The role of young age and inflicted injury. *Journal of Neurotrauma, 24*,
75–86.

Shum, D., Jamieson, E., Bahr, M., & Wallace, G. (1999). Implicit and explicit memory in children with
traumatic brain injury. *Journal of Clinical and Experimental Neuropsychology, 21*, 149–158.

Sigmund G. A., Tong, K. A., Nickerson, J. P., Wall, C. J., Oyoyo, U., & Ashwal, S. (2007). Multimodality
comparison of neuroimaging in pediatric traumatic brain injury. *Pediatric Neurology, 36*, 217–226.

Slomine, B. S., Gerring, J. P., Grados, M. A., Vasa, R., Brady, K. D., Christensen, J. R., et al. (2002).
Performance on measures of executive function following pediatric traumatic brain injury. *Brain
Injury, 16*, 759–772.

Stallings, G. A., Ewing-Cobbs, L., Francis, D. J., & Fletcher, J. M. (1996). Prediction of academic placement after pediatric head injury using neurological, demographic, and neuropsychological variables. *Journal of the International Neuropsychological Society, 2*, 39.

Stancin, T., Drotar, D., Taylor, H. G., Yeates, K. O., Wade, S. L., & Minich, N. M. (2002). Health-related
quality of life of children and adolescents after traumatic brain injury. *Pediatrics, 109*. Retrieved
from *www.pediatrics.org/cgi/content/full/109/2/e34*

Statler, K. D. (2006). Pediatric posttraumatic seizures: Epidemiology, putative mechanisms of epilepto-
genesis and promising investigational progress. *Developmental Neuroscience, 28*, 354–363.

Taylor, H. G. (2004). Research on outcomes of pediatric traumatic brain injury: Current advances and
future directions. *Developmental Neuropsychology, 25*, 199–225.

Taylor, H. G. (in press). Neurobehavioral outcomes of pediatric traumatic brain injury. In V. A. Anderson & K. O. Yeates (Eds.), *Pediatric traumatic brain injury: New directions in clinical and translational
research*. New York: Oxford University Press.

Taylor, H. G., & Alden, J. (1997). Age-related differences in outcome following childhood brain injury:
An introduction and overview. *Journal of the International Neuropsychological Society, 3*, 555–567.

Taylor, H. G., Drotar, D., Wade, S., Yeates, K. O., Stancin, T., & Klein, S. (1995). Recovery from TBI in
children: The importance of the family. In S. H. Broman & M. E. Michel (Eds.), *Traumatic head
injury in children* (pp. 188–218). New York: Oxford University Press.

Taylor, H. G., Yeates, K. O., Wade, S. L., Drotar, D., Klein, S. K., & Stancin, T. (1999). Influences on
first-year recovery from traumatic brain injury in children. *Neuropsychology, 13*, 76–89.

Taylor, H. G., Yeates, K. O., Wade, S. L., Drotar, D., Stancin, T., & Minich, N. (2002). A prospective
study of long- and short-term outcomes after traumatic brain injury in children: Behavior and
achievement. *Neuropsychology, 16*, 15–27.

Taylor, H. G., Yeates, K. O., Wade, S. L., Drotar, D., Stancin, T., & Montpetite, M. (2003). Long-term
educational interventions after traumatic brain injury in children. *Rehabilitation Psychology, 48*,
227–236.

Teasdale, G., & Jennett, B. (1974). Assessment of coma and impaired consciousness: A practical scale.
Lancet, ii, 81–84.

Tenovuo, O. (2006). Pharmacological enhancement of cognitive and behavioral deficits after traumatic
brain injury. *Current Opinion in Neurology, 19*, 528–533.

Thompson, N. M., Francis, D. J., Stuebing, K. K., Fletcher, J. M., Ewing-Cobbs, L., Miner, M. E., et al.
(1994). Motor, visual–spatial, and somatosensory skills after TBI in children and adolescents: A
study of change. *Neuropsychology, 8*, 333–342.

Van't Hooft, I. (in press). Neuropsychological rehabilitation in children with traumatic brain injuries. In
V. A. Anderson & K. O. Yeates (Eds.), *Pediatric traumatic brain injury: New directions in clinical and
translational research*. New York: Oxford University Press.

Vasa, R. A., Gerring, J. P., Grados, M., Slomine, B., Christensen, J. R., Rising, W., et al. (2002). Anxiety after severe pediatric closed head injury. *Journal of the American Academy of Child and Adolescent Psychiatry, 41,*148–156.

Verger, K., Junque, C., Jurado, M. A., Tresserras, P., Bartumeus, F., Noques, P., et al. (2000). Age effects on long-term neuropsychological outcome in paediatric traumatic brain injury. *Brain Injury, 14,* 495–503.

Wade, S. L. (in press). Psychosocial treatments for pediatric traumatic brain injury. In V. A. Anderson & K. O. Yeates (Eds.), *Pediatric traumatic brain injury: New directions in clinical and translational research.* New York: Oxford University Press.

Wade, S. L., Taylor, H. G., Walz, N. C., Salisbury, S., Stancin, T., Bernard, L. A., et al. (2008). Parent–child interactions during the initial weeks following brain injury in young children. *Rehabilitation Psychology, 53,* 180–190.

Wade, S. L., Taylor, H. G., Yeates, K. O., Drotar, D., Stancin, T., Minich, N. M., et al. (2006). Long-term parental and family adaptation following pediatric brain injury. *Journal of Pediatric Psychology, 31,* 1072–1083.

Ward, H., Shum, D., Dick, B., McKinlay, L., & Baker-Tweney, S. (2004). Interview study of the effects of paediatric traumatic brain injury on memory. *Brain Injury, 18,* 471–495.

Ward, H., Shum, D., McKinlay, L., Baker, S., & Wallace, G. (2007). Prospective memory and pediatric traumatic brain injury: Effects of cognitive demand. *Child Neuropsychology, 13,* 219–239.

Ward, H., Shum, D., Wallace, G., & Boon, J. (2002). Pediatric traumatic brain injury and procedural memory. *Journal of Clinical and Experimental Neuropsychology, 24,* 458–470.

Warschausky, S., Cohen, E. H., Parker, J. G., Levendosky, A. A., & Okun, A. (1997). Social problem-solving skills of children with traumatic brain injury. *Pediatric Rehabilitation, 1,* 77–81.

Warschausky, S., Kewman, D., & Kay, J. (1999). Empirically supported psychological and behavioral therapies in pediatric rehabilitation of TBI. *Journal of Head Trauma Rehabilitation, 14,* 373–383.

Wilde, E. A., Bigler, E. D., Hunter, J. V., Fearing, M. A., Scheibel, R. S., Newsome, M. R., et al. (2007). Hippocampus, amygdala, and basal ganglia morphometrics in children after moderate-to-severe traumatic brain injury. *Developmental Medicine and Child Neurology, 49,* 294–299.

Wilde, E. A., Chu, Z., Bigler, E. D., Hunter, J. V., Fearing, M. A., Hanten, G., et al. (2006). Diffusion tensor imaging in the corpus callosum in children after moderate to severe traumatic brain injury. *Journal of Neurotrauma, 23,* 1412–1426.

Wilde, E. A., Hunter, J. V., Newsome, M. R., Scheibel, R. S., Bigler, E. D., Johnson, J. L., et al. (2005). Frontal and temporal morphometric findings on MRI in children after moderate to severe traumatic brain injury. *Journal of Neurotrauma, 22,* 333–344.

Winogron, H. W., Knights, R. M., & Bawden, H. N. (1984). Neuropsychological deficits following head injury in children. *Journal of Clinical Neuropsychology, 6,* 269–286.

Yeates, K. O. (2000). Closed-head injury. In K. O. Yeates, M. D. Ris, & H. G. Taylor (Eds.), *Pediatric neuropsychology: Research, theory, and practice* (pp. 92–116). New York: Guilford Press.

Yeates, K. O., Armstrong, K., Janusz, J., Taylor, H. G., Wade, S., Stancin, T., et al. (2005). Long-term attention problems in children with traumatic brain injury. *Journal of the American Academy of Child and Adolescent Psychiatry, 44,* 574–584.

Yeates, K. O., Bigler, E. D., Dennis, M., Gerhardt, C. A., Rubin, K. H., Stancin, T., et al. (2007). Social outcomes in childhood brain disorder: A heuristic integration of social neuroscience and developmental psychology. *Psychological Bulletin, 133,* 535–556.

Yeates, K. O., Blumenstein, E., Patterson, C. M., & Delis, D. C. (1995a). Verbal learning and memory following pediatric TBI. *Journal of the International Neuropsychological Society, 1,* 78–87.

Yeates, K. O., & Enrile, B. G. (2005). Implicit and explicit memory in children with congenital and acquired brain disorder. *Neuropsychology, 19,* 618–628.

Yeates, K. O., Luria, J., Bartkowski, H., Rusin, J., Martin, L., & Bigler, E. D. (1999). Post-concussive symptoms in children with mild closed-head injuries. *Journal of Head Trauma Rehabilitation, 14,* 337–350.

Yeates, K. O., Patterson, C. M., Waber, D. P., & Bernstein, J. H. (2003). Constructional and figural memory skills following pediatric closed-head injury: Evaluation using the ROCF. In J. A. Knight

& E. Kaplan (Eds.), *The handbook of Rey–Osterrieth Complex Figure usage: Clinical and research applications* (pp. 83–93). Lutz, FL: Psychological Assessment Resources.

Yeates, K. O., Ris, M. D., & Taylor, H. G. (1995b). Hospital referral patterns in pediatric neuropsychology. *Child Neuropsychology, 1,* 56–62.

Yeates, K. O., Swift, E., Taylor, H. G., Wade, S. L., Drotar, D., Stancin, T., et al. (2004). Short- and long-term social outcomes following pediatric traumatic brain injury. *Journal of the International Neuropsychological Society, 10,* 412–426.

Yeates, K. O., & Taylor, H .G. (2005). Neurobehavioral outcomes of mild head injury in children and adolescents. *Pediatric Rehabilitation, 8,* 5–16.

Yeates, K. O., & Taylor, H. G. (2006). Behavior problems in school and their educational correlates among children with traumatic brain injury. *Exceptionality, 14,* 141–154.

Yeates, K. O., Taylor, H. G., Barry, C. T., Drotar, D., Wade, S. L., & Stancin, T. (2001). Neurobehavioral symptoms in childhood closed-head injuries: Changes in prevalence and correlates during the first year post-injury. *Journal of Pediatric Psychology, 26,* 79–91.

Yeates, K. O., Taylor, H. G., Drotar, D., Wade, S., Klein, S., & Stancin, T. (1997). Premorbid family environment as a predictor of neurobehavioral outcomes following pediatric TBI. *Journal of the International Neuropsychological Society, 3,* 617–630.

Yeates, K. O., Taylor, H. G., Rusin, J., Bangert, B., Dietrich, A., Nuss, K., et al. (2009). Longitudinal trajectories of post-concussive symptoms in children with mild traumatic brain injuries and their relationship to acute clinical status. *Pediatrics, 123,* 735–743.

Yeates, K. O., Taylor, H. G., Wade, S. L., Drotar, D., Stancin, T., & Minich, N. (2002). A prospective study of short- and long-term neuropsychological outcomes after traumatic brain injury in children. *Neuropsychology, 16,* 514–523.

Ylvisaker, M., Adelson, D., Braga, L. W., Burnett, S. M., Glang, A., Feeney, T., et al. (2005a). Rehabilitation and ongoing support after pediatric TBI: Twenty years of progress. *Journal of Head Trauma Rehabilitation, 20,* 90–104.

Ylvisaker, M., Todis, B., Glang, A., Urbanczyk, B., Franklin, C., DePompei, R., et al. (2001). Educating students with TBI: Themes and recommendations. *Journal of Head Trauma Rehabilitation, 16,* 76–93.

Ylvisaker, M., Turkstra, L. S., & Coelho, C. (2005b). Behavioral and social interventions for individuals with traumatic brain injury: A summary of the research with clinical implications. *Seminars in Speech and Language, 26,* 256–267.

Ylvisaker, M., Turkstra, L., Coehlo, C., Yorkston, K., Kennedy, M., Sohlberg, M. M., et al. (2007). Behavioural interventions for children and adults with behaviour disorders after TBI: A systematic review of the evidence. *Brain Injury, 21,* 769–805.

Yuan, W., Holland, S. K., Schmithorst, V. J., Walz, N. C., Cecil, K. M., Jones, B. V., et al. (2007). Diffusion tensor MR imaging reveals persistent white matter alteration after traumatic brain injury experienced during early childhood. *American Journal of Neuroradiology, 28,* 1919–1925.

CHAPTER 6

Acute Disseminated Encephalomyelitis and Childhood Multiple Sclerosis

VICKI ANDERSON
BENJAMIN J. DEERY
RANI JACOBS
ANDREW J. KORNBERG

Multiple sclerosis (MS) and acute disseminated encephalomyelitis (ADEM) are auto-immune conditions characterized by inflammatory demyelinating processes within the central nervous system (CNS). MS is the most common neurological condition that affects young adults, with clinical onset typically occurring between the ages of 20 and 40 years. Childhood MS is considered rare; indeed, many clinicians are unaware that it may be manifested in childhood, and thus MS is often incorrectly diagnosed for many years. In contrast, ADEM is a condition of young children and adolescents, with unknown prevalence. ADEM is typically a monophasic condition with good medical recovery and prognosis, whereas MS has a multiphasic course with poorer long-term recovery and a much less favorable prognosis.

HISTORICAL OVERVIEW

Reports of childhood MS first emerged in the scientific literature in the late 19th century (Hanefeld, 2007). Pierre Marie (1895) described 13 cases of childhood MS, although he later gave some other diagnoses as being more likely for several. In 1888, an autopsy-confirmed case of so-called "disseminated/insular sclerosis" was reported in a 7-year-old by Sir William Gowers. Gall, Hayles, Siekert, and Keith (1958) described 40 cases of MS with

147

childhood onset. Cases of childhood MS have been diagnosed as early as 10 months of age (Ruggieri, Polizzi, Pavone, & Grimaldi, 1999; Shaw & Alvord, 1987), although a dissertation by Totzke (1893, cited in Compston, 1998) described two cases with symptoms at birth. Only in the last decade has childhood MS received recognition, with growing research, media reports, and funding for pediatric MS centers in the United States and Canada.

ADEM was first described by Clifton in 1724, and occurred in the context of smallpox vaccination (Turnball & McIntosh, 1926). However, ADEM has attracted increasing recognition and research, tied to the rise of childhood MS. In particular, differentiating these two conditions is seen as critical for accurate diagnosis and correct treatment. Even now, diagnostic criteria vary; however, detection is more likely in pediatric hospitals, where knowledge of these emerging disease entities is greater. Improved diagnosis of ADEM and childhood MS is largely due to advances in imaging techniques.

In their acute phases, ADEM and childhood MS share many clinical symptoms and pathological/radiological features. Some researchers have even argued that the two diseases reflect different ends of the same disease spectrum. To date, however, it remains unknown why children with ADEM usually suffer a single demyelinating episode, while those with MS have multiple episodes.

EPIDEMIOLOGY

Childhood Multiple Sclerosis

MS in childhood is rare, and the exact prevalence is unclear, but it is estimated that about 2.7–5% of all persons with MS have onset before age 16, with some investigators reporting figures as high as 10% (Knox & Hader, 2004; Simone et al., 2002). One study of over 400 cases showed that 17% of patients had their first MS episode by 21 years of age (Pinhaus-Hamiel, Barak, Siev-Ner, & Achiron, 1998); other reports have documented that 5% of all individuals with MS have onset prior to 18 years, with this rate decreasing to 0.2% for prepuberty onset (Duquette et al., 1987; Koch-Henriksen, 1999; Ruggeri et al., 1999). Currently it is estimated that there are approximately 10,000 children with a diagnosis of MS in the United States alone. A further 10,000–15,000 children have experienced at least one episode of demyelination, and some of these youth will go on to develop MS at a later stage.

The overall prevalence of MS varies with geographical location, becoming more prevalent in temperate climates. High-risk regions include Canada, the northern United States, northern Europe, southern Australia, and New Zealand. Low-risk regions with a prevalence of less than 5 per 100,000 include Africa, Asia, and the tropics (Compston, 1999; Kurtzke, Beebe, & Norman, 1985; Sadovnick & Ebers, 1993). Rates of childhood MS according to geographical location, ethnicity, or race have yet to be systematically studied; however, Krupp et al. (2004) report anecdotal evidence of higher rates in certain minority groups, such as African Americans and Hispanics.

Genetic factors are also relevant. Individuals with MS are more likely to carry specific human leukocyte antigens (HLAs) (Barcellos et al., 2003; Masterman et al., 2000; Sadovnick & Ebers, 1995). One study found that patients with HLA-DR15 had earlier onset of MS than those not carrying this allele (Barcellos, 2003). Increased risk among families with a member affected by MS also points to a genetic component in MS (Compston, 1999; Sadovnick, Dircks, & Ebers, 1999). First-degree relatives have a lifetime risk of nearly 5%, compared with 0.2% in the general population (Compston, 1999; Sadovnick et al., 1993, 1999). Concordance in monozygotic twins is 30%, which is higher than that found in dizygotic twins (2–5%). Familial risk increases with younger age at onset of the probands affected by MS. However, the risk of MS in relatives of children affected by MS remains unknown.

MS is also associated with an overrepresentation of females versus males (Noseworthy, Lucchinetti, Rodriguez, & Weinshenker, 2000). The 2:1 female-to-male ratio in adults is mirrored in childhood MS, although it does vary with age. In children under 12 years, the gender bias is weakest, with almost even ratios reported. This changes for 13- to 15-year-olds, where the female MS bias is even stronger than that seen in adult MS, as illustrated in Figure 6.1 (Boiko, Vorobeychik, Paty, Devonshire, & Sadovnick, 2002b). This change in gender bias suggests a lower female predominance in prepubescent children, and points to a role for female sex hormones, as evidenced by a spike in ratios coinciding with the onset of puberty in children (Haliloglu et al., 2002).

Acute Disseminated Encephalomyelitis

As for childhood MS, the exact incidence of ADEM remains unknown, but is estimated to be 0.8 per 100,000 per year (Leake et al., 2004). In contrast to MS, no gender bias has been reported. In 50–70% of cases, ADEM occurs following infection (e.g., measles, chickenpox, rubella), but it may also occur after vaccination (Hynson et al., 2001; Murthy, Faden, Cohen, & Bakshi, 2002; Tenembaum, Chamoles, & Fejerman, 2002). In developed countries, with their tighter control of infectious diseases and more advanced vaccination procedures, ADEM is most commonly seen following a nonspecific upper respiratory tract infection, where the infective agent remains unknown. In poor and developing countries, where immunization programs are less advanced, ADEM following infection or vaccination is more frequent. Of note, the risk of postimmunization ADEM following measles vac-

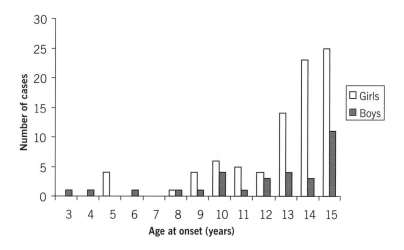

FIGURE 6.1. Distribution of patients with early onset MS according to age at onset and sex. White bars = girls; gray bars = boys. From Boiko et al., 2002b. Copyright 2002 by Walters Kluwer. Reprinted with permission.

cination, for example, is 20 times lower than the risk of developing postinfectious ADEM from the measles infection itself (Fenichel, 1982; Murthy, Yangala, Meena, & Reddy, 1999; Nalin, 1989).

In one of the few immunogenetic studies of ADEM, a Russian group (Idrissova et al., 2003) found that ADEM was associated with the HLA-DRB1*01 and HLA-DRB*17 alleles. These findings are interesting, given a previous Russian group's finding that patients with MS and HLA-DRB*17 had a less severe form of MS. It is possible that HLA-DRB*17 may be associated with less severe forms of demyelinating disease, and that ADEM, childhood MS, and adult MS may indeed represent different points on the same disease spectrum (Boiko et al., 2002a; Gusev, Demina, & Boiko, 1997).

ETIOLOGY AND PATHOGENESIS

Both environmental and genetic factors are implicated in the etiology and pathogenesis of childhood MS and ADEM. Migrational studies show that, if individuals shift from a low-MS-risk country to a high-MS-risk country (or vice versa) before puberty or during early adolescence, they adopt the risk of their new country of residence, overriding the risk of their native country (Compston, 1999; Sadovnick & Ebers, 1993, 1995). This "age at migration" effect has led to the hypothesis that environmental exposure, most likely via viral infection during childhood, is important for developing MS. During childhood, the body's immune system is maturing and may be vulnerable to becoming overactive or autoreactive later in life. Because MS appears related to some environmental exposure in childhood, it has been suggested that an "incubation" period is needed before the disease expresses itself (Kurtzke et al., 1985). However, this hypothesis fails to account fully for childhood MS.

Many viral/bacterial antigens and vaccines have been studied for connections to ADEM and MS. Although most cases of ADEM are preceded by viral or bacterial infections or by vaccination, the most common single preceding illness in developed countries remains a nonspecific upper respiratory tract infection, as noted above (Hynson et al., 2001; Leake et al., 2004; Tenembaum et al., 2002). Many of the infectious illnesses implicated in ADEM have also been linked to MS, but the long latency between exposure and clinical onset of adult MS means that any such relationship will be difficult to detect. Even in childhood MS, where the latency between exposure and clinical onset is theoretically shorter, few causal antigens have been positively identified. Epstein–Barr virus has received the most attention in the onset of childhood and adult MS, with interesting results (Alotaibi, Kennedy, Tellier, Stephens, & Banwell, 2004; Ascherio et al., 2001); however, as most children will be exposed to this virus at some stage, more research is needed to clarify its potential role and other possible viral antigens in MS etiology.

The characteristic pathological findings of both MS and ADEM are inflammatory demyelinating lesions in the white matter, with infiltration of lymphocytes and macrophages (derivatives of white blood cells typically involved in an immune response to damage or infection), and infrequent involvement of deep gray matter. Traditionally, MS was thought to involve only damage to white matter; however, recent studies have demonstrated damage to the underlying axons, and to areas of brain remote from lesions that appear normal on conventional imaging, often termed *normal-appearing brain tissue* (NABT; Filippi et al., 2000). These pathological findings are similar to those seen in experimental allergic encephalomyelitis, an experimental animal model used to study MS and ADEM (Lipton, 1975; Owens & Sriram, 1995; Rivers, Sprunt, & Berry, 1933; Wisniewski & Keith, 1977).

This model has led to two hypotheses regarding the pathogenesis of MS and ADEM, which is essentially consistent across conditions. The *inflammatory cascade* hypothesis (Menge et al., 2005) postulates that the CNS reacts directly against an infective pathogen, resulting in tissue damage and release of CNS-confined autoantigens, due to a breakdown in the blood–brain barrier. Once autoantigens are released, there is an autoreactive T-cell response, in which T cells infiltrate the CNS and cause further inflammation and tissue damage. The second, more widely accepted hypothesis, *molecular mimicry* (Davies, 1997; Fujinami & Oldstone, 1985), is based on the notion that the inciting pathogen shares structural similarity with CNS myelin proteins, although the similarity is not sufficient for the pathogen to be recognized and tolerated. Once the pathogen is introduced, T and B cells are activated and enter the CNS to detect the pathogen. CNS damage is caused by an auto-immune response that mistakes myelin for the inciting pathogen and starts to attack the myelin. A possible genetic predisposition may explain why some children develop ADEM or MS following viral/bacterial infection or vaccination, while others do not, although this possibility has yet to be systematically examined.

CLINICAL FEATURES, PRESENTATION, AND ILLNESS COURSE

The clinical features and presentation of childhood MS and ADEM are so similar that it is often impossible to differentiate the two at onset.

MS is characterized by multiple episodes of neurological dysfunction, which occur secondary to inflammation and demyelination of the CNS, and which target white matter predominantly. ADEM is generally characterized by a single such episode. Although the presenting symptoms of childhood MS are similar to those of adult MS, children are more likely to show systemic symptoms such as fever, vomiting, headache, malaise, and lethargy, followed by poorly localized neurological symptoms. In ADEM, symptoms usually appear between 4 and 13 days after infection or vaccination. Neurological signs are typically multifocal and involve altered consciousness or cognitive impairment, as well as pyramidal tract dysfunction (e.g., monoparesis, hemiparesis, ataxia, optic neuritis, cranial nerve palsy). Seizures and meningismus (irritation of the meninges with absence of infection or inflammation) can also be seen. Optic neuritis, involving deteriorating vision and painful eye movements, is a common presenting symptom in both childhood MS and ADEM; it is typically bilateral in ADEM, in contrast to a unilateral presentation in MS (Jan, 2005). Its presence in the clinical profile substantially increases the risk of later MS diagnosis (Lucchinetti et al., 1997; Morales, Slatkowski, Howard, & Warman, 2000). Neurological symptoms generally develop and peak within a matter of days. Recovery is sometimes rapid, but typically occurs over weeks to months. Full neurological recovery is seen in the majority of patients with ADEM and in the initial stages of childhood MS. Mortality rates for ADEM were once high (10–30%), but better detection and treatment have reduced these figures considerably. Poorer recovery in ADEM has been associated with the inciting agent (e.g., rubella vs. varicella infection) and aggressiveness of initial symptoms. Although factors associated with recovery in childhood MS are unknown, recovery in adult MS has been related to degree of recovery from the first episode, time between the first and second episodes, age at onset, and gender (Hammond, McLeod, Macaskill, & English, 2000; Idrissova et al., 2003; Levic et al., 1999; Noseworthy et al., 2000).

Most children and adults with MS present with relapsing–remitting MS (RRMS), characterized by episodes of neurological dysfunction (relapses) from which the patients either completely or partially recover, with no progression between relapses. Because recovery may be incomplete, residual deficits may accumulate over a period of time. Approximately one-quarter of children with RRMS will develop secondary–progressive MS (SPMS), characterized by an initial RRMS course followed by progressive neurological impairment. SPMS is less common in childhood MS than in adults, suggesting that childhood MS may represent a less aggressive form of the disease. However, because children are diagnosed earlier than adults, they are more likely to reach a more severe level of disability at a younger age.

The majority of children with ADEM have a monophasic course (90%), with no further episodes and no new pathology within 3 months of the initial clinical event. Relapsing cases of ADEM have been reported, generally occurring 4–8 weeks after treatment. Multiphasic disseminated encephalomyelitis (MDEM) has also been documented; this typically involves recurrences 4–8 weeks after treatment, but can occur years later, generally with different symptoms or new, atypical MS-type lesions. The concept of MDEM is somewhat controversial and not easily differentiated from MS. To illustrate the complexities of early diagnosis in this field, approximately 25% of children initially diagnosed with ADEM will later go on to receive a diagnosis of MS.

DIAGNOSIS AND INVESTIGATIONS

MS diagnosis requires evidence of two or more episodes of neurological dysfunction; at least two episodes of functionally significant symptoms lasting longer than 24 hours and separated by at least 30 days; and white matter lesions identified in at least two distinct CNS regions (Paty, Noseworthy, & Ebers, 1998). The diagnostic criteria for ADEM are less well defined, but a diagnosis should be considered in the context of a subacute, polysymptomatic onset of neurological symptoms suggestive of CNS involvement, with evidence of a recent infection or vaccination. The diagnosis of these conditions is fraught with difficulty, and may be delayed because a child is unable to describe symptoms (e.g., limb weakness, blurred vision) in a way that can be easily related to disease criteria. Commonly, children who later receive a diagnosis of MS were initially diagnosed with ADEM.

No single biological marker is sufficient for the definite diagnosis of childhood MS or ADEM, and the diagnosis remains a clinical one, involving the exclusion of other conditions. Neurological examination, clinical history, and radiological data are routine, but testing for abnormalities in cerebrospinal fluid, and for lesions in the optic pathways or spinal cord (via visual and somatosensory evoked potentials), is also common practice (Boutin et al., 1988; Gronseth & Ashman, 2000; Miller, 1998; Paty et al., 1998).

Neuroimaging

Specific diagnostic criteria for magnetic resonance imaging (MRI) of childhood MS and ADEM have yet to be established. Changes in the white matter associated with MS are most easily detected on T2-weighted scans and fluid-attenuated inversion recovery sequences, and appear as patchy areas of increased signal intensity. Serial scans showing new gadolinium-enhancing lesions, or new T2-weighted lesions, can be used to show distinct demyelinating episodes separated in space and time. Children with MS generally show the characteristic pattern of demyelination seen in adults, including lesions in the periventricular, juxtacortical, subcortical, infratentorial, and spinal cord white matter (Ebner, Millner, & Justich, 1990; Balassy et al., 2001; Fazekas et al., 1999). A recent study of children with MS demonstrated a decreased frequency of hypointense lesions on T1-weighted MRI, as well as lower rates of brain atrophy, when compared to adults (Balassy et al., 2001). These findings suggest that childhood MS may involve a less aggressive pathological process. Children with MS also show atypical patterns of demyelination, including large or nodular demyelinating lesions that can be mistaken for tumors. Resolution of lesions in the early stages of MS can be complete or partial, suggesting that the CNS has some ability to remyelinate; however, this ability becomes exhausted as the disease progresses, and decreasing resolution of lesions is seen with disease duration (see Figure 6.2).

Gray matter pathology is more likely in ADEM, with deep structures such as the basal ganglia and thalamus involved in up to 40% of cases (Hynson et al., 2001; Schwarz, Mohr, Knauth, Wildemann, & Storch-Hagenlocher, 2001; Tenembaum et al., 2002). Tumor-like lesions can also be found, with complete or partial resolution of these lesions in about three-quarters of all patients with ADEM (Dale et al., 2000; Hynson et al., 2001; Tenembaum et al., 2002). To support a diagnosis of ADEM, lesions are required to be of the same "age" on MRI, with no new lesions on subsequent scans. If new lesions appear, a diagnosis of childhood MS is likely. In contrast, periventricular and callosal changes are more characteristic of MS.

MS and ADEM have also been studied with nonconventional imaging techniques. Proton magnetic resonance spectroscopy has been employed in MS to detect and quantify abnormal chemical changes in normal-appearing white matter. N-acetylaspartate (NAA), used to detect axonal damage, has been of particular interest; findings indicate reduced levels of NAA in NABT in areas adjacent to existing lesions, and in areas that later become sites for MS lesions. Levels of NAA also differ according to disease stage (De Stefano, Matthews, & Arnold, 1995; Falini et al., 1998). Although this technique has yet to be used widely in ADEM and childhood MS, it has the potential to improve diagnostic accuracy. In addition, whole-brain magnetization transfer ratio (MTR), suggested to reflect damage to either myelin or axons, is found to be lower in patients with MS; reduced MTR has also been found in the NABT of patients with MS, again in some regions that precede later lesion formation on conventional MRI. MTR histograms provide a variety of measures taken to reflect MS pathology and correlate more strongly than conventional MRI with disability and cognitive impairment (Filippi et al., 2000).

Mezzapesa et al. (2004) used magnetization transfer imaging to assess axonal damage in 13 patients with childhood MS and found that the NABT of these patients did not differ significantly from that of healthy controls. These results contrast with those from adult studies, demonstrating diffuse NABT injury, and suggesting that childhood MS may have a slower rate of diffuse brain atrophy and a more favorable clinical course than that of adults. These authors also performed diffusion tensor imaging and reported that compared to controls, and indeed to adults described in the literature, children with MS showed a modest increase in $\overline{D}$ (a measure of degree of tissue damage) for NABT. More importantly, in a further study they found that patients with ADEM did not differ from controls on

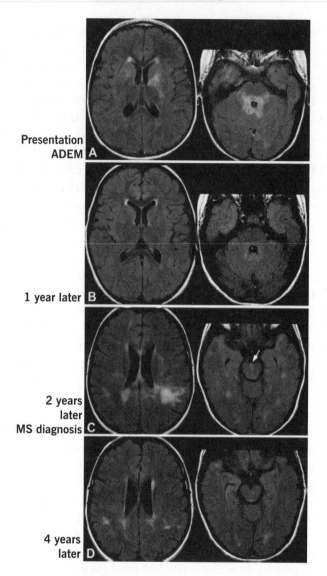

Presentation ADEM A

1 year later B

2 years later MS diagnosis C

4 years later D

FIGURE 6.2. Capacity for dramatic MRI resolution of white matter lesions in children with multiple sclerosis (MS). (A) Axial fluid-attenuated inversion recovery (FLAIR) images of an 8-year-old girl presenting with acute encephalopathy, ataxia, and tremor, diagnosed as acute disseminated encephalomyelitis. Images show ill-defined increased signal in the white matter of the brainstem and cerebellum as well as the deep gray matter. (B) Axial FLAIR images of the same child obtained 1 year later. The patient was clinically well. Near complete resolution of the prior lesions in the brainstem, cerebellum, and deep white matter is noted. No new white matter lesions are present. (C) Axial FLAIR images 2 years after her initial presentation demonstrate new lesions in the brainstem (arrow), periventricular white matter, and splenium of the corpus callosum. The patient presented with new neurologic deficits (without encephalopathy) and was diagnosed with MS. (D) Axial FLAIR images obtained 4 years after her initial presentation (2 years after the MRI shown in C). Although there has been considerable resolution of some of the prior lesions, improvement is not as dramatic as the near-complete MRI lesion resolution noted in B, suggesting that remyelination capacity may diminish either with increasing disease duration or with increasing age. The child has experienced four MS relapses, and the MRI shown in D was obtained with the child on therapy with glatiramer acetate. From Banwell et al., 2007. Copyright 2007 by Wolters Kluwer. Reprinted by permission.

any $\overline{D}$ measures (Inglese et al., 2002). Together, these findings suggest that the widespread pathology found in adult MS is not present in childhood MS or ADEM.

Differential Diagnosis: ADEM or Childhood MS?

Several studies have proposed clinical differences between these two conditions. Features suggestive of ADEM are recent infection or vaccination; systemic features at presentation (e.g., fever or headache); signs of encephalopathy or seizures; and involvement of deep gray matter, such as the basal ganglia or thalamus. Features more specific to childhood MS are less severe illness; optic neuritis; presence of oligoclonal bands, suggestive of CNS damage/disease in cerebrospinal fluid (proteins); periventricular and corpus callosum involvement; and new lesions indicated clinically or on MRI. In practice, the decision is not always clear-cut. Moreover, differentiating ADEM and childhood MS from other conditions may prove challenging, given that there are often nonspecific initial clinical profiles. CNS infections such as viral or bacterial meningoencephalitis, herpes simplex encephalitis, Lyme disease, West Nile virus, HIV, brucellosis, and syphilis, as well as neoplasms and CNS metastasis, all have similar presenting symptoms—as do less common conditions, including mitochondrial encephalopathy with lactic acidosis and stroke-like episodes, as well as adrenoleukodystrophy. A number of other conditions may also present similarly to childhood MS: Schilder disease, Devic disease or optic neuromyelitis, and Balò concentric sclerosis.

CURRENT AND FUTURE TREATMENTS

Acute Episodes/Relapses

There have been few controlled clinical trials for the treatment of ADEM and acute MS. Both are typically treated with high-dose intravenous steroids, such as methylprednisolone, based on evidence that they are caused by some sort of abnormal autoimmune response. Treatments aim to shorten and/or suppress this response and to quicken recovery. Case reports and small case series suggest corticosteroid treatment as the most effective first-line treatment, with approximately two-thirds of patients benefiting (Schwarz et al., 2001; Weinstock-Guttman & Cohen, 1996). Although steroids do not appear to improve the degree of recovery, they do shorten the length of the attack and quicken symptom recovery, and may also decrease the risk of relapse (Anlar et al., 2003). Depending on treatment response, corticosteroids will either be ceased or tapered off after hospital discharge, with some patients experiencing recurrence of symptoms during the tapering regimen. In patients who do not respond well to high-dose intravenous steroids or who develop recurrent symptoms with treatment withdrawal/tapering, other forms of therapy, such as intravenous immunoglobulin or plasmapheresis, may be particularly effective. Immunosuppressive therapies, such as cyclophosphamide or mitoxantrone, may also be considered in very severe/refractory cases.

Disease-Modifying Treatments

Several immunomodulatory drugs appear to modify the MS disease process: interferon beta-1a (Avonex or Rebif), interferon beta-1b (Betaseron), and glatiramer acetate (Copaxone).

Research (mainly case series reports) into the effectiveness and efficacy of these treatments has shown a reduction in the frequency of MS relapses (approximately 30%) and the number of new and enlarging lesions on MRI. Interferon beta-1a (Avonex and Rebif) has been shown to slow disease evolution as measured by disability progression, and to slow the rate of brain atrophy.

Symptomatic Treatments

MS is associated with a variety of symptoms that persist between relapses and have an impact on quality of life. Fatigue is one of the most common complaints, leading to problems at school, cognitive dysfunction, and emotional lability. Although education and counseling support may be important in the treatment of fatigue, children also respond to medications such as modafinil (a stimulant/wakefulness-promoting medication) and amantadine (an antiviral drug that is also used to treat Parkinson disease and has dopaminergic properties, among others) (Banwell, 2004; Banwell & Anderson, 2005; Cohen & Fisher, 1989; Rammohan et al., 2002).

Immunoablation and Future Treatments

Immunoablative treatments are thought to "reset" the body's immune system by killing off the autoreactive T and B cells, whereupon the rebuilt immune system "forgets" to start attacking itself again. Use of this procedure is based on a small number of patients with MS and comorbid leukemia, whose MS was seen to stabilize or improve after treatment with chemotherapy and hematopoietic stem cell transplantation (HSCT), and also on experimental animal models of MS following immunoablation (Comi et al., 2000; McAllister, Beatty, & Rose, 1997). Due to the mortality and morbidity rate associated with chemotherapy, this treatment has mainly been used in severe cases that are refractory to most other treatments, and is rarely used in children.

In our clinic, we followed a 14-year-old patient (JD) who was diagnosed with MS and concurrent Hodgkin lymphoma, and treated using chemotherapy without HSCT. In addition to the successful treatment of the Hodgkin lymphoma, JD's MS went into remission, with no further relapses reported since 2000. Prior to chemotherapy, JD used a wheelchair, had severe speech difficulties, was restricted in activities of daily living (ADLs), and exhibited declining intellectual functioning, together with MS relapses and highly active demyelination on MRI. Since his treatment, JD has shown remarkable recovery in multiple areas of functioning and behavior, with no new lesions on imaging. He can now play sports and manage routine ADLs; his speech has also shown significant improvement, as have his self-monitoring and self-control.

PROGNOSIS AND PREDICTORS

Although the long-term outcome following ADEM was initially considered poor, good outcome is now expected in the majority (70%) of cases (Anlar et al., 2003; Hynson et al., 2001) within 6 months of onset. This is due to two factors: First, effective immunization programs have decreased the rates of bacterial/viral infections, which had been related to poorer outcome; and, second, the use of high-dose steroids reduces the duration of neuro-logical symptoms and halts disease progression. Residual deficits occur in 10–30% of cases (Idrissova et al., 2003; Tenembaum et al., 2002) and are associated with sudden onset and greater symptom severity at presentation. In our own series of 31 children with ADEM (Hynson et al., 2001), 81% showed complete recovery, while 16% showed only mild neuro-logical sequelae. In another study, almost 25% of cases had at least one recurrent episode, while approximately 15% had three or more recurrent episodes (Cohen et al., 2001).

In adult MS, eventually over 70% of patients with RRMS will develop SPMS; that is, as noted earlier, they will experience progression of symptoms without a definable recovery. In 50% of cases, the time from first MS episode to development of SPMS is 10 years, extended to 15 years when onset was before 16 years (Boiko et al., 2002b), supporting the view that childhood MS appears to be less severe. In contrast, Confavreux, Vukusic, and Adeleine (2003) found that children with MS had a less aggressive clinical course, but that once they reached a threshold of irreversible disability in adulthood, they progressed to more severe levels of disability at the same rate as adult-onset patients. On the basis of such reports, it has been suggested that MS is a two-stage disease, with an initial stage of variable duration influenced by such factors as age of onset, gender, relapsing–remitting course, good recovery from first episode, optic neuritis as an initial symptom, number of relapses and length of time in between. The second, later stage has an invariant preprogrammed sequence and progresses at the same rate for all, regardless of age at onset, number of relapses, and other clinical variables. This "final common pathway" as described by Confavreux et al. (2003) is thought to reflect the chronic, diffuse CNS-degenerative component of MS, and corre-sponds to the progressive phase of the disease; the first stage appears to coincide consider-ably with the relapsing–remitting phase of the disease.

NEUROPSYCHOLOGICAL CONSEQUENCES

Because children typically recover well "physically" from ADEM and from initial episodes of childhood MS, cognitive symptoms may be neglected, and children often return to home and school with unrealistic expectations. This course of acute recovery is not dissimilar to that seen in other childhood conditions where white matter is involved (e.g., traumatic brain injury, hydrocephalus, cranial irradiation), where a child appears physically and medi-cally normal but is at risk for subtle deficits consistent with white matter pathology (e.g., slowed processing speed and attentional deficits).

MS and Cognition

The cognitive consequences of adult MS have only recently been well established, and they can occur early in the disease, before any marked physical disability. Between 40% and 70% of adults with MS display some cognitive dysfunction, most commonly in mem-ory, information processing, attention, and executive functions (Rao, Leo, Bernardin, & Unverzagt, 1991). In one of the earliest studies to examine cognitive function in childhood MS, Bye, Kendall, and Wilson (1985) found participants to have IQs less than 80, with declines on follow-up testing, and interpreted these results as evidence of a "dementing process." Iannetti et al. (1996) and Cole and Stuart (1995) revisited this conclusion, finding less consistent impairment on neuropsychological testing. These early studies were limited by small samples and nonspecific cognitive measures.

With increasing recognition of the existence of childhood MS and potential vulnerability of children to CNS insults, there has been an increase in both case reports and group studies, although case–control studies are few (Anderson & Moore, 1995; MacAllister, Christodoulou, Milazzo, & Krupp, 2007; McCann, Farmer, & Patel, 2004). In one of the first comprehensive studies of cognitive outcome in childhood MS, Kalb et al. (1999) highlighted the degree of subject variability on cognitive performances compared to normative data. As a group, the children with MS generally fell within normal limits, but on a case-by-case basis, high rates of cognitive and academic impairments were identified. Furthermore, Banwell and Anderson (2005) found that all 10 children with MS that they studied had impairments in at least one cognitive domain relative to age norms, with some children displaying deficits in most or all areas assessed. Deficits were most common for processing speed, working memory, and executive function. Earlier age of onset and longer disease duration were related to more severe and widespread cognitive dysfunction. Of note, participants were reported to have little evidence of physical disability; this finding indicates that, like adults with MS, children may appear well but experience significant cognitive impairments.

In the largest study of cognitive functioning to date, MacAllister et al. (2005) assessed 37 participants with childhood MS, identifying deficits in complex attention and memory. Confrontation naming was also impaired, which is interesting, given that this function is usually intact in adult MS. Approximately one-third of children required educational assistance, and almost half had a psychiatric diagnosis (e.g., major depression, anxiety). At a 2-year follow-up, cognitive decline was common and was related to baseline neurological impairment and total relapses (MacAllister et al., 2007). This pattern of cognitive decline in childhood MS has been replicated in a longitudinal study from our lab (Deery, 2008).

In summary, research examining neuropsychological sequelae in childhood MS is scarce, with available studies reporting data on small samples, and often with no reference to normative expectations. Despite these limitations, the severity and global nature of the impairments reported are compelling. Further larger-scale research is required, however, to better document these findings and to track their trajectory over time.

ADEM and Cognition

Only a handful of studies have investigated the impact of ADEM on cognition. Case reports have described ADEM presenting as a psychotic state, or with communication and cognitive deficits. A study of four adults with ADEM reported that patients had ongoing problems with memory, insight, judgment, initiative, spatial skills, and social function, even 3 years after disease onset (Sunnerhagen, Johansson, & Ekholm, 2003). Idrissova et al. (2003) found increased rates of attention-deficit/hyperactivity disorder, isolated cognitive dysfunction, and neurological symptoms in children after ADEM. Cognitive impairment was found to be associated with severity of disease onset and with degree of demyelination. Hahn et al. (2003) found that although group scores were within the normal range, all their participants displayed one or more cognitive deficits, most commonly in processing speed,

short-term verbal memory, attention, and executive functions; behavioral problems were
also detected. These findings held true regardless of clinical and radiological recovery.

In our own lab, we investigated intellectual, attentional, and social functioning in 19
children with ADEM, ages 5–16 years at time of assessment and at least 12 months post-
diagnosis, and compared their abilities to those of an age-matched, healthy control group.
The clinical group was identified through medical record audit, which minimized the
recruitment biases inherent in using clinic-based referrals. We found deficits in psychomotor speed, information processing, and attention. Deficits were more apparent on complex
attention and processing tasks, particularly those requiring working memory. Of interest,
emotional problems, particularly anxiety-related symptoms, were of greatest concern, and
more frequent in children with onset prior to 5 years (Jacobs, Anderson, Neale, Shield, &
Kornberg, 2004) (see Figure 6.3).

Comparing Cognition in ADEM and Childhood MS

Due to inherent differences between the natural course of childhood MS and that of
ADEM, there are likely to be differences in cognitive outcomes. Research suggests that
post-ADEM neuropsychological impairments may represent specific cognitive delays, consistent with white matter disruption (e.g., slowed processing, attentional problems), from
which children will eventually recover. In contrast, the multiple insults that occur in childhood MS may render these children vulnerable to persistent, global, and increasing cognitive impairments, with the full extent of these not apparent until these skills are expected
to mature. Findings from our lab support this view. We recently compared the neuropsychological profiles of two groups: children with ADEM (*n* = 9) and with childhood MS (*n* = 9),
matched with respect to demographic variables (Deery, 2008). Although both groups were
impaired relative to normative expectations, children with MS demonstrated more severe
impairments across multiple cognitive domains, with boys with MS recording particularly

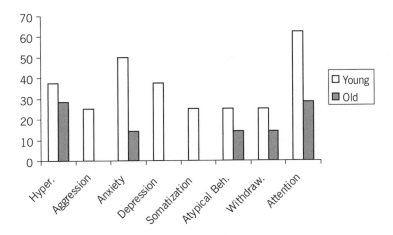

FIGURE 6.3. Proportion of children with T scores in the clinically significant range according to age at illness onset. Hyper.: hyperactivity; Atypical Beh.: atypical behaviour; Withdraw.: withdrawal. From Jacobs et
al., 2004. Copyright 2004 by Elsevier. Reprinted by permission.

poor performances. This gender difference has also been reported in adult MS, and may be related to higher levels of white matter in males and of neuroprotective and myelin-promoting hormones in females. We followed both groups over time and demonstrated that the children with MS showed global deterioration in cognitive abilities. In contrast, those with ADEM improved to normal levels on measures of simple attention and information processing, and only experienced continuing weaknesses on complex processing tasks (Deery, 2008).

Because research documenting the consequences of these conditions is in its infancy, risk factors for poorer outcome remain unclear. Although some studies have noted relationships between factors such as severity of symptoms at presentation, rapidity of onset, radiological/neurological indices, and treatment methods, sample sizes have generally been too small to confirm these suggestions. Further large-scale studies are needed to extend knowledge in these areas.

A potential explanation for cognitive deficits in children with ADEM and MS relates to the immaturity of the CNS, particularly white matter, which appears to be the primary target for pathology for both conditions. Damage to white matter can increase the risk of cognitive impairment by interfering with efficient transmission of impulses between brain regions, resulting in reduced information processing, attentional impairments, slowed response speed, and learning difficulties. During childhood, white matter development is rapid, with myelination not fully complete until well into late adolescence/early adulthood (Blakemore & Choudhury, 2006; Hudspeth & Pribram, 1990). Hence early brain insult in ADEM and childhood MS may not only cause damage to existing myelin, but may also interfere with normal white matter development (Hermann et al., 2002). Frontal regions may be especially vulnerable, as they are among the last to become myelinated, and rely on effective "communication" from posterior and subcortical regions for adequate function (Klinberg, Vaidyn, Gabrieli, Moseley, & Heidehus, 1999). Similarly, damage to existing white matter and future myelination may also have an effect on the development and establishment of cortical neural networks that are being laid down and refined during childhood and adolescence. As a consequence of these neural disruptions, deficits in information processing, and in attention and executive functions, are likely (and have been documented) to occur. If sufficiently severe, these impairments are likely to have a cumulative impact on a child's capacity to acquire new skills and knowledge, potentially explaining the cognitive decline observed by some researchers and clinicians. Although children with MS do not appear to show the diffuse NABT damage found in adult MS, they may do so when they themselves reach adulthood. Because these children may have already acquired cognitive deficits and reduced cognitive reserves during childhood, increasing disease burden later in life may leave them at particular risk of further cognitive impairment.

PSYCHOSOCIAL IMPACT AND OUTCOMES

Childhood MS and ADEM can result in social and psychological sequelae that have the potential to affect quality of life. Studies show that adults with MS are more likely to be unemployed, to need help with personal care and routine household tasks, to be less socially active, and to have severely affected ADLs than adults without MS. Adults with MS are also more likely to be depressed or suffer from bipolar disorder, and are much more likely to be divorced, than the general population (Murray, 1995). The consequences of interrupted cognitive, social, and behavioral development in childhood are likely to be even more serious than those of adult-onset MS.

Symptoms of ADEM, and more often childhood MS, are pervasive. In the more severe cases, physical and cognitive impairments can affect children's home life, interactions with peers, functioning in the classroom, and ability to participate in sports and leisure activities. For children, the ability to participate successfully in such activities has a huge impact on their development of self-worth and confidence. Ongoing difficulties due to ADEM, or a diagnosis of MS, may add further psychosocial burden. Kalb et al. (1999) have assessed the impact of childhood MS on social and emotional functioning. They found that children with MS did not perceive themselves as different from their peers in terms of scholastic competence, athletic competence, physical appearance, behavioral conduct, romantic appeal, or global self-worth. However, the authors noted that the children appeared to lack a realistic or accurate picture of MS or its potential impact. They suggested that many children appeared to display a "healthy" denial, which allowed them to cope with day-to-day life. Results from our lab do not necessarily support these findings. We found higher-than-expected rates of parent-reported depression and anxiety for children after ADEM, with many children, particularly those diagnosed at a younger age, requiring ongoing clinical management for these problems. Furthermore, children who are younger at disease onset may be most vulnerable to low self-esteem and reduced confidence, coupled with more severe and widespread cognitive and behavioral problems.

This area is clearly underresearched, and although we may draw inferences from studies addressing the psychosocial impact of other brain diseases or chronic illnesses of childhood, the unique aspects of these conditions warrants further investigation so that appropriate treatment and management can be provided.

FUTURE DIRECTIONS

ADEM and childhood MS are relatively "new" diagnoses, with only minimal research available to guide practitioners in the care and follow-up of children presenting with these conditions. Uncertainty exists at all levels: Diagnostic criteria remain poorly defined; treatment approaches are yet to be rigorously evaluated; medical and behavioral outcomes are variable at best; and key risk factors are yet to be definitively established. Furthermore, it remains unclear whether these diseases are unique, or whether they in fact fall along a continuum.

Although it may be argued that there is some potential to extrapolate from adult data, at least in the case of MS, research findings (from both neuroimaging and behavioral domains) and theoretical models lead us to caution against this approach, emphasizing that damage to the developing brain may lead to substantially different consequences from those documented in the adult brain. Indeed, this has already been highlighted for ADEM and childhood MS, where reported impairments appear more generalized and severe than those described in adult samples, despite the identification of less pathology on neuroimaging.

To make progress in this area, a number of steps are necessary. First, due to the low incidence and prevalence of these conditions, multicenter trials will be critical to ensure samples of sufficient size for answering key questions regarding effective treatments, long-term consequences, and potential risk factors. Second, almost all studies investigating neurocognitive outcome have highlighted the need for longitudinal investigation, in response to the apparent risk of cognitive decline over time. It will be of great interest to determine whether this decline holds up in larger samples, and whether it represents a delayed developmental trajectory associated with eventual catch-up, or a more permanent disability. Such studies also have the potential to contribute to theoretical models addressing the impact of early brain damage and potential risk and resilience factors more generally.

A further challenge to consider is how to take advantage of recent neuroimaging advances. In other areas, researchers have begun to report fascinating findings, linking quantitative and qualitative neuroimaging data with behavioral outcome measures. Although routine MRI approaches are limited, in part by their poor pathological specificity, nonconventional neuroimaging techniques (e.g., positron emission tomography, functional MRI, proton magnetic resonance spectroscopy, magnetization transfer imaging, diffusion-weighted imaging, tractography) have the potential to overcome these limitations by being able to better detect and characterize the different pathological processes operating in MS and ADEM, and also to quantify their severity.

In conclusion, only large-scale, multidisciplinary studies, preferably employing longitudinal designs and incorporating medical, radiological, and behavioral methodologies, will assist in furthering our knowledge of the consequences and risk factors for these rare and complex conditions.

REFERENCES

Alotaibi, S., Kennedy, J., Tellier, R., Stephens, D., & Banwell, B. (2004). Epstein–Barr virus in pediatric multiple sclerosis. *Journal of the American Medical Association, 291*(15), 1875–1879.

Anderson, V., & Moore, C. (1995). Age at injury as a predictor of outcome following pediatric head injury: A longitudinal perspective. *Child Neuropsychology, 1*, 187–202.

Anlar, B., Basaran, C., Kose, G., Guven, A., Haspolat, S., Yakut, A., et al. (2003). Acute disseminated encephalomyelitis in children: Outcome and prognosis. *Neuropediatrics, 34*, 194–199.

Ascherio, A., Munger, K. L., Lennette, E. T., Spiegelman, D., Hernan, M. A., Olek, M. J., et al. (2001). Epstein–Barr virus antibodies and risk of multiple sclerosis: A prospective study. *Journal of the American Medical Association, 286*, 3083–3088.

Balassy, C., Bernet, G., Wober-Bongol, C., Csapo, B., Szeles, J., Fleischmann, D., et al. (2001). Long-term MRI observations of childhood-onset relapsing--remitting multiple sclerosis. *Neuropediatrics, 32*, 28–37.

Banwell, B. (2004). Pediatric multiple sclerosis. *Current Neurology and Neuroscience Reports, 4*, 245–252.

Banwell, B. L., & Anderson, P. E. (2005). The cognitive burden of multiple sclerosis in children. *Neurology, 64*, 891–894.

Banwell, B. L., Shroff, M., Ness, J. M., Jeffrey, D., Schwid, S., & Weinstock-Guttman, B. (2007). MRI features of pediatric multiple sclerosis. *Neurology, 68*(Suppl. 2), S46–S53.

Barcellos, L. F., Oksenberg, J. R., Begovich, A. B., Martin, E. R., Schmidt, S., Vittinghoff, E., et al. (2003). HLA-DR2 dose effect on susceptability to multiple sclerosis and influence on disease course. *American Journal of Human Genetics, 72*, 710–716.

Blakemore, S., & Choudhury, S. (2006). Development of the adolescent brain: Implications for executive function and social cognition. *Journal of Child Psychology and Psychiatry, 47*, 296–312.

Boiko, A. N., Gusev, E. I., Sudomoina, M. A., Alekseenkov, A. D., Kulakova, O. G., Bikova, O. V., et al. (2002a). Association and linkage of juvenile MS with HLA-DR2 (15) in Russians. *Neurology, 58*, 658–660.

Boiko, A., Vorobeychik, G., Paty, D., Devonshire, V., & Sadovnick, D. (2002b). Early onset multiple sclerosis: A longitudinal study. *Neurology, 59*(7), 1006–1010.

Boutin, B., Esquivel, E., Mayer, M., Chaumet, S., Ponsot, G., & Arthuis, M. (1988). Multiple sclerosis in children: Report of clinical and paraclinical features of 19 cases. *Neuropediatrics, 19*, 118–123.

Bye, A. M. E., Kendall, B., & Wilson, J. (1985). Multiple sclerosis in childhood: A new look. *Developmental Medicine and Child Neurology, 27*, 215–222.

Cohen, O., Steiner-Birmanns, B., Biran, I., Abramsky, O., Honigman, S., & Steiner, I. (2001). Recurrence of acute disseminated encephalomyelitis at the previously affected brain site. *Archives of Neurology, 58*(5), 797–801.

Cohen, R. A., & Fisher, M. (1989). Amantadine treatment of fatigue associated with multiple sclerosis. *Archives of Neurology, 46*, 676–680.

Cole, G. F., & Stuart, C. A. (1995). A long perspective on childhood multiple sclerosis. *Developmental Medicine and Child Neurology, 37*, 661–666.

Comi, G., Kappos, L., Clanet, M., Ebers, G., Fassas, A., Fazekas, F., et al. (2000). Guidelines for autologous blood and marrow stem cell transplantation in multiple sclerosis: A consensus report. *Journal of Neurology, 247*, 376–382.

Compston, A. (1998). The story of multiple sclerosis. In *McAlpine's multiple sclerosis* (3rd ed.). London: Churchill Livingstone.

Compston, A. (1999). The genetic epidemiology of multiple sclerosis. *Philosophical Transactions of the Royal Society of London, Series B, Biological Sciences, 345*, 1623–1634.

Confavreux, C., Vukusic, S., & Adeleine, P. (2003). Early clinical predictors and progression of irreversible disability in multiple sclerosis: An amnesic process. *Brain, 126*, 770–782.

Dale, R. C., de Sousa, C., Chong, W. K., Cox, T. C., Harding, B., & Neville, B. G. (2000). Acute disseminated encephalomyelitis, multiphasic disseminated encephalomyelities and multiple sclerosis in children. *Brain, 123*, 2407–2422.

Davies, J. M. (1997). Molecular mimicry: Can epitope mimicry induce autoimmune disease? *Immunology and Cell Biology, 75*, 113–126.

Deery, B. (2008). *Childhood MS and ADEM: Longitudinal investigation and comparison of neurocognitive features in children.* Doctoral dissertation, University of Melbourne.

De Stefano, N., Matthews, P. M., & Arnold, D. L. (1995). Reversible decreases in N-acetylaspartate after acute brain injury. *Magnetic Resonance in Medicine, 34*, 721–727.

Duquette, P., Murray, T. J., Pleines, J., Ebers, G. C., Sadovnick, D., Weldon, P., et al. (1987). Multiple sclerosis in childhood: Clinical profile in 125 patients. *Journal of Pediatrics, 111*(3), 359–363.

Ebner, F., Millner, M. M., & Justich, E. (1990). Multiple sclerosis in children: Value of serial MR studies to monitor patients. *American Journal of Neuroradiology, 11*, 1023–1027.

Falini, A., Calabrese, G., Filippi, M., Origgi, D., Lipari, S., Colombo, B., et al. (1998). Benign versus secondary progressive multiple sclerosis: The potential role of 1H MR spectroscopy in defining the nature of disability. *American Journal of Neuroradiology, 19*, 223–229.

Fazekas, F., Barkhof, F., Filippi, M., Grossman, R. I., Li, D. K. B., McDonald, W. I., et al. (1999). The contribution of magnetic resonance imaging to the diagnosis of multiple sclerosis. *Neurology, 53*, 448–456.

Fenichel, G. M. (1982). Neurological complications of immunization. *Annals of Neurology, 12*, 119–128.

Filippi, M., Tortorella, C., Rovaris, M., Bozzali, M., Possa, F., Sormani, M. P., et al. (2000). Changes in the normal appearing brain tissue and cognitive impairment in multiple sclerosis. *Journal of Neurology, Neurosurgery and Psychiatry, 68*, 157–161.

Fujinami, R. S., & Oldstone, M. B. (1985). Amino acid homology between the encephalitogenic site of myelin basic protein and virus: Mechanism for autoimmunity. *Science, 230*, 1043–1045.

Gall, J. C., Hayles, A. B., Siekert R. G., & Keith, H. M. (1958). Multiple sclerosis in children: A clinical study of 40 cases with onset in childhood. *Pediatrics, 21*(5), 703–709.

Gowers, W. R. (1888). *A manual of disease of the nervous system.* London: J. & A. Churchill.

Gronseth, G. S., & Ashman, E. J. (2000). Practice parameter: The usefulness of evoked potentials in identifying clinically silent lesions in patients with suspected multiple sclerosis (an evidence-based review). Report of the Quality Standards Subcommittee of the American Academy of Neurology. *Neurology, 54*, 1720–1725.

Gusev, E. I., Demina, T. L., & Boiko, A. N. (1997). *Multiple sclerosis.* Moscow: Medicine.

Hahn, C. D., Miles, B. S., MacGregor, D. L., Blaser, S. I., Banwell, B. L., & Hetherington, C. R. (2003). Neurocognitive outcome after acute disseminated encephalomyelitis. *Pediatric Neurology, 29*, 117–123.

Haliloglu, G., Anlar, B., Aysun, S., Topcu, M., Topaloglu, H., Turanli, G., et al. (2002). Gender prevalence in childhood multiple sclerosis and myasthenia gravis. *Journal of Child Neurology, 17*, 390–392.

Hammond, S. F., McLeod, J. G., Macaskill, P., & English, D. R. (2000). Multiple sclerosis in Australia: Prognostic factors. *Journal of Clinical Neuroscience, 7*, 16–19.

Hanefeld, F. (2007). Pediatric multiple sclerosis: A short history of a long story. *Neurology, 68*(Suppl. 2), S3–S6.

Hermann, B., Seidenberg, M., Bell, B., Rutecki, P., Sheth, R., Ruggles, K., et al. (2002). The neurodevelopmental impact of childhood-onset temporal lobe epilepsy on brain structure and function. *Epilepsia, 43*(9), 1062–1071.

Hudspeth, W., & Pribram, K. (1990). Stages of brain and cognitive maturation. *Journal of Educational Psychology, 82*, 881–884.

Hynson, J. L., Kornberg, A. J., Coleman, L. T., Shield, L., Harvey, A. S., & Kean, M. J. (2001). Clinical and neuroradiologic features of acute disseminated encephalomyelitis in children. *Neurology, 56*, 1308–1312.

Iannetti, P., Marciani, M. G., Spalice, A., Raucci, U., Trasimeni, G., Gualdi, G. F., et al. (1996). Primary CNS demyelinating diseases in childhood: Multiple sclerosis. *Child's Nervous System, 12*, 149–154.

Idrissova, Z. R., Boldyreva, M. N., Dekonenko, E. P., Malishev, N. A., Leontyeva, I. Y., Martinenko, I. N., et al. (2003). Acute disseminated encephalomyelitis in children: Clinical features and HLA-DR linkage. *European Journal of Neurology, 10*, 537–546.

Inglese, M., Salvi, F., Iannucci, G., Mancardi, G. L., Mascalchi, M., & Filippi, M. (2002). Magnetization transfer and diffusion tensor MR imaging of acute disseminated encephalomyelitis. *American Journal of Neuroradiology, 23*, 267–272.

Jacobs, R., Anderson, V., Neale, J., Kornberg, A., & Shield, L. (2004). Neuropsychological outcome following ADEM in childhood: Impact of age at illness onset. *Pediatric Neurology, 31*(3), 191–197.

Jan, M. M. S. (2005). Childhood multiple sclerosis. *Journal of Pediatric Neurology, 3*, 131–136.

Kalb, R. C., Di Lorenzo, T. A., La Rocca, N. G., Caruso, L. S., Shawaryn, M. A., Elkin, R., et al. (1999). The impact of early-onset multiple sclerosis on cognitive and psychosocial indices. *International Journal of MS Care, 1*(1), 2–17.

Klinberg, T., Vaidyn, C. J., Gabrieli, J. D. E., Moseley, M. E., & Heidehus, M. (1999). Myelination and organization of the frontal white matter in children: A diffusion tensor MRI study. *NeuroReport, 10*, 2817–2821.

Knox, K., & Hader, W. J. (2004). Paediatric multiple sclerosis: A population based study. *Neurology, 62*(Suppl. 5), A230. [Abstract]

Koch-Henriksen, N. (1999). The Danish Multiple Sclerosis Registry: A 50-year follow-up. *Multiple Sclerosis, 5*(4), 293–296.

Krupp, L. B., MacAllister, W. S., Milazzo, M., Belman, A. L., Christodoulou, C., & Melville, P. (2004). Unexpected demographic profile in pediatric MS. *Annals of Neurology, 56*, S56–S56.

Kurtzke, J. F., Beebe, G. W., & Norman, J. E. (1985). Epidemiology of multiple sclerosis in United States veterans: III. Migration and the risk of MS. *Neurology, 35*(5), 672–678.

Leake, J. A. D., Albani, S., Kao, A. S., Senac, M. O., Billman, G. F., Nespeca, M. P., et al. (2004). Acute disseminated encephalomyelitis in childhood: Epidemiologic, clinical and laboratory features. *Pediatric Infectious Disease Journal, 23*, 756–764.

Levic, Z. M., Dujmovic, I., Pekmezovic, T., Jarebinski, M., Marinkovic, J., Stojsavljevic, N., et al. (1999). Prognostic factors for survival in multiple sclerosis. *Multiple Sclerosis, 5*, 171–178.

Lipton, H. L. (1975). Theiler's virus infection in mice: An unusual biphasic disease process leading to demyelination. *Infection and Immunity, 11*, 1147–1155.

Lucchinetti, C. F., Kiers, L., O'Duffy, A., Gomez, M. R., Cross, S., Leavitt, J. A., et al. (1997). Risk factors for developing multiple sclerosis after childhood optic neuritis. *Neurology, 49*, 1413–1418.

MacAllister, W. S., Belman, A. L., Milazzo, M., Weisbrot, D. M., Christodoulou, C., Scherl, W. F., et al. (2005). Cognitive functioning in children and adolescents with multiple sclerosis. *Neurology, 64*, 1422–1425.

MacAllister, W. S., Christodoulou, C., Milazzo, M., & Krupp, L. B. (2007). Longitudinal neuropsychological assessment in pediatric multiple sclerosis. *Developmental Neuropsychology, 32*(2), 625–644.

Marie, P. (1895). *Lectures on diseases of the spinal cord*. London: New Sydenham Society.

Masterman, T., Ligers, A., Olsson, T., Andersson, M., Olerup, O., & Hillert, J. (2000). HLA-DR15 is associated with lower age at onset in multiple sclerosis. *Annals of Neurology, 48*, 41–48.

McAllister, L. D., Beatty, P. G., & Rose, J. (1997). Allogenic bone marrow transplant for chronic myelogenous leukemia in a patient with multiple sclerosis. *Bone Marrow Transplantation, 19*, 395–397.

McCann, K. K., Farmer, J. E., & Patel, N. (2004). Childhood-onset multiple sclerosis and mood disorders: A case study. *Child Neuropsychology, 10*(2), 102–116.

Menge, T., Hemmer, B., Nessler, S., Wiendl, H., Neuhaus, O., Hartung, H., et al. (2005). Acute disseminated encephalomyelitis: An update. *Archives of Neurology, 62*, 1673–1680.

Mezzapesa, D. M., Rocca, M. A., Falini, A., Rodegher, M. E., Ghezzi, A., Comi, G., et al. (2004). A preliminary diffusion tensor and magnetization transfer magnetic resonance imaging study of early-onset multiple sclerosis. *Archives of Neurology, 61*, 366–368.

Miller, A. (1998). Diagnosis of multiple sclerosis. *Seminars in Neurology, 18*, 309–316.

Morales, D. S., Slatkowski, R. M., Howard, C. W., & Warman, R. (2000). Optic neuritis in children. *Journal of Pediatric Ophthalmology and Strabismus, 37*, 254–259.

Murray, T. J. (1995). The psychosocial aspects of multiple sclerosis. *Neurologic Clinics, 13*, 197–223.

Murthy, J. M., Yangala, R., Meena, A. K., & Reddy, J. J. (1999). Acute disseminated encephalomyelitis: Clinical and MRI study from South India. *Journal of the Neurological Sciences, 165*, 133–138.

Murthy, S. N., Faden, H. S., Cohen, M. E., & Bakshi, R. (2002). Acute disseminated encephalomyelitis in children. *Pediatrics, 110*, e21.

Nalin, D. R. (1989). Mumps, measles and rubella vaccination and encephalitis [Letter]. *British Medical Journal, 299*, 1219.

Noseworthy, J. H., Lucchinetti, C., Rodriguez, M., & Weinshenker, B. G. (2000). Multiple sclerosis. *New England Journal of Medicine, 343*, 938–952.

Owens, T., & Sriram, S. (1995). The immunology of multiple sclerosis and its animal model: Experimental allergic encephalomyelitis. *Neurologic Clinics, 13*, 51–73.

Paty, D. W., Noseworthy, J. H., & Ebers, G. C. (1998). Diagnosis of multiple sclerosis. In D. W. Paty & G. C. Ebers (Eds.), *Multiple sclerosis*. Philadelphia: F.A. Davis.

Pinhaus-Hamiel, O., Barak, Y., Siev-Ner, I., & Achiron, A. (1998). Juvenile multiple sclerosis: Clinical features and prognostic characteristics. *Journal of Pediatrics, 132*, 735–737.

Rammohan, K. W., Rosenberg, J. H., Lynn, D. J., Blumenfeld, A. M., Pollak, C. P., & Nagaraja, H. N. (2002). Efficacy and safety of modafinil (Provigil) for the treatment of fatigue in multiple sclerosis: A two centre phase 2 study. *Journal of Neurology, Neurosurgery and Psychiatry, 72*, 179–183.

Rao, S. M., Leo, G. J., Bernardin, L., & Unverzagt, F. (1991). Cognitive dysfunction in multiple sclerosis: I. Frequency, patterns, and predictors. *Neurology, 41*, 685–691.

Rivers, T. M., Sprunt, D. H., & Berry, G. P. (1933). Observations on attempts to produce acute disseminated encephalomyelitis. *Journal of Experimental Medicine, 58*, 39–53.

Ruggieri, M., Polizzi, A., Pavone, L., & Grimaldi, L. M. (1999). Multiple sclerosis in children under 6 years of age. *Neurology, 53*(3), 478–484.

Sadovnick, A. D., Armstrong, H., Rice, G. P. A., Bulman, D., Hashimoto, L., Paty, D. W., et al. (1993). A population-based study of multiple sclerosis in twins: Update. *Annals of Neurology, 33*, 281–285.

Sadovnick, A. D., Dircks, A., & Ebers, G. C. (1999). Genetic counselling in multiple sclerosis: Risks to sibs and children of affected individuals. *Clinical Genetics, 56*, 118–122.

Sadovnick, A. D., & Ebers, G. C. (1993). Epidemiology of multiple sclerosis: A critical overview. *Canadian Journal of Neurological Sciences, 20,* 17–29.

Sadovnick, A. D., & Ebers, G. C. (1995). Genetics of multiple sclerosis. *Neurologic Clinics, 13,* 99–118.

Schwarz, S., Mohr, A., Knauth, M., Wildemann, B., & Storch-Hagenlocher, B. (2001). Acute disseminated encephalomyelitis: A follow-up study of 40 adult patients. *Neurology, 56,* 1313–1318.

Shaw, C. M., & Alvord, E. C., Jr. (1987). Multiple sclerosis beginning in infancy. *Journal of Child Neurology, 2,* 252–256.

Simone, I. L., Carrara, D., Tortorella, C., Liquori, M., Lepore, V., Pelligrini, F., et al. (2002). Course and prognosis in early onset MS. Comparison with adult-onset forms. *Neurology, 59,* 1922–1928.

Sunnerhagen, K. S., Johansson, K., & Ekholm, S. (2003). Rehabilitation problems after acute disseminated encephalomyelitis: Four cases. *Journal of Rehabilitation Medicine, 35,* 20–25.

Tenembaum, S., Chamoles, N., & Fejerman, N. (2002). Acute disseminated encephalomyelitis: A long-term follow-up study of 84 pediatric patients. *Neurology, 59,* 1224–1231.

Turnball, H. M., & McIntosh, J. (1926). Encephalomyelitis following vaccination. *British Journal of Experimental Pathology, 7,* 181–222.

Weinstock-Guttman, B., & Cohen, J. A. (1996). Emerging therapies for multiple sclerosis. *The Neurologist, 2,* 342–355.

Wisniewski, H. M., & Keith, A. B. (1977). Chronic experimental allergic encephalomyelitis: An experimental model of multiple sclerosis. *Annals of Neurology, 1,* 144–148.

CHAPTER 7

Tuberous Sclerosis Complex

Anna W. Byars

BRIEF HISTORICAL OVERVIEW AND DIAGNOSTIC CRITERIA

According to Gomez, Sampson, and Whittemore (1990), tuberous sclerosis complex (TSC) was first described in 1862 by Von Recklinghausen and later elaborated on by Bourneville in the 1880s, who used the term *sclerose tubereuse* to reflect the potato-like appearance of the cortical tubers that characterized the disorder. Several years later, Vogt focused on facial angiofibromas, seizures, and mental retardation as cardinal features of the disorder (Gomez et al., 1999), which were thought to be necessary for the diagnosis until relatively recently. In 1998, a consensus conference on TSC was sponsored by the National Institutes of Health and the National Tuberous Sclerosis Association (Hyman & Whittemore, 2000), and resulted in the publication of revised diagnostic criteria for TSC (Roach, Gomez, & Northrup, 1998; see Table 7.1). These diagnostic criteria (Roach et al., 1998) are complex; the classic triad of seizures, mental retardation, and adenoma sebaceum (facial angiofibroma) described by Vogt in 1908 is actually present in only 29% of cases (Gomez, 1988).

PATHOLOGICAL FEATURES

TSC affects multiple organ systems, including skin (Webb, Clarke, Fryer, & Osborne, 1996), heart (Webb, Thomas, & Osborne, 1993), kidney (O'Callaghan, Noakes, Martyns, & Osborne, 2004b), lungs (Castro, Shepherd, Gomez, Lie, & Ryu, 1995), and brain (DiMario, 2004).

TABLE 7.1. Revised Diagnostic Criteria for Tuberous Sclerosis Complex (TSC)

Major features	Minor features
Facial angiofibromas or forehead plaque	Multiple pits in dental enamel
Nontraumatic ungula or periungual fibroma	Hamartomatous rectal polyps
Hypomelanotic macules (more than three)	Bone cysts
Shagreen patch (connective tissue nevus)	Cerebral white matter radial migration lines
Multiple retinal nodular hamartoma	Gingival fibromas
Cortical tuber	Nonrenal hamartoma
Subependymal nodule	Retinal achromic patch
Subependymal giant cell astrocytoma	"Confetti" skin lesions
Cardiac rhabdomyoma, single or multiple	Multiple renal cysts
Lymphangiomyomatosis	
Renal angiomyolipoma	

Definite TSC: Either two major features or one major feature plus two minor features
Probable TSC: One major plus one minor feature
Possible TSC: Either one major feature or two or more minor features

Note. From Roach, Gomez, and Northrup (1998). Copyright 1998 by SAGE Publications. Reprinted by permission.

Skin

The cutaneous features of TSC are common and may be the first sign of disease. The most distinctive of these are the facial angiofibromas, which typically appear in middle childhood and may progress during puberty and adolescence. They are potentially disfiguring. Various other skin findings may be present from birth, including ash leaf spots or hypomelanotic macules, shagreen patches, and ungual fibromas.

Heart

The primary cardiac manifestation of TSC is cardiac rhabdomyoma, a benign tumor that is typically clinically asymptomatic. However some patients have difficulty with the function of cardiac valves that may be affected, or with arrhythmia or cardiomyopathy. These lesions develop prenatally and usually involute or resolve with age.

Kidney

Renal angiomyolipomas and renal cysts are the typical kidney manifestations of TSC. Symptomatic renal involvement is not common in childhood (Franz, 1998).

Brain

Structural Characteristics

The abnormality in brain development occurs during embryogenesis and results in cortical tubers, subependymal nodules, subcortical heterotopias, cortical dysplasia, and subependymal giant cell astrocytomas. The cortical tubers (or, more precisely, the surrounding tissues) frequently act as the focus for epileptiform discharges. See Figure 7.1 for a magnetic resonance imaging (MRI) scan of a severely affected brain.

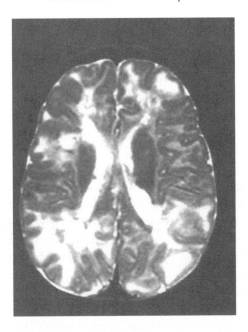

FIGURE 7.1. T2-weighted MRI scan of a brain severely affected by TSC, showing multiple cortical tubers as well as subependymal nodules characteristic of TSC.

Epilepsy

As many as 80–90% of individuals with TSC will develop epilepsy (Gomez et al., 1999), which commonly begins in infancy. The seizures that begin in the first year of life usually resemble infantile spasms; partial seizures may also occur. The partial seizures may precede (usually identified in retrospect after the development of spasms), co-occur with, or evolve from the infantile spasms (Curatolo, Seri, Verdecchia, & Bombardieri, 2001). Various other seizure types may be seen in TSC as well; typical absence seizures are the only type that have not been observed (Thiele, 2004). Epilepsy associated with TSC is usually difficult to treat, and in many patients it is medically intractable.

EPIDEMIOLOGY AND GENETICS

TSC is an autosomal dominant disease with an incidence estimated at between 1 in 6,000 and 1 in 9,000 (Osborne, Fryer, & Webb, 1991; Hyman & Whittemore, 2000). These estimates put the incidence of TSC on a par with that of more frequently recognized inherited pediatric diseases, such as cystic fibrosis (Franz, 1998). It is characterized by high-penetrance involvement of multiple organ systems and by considerable variability and expression (Gomez, 1988), as well as a high rate of spontaneous mutation. TSC is due to mutation in either the TSC1 gene (9q34), identified in 1997 (van Slegtenhorst et al., 1997), or the TSC2 gene (16p13.3), discovered in 1993 (European Chromosome 16 Tuberous Sclerosis Consortium, 1993). These genes code for the proteins hamartin and tuberin, respectively, which act as tumor suppressors and normally prevent the development of tumors or other forms of excessive cell growth, such as cortical tubers. The actual manifestation of symptoms seems to depend on "second-hit" mutations that knock out the normal allele and result in abnormalities in cell differentiation and migration. In addition, hamartin and tuberin interact to form a complex that acts to decrease activity of mammalian target of rapamycin (mTOR), which regulates the synthesis of proteins important for cell proliferation, growth, and survival (see Holmes, Stafstrom, & the Tuberous Sclerosis Study Group, 2007, or Curatolo, Bombardieri, & Jozwiak, 2008, for a discussion). These relatively recently identified molecular mechanisms have led to speculation about potential treatment avenues, which are described below.

In some studies examining the relationship between genotype and phenotype, the clinical symptoms associated with TSC2 appeared to be more severe and more likely to include mental retardation (Dabora et al., 2001; Jones et al., 1999); another study, however, found no differences in the type or degree of symptoms associated with TSC1 and TSC2 (van Slegtenhorst, Verhoef, Tempelaars, et al., 1999). de Vries and Bolton (2000), based on data they obtained from a mail survey of 510 families of individuals with TSC, concluded that the phenotype differences between TSC1 and TSC2 disease are related to severity rather than to the specific symptoms involved in either. A recent study has confirmed the association between TSC2 mutations and poorer cognitive performance, as well as earlier age of seizure onset and the presence of more cortical tubers (Jansen et al., 2008a). Jansen et al. have emphasized, however, that there is considerable overlap in both neurological and cognitive phenotype in patients with TSC1 and TSC2 mutations.

NEUROPATHOLOGICAL SUBSTRATE

TSC is a disorder of cellular differentiation, proliferation, and neuronal migration (Mizuguchi & Takashima, 2001). The characteristic findings on brain imaging are cortical tubers, which can occur throughout the brain and can be described as discrete areas of disorganization of cortical lamination (Ess, 2006). Subependymal nodules are also common. These can grow into subependymal giant cell astrocytomas, which may require surgical intervention. Understanding of the neuropathology of TSC has evolved in concert with the development of more sensitive imaging techniques (Franz, 1998; Inoue et al., 1998). Early studies relied on computed tomography (Clarke, Cook, & Osborne, 1996; Menor, Marti-Bonmati, Mulas, Poyatos, & Cortina, 1992; Webb, Thomson, & Osborne, 1991b), which does not adequately identify the cortical malformations and tubers that are prevalent in TSC. Advances in MRI (increased field strength of the magnets used for routine clinical scanning, together with refined imaging protocols) have allowed for more precise counting of cortical tubers, as well as calculation of tuber volumes (*tuber–brain proportion*) (Jansen et al., 2008a) and better identification of subtle cortical malformations.

NEUROPSYCHOLOGICAL AND
NEUROBEHAVIORAL CONSEQUENCES

The population with TSC is particularly interesting from a neurobehavioral standpoint, because several mechanisms may be hypothesized to underlie the deficits that are observed. These mechanisms include the cortical tubers, infantile spasms, chronic seizure activity, and other neurological findings that are characteristic of TSC. The neurobehavioral symptoms associated with TSC include mental retardation and autism or autistic features (Asato & Hardan, 2004). Sleep disturbance and extreme hyperactivity have also been noted (Hunt, 1993).

Intellectual Impairment

The most common neuropsychological consequence of TSC is mental retardation. It was initially thought to be universally present; however, with improved identification and diagnosis, it is clear that approximately only 50% of people with TSC will have mental retardation (Joinson et al., 2003). In an epidemiological sample of 108 individuals with TSC, Joinson et al. (2003) used standardized tests and comparisons with siblings to demonstrate that IQ was bimodally distributed: 44% of the patients with TSC had an IQ below 70. Those with normal-range intelligence had a mean IQ (94) that was significantly lower than that of unaffected siblings (106). There were no data presented to suggest that some abilities might be weak despite average overall IQ. Another study of patients with TSC recruited from a variety of clinical settings, rather than on an epidemiological basis, documented an IQ below 70 in 55% of their 98 cases (Lewis, Thomas, Murphy, & Sampson, 2004).

There are two risk factors for intellectual impairment in patients with TSC: *tuber burden*, or the number of tubers an individual has, and a history of infantile spasms. The two factors generally co-occur (Doherty, Goh, Young Poussaint, Erdag, & Thiele, 2005). Shepherd, Houser, and Gomez (1995) demonstrated a relationship between the number of tubers and mental disability. They also found that children with mental disability had seizures or a history of seizures; those children without such disability had no history of seizures. The degree to which tuber burden or epilepsy is more responsible for cognitive impairment on either a group or an individual-patient basis is not known. The degree of intellectual impairment has been associated with the number of tubers in an individual (O'Callaghan et al., 2004a; Shepherd et al., 1995), the number of lobes involved (Weber, Egelhoff, McKellop, & Franz, 2000), and whether or not tubers are distributed unilaterally or bilaterally (Zaroff et al., 2006).

A meta-analysis (Goodman et al., 1997) of a small number of studies with varying methodologies suggested that the total number of cortical tubers is a marker for overall neurological severity of TSC in individual patients, defined as the degree of mental retardation. Some have questioned the strength of this finding (Doherty et al., 2005) because of the few studies included and the different methodologies used in these studies. Humphrey, Higgins, Yates, and Bolton (2004) reported on a pair of monozygotic twins with TSC who had differing degrees of developmental delay. The more severely affected twin had a smaller number of tubers, but they were large and resulted in extensive brain involvement, along with mental retardation and autism; the less severely affected twin had more tubers, but they were small, and he did not meet the criteria for mental retardation or autism.

The presence of mental retardation is also strongly associated with a history of infantile spasms in particular and epilepsy in general (Goh, Kwiatkowski, Dorer, & Thiele, 2005; Hunt, 1993; Joinson et al., 2003; Jozwiak, Goodman, & Lamm, 1998; O'Callaghan et al., 2004a; Shepherd & Stephenson, 1992). Early onset of seizures has also been shown to be associated with poor developmental and intellectual outcome (Gomez et al., 1999; Zaroff et al., 2006), although it has been suggested that this association is a result of the age distribution of infantile spasms (Jozwiak et al., 1998). A small prospective study of children with TSC born to families already identified with TSC (Webb, Fryer, & Osborne, 1991a) showed that the children who experienced developmental delay and subsequent mental retardation (38% of their sample of 26 patients) all had seizures at a young age (a mean onset of 10 months of age). The individuals with unimpaired cognitive development attended normal school or were gainfully employed.

Neuropsychological Deficits

Prather and de Vries (2004) noted that there are few data concerning the cognitive and behavioral characteristics of individuals with TSC but without mental retardation. Early studies sought to identify specific patterns of neuropsychological impairment that might be associated with particular tuber locations, but were largely unsuccessful in this regard (Jambaque et al., 1991; Weber, Egelhoff, & Franz, 1996). Global impairment across neuropsychological domains was the most frequent finding in these studies. Weber et al. (1996) found no differences in the pattern of neuropsychological deficit among patients with varying tuber locations. Jambaque et al. (1991) studied 23 patients with TSC; their assessments included measures of naming, visual-constructive ability, and memory, but the analyses focused only on IQ scores from at least four different IQ tests. Of the 23 patients, 16 had IQ scores in the mentally retarded range, with 8 of them having IQ scores below 40. In the 7 patients with IQ scores in the average range, various isolated deficits were described, including dyspraxia, speech delay, visual–spatial deficit, memory impairment, and dyscalculia (each in one patient), as well as behavior problems, including hyperactivity and aggression (each in one patient). There was a specific functional anatomical relationship between neuropsychological profile and tuber location in only one case: that of a patient with average IQ, constructional dyspraxia, and a single left parietal tuber. They also found that transient spasms or late-onset partial seizures were the only seizure types occurring in their patients who had normal intelligence. The majority of their sample with mental retardation had multiple bilateral cortical tubers.

With the increasing identification of patients who have TSC but no intellectual deficit, a few studies of neuropsychological profiles have been carried out (Prather & de Vries, 2004). Specific deficits in attention (de Vries & Watson, 2008; Harrison, O'Callaghan, Hancock, Osborne, & Bolton, 1999) and executive functions (Harrison et al., 1999) have been documented in patients with TSC and normal intelligence. Harrison et al. (1999) compared seven patients with TSC and normal intelligence to nine healthy control participants, using primarily computerized measures of memory and problem solving (the Cambridge Neuropsychological Test Automated Battery, or CANTAB). The group means of the patients and controls did not differ for any of the measures, including the Mini-Mental State Exam, Raven's Progressive Matrices, the National Adult Reading Test, and the National Adult Reading Test in addition to the CANTAB subtests. However, examination of the presence of impaired scores in each group did show a difference: None of the control participants produced an impaired performance, but five of the seven patients with TSC scored at or below the 5th percentile on one or more of the tests. The authors appropriately concluded, however, that the small sample size precluded definitive statements regarding the relationship of lesion location and neuropsychological deficit. Jansen et al. (2008b) have noted, however, that specific deficits in memory and learning in their patient sample were consistent with general intellectual function.

One of the ongoing problems with the TSC literature is that studies measuring only global intellectual function—that is, relying on IQ or developmental quotient (DQ) scores (Jambaque et al., 1991; Winterkorn, Pulsifer, & Thiele, 2007)—are characterized as measuring neuropsychological status. For example, Winterkorn et al. (2007) noted that their study was one with quantitative neuropsychiatric data on a large sample. They reviewed the medical records of 107 patients seen in their TSC clinic who had undergone neuropsychiatric assessment. They observed the typical bimodal distribution of IQ scores in these patients, with 57% of their sample having normal-range IQ or DQ scores. They also found that IQ/DQ scores were lower for those patients with refractory epilepsy and documented TSC2 mutations. No data about specific neuropsychological deficits, were presented, however.

Autism/Other Pervasive Developmental Disorders

Autism and other pervasive developmental disorders (PDD) are much more common in patients with TSC than in the general population (Asano et al., 2001; Baker, Piven, & Sato, 1998; Gillberg, Gillberg, & Ahlsen, 1994; Hunt & Shepherd, 1993). Rates of autism specifically are estimated to be approximately 25% in the population with TSC, and as many as 40–50% of patients with TSC meet criteria for autism spectrum disorders (ASD) or PDD in general (Gutierrez, Smalley, & Tanguay, 1998; Wiznitzer, 2004). The mechanism for this association is not understood. It may be related to common genetic factors, to generalized brain dysfunction, or to specific regions disrupted by tubers or seizures that play a role in autism. It is clear that of all the genetic syndromes that may lead to mental retardation, TSC is the most strongly associated with autism, and therefore may be the most likely to provide clues about its causes.

A number of studies have sought to characterize children with autism and TSC. An early study (Smalley, Tanguay, Smith, & Gutierrez, 1992), using the Autism Diagnostic Interview compared 13 children with TSC to 14 children with autism. Seven of the patients with TSC met the criteria for autism; they had fewer preoccupations, compulsions, or unusual attachments to objects than did the patients with autism but without TSC. The groups did not differ on the frequency of stereotypies or sensory responses. In comparing the patients with TSC and autism to the patients with TSC but without autism, Smalley et al. found more males than females and more mental retardation. The groups were not significantly different with respect to a history of seizures, although there were more seizures in individuals with TSC and autism than in those with TSC without autism. More recently, Jeste, Sahin, Bolton, Ploubidis, and Humphrey (2008) prospectively followed a group of 20 children with TSC with and without autism who were referred to a TSC clinic. They used the Autism Diagnostic Observation Schedule and assessed the children's cognition and language at 18, 24, 36, and 60 months of age. They found that the children with TSC and autism had greater cognitive impairment than those with TSC but without autism.

Mental retardation and infantile spasms have been identified as risk factors for autism in TSC (Gutierrez et al., 1998; Hunt & Dennis, 1987; Riikonen & Simell, 1990). Most studies are retrospective in nature and report on the prevalence of mental retardation and infantile spasms in children who meet the criteria for autism. Humphrey, Neville, Clarke, and Bolton (2006) prospectively followed an infant with standardized measures of development from before the onset of seizures until he had developed both epilepsy (infantile spasms and complex partial seizures) and autism and mental retardation. They were able to document a temporal relationship between the onset of seizures at 21 months of age and the development of autistic behavior.

A few studies have investigated the possible link between autistic behavioral symptoms and tuber location or number. Some studies (Bolton & Griffiths, 1997; Bolton, Park, Higgins, Griffiths, & Pickles, 2002) have found higher numbers of temporal lobe tubers in patients with TSC and autism/PDD than in patients with TSC but without autism/PDD, although another study found that tuber location was not associated with a *Diagnostic and Statistical Manual of Mental Disorders*, fourth edition (DSM-IV) diagnosis of autistic disorder (Walz, Byars, Egelhoff, & Franz, 2002). This discrepancy may have had to do with the differences in diagnostic criteria for autism/PDD versus DSM-IV autistic disorder. In another study, the severity of autistic features was related to the presence of cerebellar tubers (Weber et al., 2000). Positron emission tomography data have suggested that autism in TSC is related to both cortical and subcortical abnormalities (Asano et al., 2001).

In addition to the high rates of autism and other PDD in TSC, other behavioral problems occur with greater frequency in TSC. Like autism and other PDD, these problems are more common among patients with mental retardation than among those without it; they include language disorder, hyperactivity, and aggression. One study showed, however, that hyperactivity and autistic features were associated with TSC at higher rates than in patients with infantile spasms without TSC (Hunt & Dennis, 1987). A more recent study highlighted the frequency of previously unrecognized anxiety disorders (Lewis et al., 2004). A questionnaire study documented high rates of anxiety symptoms (40%), depressed mood (23%), and aggressive behavior (58%) in 265 children and adolescents with TSC (de Vries, Hunt, & Bolton, 2007). These problems were equally endorsed by parents of patients with and without mental retardation. Similar rates of these symptoms were found in a clinic-based study of 241 children and adults with TSC (Muzykewicz, Newberry, Danforth, Halpern, & Thiele, 2007), with some form of psychiatric symptomatology occurring at an overall rate of 66%. A recent study (Raznahan, Joinson, O'Callaghan, Osborne, & Bolton, 2006) used structured diagnostic interviews with 60 adults with TSC (42 with epilepsy and 25 with IQ below 70) and found that 40% of them had had mental illness. The most common diagnoses were major depression, alcoholism, and anxiety disorders. Only one person had a diagnosis of schizophrenia.

RECOMMENDATIONS FOR ASSESSMENT OF COGNITIVE AND BEHAVIORAL PROBLEMS

The Behavioral and Psychiatric Panel at the consensus conference described earlier (Hyman & Whittemore, 2000) recommended regular assessment of cognition and behavior at specific time points for patients with TSC. These time points include the time of diagnosis and at school entry, as well as any point at which specific cognitive or behavioral difficulties are recognized. A subsequent consensus conference sponsored by the Tuberous Sclerosis Association (United Kingdom) and the Tuberous Sclerosis Alliance (United States) was held in the United Kingdom in 2003, and produced clinical guidelines for assessment of cognitive and behavioral difficulties in TSC (de Vries et al., 2005). These guidelines provide a good summary of the general purposes of assessment and areas of special concern in TSC at each time point, and they are outlined in Table 7.2.

TREATMENTS THAT AFFECT COGNITION AND BEHAVIOR

Treatment of TSC is aimed at treating the affected organ systems. From a neurological standpoint, the most common treatment is the use of antiepileptic drugs (AEDs) to treat seizures. The effects of AED therapy on cognition and behavior have long been recognized (see Loring, Marino, & Meador, 2007 for a review), and these effects are manifest in patients with TSC. There are also some considerations of treatment specific to TSC. For example, the antiepileptic drug vigabatrin has been shown to have marked efficacy in control of infantile spasms, particularly in children with TSC (Chiron, Dulac, & Luna, 1990; Curatolo, 1994). Because vigabatrin has been associated with the development of visual field defects, it has not been approved by the Food and Drug Administration and is therefore not widely used in the United States. Children who are treated early and with good seizure control may subsequently have a better developmental course (Franz, 1998; Jambaque, Chiron, Dumas, Mumford, & Dulac, 2000). Some have questioned whether the small risk of visual field defects outweighs the possible benefit of preventing mental retardation and autism (Humphrey et al., 2006).

Although epilepsy in TSC is generally medically refractory, patients with TSC were long thought to be poor candidates for epilepsy surgery, because they generally have multifocal epileptiform activity and multiple tubers (Weiner, Ferraris, LaJoie, Miles, & Devinsky,

TABLE 7.2. Common Cognitive and Behavioral Problems in TSC: Typical Ages at Presentation and Appropriate Interventions

Age (years)	Most likely cognitive or behavioral problem presenting at this age	Appropriate intervention
0–3	Global intellectual impairment	Individual education plan
	Autism spectrum disorders	Early intervention programs for autism
3–8	Impulsivity	Provide structure/coaching + psychopharmacology
	ADD/ADHD	
8–12	Organizational impairment	Provide structure/coaching + psychopharmacology
	ADD/ADHD	
12–18	Independent living skills	Coaching
	Affect-regulation and judgement	Coaching
	Anxiety disorders and depressive disorders	Cognitive behavioral therapy + psychopharmacology
18+	Anxiety disorders and depressive disorders	Cognitive behavioral therapy + psychopharmacology

Note. From deVries et al. (2005). Copyright 2005 by Springer Science+Business Media. Reprinted by permission.

2004). It was assumed that if one epileptogenic tuber were resected and seizures were thereby reduced or eliminated, another tuber might become an active focus. However, good outcome following epilepsy surgery has been demonstrated in patients with TSC who were carefully evaluated and selected (Avellino, Berger, Rostomily, Shaw, & Ojemann, 1997; Bebin, Kelly, & Gomez, 1993; Weiner et al., 2006). A review of 25 papers that reported on postsurgery seizure outcome in 177 patients with TSC characterized epilepsy surgery as very successful in patients with TSC; seizure freedom or improvement was not as good as that for straightforward temporal lobe epilepsy surgery, but was better than that for extratemporal epilepsy surgery (Jansen, van Huffelen, Algra, & van Nieuwenhuizen, 2007). A case report noted some improvement in behavior as well as seizures after epilepsy surgery in two young boys (Gillberg, Uvebrant, Carlsson, Hedstrom, & Silfvenius, 1996).

RESEARCH LIMITATIONS AND FUTURE DIRECTIONS

There has been extraordinary progress in the understanding of the genetic and molecular bases of TSC over the past 20 years (Au, Williams, Gambello, & Northrup, 2004), as well as in the recognition and description of neurobehavioral problems associated with TSC (Prather & de Vries, 2004; Zaroff et al., 2005). Several weaknesses characterized early research in this area, including a lack of standardized measures of intelligence and neuropsychological function, overreliance on the reports of parents or the impressions of physicians, the use of retrospective study designs. A significant ascertainment bias also existed in earlier studies, in that the more severely affected cases were included. This bias has diminished over the years with the development of specific diagnostic criteria, increased recognition of the variable expression of the disease, and wide availability of genetic tests. Future studies should include standardized and validated assessments of cognitive and behavioral outcomes, in order to base treatment goals and strategies on the most reliable data.

Future research should certainly make use of prospective designs for descriptive studies clarifying the natural course of the disorder and the extent of its variability in expression of cognitive and behavioral symptoms, as well as for clinical trials of promising treatments. One such treatment is the use of rapamycin, an immunosuppressant used to treat transplant patients. It is an mTOR inhibitor that has been shown to reduce the volume of subependymal giant cell astrocytomas (Franz et al., 2006) and renal angiomyolipomas (Bissler et al., 2008). A recent study in an animal model of TSC has shown improvement of learning deficits with administration of rapamycin (Ehninger et al., 2008), which may provide an avenue of treatment for the cognitive symptoms of TSC as well.

REFERENCES

Asano, E., Chugani, D. C., Muzik, O., Behen, M., Janisse, J., Rothermel, R., et al. (2001). Autism in tuberous sclerosis complex is related to both cortical and subcortical dysfunction. *Neurology, 57,* 1269–1277.
Asato, M. R., & Hardan, A. Y. (2004). Neuropsychiatric problems in tuberous sclerosis complex. *Journal of Child Neurology, 19,* 241–249.
Au, K.-S., Williams, A. T., Gambello, M. J., & Northrup, H. (2004). Molecular genetic basis of tuberous sclerosis complex. *Journal of Child Neurology, 19,* 699–709.

Avellino, A. M., Berger, M. S., Rostomily, R. C., Shaw, C. M., & Ojemann, G. A. (1997). Surgical treatment and seizure outcome in patients with tuberous sclerosis. *Journal of Neurosurgery, 87*, 391–396.

Baker, P., Piven, J., & Sato, Y. (1998). Autism and tuberous sclerosis complex: Prevalence and clinical features. *Journal of Autism and Developmental Disorders, 28*, 279–285.

Bebin, E. M., Kelly, P. J., & Gomez, M. R. (1993). Surgical treatment for epilepsy in cerebral tuberous sclerosis. *Epilepsia, 34*, 651–657.

Bissler, J. J., McCormack, F. X., Young, L. R., Elwing, J. M., Chuck, G., Leonard, J. M., et al. (2008). Sirolimus for angiomyolipoma in tuberous sclerosis complex or lymphangioleiomyomatosis. *New England Journal of Medicine, 358*, 140–151.

Bolton, P., & Griffiths, P. D. (1997). Association of tuberous sclerosis of temporal lobes with autism and atypical autism. *Lancet, 349*, 392–395.

Bolton, P. F., Park, R. J., Higgins, J. N., Griffiths, P. D., & Pickles, A. (2002). Neuroepileptic determinants of autism spectrum disorders in tuberous sclerosis complex. *Brain, 125*, 1247–1255.

Castro, M., Shepherd, C. W., Gomez, M. R., Lie, J. T., & Ryu, J. H. (1995). Pulmonary tuberous sclerosis. *Chest, 107*, 189–195.

Chiron, C., Dulac, O., & Luna, D. (1990). Vigabatrin in infantile spasms. *Lancet, 335*, 363–364.

Clarke, A., Cook, P., & Osborne, J.P. (1996). Cranial computer tomographic findings in tuberous sclerosis are not affected by sex. *Developmental Medicine and Child Neurology, 38*, 139–145.

Curatolo, P. (1994). Vigabatrin for refractory partial seizures in children with tuberous sclerosis. *Neuropediatrics, 25*, 55.

Curatolo, P., Bombardieri, R., & Jozwiak, S. (2008). Tuberous sclerosis. *Lancet, 372*, 657–668.

Curatolo, P., Seri, S., Verdecchia, M., & Bombardieri, R. (2001). Infantile spasms in tuberous sclerosis complex. *Brain and Development, 173*, 502–507.

Dabora, S. L., Jozwiak, S., Franz, D. N., Roberts, P. S., Nieto, A., Chung, J., et al. (2001). Mutational analysis in a cohort of 224 tuberous sclerosis patients indicates increased severity of TSC2, compared with TSC1, disease in multiple organs. *American Journal of Medical Genetics, 68*, 64–80.

de Vries, P. J., & Bolton, P. (2000). Genotype–phenotype correlations in tuberous sclerosis. *Journal of Medical Genetics, 37*, E3.

de Vries, P. J., Humphrey, A., McCartney, D., Prather, P., Bolton, P., & Hunt, A. (2005). Consensus clinical guidelines for the assessment of cognitive and behavioural problems in tuberous sclerosis. *European Journal of Child and Adolescent Psychiatry, 14*, 183–190.

de Vries, P. J., Hunt, A., & Bolton, P. F. (2007). The psychopathologies of children and adolescents with tuberous sclerosis complex (TSC). *European Journal of Child and Adolescent Psychiatry, 16*, 16–24.

de Vries, P. J., & Watson, P. (2008). Attention deficits in tuberous sclerosis complex (TSC): Rethinking the pathways to the endstate. *Journal of Intellectual Disability Research, 52*, 348–357.

DiMario, F. J. (2004). Brain abnormalities in tuberous sclerosis complex. *Journal of Child Neurology, 19*, 650–657.

Doherty, C., Goh, S., Young Poussaint, T., Erdag, N., & Thiele, E. A. (2005). Prognostic significance of tuber count and location in tuberous sclerosis complex. *Journal of Child Neurology, 20*, 837–841.

Ehninger, D., Han, S., Shilyansky, C., Zhou, Y., Li, W., Kwiatkowski, D. J., et al. (2008). Reversal of learning deficits in a Tsc2+/– mouse model of tuberous sclerosis. *Nature Medicine, 14*, 843–848.

Ess, K. C. (2006). The neurobiology of tuberous sclerosis complex. *Seminars in Pediatric Neurology, 13*, 37–42.

European Chromosome 16 Tuberous Sclerosis Consortium. (1993). Identification and characterization of the tuberous sclerosis gene on chromosome 16. *Cell, 75*, 1–11.

Franz, D. N. (1998). Diagnosis and management of tuberous sclerosis complex. *Seminars in Pediatric Neurology, 5*, 253–268.

Franz, D. N., Leonard, J., Tudor, C., Chuck, G., Care, M., Sethuraman, G., et al. (2006). Rapamycin causes regression of astrocytomas in tuberous sclerosis complex. *Annals of Neurology, 59*, 490–498.

Gillberg, C., Uvebrant, P., Carlsson, G., Hedstrom, A., & Silfvenius, H. (1996). Autism and epilepsy (and tuberous sclerosis?) in two pre-adolescent boys: Neuropsychiatric aspects before and after epilepsy surgery. *Journal of Intellectual Disability Research, 40*, 75–81.

Gillberg, I. C., Gillberg, C., & Ahlsen, G. (1994). Autistic behaviour and attention deficits in tuberous sclerosis. *Developmental Medicine and Child Neurology, 36,* 50–56.

Goh, S., Kwiatkowski, D. J., Dorer, D. J., & Thiele, E. A. (2005). Infantile spasms and intellectual outcomes in children with tuberous sclerosis complex. *Neurology, 65,* 235–238.

Gomez, M. R. (1988). Neurologic and psychiatric features. In M. R. Gomez (Ed.), *Tuberous sclerosis* (pp. 21–36). New York: Raven Press.

Gomez, M. R., Sampson, J. R., & Whittemore, V. H. (1999). *Tuberous sclerosis complex.* New York: Oxford University Press.

Goodman, M., Lamm, S. H., Engel, A., Shepherd, C. W., Houser, O. W., & Gomez, M. R. (1997). Cortical tuber count: A biomarker indicating neurologic severity of tuberous sclerosis complex. *Journal of Child Neurology, 12,* 85–90.

Gutierrez, G. C., Smalley, S. L., & Tanguay, P. E. (1998). Autism in tuberous sclerosis complex. *Journal of Autism and Developmental Disorders, 28,* 97–103.

Harrison, J. E., O'Callaghan, F. J., Hancock, E., Osborne, J. P., & Bolton, P. F. (1999). Cognitive deficits in normally intelligent patients with tuberous sclerosis. *American Journal of Medical Genetics, 88,* 642–646.

Holmes, G. L., Stafstrom, C. E., & the Tuberous Sclerosis Study Group. (2007). Tuberous sclerosis complex and epilepsy: Recent developments and future challenges. *Epilepsia, 48,* 617–630.

Humphrey, A., Higgins, J. N., Yates, J. R., & Bolton, P. F. (2004). Monozygotic twins with tuberous sclerosis discordant for the severity of developmental deficits. *Neurology, 62,* 795–798.

Humphrey, A., Neville, B. G., Clarke, A., & Bolton, P. F. (2006). Autistic regression associated with seizure onset in an infant with tuberous sclerosis. *Developmental Medicine and Child Neurology, 48,* 609–611.

Hunt, A. (1993). Development, behaviour, and seizures in 300 cases of tuberous sclerosis. *Journal of Intellectual Disability Research, 37,* 41–51.

Hunt, A., & Dennis, J. (1987). Psychiatric disorder among children with tuberous sclerosis. *Developmental Medicine and Child Neurology, 29,* 190–198.

Hunt, A., & Shepherd, C. (1993). A prevalence study of autism in tuberous sclerosis. *Journal of Autism and Developmental Disorders, 23,* 323–339.

Hyman, M. H., & Whittemore, V. H. (2000). National Institutes of Health consensus conference: Tuberous sclerosis complex. *Archives of Neurology, 57,* 662–665.

Inoue, Y., Nemoto, Y., Murata, R., Tashiro, T., Shakudo, M., Kohno, K., et al. (1998). CT and MR imaging of cerebral tuberous sclerosis. *Brain and Development, 20,* 209–221.

Jambaque, I., Chiron, C., Dumas, C., Mumford, J., & Dulac, O. (2000). Mental and behavioral outcome of infantile epilepsy treated by vigabatrin in tuberous sclerosis patients. *Epilepsy Research, 38,* 151–160.

Jambaque, I., Cusmai, R., Curatolo, P., Cortesi, F., Perrot, C., & Dulac, O. (1991). Neuropsychological aspects of tuberous sclerosis in relation to epilepsy and MRI findings. *Developmental Medicine and Child Neurology, 33,* 698–705.

Jansen, F. E., Braams, O., Vincken, K. L., Algra, A., Anbeek, P., Jennekens-Schinkel, A., et al. (2008a). Overlapping neurologic and cognitive phenotypes in patients with TSC1 or TSC2 mutations. *Neurology, 70,* 908–915.

Jansen, F. E., van Huffelen, A. C., Algra, A., & van Nieuwenhuizen, O. (2007). Epilepsy surgery in tuberous sclerosis: A systematic review. *Epilepsia, 48,* 1477–1484.

Jansen, F. E., Vincken, K. L., Algra, A., Anbeek, P., Braams, O., Nellist, M., et al. (2008b). Cognitive impairment in tuberous sclerosis complex is a multifactorial condition. *Neurology, 70,* 916–923.

Jeste, S. S., Sahin, M., Bolton, P., Ploubidis, G. B., & Humphrey, A. (2008). Characterization of autism in young children with tuberous sclerosis complex. *Journal of Child Neurology, 23,* 520–525.

Joinson, C., O'Callaghan, F. J., Osborne, J. P., Martyn, C., Harris, T., & Bolton, P. (2003). Learning disability and epilepsy in an epidemiological sample of individuals with tuberous sclerosis complex. *Psychological Medicine, 33,* 335–344.

Jones, A. C., Shyamsundar, M. M., Thomas, M. W., Maynard, J., Idziaszczyk, S., Tomkins, S., et al.

(1999). Comprehensive mutation analysis of TSC1 and TSC2-and phenotypic correlations in 150 families with tuberous sclerosis. *American Journal of Human Genetics, 64,* 1305–1315.

Jozwiak, S., Goodman, M., & Lamm, S. H. (1998). Poor mental development in patients with tuberous sclerosis complex: Clinical risk factors. *Archives of Neurology, 55,* 379–384.

Lewis, J. C., Thomas, H. V., Murphy, K. C., & Sampson, J. R. (2004). Genotype and psychological phenotype in tuberous sclerosis. *Journal of Medical Genetics, 41,* 203–207.

Loring, D. W., Marino, S., & Meador, K. J. (2007). Neuropsychological and behavioral effects of antiepilepsy drugs. *Neuropsychology Review, 17,* 413–425.

Menor, F., Marti-Bonmati, L., Mulas, F., Poyatos, C., & Cortina, H. (1992). Neuroimaging in tuberous sclerosis: A clinicoradiological evaluation in pediatric patients. *Pediatric Radiology, 22,* 485–489.

Mizuguchi, M., & Takashima, S. (2001). Neuropathology of tuberous sclerosis. *Brain and Development, 23,* 508–515.

Muzykewicz, D. A., Newberry, P., Danforth, N., Halpern, E. F., & Thiele, E. A. (2007). Psychiatric comorbid conditions in a clinic population of 241 patients with tuberous sclerosis complex. *Epilepsy and Behavior, 11,* 506–513.

O'Callaghan, F. J. K., Harris, T., Joinson, C., Bolton, P., Noakes, M., Presdee, D., et al. (2004a). The relation of infantile spasms, tubers, and intelligence in tuberous sclerosis complex. *Archives of Disease in Childhood, 89,* 530–533.

O'Callaghan, F. J., Noakes, M. J., Martyn, C. N., & Osborne J. P. (2004b). An epidemiological study of renal pathology in tuberous sclerosis complex. *BJU International, 94,* 853–857.

Osborne, J. P., Fryer, A., & Webb, D. (1991). Epidemiology of tuberous sclerosis. *Annals of the New York Academy of Sciences, 615,* 125–127.

Prather, P., & de Vries, P. J. (2004). Behavioral and cognitive aspects of tuberous sclerosis complex. *Journal of Child Neurology, 19,* 666–674.

Raznahan, A., Joinson, C., O'Callaghan, F., Osborne, J. P., & Bolton, P. F. (2006). Psychopathology in tuberous sclerosis: An overview and findings in a population-based sample of adults with tuberous sclerosis. *Journal of Intellectual Disability Research, 50,* 561–569.

Riikonen, R., & Simell, O. (1990). Tuberous sclerosis and infantile spasms. *Developmental Medicine and Child Neurology, 32,* 203–209.

Roach, E. S., Gomez, M. R., & Northrup, H. (1998). Tuberous sclerosis complex consensus conference: Revised clinical diagnostic criteria. *Journal of Child Neurology, 13,* 624–628.

Shepherd, C. W., Houser, O. W., & Gomez, M. R. (1995). MR findings in tuberous sclerosis complex and correlation with seizure development and mental impairment. *American Journal of Neuroradiology, 16,* 149–155.

Shepherd, C. W., & Stephenson, J. B. P. (1992). Seizures and intellectual disability associated with tuberous sclerosis complex in the west of Scotland. *Developmental Medicine and Child Neurology, 34,* 766–774.

Smalley, S. L., Tanguay, P. E., Smith, M., & Gutierrez, G. (1992). Autism and tuberous sclerosis. *Journal of Autism and Developmental Disorders, 22,* 339–355.

Thiele, E. A. (2004). Managing epilepsy in tuberous sclerosis complex. *Journal of Child Neurology, 19,* 680–686.

van Slegtenhorst, M., de Hoogt, R., Hermans, C., Nellist, M., Janssen, B., Verhoef, S., et al. (1997). Identification of the tuberous sclerosis gene TSC1 on chromosome 9q34. *Science, 277,* 805–808.

van Slegtenhorst, M., Verhoef, S., Tempelaars, A., Bakker, L., Wang, Q., Wessels, M., et al. (1999). Mutational spectrum of the TSC1 gene in a cohort of 225 tuberous sclerosis complex patients: No evidence for genotype-phenotype correlation. *Journal of Medical Genetics, 36,* 285–289.

Walz, N. C., Byars, A. W., Egelhoff, J. C., & Franz, D. N. (2002). Supratentorial tuber location and autism in tuberous sclerosis complex. *Journal of Child Neurology, 17,* 830–832.

Webb, D. W., Clarke, A., Fryer, A., & Osborne, J. P. (1996). The cutaneous features of tuberous sclerosis: A population study. *British Journal of Dermatology, 135,* 1–5.

Webb, D. W., Fryer, A. E., & Osborne, J. P. (1991a). On the incidence of fits and mental retardation in tuberous sclerosis. *Journal of Medical Genetics, 28,* 395–397.

Webb, D. W., Fryer, A. E., & Osborne, J. P. (1996b). Morbidity associated with tuberous sclerosis: A population study. *Developmental Medicine and Child Neurology, 38,* 146–155.

Webb, D. W., Thomas, R. D., & Osborne, J. P. (1993). Cardiac rhabdomyomas and their association with tuberous sclerosis. *Archives of Disease in Childhood, 68,* 367–370.

Webb, D. W., Thomson, J. L. G., & Osborne, J. P. (1991b). Cranial magnetic resonance imaging in patients with tuberous sclerosis and normal intellect. *Archives of Disease in Childhood, 66,* 1375–1377.

Weber, A. M., Egelhoff, J. C., & Franz, D. N. (1996, September). *Correlation of neuropsychologic and neuroimaging findings in tuberous sclerosis.* Paper presented at the international Biannual Tuberous Sclerosis International Research Symposium, Bath, UK.

Weber, A. M., Egelhoff, J. C., McKellop, J. M., & Franz, D. N. (2000). Autism and the cerebellum: Evidence from tuberous sclerosis. *Journal of Autism and Developmental Disorders, 30,* 511–517.

Weiner, H. L., Carlson, C., Ridgway, E. B., Zaroff, C. M., Miles, D., LaJoie, J., et al. (2006). Epilepsy surgery in young children with tuberous sclerosis: Results of a novel approach. *Pediatrics, 117,* 1494–1502.

Weiner, H. L., Ferraris, N., LaJoie, J., Miles, D., & Devinsky, O. (2004). Epilepsy surgery for children with tuberous sclerosis complex. *Journal of Child Neurology, 19,* 687–689.

Winterkorn, E. B., Pulsifer, M. B., & Thiele, E. A. (2007). Cognitive prognosis of patients with tuberous sclerosis complex. *Neurology, 68,* 62–64.

Wiznitzer, M. (2004). Autism and tuberous sclerosis. *Journal of Child Neurology, 19,* 675–679.

Zaroff, C. M., Barr, W. B., Carlson, C., LaJoie, J., Madhaven, D., Miles, D. K., et al. (2006). Mental retardation and relation to seizure and tuber burden in tuberous sclerosis complex. *Seizure, 15,* 558–562.

Zaroff, C. M., Morrison, C., Ferraris, N., Weiner, H. L., Miles, D. K., & Devinsky, O. (2005). Developmental outcome of epilepsy surgery in tuberous sclerosis complex. *Epileptic Disorders, 7,* 321–326.

CHAPTER 8

Perinatal Stroke

JOAN STILES
RUTH D. NASS
SUSAN C. LEVINE
PAMELA MOSES
JUDY S. REILLY

Perinatal stroke (PS) is a cerebrovascular event that occurs in the period just before birth or immediately after, and is usually observed among infants born at term (Lynch & Nelson, 2001). The prevalence rate of PS is estimated at 1 in 4,000, but it is widely believed that this estimate is low, reflecting only those cases that present with identifiable symptoms. The prevalence and clinical significance of PS have become more apparent with the advent of modern neuroimaging techniques, making the understanding of its consequences and outcomes a clinical priority.

PSs most commonly involves the middle cerebral artery distribution, creating large lesions that compromise much of one cerebral hemisphere. In adults, such lesions result in significant deficits; the specific patterns of these differ, depending on the side and site of the injury. However, children with such large lesions often achieve considerably better function than their adult counterparts across a range of physical, cognitive, and affective domains. These developmental differences probably reflect fundamental properties of human brain development. Typical brain development is dynamic and relies upon both genetic cues and appropriate input (Stiles, 2008). In the late prenatal period, and for an extended time postnatally, normal brain development is characterized by the emergence and subsequent retraction of exuberant neural resources as the developing brain adapts to the contingencies of the world (Huttenlocher & Dabholkar, 1997; Huttenlocher, 2002). Principles of *competition* and *functional optimization* have been used to describe these important aspects of late prenatal and postnatal brain development (Changeux & Danchin, 1976; Cowan, Fawcett,

O'Leary, & Stanfield, 1984; Greenough, Hwang, & Gorman, 1985; Quartz & Sejnowski, 1997). The characterization of brain development as dynamic and adaptive has important implications for the study of brain development following PS.

Early injury constitutes a perturbation of basic neurodevelopmental processes: It reduces available neural resources, and it alters both the typical development of the neurobiological system and the capacity of the neural system to process input. However, because the injury occurs during a period of adaptive exuberance, the insult itself becomes a part of the developmental dynamic. Injury is never beneficial, and extensive injury during this period may exceed the adaptive capacity of the developing brain. But when injury is more localized (as in the case of stroke), it alters, but does not fundamentally disrupt, the development of neural networks. Rather, the developing brain can adapt, within limits, to the effects of injury. When a circumscribed region of cortex is lost, the remaining cortex may organize differently and preserve function. The study of children with PS provides an important opportunity to examine more closely questions concerning both the extent and limits of neural plasticity in humans.

This chapter examines the medical and neuropsychological effects of PS. It begins with an overview of the mechanisms and suspected causes of stroke in the perinatal period, and considers the medical consequences for the physical development of the motor and sensory systems. The remainder of the chapter focuses on the behavioral consequences of PS. The discussion of neuropsychological effects includes an overview of research using standardized measures of behavioral development, as well as a summary of experimental studies that examine specific aspects of development in greater detail. Finally, we review some very recent functional neuroimaging studies designed to examine alternative patterns of brain organization that can emerge after PS.

MECHANISMS AND MEDICAL CONSEQUENCES

PS generally occurs during the third trimester, during labor and delivery, or during the neonatal period. The majority of perinatal strokes involve the left hemisphere (LH)—a finding attributable to anatomical or hemodynamic differences between the left and right common carotid arteries (Volpe, 2001). Term infants generally have large strokes involving the main branch of the middle cerebral artery, damaging both cortical and subcortical regions (Figure 8.1; Bax, Tydeman, & Flodmark, 2006; Wu, Croen, Shah, Newman, & Najjar, 2006). Middle cerebral artery branch occlusions, basal ganglia infarcts, cerebellar infarcts, and internal capsule lacunes are occasionally reported (Govaert et al., 2000; Kwong, Wong, Fong, Wong, & So, 2004). Some preterm infants have multifocal arterial strokes involving branches of cortical or lenticulostriate arteries (Bax et al., 2006; de Vries et al., 1997). But most preterm infants have periventricular hemorrhagic infarctions, resulting in porencephalic cysts and white matter changes (periventricular leukomalacia) (Bax et al., 2006; Volpe, 2001; Wu et al., 2006).

A number of maternal and fetal/neonatal risk factors and associated features for stroke in the term infant have been documented (see Table 8.1; Lee et al., 2005a; Mercuri et al., 2001; Nelson & Lynch, 2004; Wu et al., 2006). Multiple independent risk factors and associated features increase the likelihood of stroke. Thromboembolic events, the most likely cause of stroke, may originate from intra- or extracranial blood vessels, the heart, or the

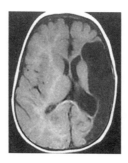

FIGURE 8.1. MRI scan at age 5 years that shows the residua of a neonatal middle cerebral artery stroke.

placenta (Pathan & Kittner, 2003). Many of the risk factors affect the placenta directly or indirectly. The placenta is a highly vascular organ that regulates its own hemostasis. Many complications of pregnancy (e.g., chorioamnionitis or preeclampsia) may tip the balance toward excessive coagulation, increasing stroke risk (Nelson & Lynch, 2004).

Clinical Presentation and Outcome

The majority of infants whose strokes occur at term present with seizures in the neonatal period (70%), whereas 75% of preterm infants whose strokes occur prenatally are diagnosed incidentally when a routine ultrasound shows a periventricular hemorrhagic infarction. Some children with PS do not present until several months of age, when decreased hand use is noted and imaging reveals an old stroke, which is presumed to have occurred in the perinatal period. Because proximal arm and leg muscles have bilateral innervation, and infants do not really start to use their hands until a few months of age, the hemiparesis is not immediately apparent. Newborns whose injury occurs during labor and delivery have acute signs of brain insult (e.g., seizures), while those whose stroke occurred even a few days before birth have "recovered" and are asymptomatic. Infants with prenatal strokes may or may not have symptoms when their stroke occurs.

TABLE 8.1. Maternal and Fetal/Neonatal Risk Factors and Associated Features for PS

Maternal	Fetal/neonatal
History of infertility	Fetal heart rate abnormalities during birth
Primiparity (first child)	Asphyxia
Vacuum extraction	Low Apgar scores
Emergency cesarean section	Resuscitation at birth
Chorioamnionitis (placental infection)	Cardiac anomalies
Prolonged rupture of membranes	Polycythemia (excess red cells)
Preeclampsia (hypertension plus kidney problems and, rarely, seizures)	Infection
	Coagulation abnormalities
Oligiohydramnious (decreased amniotic fluid)	Smallness for gestational age
Infection during pregnancy, especially urinary tract	
Coagulation abnormalities	
Autoimmune disorders	
Twin gestation	
Advanced maternal age	

Note. Data from Mercuri et al. (2001); Nelson and Lynch (2004); Lee et al. (2005); and Wu et al. (2006).

Neonatal seizures are routinely evaluated with an electroencephalogram (EEG) to assess abnormal brain electrical activity, and X-ray computed tomography and/or magnetic resonance imaging (MRI) to detect anatomical abnormality. Imaging of children presenting with hemiparesis during the first year documents the extent of the lesions and confirms the unilaterality of the pathology. The medical workup at all ages includes an assessment of the heart, studies of blood clotting, and studies evaluating for metabolic/genetic problems that can cause stroke. Between 30% and 50% of children who had a neonatal stroke are grossly neurologically normal (Lee et al., 2005b; Nelson & Lynch, 2004). Cerebral palsy (CP) occurs in 40–60%, epilepsy in about 40%, visual problems in 25%, and behavior problems in 20%. About 80% have an abnormality in at least one domain. Risk factors for poor outcome include abnormal exam at discharge from the nursery, neonatal seizures, abnormal EEG, blood clotting abnormalities, and late presentation of CP (Bax et al., 2006; Mercuri et al., 1999, 2001; Sreenan, Bhargava, & Robertson, 2000; Wu et al., 2004). Site, side, and timing of stroke may also affect outcome (Kwong et al., 2004; Nass, Peterson, & Koch, 1989; Staudt et al., 2004).

Neonatal seizures occurring concurrently with the stroke are generally few in number and easy to control. However, abnormal neonatal EEG predicts poorer outcome at 15 months (Mercuri et al., 1999). Most children who have seizures as newborns never have them again, and about 25–40% have recurrent seizures later in life that are easily controlled with medication. Some have persistent seizures, and some develop intractable seizures. Rarely, surgery is required to control the seizures. Epilepsy in the population with PS tends to lower IQ or overall cognitive abilities (Carlsson, Hagberg, & Olsson, 2003; Isaacs, Christie, Vargha-Khadem, & Mishkin, 1996; Muter, Taylor, & Vargha-Khadem, 1997; Vargha-Khadem, Isaacs, van der Werf, Robb, & Wilson, 1992).

Motor Function

Studies of motor outcome have focused on the type and degree of motor deficits, effects of lesion location, patterns of motor pathway reorganization, and features of mirror movements. Hemiplegic CP can affect both arm and leg—often to different degrees, depending on the location of the lesion. Some studies have addressed the leg and gait difficulties, but most have focused on the hand because it is generally more involved. Motor deficits in hemiplegic CP manifest themselves not only as weakness, spasticity, and impaired dexterity, but also as higher-order movement-planning difficulties (*apraxia*). Imaging studies have shown that children whose stroke involved the internal capsule, basal ganglia, and cerebral cortex had hemiplegia (Boardman et al., 2005; de Vries et al., 1997; Humphreys, Whiting, & Pham, 2000) both at 15 months (Mercuri et al., 1999) and at follow-up in the school-age period (Mercuri et al., 2004). Children with hemiplegic CP who have a normal MRI are likely to outgrow the hemiparesis by age 3 (Nelson & Ellenberg, 1982; Wu et al., 2006). Degree of hemiplegia has been found to correlate significantly with IQ in children with PS (Levine, Huttenlocher, Banich, & Duda, 1987).

The gait in hemiplegic CP is described as *circumducting*; that is, body position is crouched, and the impaired leg lifts and swings rather than moving straight forward because of increased tone/spasticity at the hip. Toe walking may also occur because of increased tone/spasticity at the ankle (Wren, Rethlefsen, & Kay, 2005). Kinematic studies demonstrate a gait similar to an inverted pendulum on the nonaffected limb and a pogo stick on the affected limb (Fonseca, Holt, Fetters, & Saltzman, 2004). Upper-limb abnormality involves spasticity (Bax et al., 2006). This is most apparent at the elbow, which tends to bend; at the wrist, which tends to flex; in the hand, which tends to droop because holding the palm up is difficult; and in the fingers, which tend to flex. Weakness is mild in about 60%, moderate in about 35%, and severe in about 5% (Bax et al., 2006). Dexterity in both the fingers and the hand is compromised even in a mildly affected hand (Brown, van Rensburg, Walsh, Lakie, & Wright, 1987; Duque et al., 2003; Eliasson & Gordon, 2000; Gordon, Lewis, Eliasson, & Duff, 2003; Krumlinde-Sundholm & Eliasson, 2002; Steenbergen, van Thiel, Hulstijn, & Meulenbroek, 2000). Apraxia occurs; movement planning is often compromised (Eliasson, Gordon, & Forssberg, 1991, 1992, 1995; Forssberg, Eliasson, Redon-Zouitenn, Mercuri, & Dubowitz, 1999; Gordon, Charles, & Duff, 1999; Gordon & Duff, 1999a, 1999b; Duff & Gordon, 2003). The temporal relationship between the different hand muscles deviates from normal (Duque et al., 2003).   Neglect of the impaired hand (Trauner, 2003) may increase performance deficits. Because of such neglect, residual motor capabilities may not be tapped to their maximum. As in adults, neglect may be more common with right-hemisphere (RH) lesions, and apraxia more common and more often bilateral with LH lesions (Steenbergen & van der Kamp, 2004; Trauner, 2003). The latter may reflect deficits of motor imagery (Steenbergen & Gordon, 2006).

Constraint therapy, which involves restraining the good arm to force the use of the impaired arm (Charles, Wolf, Schneider, & Gordon, 2006), has been used to counter the tendency not to use the impaired hand. Other work has shown that with practice, children with CP improve their motor execution skills for grip–lift synergy, as well as their ability to sense the weight and texture of novel objects (Duff & Gordon, 2003).

Minor motor deficits have been documented in the putatively uninvolved arm and hand (Steenbergen & van der Kamp, 2004). Dexterity scores for this arm and hand are lower than those of controls, and motor planning is affected (Steenbergen & Meulenbroek, 2006). Performing tasks of everyday life occurs in a step-by-step rather than continuous fashion, and the uninvolved hand does not achieve "end posture comfort" (i.e., the action that is performed after an object has been picked up, such as drinking from a glass; Mutsaarts, Steenbergen, & Bekkering, 2005).

Bimanual coordination problems are also reported and reflect both poor dexterity in the impaired hand and higher-order motor planning problems. But bimanual coordination is affected even if the impaired hand is dexterous. Moreover, deficits are reciprocal; the intact hand affects the impaired hand and vice versa (Hung, Charles, & Gordon, 2004; Punt, Riddoch, & Humphreys, 2005; Utley, Steenbergen, & Sugden, 2004).

In typical development, corticospinal tracts originate in the motor cortex, and the vast majority of fibers cross in the medullary pyramids and control the contralateral limb. In hemiplegic CP, three reorganization patterns are described (Figure 8.2; Carr, Harrison, Evans, & Stephens, 1993; Maegaki et al., 1997; Nezu, Kimura, Takeshita, & Tanaka, 1999; Staudt et al., 2002a). Patients with small lesions and minor hand impairment have intact crossed corticospinal connections from the damaged hemisphere to the paretic hand, whereas those with large lesions and more severe hand impairments depend on an uncrossed corticospinal tract from the intact hemisphere to the paretic hand. Patients with intermediate-sized lesions have features of both the small and large lesion groups (Staudt et al., 2002a). Ipsilateral reorganization of the primary motor type (Farmer, Harrison, Ingram, & Stephens, 1991; Carr et al., 1993; Macdonell et al., 1999; Maegaki et al., 1997; Nezu et

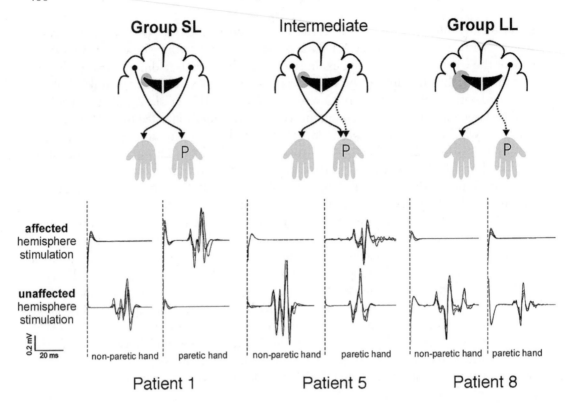

FIGURE 8.2. Schematic illustration of corticospinal tract organization in the three subgroups of patients (P, paretic hand) and transmagnetic stimulation (TMS) results for one representative patient from each group. TMS activates working motor cortex. The vertical dashed line indicates time of the TMS stimulus. Patients with small lesions (SL) and minor hand impairment have intact crossed corticospinal connections from the damaged hemisphere to the paretic hand (premotor type; i.e., without ipsilateral motor projections but with significant activation of ipsilateral premotor areas), whereas those with large lesions (LL) and more severe hand impairments depend on an uncrossed corticospinal tract from the intact hemisphere to the paretic hand (primary motor type; i.e., with abnormal ipsilateral corticospinal projections to the paretic hand). Patients with intermediate-sized lesions have features of both the small and large lesion groups—a combined type with partial integrity of the crossed corticospinal tract (as in the small-lesion premotor group) and the presence of abnormal, ipsilateral projections (as in the large-lesion group). From Staudt et al. (2002a). Copyright 2002 by Oxford University Press. Reprinted by permission.

al., 1999; Nirkko et al., 1997; Thickbroom, Byrnes, Archer, Nagarajan, & Mastaglia, 2001) seems to be specific to early brain damage (Carr et al., 1993; Maegaki et al., 1997; Nezu et al., 1999; Staudt et al., 2002a). Functional MRI (fMRI) can be used to define task-related regions of brain activity. An fMRI study of six patients with unilateral damage in the perinatal period revealed significant activation of the intact hemisphere during movement of the contralateral as well as the ipsilateral (hemiparetic) hand. This contrasted with the pattern observed in right-handed controls, who exhibited little if any ipsilateral activation. These findings suggest that the motor functions of the human brain exhibit functional plasticity following early unilateral brain injury (Cao, Vikingstad, Huttenlocher, Towle, & Levin, 1994).

Mirror movements occur during normal development, but disappear at about age 10 years (Connolly & Stratton, 1968). In children with hemiplegic CP, mirror movements are prominent and persistent (Nass, 1985; Woods & Teuber, 1978). The exaggerated mirror movements in hemiplegic CP probably reflect compensatory elaboration of ipsilateral motor tracts from the intact hemisphere to the impaired hand. The most marked mirror movements are described in those with ipsilateral reorganization of the primary motor type (Carr et al., 1993; Farmer et al., 1991; Macdonell et al., 1999; Maegaki et al., 1997; Nirkko et al., 1997; Nezu et al., 1999; Staudt et al., 2002a; Thickbroom et al., 2001). Mirror movements can interfere with bimanual activities (Kuhtz-Buschbeck, Sundholm, Eliasson, & Forssberg, 2000). Clearly, mirror movements are an example of "plasticity at a price."

Sensory Function

Cortical sensory deficits occur in about 50% of children with hemiplegic CP (Himmelmann, Beckung, Hagberg, & Uvebrant, 2006; Van Heest, House, & Putnam, 1993; Yekutiel, Jariwala, & Stretch, 1994). Deficits in two-point discrimination and *stereognosis* (recognition of objects by touch) are common. Obvious bilateral sensory deficits occur even after unilateral insults (Cooper, Majnemer, Rosenblatt, & Birnbaum, 1995; Lesny, Stehlik, Tomasek, Tomankova, & Havlicek, 1993). Functional imaging studies demonstrate little plasticity in sensory cortex (Cao et al., 1994; Chu, Huttenlocher, Levin, & Towle, 2000). Unlike the motor system, in which an ipsilateral pathway from the intact hemisphere to the impaired hand often develops, the crossed sensory pathways remain dominant (Staudt et al., 2002a; Thickbroom et al., 2001). Because of the timing of at least periventricular injury, actively developing thalamocortical somatosensory projections can bypass the lesion to reach their original cortical destination (Staudt et al., 2006). Impairment of sensory–motor integration at the cortical level could result from the discrepancy between the presence of reorganization in the motor system and its absence in the sensory system (Thickbroom et al., 2001).

MRI-Based Measures of Brain Development after Early Injury

Historically, studies of cognitive development following early brain injury have been accompanied by neuroanatomical assessments reporting the size and extent of the lesions. Careful documentation of lesion sites in relationship to cognitive impairments is essential for brain mapping; however, the PS brain–behavior studies to date suggest that the key to understanding postlesion resiliency lies in the examination of alternative patterns of development in the intact regions of the brain.

MRI provides a means for investigating the pattern of development in uninjured portions of the brain by quantitative image analysis and measurement of the size of gray and white matter structures. Two MRI-based studies have examined the macroanatomical growth of intact brain regions in children with PS. The studies were designed to determine whether there are patterns of under- or overgrowth in the uninjured hemisphere or intact portions of the injured hemisphere. Measurement of the corpus callosum, the primary fiber tract projecting between the injured and uninjured hemispheres, was used to examine possible interhemispheric effects (Moses et al., 2000). The cross-sectional area of the callosum was reduced in children with early injury relative to controls with typical development

(TD). The cortical projections that comprise the corpus callosum connect homologous regions along the anterior–posterior extent of the two cerebral hemispheres. In all subjects, measurement of five callosal subregions showed region-specific thinning that corresponded to the site of injury. This finding introduced the possibility of abnormalities in the uninjured hemisphere as well.

The second study focused on the volume of cerebral gray and white matter in lobar divisions of the uninjured and injured hemispheres (Moses, 1999). The intact hemisphere in children with PS showed normal gray matter, but low white matter volume, relative to peers with TD. Furthermore, the white matter reduction was specific to the lobar region contralateral to the original injury. Whereas the degree of callosal thinning correlated with the estimated lesion size, the contralesional cerebral white matter reduction did not correspond to lesion size. The uncoupling of lesion size and the degree of white matter reduction in the contralesional lobe indicates that in addition to a direct loss of transcallosal axons to and from the injury site, there may be a secondary effect in the intact hemisphere, such as a postlesion increase in intrahemispheric connectivity that partially (but not completely) compensates for the direct loss of white matter fibers.

Assessment of the injured hemisphere concentrated on a subgroup of children with pericentral lesions that left the frontal lobe, the occipital lobe, or both intact (Moses, 1999). In these cases, white matter volumes were low in the occipital lobe. The posterior white matter abnormality may be attributable to disruption of the two major fiber bundles—the superior longitudinal fasciculus and the occipitofrontal fasciculus—that arise from the posterior cortex and converge in the pericentral region where the lesions were located. Even a small lesion in the region surrounding the central sulcus, where the fiber tracts are most tightly bundled, may have an impact on the posterior lobar white matter volume.

The MRI studies show that PS is accompanied by white matter abnormalities, which may be accounted for by direct damage to fibers normally projecting to and from the lesion site. The reduction of callosal cross-sectional area, contralesional white matter volume, and ipsilesional occipital lobe white matter, relative to those of controls, conforms to the projection pathways of the lesions studied. In addition, the lack of a systematic relationship between the amount of contralesional white matter volume reduction and the lesion size raises the possibility of a secondary effect of increased local, intrahemispheric connections in lieu of transcallosal connectivity.

RESEARCH USING STANDARDIZED MEASURES OF INTELLECTUAL DEVELOPMENT

Studies of the IQ levels of children with PS generally provide only a snapshot of their cognitive functioning, as IQ tests are usually given at only one developmental time point. These studies leave us with a somewhat mixed pattern of results: Some report that the average IQ of children in this population is more than one standard deviation below that of control children (Levine et al., 1987; Perlstein & Hood, 1955; St. James-Roberts, 1981; Woods, 1980), whereas others report no significant IQ deficit (e.g., Aram & Ekelman, 1986; Bates, Vicari, & Trauner, 1999; Nass et al., 1989). A recent longitudinal study suggests that this discrepancy may reflect differences in the age of the children at the time of assessment (Levine, Kraus, Alexander, Suriyakham, & Huttenlocher, 2005). Studies that report little or no impact on IQ tend to assess children at earlier time points than those that report IQ deficits. In the Levine et al. (2005) study, children with PS were administered an IQ test at two different time points (before and after age 7). Results showed that the children with PS had significantly lower Verbal and Performance IQ levels at the later time point. Importantly, the lower IQ levels at the later assessment time point did not reflect a loss of skills, but slower acquisition of knowledge (Banich, Levine, Kim, & Huttenlocher, 1990).

It is possible that the increasing IQ gap between children with PS and TD reflects maturational changes in the developing brain. That is, particular brain regions may only contribute to task performance of children with TB once they have reached a sufficient level of maturity. If these regions are damaged and fail to develop normally in the children with PS, an IQ gap may become increasingly apparent over time. The decline in IQ in children with brain injury can also be thought of as reflecting limitations that early lesions place on the brain's processing capacities. If we assume that these processing capacities are more taxed as task demands increase, the gap between the IQ levels of children with TD and PS may be expected to widen over time. Thus the degree of functional plasticity observed after an early lesion may depend on the age of the child at the time of assessment. It may also depend on the specific domain of functioning being examined. Since IQ tests were designed to assess overall levels of functioning rather than functioning in particular domains, it is important to examine performance with tasks that tap specific aspects of functioning in order to address this question (Levine et al., 2005).

EXPERIMENTAL STUDIES OF BEHAVIORAL DEVELOPMENT

The study of the effects of stroke in adults has made substantial contributions to our understanding of mature patterns of brain organization for higher cognitive functions. These studies use a logic of subtraction and dissociation, in that their goal is to understand which functional *loss* is uniquely associated with injury to a particular brain region. However, such logic fails in studies of children with PS, because the children's injuries occur prior to their acquisition of most higher cognitive functions. Instead, the key questions in studies of the effect of stroke in children center on delineating the mechanisms that underlie the dynamic features of cognitive and neural development. Rather than identifying a *typical* profile of functional organization, the goal is to identify the multiple, *alternative* patterns of brain organization that can arise following early injury to the developing brain. Four questions are central to the study of cognitive and affective development in children with PS:

1. Is there evidence of cognitive deficit early in development?
2. Are the associations between patterns of behavioral deficit and sites of brain injury among children comparable to the associations observed among adults?
3. Do behavioral deficits persist over time?
4. What is the nature of the change and how does this change, occur?

These questions are examined within the context of data from three behavioral domains: language, visual–spatial processing, and affect. Interestingly, the answers to the four questions differ across these basic behavioral domains, suggesting that the developmental trajectories and capacity for plastic adaptation may vary by behavioral function.

These contrasting profiles have important implications for understanding the development of brain–behavior relations.

Language Development

The study of adult patterns of brain organization for language began more than 160 years ago, with Paul Broca's original study of a patient with aphasia who was found to have significant injury to anterior regions of the LH. Subsequent work has largely confirmed the early findings. For 95–98% of adults, core aspects of language (phonology, morphology, and syntax) are mediated by the LH. Other work has shown that the RH also plays a role in pragmatics, or the ways language is used. Adults with injury to the RH often have difficulty with nonliteral language (e.g., humor, metaphor, and sarcasm). They are also impaired in discourse cohesion (e.g., running on, failing to convey the point or "gist" of a story.)

Studies of early language acquisition in children with PS have all noted a delay in language onset, with subsequent progress that follows the typical sequence of language development. Unlike the profile of adults with strokes, language delays are observed among children with lesions to either the LH or RH. Marchman, Miller, and Bates (1991) examined the phonological development in children with PS, and found delay in the onset of babbling; once it emerged, however, development followed the normal trajectory. In a large cross-sectional study of language acquisition, Bates et al. (1997) used the MacArthur Communicative Development Inventories (MCDI), a parental report battery (Fenson et al., 1993), to chronicle early language development. They report that the group with PS as a whole was delayed for the onset of language. Within this context of delay, they found that among 8- to 16-month-old children with PS, early RH injury resulted in the greatest deficits in comprehension. At somewhat later ages (20–48 months) left posterior temporal damage was associated with deficits in word and grammatical *production*—a finding that contrasts with the typical finding of *comprehension* deficits in adult stroke patients with such lesions. Complementing the parental report data, Bates et al. (1997) analyzed spontaneous language samples. They found a similar profile for mean length of utterance: Children with left posterior damage used shorter utterances than controls or children with injury to other brain regions.

These findings have been broadly confirmed by other groups, including those studying other languages. Using an Italian version of the MCDI, Vicari et al. (2000) also noted early delay in language onset with some site-specific profiles: Children with LH injury were more delayed than those with RH injury in early lexical production. Another study of Italian children with PS (Chilosi, Cipriani, Bertuccelli, Pfanner, & Cioni, 2001) reported similar findings. Looking at productive vocabulary longitudinally, Feldman and colleagues (Feldman, 1994; Feldman, Holland, Kemp, & Janosky, 1992) found initial delay in the group overall; they also found wide variability, with some children performing in the normal range and others delayed. However, after the initial delay, most of the children showed steady progress. On the Index of Productive Syntax, a measure of emergent syntax, half their group with LH injury fell well below the norm, as did half of those with RH injury. A longitudinal study of free-speech data (Thal, Reilly, Seibert, Jeffries, & Fenson, 2004) reported similar findings, with no site-specific profiles. These data are consistent with and are complemented by a large longitudinal study of children with PS (Brasky, Nikolas, Meanwell, Levine, & Goldin-Meadow, 2005; Levine et al., 2005): The investigators found overall delay in the onset of language, but also found that lesion size rather than site modulated the developmental trajectory for both productive vocabulary and syntactic development. Together, these data suggest that early brain injury to either hemisphere will delay the emergence of language, and that acquiring language, unlike maintaining an adult language system, requires both hemispheres of the brain.

By age 4, children with TD have mastered the majority of the grammatical structures of their language; language development after age 5, in addition to a growing vocabulary, reflects the increasingly flexible use of those grammatical structures for different discourse genres. Using a biographical interview, Bates et al. (2001) compared the productive language of children with PS (ages 5–8) to that of adults with homologous lesions. In this discourse context, where a child (or adult) must respond to an experimenter's questions, the adults displayed the predicted profile of lesion-specific deficits. Among the children with PS, however, spontaneous language was comparable to that of controls with respect to morphological errors and use of complex syntax; as such, the earlier site-specific differences had resolved. For morphosyntax, the language of the group with PS was comparable to that of peers with TD. In this same data set, *anaphora*, or the use of pronouns, was also examined. Adults with RH injury often have difficulty with discourse coherence. Pronouns represent one linguistic means to connect utterances (Halliday & Hasan, 1976), because they serve as links to preceding noun phrases. Examination of the children's use of pronouns (Dardier, Reilly, Bates, Delaye, & Laurent-Vannier, 2005) revealed that both children with TD and children with PS had many pronouns for which the referent was unclear. However, young children (ages 5–6) with RH injury had significantly more ambiguous pronouns than either children with TD or children with LH injury. Interestingly, this difference had resolved by 8 years of age. These findings suggest that although the acquisition of linguistic structures requires a bilateral brain network, the group with PS is making good progress in acquiring such structures. How children actually use and recruit such structures for discourse may be mediated by the RH, as is typical in the adult model.

To better understand language development in school-age children, Reilly and colleagues (Reilly, Bates, & Marchman, 1998; Reilly, Losh, Bellugi, & Wulfeck, 2004) focused on a more challenging discourse genre—narratives. The task required children to tell a story based upon a wordless picture book by Mayer (1969), *Frog, Where Are You?* At 4–6 years of age, all of the children with PS told shorter stories, made more morphological errors, and used fewer complex sentences than controls; however, there were no significant side- or site-specific differences. It is important to note that the morphological errors of the children with PS were similar to those of younger controls, suggesting that language acquisition follows a similar course in the group with PS, even though it is mediated by different brain structures. By middle school ages (7–12 years), the group with PS performed in the low-normal range on all morphosyntactic as well as narrative measures, including having the same number of episodes in their stories and inferring the theme of the story. Although no side-specific differences were found in the morphosyntactic measures, there was a trend reflecting less frequent use of complex sentences in those with RH than in those with LH injury (Reilly, Stiles, Wulfeck, & Nass, 2005b). One function of complex sentences in a narrative is to link the episodes of the story (e.g., "*When the boy was sleeping,* the frog escaped!") or to integrate the local event with the theme of the narrative—in this case, searching for the lost frog (e.g., "He looked in the hole *to try and find his frog.*"). It is likely that the decreased use of complex syntax in narratives reflects an impairment in the use of language for discourse cohesion. This profile is reminiscent of that of adults with RH injury. However, the early pronominal impairment appears to resolve with age in the children, and we expect that this is the case with complex syntax as well.

In telling a story and in responding to questions in an interview, children have choices about the vocabulary and the linguistic structures they use. Alternative methods of assessing language include standardized tests, as well as online measures of comprehension and grammaticality, which may be more sensitive measures of morphosyntactic abilities. Two studies (Ballantyne, Spilkin, & Trauner, 2007; MacWhinney, Feldman, Sacco, & Valdes-Perez, 2000) using the Clinical Evaluation of Language Function—Revised, reported that the group with PS performed significantly worse overall than controls with TD. However, on some subtests, MacWhinney et al. found that the children with LH injury matched the controls' performance, and Ballantyne et al. reported that children with seizures performed significantly more poorly than the rest of the group with PS. Seizure status as a factor in mediating performance has also been noted by other researchers (e.g., Dall'Oglio, Bates, Volterra, Di Capua, & Pezzini, 1994).

Online measures assess not only accuracy but also reaction time (RT), an index of processing speed. MacWhinney et al. (2000) administered an online battery of detection, recognition and word repetition, and picture-naming tasks; they found that overall, the group with PS showed slight impairments and slower RTs than controls, although these differences resolved with age. Looking at more complex language, Dick, Wulfeck, Krupa-Kwiatkowski, and Bates (2004) assessed sentence interpretation in children with PS. For the simpler constructions (active sentences and subject clefts), the group with PS performed comparably to controls; however, they were less accurate on more complex constructions (passive sentences and object clefts). This profile was mirrored in their RTs. An additional study focused on school-age children's knowledge of the language by asking children to make grammaticality judgments on grammatical or ungrammatical sentences, including determiner or auxiliary verb violations (Wulfeck, Bates, Krupa-Kwiatkowski, & Saltzman, 2004). Grammatical sensitivity of the group with PS was somewhat below that of the controls, but well above chance; also, and similar to the group with TD, the group with PS improved with age. Together, these studies present a picture of subtle impairments in the group with PS in the processing of complex language. Many of the differences resolve with age, suggesting catch-up in individual aspects of language learning. Interestingly, the performance of children with PS on these online tasks was similar to that of younger healthy controls. The similarity of the error patterns and responses to those of younger children with TD suggest that in spite of differences in neural mediation, all of these children approach the problem of acquiring a language in a similar manner, and that the process of language acquisition is constrained.

In summary, children with PS do surprisingly well in acquiring the grammatical structures of their language. Unlike adults with homologous damage, children with *either* RH or LH injury show initial delay. However, once language emerges, the development of language structures follows the same patterns evident in children with TD. Early site-specific profiles resolve, and by middle school age the group with PS performs in the low-normal range. But language acquisition is not just a matter of "catching up"; rather, at each new level of linguistic challenge, these children exhibit initial delay and subsequent development in mastering grammatical structures. Regarding pragmatics, or how the group with PS *uses* language, there is emerging evidence that the RH may play an early role in integrating discourse; children with RH injury mirror the profile of adults with similar injury, but in a more subtle manner. Furthermore, similar to the acquisition of linguistic structures, there is evidence of an iterative profile (wherein early deficits resolve with age but are again revealed in more challenging discourse contexts).

Visual Pattern Processing

Studies of spatial cognitive development in children with PS have focused on the analysis of visual pattern information. In adults, the neural system for processing visual pattern information—the so-called "what" system—is a bilateral occipitotemporal (OT) network. Within this network, the two cerebral hemispheres play complementary processing roles: The left OT region is dominant for processing parts or features, and the right OT region is dominant in processing pattern configuration. Among adult patients after stroke, left OT injury impairs processing of the parts of a spatial array, whereas right OT injury compromises configural processing (e.g., Delis, Robertson, & Efron, 1986; McFie & Zangwill, 1960; Piercy, Hecaen, & De Ajuriaguerra, 1960; Robertson & Delis, 1986; Robertson & Lamb, 1991; Swindell, Holland, Fromm, & Greenhouse, 1988; Warrington, James, & Kinsbourne, 1966). Data from children with PS suggest that the basic organization of the OT system is established early, but is capable of at least limited adaptive organization. The pattern of deficits associated with RH or LH injury is similar in adults and children, but the children's deficits are milder, and they appear to be better able to compensate for their deficits. Studies examining visual pattern processing among children ranging in age from the preschool period through adolescence provide supporting evidence for subtle, persistent, lesion-specific deficits (Stiles & Nass, 1991; Stiles, Paul, & Hesselink, 2006; Stiles, Reilly, Paul, & Moses, 2005; Stiles, Stern, Trauner, & Nass, 1996; Stiles-Davis, 1988; Stiles-Davis, Janowsky, Engel, & Nass, 1988; Stiles-Davis, Sugarman, & Nass, 1985).

Studies using *hierarchical* pattern stimuli have provided extensive data on visual pattern analysis in both typical and atypical populations. Hierarchical patterns are large "global-level" forms composed of appropriately arranged "local-level" elements (e.g., a global-level triangle made up of smaller local-level squares). When asked to copy such patterns from memory, adults with RH injury have difficulty with the global-level forms, whereas local-level processing is impaired by LH injury (Delis et al., 1986; Delis, Kiefner, & Fridlund, 1988). Children with RH and LH injury show similar patterns of deficits, as shown by data from a study of 5- to 12-year-old children with PS (Stiles et al., 2008). Reproduction accuracy for the global-level, but not local-level, forms was significantly lower than that of controls for children with RH injury; the reverse pattern was observed for children with LH injury. Furthermore, whereas accuracy improved for all groups with development, the pattern of deficit persisted for both groups with PS.

Other studies of visual–spatial processing confirm the early patterns of impairment, but also suggest that children may compensate for their deficits by adopting alternative processing strategies. A study of block construction among preschool-age children with PS documents the importance of examining both *what* children produce when they are given a spatial task, and *how* they approach the problem—that is, what strategies or procedures they use to complete the task (Stiles et al., 1996; Vicari, Stiles, Stern, & Resca, 1998). In this study, 4- to 6-year-old children were presented with a series of simple block models (e.g., a line of blocks or a double arch) and asked to reproduce them. The accuracy measure assessed the quality of the final product, while the process measure examined how a child approached the problem of construction. Children with LH injury were initially delayed on the task, producing overly simplified constructions. By age 4, they showed an interesting dissociation between product and process. When accuracy of performance was assessed, the performance of the children with LH injury was high, comparable to that of age-matched controls. However, when process was examined, performance diverged from that of the group with TD. The procedures they used to copy the models were greatly simplified. Specifically, the procedures the children adopted were typical of those observed among younger children at a point in development when they are unable to reproduce the models accurately. This developmental dissociation between product and process persisted at least through age 6. Children with RH injury were also initially delayed on this task, producing only simplified constructions. At age 4, the accuracy of their construction was very poor; their constructions were poorly configured. However, at this time, the procedures they used to generate these ill-formed constructions were comparable those of to age-matched controls. Thus, at age 4, the performance dissociation for the children with RH injury was the opposite of that observed for the children with LH injury: They could employ sophisticated construction strategies, but with very poor results. By age 6, children with RH injury were able to copy the target constructions accurately, but like their LH-injured peers, they now used simpler construction procedures. It appears that by adopting a less complicated construction strategy, the children with RH injury were able to compensate for spatial deficits and succeed in generating accurate constructions. This study suggests that there is impairment in spatial processing following early injury, and that there is compensation with development. However, closer examination of how spatial constructions are generated suggests persistent, subtle deficits.

Evidence for the use of alternative strategies is also observed among older children using a more difficult construction task, the Rey–Osterrieth Complex Figure (ROCF). The ROCF was developed to evaluate spatial planning in adult patients. The figure is organized around a central rectangle that is divided symmetrically with bisecting lines; pattern details are positioned within and around the core rectangle. The most efficient, though demanding, copying strategy is to begin with the core rectangle and bisectors, and then add details. School-age children with TD do not use this advanced strategy; rather, they parse the figure into smaller units. The size of the unit increases with age, such that 6- to 7-year-olds use a very piecemeal strategy, while older children use progressively larger subunits (quadrants, halves) until finally, by 12 years, the advanced strategy is dominant.

The ROCF is challenging for children with PS (Akshoomoff, Feroleto, Doyle, & Stiles, 2002; Akshoomoff & Stiles, 2003), as illustrated in a longitudinal study of 6- to 13-year-olds. Two versions of the task were administered: copying with the model present, and an immediate memory task. On the copying task, the children with RH or LH injury performed worse than controls. Deficits were particularly evident among the youngest children (age 6), but did not differ by side of lesion. Performance improved in such a manner that by 10 years the children's copies were accurate, but they were produced by using the most immature and piecemeal strategy. The failure to find differences between the groups with RH and LH injury probably reflects underlying task demands that place equal emphasis on segmentation and integration. Thus a deficit in either process would disrupt performance on the task.

In contrast to the findings from the copying task, the memory task did distinguish between the lesion groups. When the copying and memory data from the oldest children in the sample were compared, few differences were observed for the children with RH injury: Under both task conditions, they produced accurate reproductions by using a piecemeal strategy. However, a dramatic shift in the strategies of the children with LH injury was observed in the memory task. Unlike on the copying task, these children organized their memory reproductions around the core rectangle and produced relatively few additional details. The demands of the memory task thus revealed the characteristic LH visual–spatial processing deficit, while the copying task captured the children's strategies for compensating for that deficit.

Coding of Spatial Location

Very few studies have examined dorsal visual stream processing in children with PS. In adults, the dorsal stream—the so-called "where" system—is a bilateral occipitoparietal network (Ungerleider & Mishkin, 1982) that is involved in several aspects of spatial processing, including spatial transformation and location processing. Lateralized differences in dorsal stream processing have been documented for coding of categorical and coordinate relations among both adults and children (e.g., Hellige & Michimata, 1989; Koenig, Reiss, & Kosslyn, 1990; Reese & Stiles, 2005). These studies indicate that the LH is dominant for categorical spatial relations (e.g., above–below), whereas the RH is dominant for coordinate spatial relations that retain precise metric information about the location of objects and the distance between objects. Further support for this distinction comes from a study by Laeng (1994). In this study, adult patients with LH damage after stroke were more impaired on categorical spatial tasks, whereas those with RH damage were more impaired on metric spatial tasks.

In a recent study, Lourenco and Levine (2009) have used a simple location task to examine whether this is also true of young children with LH and RH lesions. Children with PS and TD (ages 3–5) were shown the locations of different toys on a long, narrow rug (5 feet by 8 inches), one at a time. The toy was then removed, and each child was asked to replicate the location of the toy. This was a one-dimensional coding task, as there was no variation in the location of the toys along the y coordinate, only along the x coordinate. On this task, young children (16–24 months) were found to use category information, making choices that were biased slightly toward the center of the space (Huttenlocher, Newcombe, & Sandberg, 1994). By 3 years of age, children with TD were extremely accurate on this task and did not show evidence of using category information. Similarly, by 3 years of age, children with early LH injury exhibited accurate metric performance. In contrast, at 3 and 4 years of age, children with RH injury showed marked category effects, representing locations that were not near the center of the space as much closer to the center than they actually were. This bias toward the center of the category was even more pronounced than that of toddlers with TD (18–24 months). However, by 5 years of age, children with both LH and RH injury could accurately code the metric location of the objects. Thus, as for the ventral stream (visual pattern) processing tasks described above, there is evidence for an early deficit that mirrors the difficulty adult patients with RH lesions have with metric coding. However, in children with PS there is also evidence for marked plasticity, as the children with RH injury show a normalization of performance by age 5. Lourenco and Levine are currently investigating whether the metric coding deficit reasserts itself on more difficult, two-dimensional location-coding tasks.

Face and Affect Processing

The majority of lesion studies from adults suggest that the RH, especially frontoparietal regions, plays a critical role in the recognition of emotions (Adolphs, Damasio, & Tranel, 2002; Adolphs, Tranel, & Damasio, 2003; Blonder, Bowers, & Heilman, 1991; Borod, 1992, 1993; Borod et al., 1998; Damasio, Adolphs, & Damasio, 2003; De Renzi, Perani, Carlesimo, & Silveri, 1994; Ley & Bryden, 1979; Stone & Valentine, 2003). Recent models of face processing propose dissociations in the neural systems responsible for processing face identity from other aspects—specifically, discrimination, labeling, and recognition of facial affect (Bowers, Bauer, Coslett, & Heilman, 1985; Bowers & Heilman, 1984; Bruce & Young, 1986; Tranel, Damasio, & Damasio, 1988). Both structural imaging and functional imaging have largely confirmed this suggestion (Adolphs, 2001; Haxby, Hoffman, & Gobbini, 2000). Studies of emotion processing in children with PS include both naturalistic and experimental studies of children from infancy through adolescence.

Faces constitute an early and frequently encountered category of visual input. They are arguably the most important social stimuli in the environment of a young child. Affective facial expressions are critical social cues conveying information about both interpersonal interaction and environmental threat. Evidence for impairment of face processing in socially and affectively neutral contexts would be likely to reflect a basic deficit in visual–spatial processing, but such impairment may also have an impact on children's behavior in social contexts. Deficits in the ability to process faces and the social and affective cues they convey have the potential to exacerbate a primary socioaffective processing deficit, creating additional challenges for the child with PS.

A large body of data has shown that infants can process faces and may even show adultlike processing biases (Cohen & Cashon, 2001; de Schonen & Mathivet, 1990; Nelson, 2001; Simion, Cassia, Turati, & Valenza, 2001; Thompson, Madrid, Westbrook, & Johnston, 2001). Early characterizations of developmental gains during the school-age period suggested that featural strategies may initially predominate in face processing (Carey & Diamond, 1977). However, later work showed that even preschool children rely on holistic and configural information, although they perhaps rely on less information than older children and adults do (Pedelty, Levine, & Shevell, 1985; e.g., Baenninger, 1994; Tanaka, Kay, Grinnell, Stansfield, & Szechter, 1998; but see Schwarzer, 2002; Pellicano & Rhodes, 2003). Face processing typically activates OT regions, including the fusiform gyrus, bilaterally (Haxby et al., 1994). Consistent with the notion that face discrimination may rely more on the holistic and configural processing capacity of the RH than on the featural processing system of the LH (Hillger & Koenig, 1991; Levine & Levy, 1986; Rhodes, 1993; Rossion et al., 2000), many imaging studies report RH bias (Kanwisher, McDermott, & Chun, 1997; McCarthy, Puce, Gore, & Allison, 1997). Face processing may thus be differentially affected by the laterality of the early brain injury.

A growing body of evidence suggests that face processing is affected by early brain injury. However, the evidence suggests that impairment is not confined to children with RH injury and can extend to children with LH injury as well. de Schonen and colleagues (de Schonen, Mancini, Camps, Maes, & Laurent, 2005; Mancini, de Schonen, Deruelle, & Massoulier, 1994) reported a series of studies examining different aspects of face processing in school-age children with PS. Deficits in face processing were common in their population of children, and as common among the children with LH injury as with RH injury. The severity of the face-processing deficits reported in this study suggests that face processing may be established very early and be less plastic than other aspects of visual–spatial processing. Data from a study of somewhat older children and adolescents with PS are consistent with these findings. Paul and colleagues (Paul et al., 2009; Stiles et al., 2006) examined RT and accuracy in a face-identity-matching task. Children and adolescents with RH injury were significantly slower and less accurate in identifying faces than controls with TD. The performance of the group with LH injury was marginally worse than that of controls but did not differ significantly from that of the RH-injured group, suggesting that early lesions to either hemisphere affect face processing, but perhaps more moderately in the case of LH lesions. Together, the data suggest that face processing is vulnerable to the effects of early injury, manifesting significant impairments that extend well into adolescence.

By their first birthday, as productive language emerges, infants with TD are already effective at communicating via emotional facial expression, vocalizations, and gestures. Naturalistic studies of emotional facial expressions in infants with PS suggest that RH injury may selectively affect expression of emotion. Reilly, Stiles, Larsen, and Traunier (1995) used the Facial Action Coding System (Ekman & Friesen, 1978) to assess frequency of infants' positive affect (smiles) in response to their mothers' bids for interaction. Although all the children smiled, both the controls with TD and the children with LH injury smiled easily and often; in contrast, those with RH injury seldom smiled. Longitudinal case studies confirmed these data, suggesting that the RH plays a significant role in emotional expression from the first year of life, and that valence (positive–negative) is a significant factor in the organization of emotions (Reilly et al., 1995). Interestingly, increased negativity in children with RH has also been reported in a toddler temperament study based on a parental questionnaire (Nass & Koch, 1987).

A complementary study of prelinguistic affective vocalizations (Reilly, Charfen, Stiles, del Guercio, & Nass, 2005a) in a larger group of infants with PS exhibited a similar profile: Both controls and infants with LH injury produced more positive than negative vocalizations. The RH-injured group produced significantly more negative vocalizations than either of the other groups, and the children with RH basal ganglia involvement most strongly exhibited this profile. Together, the face and vocalization findings suggest that the neural substrates for emotion are established early, and that the profile of deficit is not modality-specific but general to the domain of emotion.

Labeling emotions, a traditional task in the emotion literature, recruits not just emotional but also spatial and linguistic abilities. Reilly et al. (2005a) collected free-labeling data from 4- to 8-year-old children with PS and controls with TD. Among the controls, slight improvement was observed with age, and the children with RH lesions performed like the controls. Surprisingly, the younger children (ages 4–5) with LH lesions fared the worst in labeling emotional expressions, but this early deficit resolved by age 6. The data present a conundrum. Early on, those with RH lesions appeared to have production impairments for emotional facial expressions; however, the labeling task suggested that the young children with LH lesions had the most difficulty. Several interpretations are possible. Given the multiple domains that labeling draws on, the performance of the LH-injured group may reflect difficulty in isolating and identifying features within a spatial array, or it may reflect a subtle linguistic deficit. Regardless of which systems are responsible in the younger group, it is important to note that, consistent with the profiles for language and spatial development, the early deficits tend to resolve with age. In contrast to the "catch-up" evident in the labeling task, side-specific deficits in facial recognition, although subtle, persist (Paul et al., 2009; Stiles et al., 2006). It may well be that with more challenging tasks—for example, using RT to assess labeling—we would see slower RTs in the group with PS on labeling as well. However, on the basis of the RT language studies (discussed above), we would not expect right–left differences; again, this highlights the differential profiles for linguistic and spatial processing.

ALTERNATIVE PATTERNS OF BRAIN ORGANIZATION: fMRI STUDIES

Over the past decade, fMRI has become a widely applied tool for defining profiles of neural organization. In the past few years, this technique has begun to be applied to studies of children with PS. This approach provides the opportunity to begin defining the alternative patterns of brain organization that can arise following early brain injury, but thus far the data are limited. The application of an imaging methodology that relies on group data for statistical robustness has been a challenge in studies of children with PS. The structural abnormalities in the brains of children with PS make anatomical normalization and averaging difficult. However, the more fundamental question is whether averaging is an optimal approach for understanding alternative patterns of organization in this population. Every lesion is unique and introduces different factors into the neurological equation. Thus greater individual variation in neural organization should be predicted for this population, and averaging of activation data may mask important findings. Thus far, most fMRI studies of children with PS have reported activation data for individual subjects. In some cases, they take the form of individual case reports; in others, individual patterns are classified into categories that capture distinctive and more general patterns of activation, thus creating meaningful subgroups. The growing body of data has the potential to make significant contributions to our understanding of the range of alternative patterns of neural organization that can emerge in the wake of early injury.

fMRI Studies of Language Processing

Initial studies of neural organization in children with early LH injury reported increased activation in RH homologues of Broca's and Wernicke's areas (e.g., Müller et al., 1999; Staudt et al., 2002b), suggesting that right lateralization would indicate better language functioning in this population. Two recent fMRI studies have tested this hypothesis. The first study (Raja et al., 2006) examined lateralization of neural activity in children with PS during a category fluency task and its correlation with level of language functioning on standardized language tests and Verbal IQ. As expected, both children with RH lesions and controls showed left lateralization in anterior and posterior regions. By contrast, children with LH lesions showed bilateral activity. Interestingly, for these children, level of language functioning was correlated with bilateral activation in posterior language regions rather than with RH activation. The second fMRI study (Saccuman et al., 2006) used two levels of syntactic complexity to explore the neural activation associated with the processing of syntactic and morphological cues used to determine the agent role in "simple" versus "complex" sentences in children and adolescents with PS. They found that the children with PS showed activations in superior temporal and inferior frontal regions comparable to those of controls. Children with LH lesions had more bilateral activation, but all children showed active clusters in the LH, including the tissue immediately adjacent to lesions. Together, these data suggest that the LH may be privileged for language processing even in the presence of large lesions, and they argue against the hypotheses of a massive "relocation" of the neural substrate for language comprehension and for more subtle plastic adaptations.

fMRI Studies of Visual–Spatial Processing

fMRI data on spatial processing are more limited than the data for language, consisting of individual case reports. The children included in these reports have comparatively small lesions that do not directly affect the ventral OT regions implicated in visual–spatial tasks. Nonetheless, their behavioral profiles reflect the typical pattern of deficit associated with the side of their injury. The anatomical data discussed earlier suggest the possibility that indirect compromise of the posterior OT brain areas can account for the patterns of impairment observed in these children.

The task used in the fMRI study of global–local processing required participants to attend, on different imaging runs, to either the global level or the local level of a hierarachial stimulus (Stiles et al., 2003). For typical adults and adolescents (Martinez et al., 1997; Moses et al., 2002), greater activation is observed in right ventral OT regions during global processing and in left ventral OT regions during local processing. The two children with PS included a 13-year-old male (K-LH) with a large lesion in the left parietal lobe and white matter volume reduction in areas posterior to the lesion, and a 15-year-old male (M-RH) with a large RH lesion in the periventricular region of the parietotemporal lobes and a white matter volume reduction posterior to the lesion. For both global and local task conditions, K-LH's activation was strongly asymmetrical and localized primarily within the uninjured right OT; M-RH's activation showed the opposite pattern, with activation localized within the uninjured left OT. These profiles of activation argue for the emergence of alternative patterns of brain organization in which the normally bilateral distribution of processing becomes consolidated within a single hemisphere.

The task used in the fMRI study of face processing required participants to judge whether a target face matched one of two reference faces. Both adults and typical 10-year-old children activate the ventral OT area, including the fusiform face area (FFA), bilaterally (Passarotti et al., 2003). The two children with PS included a 12-year-old male (A-RH) with a large right perisylvian lesion (posterior inferior frontal, inferior pre- and postcentral, and supramarginal gyri), and a 14-year-old male (L-LH) with a porencephaly in the left cerebral hemisphere (affecting the deep white matter of the superior and inferior frontal gyri, precentral gyrus [including the corticospinal and corticobulbar tracts], and corpus callosum). Both of these children with PS had bilateral activation of the FFA similar to that of controls, suggesting that basic organization for face processing can emerge following early insult. This is surprising, given the results from the global–local task described above, and it suggests an early precedence for face processing. However, enhanced activation was also observed for the children with PS in more superior regions of the left fusiform. It has been shown (Gerlach, Law, Gade, & Paulson, 1999; Joseph & Gathers, 2003) that activity in this region may be associated with difficult visual discrimination tasks. Thus the enhanced activation for the children with PS may reflect demands associated with their subtle, but persistent, spatial processing deficits.

SUMMARY AND CONCLUSIONS

Work in developmental neurobiology has provided an extensive body of evidence laying out the fundamental principles of neural development. This work has redefined ideas about the role of plasticity in early neural development, and it has important implications for the study of human brain development both in typical populations and in populations of children with brain disorders. The older pediatric clinical literature portrayed early brain plasticity as a secondary system that is recruited in the wake of early injury. However, the emerging view of the developing brain as dynamic and constantly adapting to endogenous biological signals and exogenous input provides a very different perspective on the nature of plasticity. The early brain injury does not recruit an ancillary adaptive function; rather, it becomes integrated into the ongoing, dynamic, and adaptive processes of brain development, which are inherently plastic. Early pathology is never optimal or beneficial, but its consequences and effects are best understood as the product of a dynamic set of processes reflecting fundamental properties of neurocognitive development.

The study of children with PS provides a unique window into the workings of these complex developmental processes. PS is medically well defined as a cerebrovascular event occurring during the last trimester or shortly after birth. The lesions in many children with PS are large, compromising much of one cerebral hemisphere. When such injury occurs in a mature individual, the effects are devastating and debilitating. Yet across a range of physiological and behavioral domains, the degree of physical and functional adaptation to insult when it occurs early in life is remarkable. There is, however, evidence that different neural systems and functions may vary in their capacity for adaptive reorganization, even when injury is early. Although basic sensory and motor systems are capable of considerable reorganization, the residual effects on function are often greater than for other domains. Within behavioral domains, level of function is consistently superior to that of adults with comparable injury, but varies by skill domain. Early-developing functions (such as those associated with face and affect processing) appear to be more vulnerable than later-developing functions (such as language). Similarly, functions such as visual–spatial processing that have a long evolutionary history and are closely linked to a specific sensory system exhibit somewhat less functional plasticity.

Furthermore, there may be subtle limits on the upper range of development. Across the spectrum of behavioral domains, there is evidence of initial developmental delay on age-appropriate tasks, followed by mastery at a later developmental period. This pattern is iterative: Within each successive developmental period, the introduction of a more challenging, age-appropriate task initially reveals evidence of subtle persistent deficit, and only later is mastery achieved. In some cases, there is evidence that children master tasks via the development of compensatory strategies that may suffice but are not optimal for the task. Finally, longitudinal studies of IQ suggest an eventual leveling, which begins in late childhood and early adolescence, in the capacity of children with PS to deal with more and more challenging cognitive and linguistic problems. Nonetheless, even with these developmental limitations, the level of function observed in children with PS is impressive and reflects the capacity of the developing human brain to adapt to the contingencies of extensive physical insult. As such, it provides a dramatic example of the adaptive and dynamic nature of human brain development.

Although the data described in this chapter provide a compelling case for the plasticity of the developing brain, a number of questions remain to be answered. One important question is this: What role do the specific experiences of an individual child play in directing development? There is ample evidence from the animal literature that specific experiences early in development can dramatically alter the neural organization. The neuroimaging data from children with PS confirm that reorganization occurs. However, those data cannot specify the particular events that underlie the emerging alternative reorganization. Data on the effects of individual experiences are extremely limited and challenging to obtain. One very recent study, however, supports the idea that the specific experiences of the individual child can affect behavioral profiles, and thus presumably neural profiles. Levine and colleagues (Rowe, Levine, Fischer, & Goldin-Meadow, 2009) have shown that children with the PS who receive more extensive language input progress more rapidly than children who receive more limited input. On measures of lexical acquisition, the effects of input are equivalent for children with PS and controls, reflecting the generalized effects of input. However, on measures of syntax acquisition the magnitude of the effects of input are significantly greater for the group with PS than for the controls. Specifically, the learning trajectories for children with PS who receive high levels of input are steeper than those of controls with TD who receive low input. These data suggest that rich input may be particularly important in the wake of early injury. These kinds of data are compelling and suggest that studies of individual differences among children with PS could be an important source of data on mechanisms of brain plasticity.

Recent advances in structural MRI offer a means of exploring these questions in greater depth. Diffusion tensor imaging (DTI) is an MRI-based technique that allows for assessment of the integrity and maturation of white matter pathways in the brain (Huppi & Dubois, 2006; Schmahmann et al., 2007). Several recent studies have demonstrated that DTI measures of individual pathway maturation can be correlated with measures of behavior, thus providing an index of the association between brain and behavioral development (e.g., Beaulieu et al., 2005; Ben-Shachar, Dougherty, & Wandell, 2007; Deutsch et al., 2005; Niogi & McCandliss, 2006; Schmithorst, Wilke, Dardzinski, & Holland, 2005). These kinds of studies have the potential to enrich our understanding of brain and cognitive development following early injury, and to further specify the role of input variation in the plasticity of the developing brain.

ACKNOWLEDGMENTS

This work was supported by the National Institute of Child Health and Human Development (Grant Nos. P01-HD040605 and R01-HD25077), National Institute of Neurological Disorders and Stroke (Grant No. P50-NS22343), and National Institute of Deafness and Communicative Disorders (Grant No. P50-DC01289). We wish to thank the parents and children for their participation in the studies presented in this chapter and to Stella F. Lourenco for helpful comments.

REFERENCES

Adolphs, R. (2001). The neurobiology of social cognition. *Current Opinion in Neurobiology, 11*, 231–239.

Adolphs, R., Damasio, H., & Tranel, D. (2002). Neural systems for recognition of emotional prosody: A 3-D lesion study. *Emotion, 2*, 23–51.

Adolphs, R., Tranel, D., & Damasio, A. R. (2003). Dissociable neural systems for recognizing emotions. *Brain and Cognition, 52*, 61–69.

Akshoomoff, N. A., Feroleto, C. C., Doyle, R. E., & Stiles, J. (2002). The impact of early unilateral brain injury on perceptual organization and visual memory. *Neuropsychologia, 40*, 539–561.

Akshoomoff, N. A., & Stiles, J. (2003). Children's performance on the ROCF and the development of spatial analysis. In J. A. Knight & E. Kaplan (Eds.), *The handbook of Rey–Osterrieth Complex Figure usage: Clinical and research applications* (pp. 393–409). Lutz, FL: Psychological Assessment Resources.

Aram, D. M., & Ekelman, B. L. (1986). Cognitive profiles of children with early onset of unilateral lesions. *Developmental Neuropsychology, 2*, 155–172.

Baenninger, M. (1994). The development of face recognition: Featural or configurational processing? *Journal of Experimental Child Psychology, 57*, 377–396.

Ballantyne, A. O., Spilkin, A., & Trauner, D. (2007). Language outcome after perinatal stroke: Does side matter? *Child Neuropsychology, 13*(6), 494–509.

Banich, M. T., Levine, S. C., Kim, H., & Huttenlocher, P. (1990). The effects of developmental factors on IQ in hemiplegic children. *Neuropsychologia, 28*, 35–47.

Bates, E., Reilly, J., Wulfeck, B., Dronkers, N., Opie, M., Fenson, J., et al. (2001). Differential effects of unilateral lesions on language production in children and adults. *Brain and Language, 79*, 223–265.

Bates, E., Thal, D., Trauner, D., Fenson, J., Aram, D., Eisele, J., et al. (1997). From first words to grammar in children with focal brain injury. *Developmental Neuropsychology, 13*, 275–343.

Bates, E., Vicari, S., & Trauner, D. (1999). Neural mediation of language development: Perspectives from lesion studies of infants and children. In H. Tager-Flusberg (Ed.), *Neurodevelopmental disorders* (pp. 533–581). Cambridge, MA: MIT Press.

Bax, M., Tydeman, C., & Flodmark, O. (2006). Clinical and MRI correlates of cerebral palsy: The European Cerebral Palsy Study. *Journal of the American Medical Association, 296*, 1602–1608.

Beaulieu, C., Plewes, C., Paulson, L. A., Roy, D., Snook, L., Concha, L., et al. (2005). Imaging brain connectivity in children with diverse reading ability. *NeuroImage, 25*, 1266–1271.

Ben-Shachar, M., Dougherty, R. F., & Wandell, B. A. (2007). White matter pathways in reading. *Current Opinion in Neurobiology, 17*, 258–270.

Blonder, L. X., Bowers, D., & Heilman, K. M. (1991). The role of the right hemisphere in emotional communication. *Brain, 114*(Pt. 3), 1115–1127.

Boardman, J. P., Ganesan, V., Rutherford, M. A., Saunders, D. E., Mercuri, E., & Cowan, F. (2005). Magnetic resonance image correlates of hemiparesis after neonatal and childhood middle cerebral artery stroke. *Pediatrics, 115*, 321–326.

Borod, J. C. (1992). Interhemispheric and intrahemispheric control of emotion: A focus on unilateral brain damage. *Journal of Consulting and Clinical Psychology, 60*, 339–348.

Borod, J. C. (1993). Cerebral mechanisms underlying facial, prosodic, and lexical emotional expression: A review of neuropsychological studies and methodological issues. *Neuropsychology, 7*, 445–463.

Borod, J. C., Cicero, B. A., Obler, L. K., Welkowitz, J., Erhan, H. M., Santschi, C., et al. (1998). Right hemisphere emotional perception: Evidence across multiple channels. *Neuropsychology, 12*, 446–458.

Bowers, D., Bauer, R. M., Coslett, H. B., & Heilman, K. M. (1985). Processing of faces by patients with unilateral hemisphere lesions: I. Dissociation between judgments of facial affect and facial identity. *Brain and Cognition, 4*, 258–272.

Bowers, D., & Heilman, K. M. (1984). Dissociation between the processing of affective and nonaffective faces: A case study. *Journal of Clinical Neuropsychology, 6*, 367–379.

Brasky, K., Nikolas, M., Meanwell, C., Levine, S. C., & Goldin-Meadow, S. (2005, June). *Language devel-*

opment in children with unilateral brain injury: Effects of lesion size. Paper presented at the Symposium on Research in Child Language Disorders, Madison, WI.

Brown, J. K., van Rensburg, F., Walsh, G., Lakie, M., & Wright, G. W. (1987). A neurological study of hand function of hemiplegic children. *Developmental Medicine and Child Neurology, 29,* 287–304.

Bruce, V., & Young, A. (1986). Understanding face recognition. *British Journal of Psychology, 77,* 305–327.

Cao, Y., Vikingstad, E. M., Huttenlocher, P. R., Towle, V. L., & Levin, D. N. (1994). Functional magnetic resonance studies of the reorganization of the human hand sensorimotor area after unilateral brain injury in the perinatal period. *Proceedings of the National Academy of Sciences USA, 91,* 9612–9616.

Carey, S., & Diamond, R. (1977). From piecemeal to configurational representation of faces. *Science, 195,* 312–314.

Carlsson, M., Hagberg, G., & Olsson, I. (2003). Clinical and aetiological aspects of epilepsy in children with cerebral palsy. *Developmental Medicine and Child Neurology, 45,* 371–376.

Carr, L. J., Harrison, L. M., Evans, A. L., & Stephens, J. A. (1993). Patterns of central motor reorganization in hemiplegic cerebral palsy. *Brain, 116*(Pt. 5), 1223–1247.

Changeux, J. P., & Danchin, A. (1976). Selective stabilisation of developing synapses as a mechanism for the specification of neuronal networks. *Nature, 264,* 705–712.

Charles, J. R., Wolf, S. L., Schneider, J. A., & Gordon, A. M. (2006). Efficacy of a child-friendly form of constraint-induced movement therapy in hemiplegic cerebral palsy: A randomized control trial. *Developmental Medicine and Child Neurology, 48,* 635–642.

Chilosi, A. M., Cipriani, P. P., Bertuccelli, B., Pfanner, P. L., & Cioni, P. G. (2001). Early cognitive and communication development in children with focal brain lesions. *Journal of Child Neurology, 16,* 309–316.

Chu, D., Huttenlocher, P. R., Levin, D. N., & Towle, V. L. (2000). Reorganization of the hand somatosensory cortex following perinatal unilateral brain injury. *Neuropediatrics, 31,* 63–69.

Cohen, L. B., & Cashon, C. H. (2001). Do 7-month-old infants process independent features or facial configurations? *Infant and Child Development, 10,* 83–92.

Connolly, K., & Stratton, P. (1968). Developmental changes in associated movements. *Developmental Medicine and Child Neurology, 10,* 49–56.

Cooper, J., Majnemer, A., Rosenblatt, B., & Birnbaum, R. (1995). The determination of sensory deficits in children with hemiplegic cerebral palsy. *Journal of Child Neurology, 10,* 300–309.

Cowan, W. M., Fawcett, J. W., O'Leary, D. D., & Stanfield, B. B. (1984). Regressive events in neurogenesis. *Science, 225,* 1258–1265.

Dall'Oglio, A. M., Bates, E., Volterra, V., Di Capua, M., & Pezzini, G. (1994). Early cognition, communication and language in children with focal brain injury. *Developmental Medicine and Child Neurology, 36,* 1076–1098.

Damasio, A., Adolphs, R., & Damasio, H. (2003). The contributions of the lesion method to the functional neuroanatomy of emotion. In R. J. Davidson, K. R. Scherer, & H. H. Goldsmith (Eds.), *Handbook of affective sciences* (pp. 66–92). Oxford: Oxford University Press.

Dardier, V., Reilly, J., Bates, E., Delaye, C., & Laurent-Vannier, A. (2005). La cohesion du discours de chez les enfants et les adolescents cerbroleses: Analyse de l'usage des pronoms et des connecteurs. *Cahiers d'Acquisition et Pathologie du Langage,* 101–114.

Delis, D. C., Kiefner, M. G., & Fridlund, A. J. (1988). Visuospatial dysfunction following unilateral brain damage: Dissociations in hierarchical hemispatial analysis. *Journal of Clinical and Experimental Neuropsychology, 10,* 421–431.

Delis, D. C., Robertson, L. C., & Efron, R. (1986). Hemispheric specialization of memory for visual hierarchical stimuli. *Neuropsychologia, 24,* 205–214.

De Renzi, E., Perani, D., Carlesimo, G. A., & Silveri, M. C. (1994). Prosopagnosia can be associated with damage confined to the right hemisphere: An MRI and PET study and a review of the literature. *Neuropsychologia, 32,* 893–902.

de Schonen, S., Mancini, J., Camps, R., Maes, E., & Laurent, A. (2005). Early brain lesions and face-processing development. *Developmental Psychobiology, 46,* 184–208.

de Schonen, S., & Mathivet, E. (1990). Hemispheric asymmetry in a face discrimination task in infants. *Child Development, 61*, 1192–1205.

Deutsch, G. K., Dougherty, R. F., Bammer, R., Siok, W. T., Gabrieli, J. D., & Wandell, B. (2005). Children's reading performance is correlated with white matter structure measured by diffusion tensor imaging. *Cortex, 41*, 354–363.

de Vries, L. S., Groenendaal, F., Eken, P., van Haastert, I. C., Rademaker, K. J., & Meiners, L. C. (1997). Infarcts in the vascular distribution of the middle cerebral artery in preterm and fullterm infants. *Neuropediatrics, 28*, 88–96.

Dick, F., Wulfeck, B., Krupa-Kwiatkowski, M., & Bates, E. (2004). The development of complex sentence interpretation in typically developing children compared with children with specific language impairments or early unilateral focal lesions. *Developmental Science, 7*, 360–377.

Duff, S. V., & Gordon, A. M. (2003). Learning of grasp control in children with hemiplegic cerebral palsy. *Developmental Medicine and Child Neurology, 45*, 746–757.

Duque, J., Thonnard, J. L., Vandermeeren, Y., Sebire, G., Cosnard, G., & Olivier, E. (2003). Correlation between impaired dexterity and corticospinal tract dysgenesis in congenital hemiplegia. *Brain, 126*, 732–747.

Ekman, P., & Friesen, W. V. (1978). *Facial Action Coding System: Investigator's guide.* Palo Alto, CA: Consulting Psychologists Press.

Eliasson, A. C., & Gordon, A. M. (2000). Impaired force coordination during object release in children with hemiplegic cerebral palsy. *Developmental Medicine and Child Neurology, 42*, 228–234.

Eliasson, A. C., Gordon, A. M., & Forssberg, H. (1991). Basic co-ordination of manipulative forces of children with cerebral palsy. *Developmental Medicine and Child Neurology, 33*, 661–670.

Eliasson, A. C., Gordon, A. M., & Forssberg, H. (1992). Impaired anticipatory control of isometric forces during grasping by children with cerebral palsy. *Developmental Medicine and Child Neurology, 34*, 216–225.

Eliasson, A. C., Gordon, A. M., & Forssberg, H. (1995). Tactile control of isometric fingertip forces during grasping in children with cerebral palsy. *Developmental Medicine and Child Neurology, 37*, 72–84.

Farmer, S. F., Harrison, L. M., Ingram, D. A., & Stephens, J. A. (1991). Plasticity of central motor pathways in children with hemiplegic cerebral palsy. *Neurology, 41*, 1505–1510.

Feldman, H. M. (1994). Language development after early brain injury: A replication study. In H. Tager-Flusberg (Ed.), *Constraints on language acquisition: Studies of atypical children* (pp. 75–90). Hillsdale, NJ: Erlbaum.

Feldman, H. M., Holland, A. L., Kemp, S. S., & Janosky, J. E. (1992). Language development after unilateral brain injury. *Brain and Language, 42*, 89–102.

Fenson, L., Dale, P. S., Reznick, J. S., Thal, D., Bates, E., Hartung, J. P., et al. (1993). *The MacArthur Communicative Development Inventories: User's guide and technical manual.* San Diego, CA: Singular.

Fonseca, S. T., Holt, K. G., Fetters, L., & Saltzman, E. (2004). Dynamic resources used in ambulation by children with spastic hemiplegic cerebral palsy: Relationship to kinematics, energetics, and asymmetries. *Physical Therapy, 84*, 344–354 (discussion, 355–358).

Forssberg, H., Eliasson, A. C., Redon-Zouitenn, C., Mercuri, E., & Dubowitz, L. (1999). Impaired grip-lift synergy in children with unilateral brain lesions. *Brain, 122*(Pt. 6), 1157–1168.

Gerlach, C., Law, I., Gade, A., & Paulson, O. B. (1999). Perceptual differentiation and category effects in normal object recognition: A PET study. *Brain, 122*, 2159–2170.

Gordon, A. M., Charles, J., & Duff, S. V. (1999). Fingertip forces during object manipulation in children with hemiplegic cerebral palsy: II. Bilateral coordination. *Developmental Medicine and Child Neurology, 41*, 176–185.

Gordon, A. M., & Duff, S. V. (1999a). Fingertip forces during object manipulation in children with hemiplegic cerebral palsy: I. Anticipatory scaling. *Developmental Medicine and Child Neurology, 41*, 166–175.

Gordon, A. M., & Duff, S. V. (1999b). Relation between clinical measures and fine manipulative control in children with hemiplegic cerebral palsy. *Developmental Medicine and Child Neurology, 41*, 586–591.

Gordon, A. M., Lewis, S. R., Eliasson, A. C., & Duff, S. V. (2003). Object release under varying task constraints in children with hemiplegic cerebral palsy. *Developmental Medicine and Child Neurology*, *45*, 240–248.

Govaert, P., Matthys, E., Zecic, A., Roelens, F., Oostra, A., & Vanzieleghem, B. (2000). Perinatal cortical infarction within middle cerebral artery trunks. *Archives of Disease in Childhood: Fetal and Neonatal Edition*, *82*, F59–F63.

Greenough, W. T., Hwang, H. M., & Gorman, C. (1985). Evidence for active synapse formation or altered postsynaptic metabolism in visual cortex of rats reared in complex environments. *Proceedings of the National Academy of Sciences USA*, *82*, 4549–4552.

Halliday, M. A. K., & Hasan, R. (1976). *Cohesion in English*. London: Longman.

Haxby, J. V., Hoffman, E. A., & Gobbini, M. I. (2000). The distributed human neural system for face perception. *Trends in Cognitive Sciences*, *4*, 223–233.

Haxby, J. V., Horwitz, B., Ungerleider, L. G., Maisog, J. M., Pietrini, P., & Grady, C. L. (1994). The functional organization of human extrastriate cortex: A PET-rCBF study of selective attention to faces and locations. *Journal of Neuroscience*, *14*, 6336–6353.

Hellige, J. B., & Michimata, C. (1989). Categorization versus distance: Hemispheric differences for processing spatial information. *Memory and Cognition*, *17*, 770–776.

Hillger, L. A., & Koenig, O. (1991). Separable mechanisms in face processing: Evidence from hemispheric specialization. *Journal of Cognitive Neuroscience*, *3*, 42–58.

Himmelmann, K., Beckung, E., Hagberg, G., & Uvebrant, P. (2006). Gross and fine motor function and accompanying impairments in cerebral palsy. *Developmental Medicine and Child Neurology*, *48*, 417–423.

Humphreys, P., Whiting, S., & Pham, B. (2000). Hemiparetic cerebral palsy: Clinical pattern and imaging in prediction of outcome. *Canadian Journal of Neurological Sciences*, *27*, 210–219.

Hung, Y. C., Charles, J., & Gordon, A. M. (2004). Bimanual coordination during a goal-directed task in children with hemiplegic cerebral palsy. *Developmental Medicine and Child Neurology*, *46*, 746–753.

Huppi, P. S., & Dubois, J. (2006). Diffusion tensor imaging of brain development. *Seminars in Fetal and Neonatal Medicine*, *11*, 489–497.

Huttenlocher, J., Newcombe, N., & Sandberg, E. H. (1994). The coding of spatial location in young children. *Cognitive Psychology*, *27*, 115–148.

Huttenlocher, P. R. (2002). *Neural plasticity: The effects of environment on the development of the cerebral cortex*. Cambridge, MA: Harvard University Press.

Huttenlocher, P. R., & Dabholkar, A. S. (1997). Regional differences in synaptogenesis in human cerebral cortex. *Journal of Comparative Neurology*, *387*, 167–178.

Isaacs, E., Christie, D., Vargha-Khadem, F., & Mishkin, M. (1996). Effects of hemispheric side of injury, age at injury, and presence of seizure disorder on functional ear and hand asymmetries in hemiplegic children. *Neuropsychologia*, *34*, 127–137.

Joseph, J. E., & Gathers, A. D. (2003). Effects of structural similarity on neural substrates for object recognition. *Cognitive, Affective, and Behavioral Neuroscience*, *3*, 1–16.

Kanwisher, N., McDermott, J., & Chun, M. M. (1997). The fusiform face area: A module in human extrastriate cortex specialized for face perception. *Journal of Neuroscience*, *17*, 4302–4311.

Koenig, O., Reiss, L. P., & Kosslyn, S. M. (1990). The development of spatial relation representations: Evidence from studies of cerebral lateralization. *Journal of Experimental Child Psychology*, *50*, 119–130.

Krumlinde-Sundholm, L., & Eliasson, A. C. (2002). Comparing tests of tactile sensibility: Aspects relevant to testing children with spastic hemiplegia. *Developmental Medicine and Child Neurology*, *44*, 604–612.

Kuhtz-Buschbeck, J. P., Sundholm, L. K., Eliasson, A. C., & Forssberg, H. (2000). Quantitative assessment of mirror movements in children and adolescents with hemiplegic cerebral palsy. *Developmental Medicine and Child Neurology*, *42*, 728–736.

Kwong, K. L., Wong, Y. C., Fong, C. M., Wong, S. N., & So, K. T. (2004). Magnetic resonance imaging in 122 children with spastic cerebral palsy. *Pediatric Neurology*, *31*, 172–176.

Laeng, B. (1994). Lateralization of categorical and coordinate spatial functions: A study of unilateral stroke patients. *Journal of Cognitive Neuroscience, 6,* 189–203.

Lee, J., Croen, L. A., Backstrand, K. H., Yoshida, C. K., Henning, L. H., Lindan, C., et al. (2005a). Maternal and infant characteristics associated with perinatal arterial stroke in the infant. *Journal of the American Medical Association, 293,* 723–729.

Lee, J., Croen, L. A., Lindan, C., Nash, K. B., Yoshida, C. K., Ferriero, D. M., et al. (2005b). Predictors of outcome in perinatal arterial stroke: A population-based study. *Annals of Neurology, 58,* 303–308.

Lesny, I., Stehlik, A., Tomasek, J., Tomankova, A., & Havlicek, I. (1993). Sensory disorders in cerebral palsy: Two-point discrimination. *Developmental Medicine and Child Neurology, 35,* 402–405.

Levine, S. C., Huttenlocher, P., Banich, M. T., & Duda, E. (1987). Factors affecting cognitive functioning of hemiplegic children. *Developmental Medicine and Child Neurology, 29,* 27–35.

Levine, S. C., Kraus, R., Alexander, E., Suriyakham, L. W., & Huttenlocher, P. R. (2005). IQ decline following early unilateral brain injury: A longitudinal study. *Brain and Cognition, 59,* 114–123.

Levine, S. C., & Levy, J. (1986). Perceptual asymmetry for chimeric faces across the life span. *Brain and Cognition, 5,* 291–306.

Ley, R. G., & Bryden, M. P. (1979). Hemispheric differences in processing emotions and faces. *Brain and Language, 7,* 127–138.

Lourenco, S. F., & Levine, S. C. (2009). *Location representation following early brain injury: Hemispheric dissocations in categorical and coordinate processing.* Manuscript in preparation.

Lynch, J. K., & Nelson, K. B. (2001). Epidemiology of perinatal stroke. *Current Opinion in Pediatrics, 13,* 499–505.

Macdonell, R. A., Jackson, G. D., Curatolo, J. M., Abbott, D. F., Berkovic, S. F., Carey, L. M., et al. (1999). Motor cortex localization using functional MRI and transcranial magnetic stimulation. *Neurology, 53,* 1462–1467.

MacWhinney, B., Feldman, H., Sacco, K., & Valdes-Perez, R. (2000). Online measures of basic language skills in children with early focal brain lesions. *Brain and Language, 71,* 400–431.

Maegaki, Y., Maeoka, Y., Ishii, S., Shiota, M., Takeuchi, A., Yoshino, K., et al. (1997). Mechanisms of central motor reorganization in pediatric hemiplegic patients. *Neuropediatrics, 28,* 168–174.

Mancini, J., de Schonen, S., Deruelle, C., & Massoulier, A. (1994). Face recognition in children with early right or left brain damage. *Developmental Medicine and Child Neurology, 36,* 156–166.

Marchman, V. A., Miller, R., & Bates, E. A. (1991). Babble and first words in children with focal brain injury. *Applied Psycholinguistics, 12,* 1–22.

Martinez, A., Moses, P., Frank, L., Buxton, R., Wong, E., & Stiles, J. (1997). Hemispheric asymmetries in global and local processing: evidence from fMRI. *NeuroReport, 8,* 1685–1689.

Mayer, M. (1969). *Frog, where are you?* New York: Dial Press.

McCarthy, G., Puce, A., Gore, J. C., & Allison, T. (1997). Face-specific processing in the human fusiform gyrus. *Journal of Cognitive Neuroscience, 9,* 605–610.

McFie, J., & Zangwill, O. L. (1960). Visual-constructive disabilities associated with lesions of the left cerebral hemisphere. *Brain, 83,* 243–259.

Mercuri, E., Barnett, A., Rutherford, M., Guzzetta, A., Haataja, L., Cioni, G., et al. (2004). Neonatal cerebral infarction and neuromotor outcome at school age. *Pediatrics, 113,* 95–100.

Mercuri, E., Cowan, F., Gupte, G., Manning, R., Laffan, M., Rutherford, M., et al. (2001). Prothrombotic disorders and abnormal neurodevelopmental outcome in infants with neonatal cerebral infarction. *Pediatrics, 107,* 1400–1404.

Mercuri, E., Rutherford, M., Cowan, F., Pennock, J., Counsell, S., Papadimitriou, M., et al. (1999). Early prognostic indicators of outcome in infants with neonatal cerebral infarction: A clinical, electroencephalogram, and magnetic resonance imaging study. *Pediatrics, 103,* 39–46.

Moses, P. (1999). *MRI-based quantitative analysis of neuroanatomical brain development following pre- and perinatal brain injury.* Unpublished manuscript, University of California, San Diego.

Moses, P., Courchesne, E., Stiles, J., Trauner, D., Egaas, B., & Edwards, E. (2000). Regional size reduction in the human corpus callosum following pre- and perinatal brain injury. *Cerebral Cortex, 10,* 1200–1210.

Moses, P., Roe, K., Buxton, R. B., Wong, E. C., Frank, L. R., & Stiles, J. (2002). Functional MRI of global and local processing in children. *NeuroImage, 16,* 415–424.

Müller, R. A., Rothermel, R. D., Behen, M. E., Muzik, O., Chakraborty, P. K., & Chugani, H. T. (1999). Language organization in patients with early and late left-hemisphere lesion: A PET study. *Neuropsychologia, 37,* 545–557.

Muter, V., Taylor, S., & Vargha-Khadem, F. (1997). A longitudinal study of early intellectual development in hemiplegic children. *Neuropsychologia, 35,* 289–298.

Mutsaarts, M., Steenbergen, B., & Bekkering, H. (2005). Anticipatory planning of movement sequences in hemiparetic cerebral palsy. *Motor Control, 9,* 439–458.

Nass, R. (1985). Mirror movement asymmetries in congenital hemiparesis: The inhibition hypothesis revisited. *Neurology, 35,* 1059–1062.

Nass, R., & Koch, D. (1987). Temperament differences in toddlers with early unilateral right- and left-brain damage. *Developmental Neuropsychology, 3,* 93–99.

Nass, R., Peterson, H. D., & Koch, D. (1989). Differential effects of congenital left and right brain injury on intelligence. *Brain and Cognition, 9,* 258–266.

Nelson, C. A. (2001). The development and neural bases of face recognition. *Infant and Child Development, 10,* 3–18.

Nelson, K. B., & Ellenberg, J. H. (1982). Children who "outgrew" cerebral palsy. *Pediatrics, 69,* 529–536.

Nelson, K. B., & Lynch, J. K. (2004). Stroke in newborn infants. *Lancet Neurology, 3,* 150–158.

Nezu, A., Kimura, S., Takeshita, S., & Tanaka, M. (1999). Functional recovery in hemiplegic cerebral palsy: Ipsilateral electromyographic responses to focal transcranial magnetic stimulation. *Brain and Development, 21,* 162–165.

Niogi, S. N., & McCandliss, B. D. (2006). Left lateralized white matter microstructure accounts for individual differences in reading ability and disability. *Neuropsychologia, 44,* 2178–2188.

Nirkko, A. C., Rosler, K. M., Ozdoba, C., Heid, O., Schroth, G., & Hess, C. W. (1997). Human cortical plasticity: Functional recovery with mirror movements. *Neurology, 48,* 1090–1093.

Passarotti, A. M., Paul, B. M., Bussiere, J. R., Buxton, R. B., Wong, E. C., & Stiles, J. (2003). The development of face and location processing: An fMRI study. *Developmental Science, 6,* 100–117.

Pathan, M., & Kittner, S. J. (2003). Pregnancy and stroke. *Currrent Neurology and Neuroscience Reports, 3,* 27–31.

Paul, B., Carapetian, S., Hesselink, J., Nass, R., Trauner, D., & Stiles, J. (2009). *Face and location processing in children with early unilateral brain injury.* Manuscript in preparation.

Pedelty, L., Levine, S. C., & Shevell, S. K. (1985). Developmental changes in face processing: Results from multidimensional scaling. *Journal of Experimental Child Psychology, 39,* 421–436.

Pellicano, E., & Rhodes, G. (2003). Holistic processing of faces in preschool children and adults. *Psychological Science, 14,* 618–622.

Perlstein, M. A., & Hood, P. N. (1955). Infantile spastic hemiplegia. *American Journal of Physical Medicine, 34,* 391–407.

Piercy, M., Hecaen, H., & De Ajuriaguerra, J. (1960). Constructional apraxia associated with unilateral cerebral lesions: Left and right sided cases compared. *Brain, 83,* 225–242.

Punt, T. D., Riddoch, M. J., & Humphreys, G. W. (2005). Don't think twice, it's all right: Contralesional dependency for bimanual prehension movements. *Neuropsychologia, 43,* 1547–1558.

Quartz, S. R., & Sejnowski, T. J. (1997). The neural basis of cognitive development: A constructivist manifesto. *Behavioral and Brain Sciences, 20,* 537–556 (discussion, 556–596).

Raja, A. C., Josse, G., Suriyakham, L. W., Fisher, J. A., Huttenlocher, P. R., Levine, S. C., et al. (2006, July). *Regional brain activation after early left and right hemisphere stroke: Relation to cognitive functioning.* Paper presented at the 12th Annual Meeting of the Organization for Human Brain Mapping, Florence, Italy.

Reese, C. J., & Stiles, J. (2005). Hemispheric specialization for categorical and coordinate spatial relations during an image generation task: Evidence from children and adults. *Neuropsychologia, 43,* 517–529.

Reilly, J., Bates, E. A., & Marchman, V. A. (1998). Narrative discourse in children with early focal brain injury. *Brain and Language, 61,* 335–375.

Reilly, J., Charfen, V., Stiles, J., del Guercio, C., & Nass, R. (2005a). Labeling emotional facial expressions in children with early brain damage. *Journal of Cognitive Neuroscience Supplement, 17*(Suppl.), 162.

Reilly, J., Losh, M., Bellugi, U., & Wulfeck, B. (2004). "Frog, where are you?": Narratives in children with specific language impairment, early focal brain injury, and Williams syndrome. *Brain and Language, 88,* 229–247.

Reilly, J., Stiles, J., Larsen, J., & Trauner, D. (1995). Affective facial expression in infants with focal brain damage. *Neuropsychologia, 33,* 83–99.

Reilly, J., Stiles, J., Wulfeck, B., & Nass, R. (2005b). Language development in children with early focal brain damage: Is there a right hemisphere profile? *Journal of Cognitive Neuroscience Supplement, 17*(Suppl.), 229.

Rhodes, G. (1993). Configural coding, expertise, and the right hemisphere advantage for face recognition. *Brain and Cognition, 22,* 19–41.

Robertson, L. C., & Delis, D. C. (1986). "Part–whole" processing in unilateral brain-damaged patients: Dysfunction of hierarchical organization. *Neuropsychologia, 24,* 363–370.

Robertson, L. C., & Lamb, M. R. (1991). Neuropsychological contributions to theories of part/whole organization. *Cognitive Psychology, 23,* 299–330.

Rossion, B., Dricot, L., Devolder, A., Bodart, J. M., Crommelinck, M., De Gelder, B., et al. (2000). Hemispheric asymmetries for whole-based and part-based face processing in the human fusiform gyrus. *Journal of Cognitive Neuroscience, 12,* 793–802.

Rowe, M. L., Levine, S. C., Fischer, J. A., & Goldin-Meadow, S. (2009). Does linguistic input play the same role in language learning for children with and without early brain injury? *Developmental Psychology, 45*(1), 90–102.

Saccuman, M. C., Dick, F., Krupa-Kwiatkowski, M., Moses, P., Bates, E., Perani, D., et al. (2006, July). *Lanugage processing in children and adolescents with early unilateral focal brain lesions: An FMRI study.* Paper presented at the 12th Annual Meeting of the Organization for Human Brain Mapping, Florence, Italy.

Schmahmann, J. D., Pandya, D. N., Wang, R., Dai, G., D'Arceuil, H. E., de Crespigny, A. J., et al. (2007). Association fibre pathways of the brain: Parallel observations from diffusion spectrum imaging and autoradiography. *Brain, 130,* 630–653.

Schmithorst, V. J., Wilke, M., Dardzinski, B. J., & Holland, S. K. (2005). Cognitive functions correlate with white matter architecture in a normal pediatric population: A diffusion tensor MRI study. *Human Brain Mapping, 26,* 139–147.

Schwarzer, G. (2002). Processing of facial and non-facial visual stimuli in 2–5-year-old children. *Infant and Child Development, 11,* 253–270.

Simion, F., Cassia, V. M., Turati, C., & Valenza, E. (2001). The origins of face perception: Specific versus non-specific mechanisms. *Infant and Child Development, 10,* 59–65.

Sreenan, C., Bhargava, R., & Robertson, C. M. (2000). Cerebral infarction in the term newborn: Clinical presentation and long-term outcome. *Journal of Pediatrics, 137,* 351–355.

St. James-Roberts, I. (1981). A reinterpretation of hemispherectomy data without functional plasticity of the brain: I. Intellectual function. *Brain and Language, 13,* 31–53.

Staudt, M., Braun, C., Gerloff, C., Erb, M., Grodd, W., & Krageloh-Mann, I. (2006). Developing somatosensory projections bypass periventricular brain lesions. *Neurology, 67,* 522–525.

Staudt, M., Gerloff, C., Grodd, W., Holthausen, H., Niemann, G., & Krageloh-Mann, I. (2004). Reorganization in congenital hemiparesis acquired at different gestational ages. *Annals of Neurology, 56,* 854–863.

Staudt, M., Grodd, W., Gerloff, C., Erb, M., Stitz, J., & Krageloh-Mann, I. (2002a). Two types of ipsilateral reorganization in congenital hemiparesis: A TMS and fMRI study. *Brain, 125*, 2222–2237.

Staudt, M., Lidzba, K., Grodd, W., Wildgruber, D., Erb, M., & Krageloh-Mann, I. (2002b). Right-hemispheric organization of language following early left-sided brain lesions: Functional MRI topography. *NeuroImage, 16*, 954–967.

Steenbergen, B., & Gordon, A. M. (2006). Activity limitation in hemiplegic cerebral palsy: Evidence for disorders in motor planning. *Developmental Medicine and Child Neurology, 48*, 780–783.

Steenbergen, B., & Meulenbroek, R. G. (2006). Deviations in upper-limb function of the less-affected side in congenital hemiparesis. *Neuropsychologia, 44*, 2296–2307.

Steenbergen, B., & van der Kamp, J. (2004). Control of prehension in hemiparetic cerebral palsy: Similarities and differences between the ipsi- and contra-lesional sides of the body. *Developmental Medicine and Child Neurology, 46*, 325–332.

Steenbergen, B., van Thiel, E., Hulstijn, W., & Meulenbroek, R. G. J. (2000). The coordination of reaching and grasping in spastic hemiparesis. *Human Movement Science, 19*, 75–105.

Stiles, J. (2008). *The fundamentals of brain development: Integrating nature and nurture*. Cambridge, MA: Harvard University Press.

Stiles, J., Moses, P., Roe, K., Akshoomoff, N. A., Trauner, D., Hesselink, J., et al. (2003). Alternative brain organization after prenatal cerebral injury: Convergent fMRI and cognitive data. *Journal of the International Neuropsychological Society, 9*, 604–622.

Stiles, J., & Nass, R. (1991). Spatial grouping activity in young children with congenital right or left hemisphere brain injury. *Brain and Cognition, 15*, 201–222.

Stiles, J., Paul, B., & Hesselink, J. (2006). Spatial cognitive development following early focal brain injury: Evidence for adaptive change in brain and cognition. In Y. Munakata & M. H. Johnson (Eds.), *Attention and performance XXI: Process of change in brain and cognitive development* (pp. 535–561). Oxford: Oxford University Press.

Stiles, J., Reilly, J., Paul, B., & Moses, P. (2005). Cognitive development following early brain injury: Evidence for neural adaptation. *Trends in Cognitive Sciences, 9*, 136–143.

Stiles, J., Stern, C., Appelbaum, M., Nass, R., Trauner, D., & Hesselink, J. (2008). Effects of early focal brain injury on memory for visuospatial patterns: Selective deficits of global–local processing. *Neuropsychology, 22*, 61–73.

Stiles, J., Stern, C., Trauner, D., & Nass, R. (1996). Developmental change in spatial grouping activity among children with early focal brain injury: Evidence from a modeling task. *Brain and Cognition, 31*, 46–62.

Stiles-Davis, J. (1988). Developmental change in young children's spatial grouping activity. *Developmental Psychology, 24*, 522–531.

Stiles-Davis, J., Janowsky, J., Engel, M., & Nass, R. D. (1988). Drawing ability in four young children with congenital unilateral brain lesions. *Neuropsychologia, 26*, 359–371.

Stiles-Davis, J., Sugarman, S., & Nass, R. (1985). The development of spatial and class relations in four young children with right-cerebral-hemisphere damage: Evidence for an early spatial constructive deficit. *Brain and Cognition, 4*, 388–412.

Stone, A., & Valentine, T. (2003). Perspectives on prosopagnosia and models of face recognition. *Cortex, 39*, 31–40.

Swindell, C. S., Holland, A. L., Fromm, D., & Greenhouse, J. B. (1988). Characteristics of recovery of drawing ability in left and right brain-damaged patients. *Brain and Cognition, 7*, 16–30.

Tanaka, J. W., Kay, J. B., Grinnell, E., Stansfield, B., & Szechter, L. (1998). Face recognition in young children: When the whole is greater than the sum of its parts. *Visual Cognition, 5*, 479–496.

Thal, D. J., Reilly, J., Seibert, L., Jeffries, R., & Fenson, J. (2004). Language development in children at risk for language impairment: Cross-population comparisons. *Brain and Language, 88*, 167–179.

Thickbroom, G. W., Byrnes, M. L., Archer, S. A., Nagarajan, L., & Mastaglia, F. L. (2001). Differences in sensory and motor cortical organization following brain injury early in life. *Annals of Neurology, 49*, 320–327.

Thompson, L. A., Madrid, V., Westbrook, S., & Johnston, V. (2001). Infants attend to second-order relational properties of faces. *Psychonomic Bulletin and Review, 8,* 769–777.

Tranel, D., Damasio, A. R., & Damasio, H. (1988). Intact recognition of facial expression, gender, and age in patients with impaired recognition of face identity. *Neurology, 38,* 690–696.

Trauner, D. A. (2003). Hemispatial neglect in young children with early unilateral brain damage. *Developmental Medicine and Child Neurology, 45,* 160–166.

Ungerleider, L. G., & Mishkin, M. (1982). Two cortical visual systems. In D. J. Ingle, M. A. Goodale, & R. J. W. Mansfield (Eds.) (pp. 549–586). *Analysis of visual behavior,* Cambridge, MA: MIT Press.

Utley, A., Steenbergen, B., & Sugden, D. A. (2004). The influence of object size on discrete bimanual coordination in children with hemiplegic cerebral palsy. *Disability and Rehabilitation, 26,* 603–613.

Van Heest, A. E., House, J., & Putnam, M. (1993). Sensibility deficiencies in the hands of children with spastic hemiplegia. *Journal of Hand Surgery (American Volume), 18,* 278–281.

Vargha-Khadem, F., Isaacs, E., van der Werf, S., Robb, S., & Wilson, J. (1992). Development of intelligence and memory in children with hemiplegic cerebral palsy: The deleterious consequences of early seizures. *Brain, 115,* 315–329.

Vicari, S., Albertoni, A., Chilosi, A. M., Cipriani, P., Cioni, G., & Bates, E. (2000). Plasticity and reorganization during language development in children with early brain injury. *Cortex, 36,* 31–46.

Vicari, S., Stiles, J., Stern, C., & Resca, A. (1998). Spatial grouping activity in children with early cortical and subcortical lesions. *Developmental Medicine and Child Neurology, 40,* 90–99.

Volpe, J. J. (2001). *Neurology of the newborn.* Philadelphia: Saunders.

Warrington, E. K., James, M., & Kinsbourne, M. (1966). Drawing disability in relation to laterality of cerebral lesion. *Brain, 89,* 53–82.

Woods, B. T. (1980). The restricted effects of right-hemisphere lesions after age one: Wechsler test data. *Neuropsychologia, 18,* 65–70.

Woods, B. T., & Teuber, H. L. (1978). Mirror movements after childhood hemiparesis. *Neurology, 28,* 1152–1157.

Wren, T. A., Rethlefsen, S., & Kay, R. M. (2005). Prevalence of specific gait abnormalities in children with cerebral palsy: Influence of cerebral palsy subtype, age, and previous surgery. *Journal of Pediatric Orthopedics, 25,* 79–83.

Wu, Y. W., Croen, L. A., Shah, S. J., Newman, T. B., & Najjar, D. V. (2006). Cerebral palsy in a term population: Risk factors and neuroimaging findings. *Pediatrics, 118,* 690–697.

Wu, Y. W., March, W. M., Croen, L. A., Grether, J. K., Escobar, G. J., & Newman, T. B. (2004). Perinatal stroke in children with motor impairment: A population-based study. *Pediatrics, 114,* 612–619.

Wulfeck, B., Bates, E., Krupa-Kwiatkowski, M., & Saltzman, D. (2004). Grammaticality sensitivity in children with early focal brain injury and children with specific language impairment. *Brain and Language, 88,* 215–228.

Yekutiel, M., Jariwala, M., & Stretch, P. (1994). Sensory deficit in the hands of children with cerebral palsy: A new look at assessment and prevalence. *Developmental Medicine and Child Neurology, 36,* 619–624.

CHAPTER 9

Environmental Toxicants

KIM N. DIETRICH

Pediatric neuropsychologists are frequently on the front lines when parents have questions regarding the cause of their children's behavioral difficulties. Now more than ever, clinicians are likely to be asked about the possible role of environmental exposures. In 1999, the California Department of Developmental Services reported that in the preceding 10 years there was a 273% increase in the number of children with autism spectrum disorders (ASD) (Byrd, 2002). This led to widespread speculation that some change in the environment was responsible for this "epidemic" of ASD (Wallis, 2007). The last two decades have also witnessed an enormous increase in the diagnosis of attention-deficit/hyperactivity disorder (ADHD) and its treatment with stimulants (Kelleher, McInerny, Gardner, Childs, & Wasserman, 2000; Safer, Zito, & Fine, 1996). As in the case of ASD, there has been much speculation about the role that environmental chemical exposures may play in the etiology of ADHD and related behavioral and learning disorders (Schettler, Stein, Reich, & Valenti, 2000; Weiss & Landrigan, 2000). Therefore, it is important for pediatric neuropsychologists to be familiar with the current research and methodological issues in this area.

The neuropsychological consequences of early exposure to environmental chemicals continue to be subjects of intense interest as well as some controversy (Grandjean & Landrigan, 2006; Plunkett, 2007). Since publication of the first edition of this chapter (Dietrich, 2000), our understanding of the developmental neurotoxicity of environmental chemicals has advanced considerably. A number of revealing new investigations using advanced research designs (e.g., prospective studies, clinical trials) have been published. Furthermore, the unique methodological challenges faced by investigators studying environmental pollutants and child neurobehavioral development have come into better focus

(Dietrich et al., 2005). The purpose of the present chapter is to provide an overview of the basic concepts in this field, as well as to update readers on the new data and their practical significance for pediatric neuropsychologists.

For the most part, this chapter focuses on environmental *toxicants* as opposed to toxins. The word *toxin* is loosely used by some medical writers to mean all poisons, but it should be reserved for its more precise definition. Toxicants are exogenous (sometimes human-made or synthetic) poisons that present a risk of death, birth defects, or disease (e.g., pesticides), whereas toxins are proteins produced by the metabolic activity of a microorganism, animal, or plant (e.g., botulism). The neurobehavioral effects of developmental exposure to drugs, tobacco, and alcohol *in utero* are also not discussed, although these exposures are often measured as potential confounders in the studies discussed here.

ENVIRONMENTAL CHEMICALS

It is estimated that there are approximately 80,000 chemicals currently in commercial use. However, few have been evaluated for their potential to produce developmental harm. Under half of these have been subjected to even the most rudimentary laboratory testing for toxicity, and only a very small subfraction of these have been tested for their developmental neurotoxicity in animal experiments (Grandjean & Landrigan, 2006). Of the thousands of known commercial compounds, only a few have been proven to cause developmental neurotoxicity in humans (Brent, 2001). As illustrated in Figure 9.1, this probably reflects a dearth of rigorous neurodevelopmental toxicity testing in the laboratory, as well as a lack of human epidemiological studies of suspect compounds. For example, the neurodevelopmental consequences of exposure to the more than 600 currently registered pesticides—chemicals specifically designed to be neurotoxic—are largely unknown (Lanphear, Vorhees, & Bellinger, 2005b), despite the fact that many of these chemicals and/or their metabolites are routinely found in the blood and bodily fluids of pregnant women and children (Centers for Disease Control and Prevention [CDC], 2005).

CHILDREN AND ENVIRONMENTAL CHEMICALS

Children are different from adults in important ways that make them more likely to ingest, absorb, and be harmed by environmental chemicals (American Academy of Pediatrics, 2003). Compared to adults, infants and children consume more grams of food per kilogram of body weight per day. This difference is more than threefold between a child under 1 year of age and an adult. Children's water requirements are also greater—about 120 mL/kg/day for an infant, compared with 40 mL for a young adult. The air intake of a resting infant is twice that of an adult under the same conditions. As a result of these accelerated rates of consumption, children receive higher doses of whatever toxicants may be present in food, beverages, or air. Infants and children also consume different types of foods than adults do. For example, breast milk and/or infant formula (reconstituted with tap water) predominate in the first year. Children also consume more vegetables, fruits, and fruit juices. These qualitative and quantitative differences in diet can result in greater exposure to water- and food-borne toxicants.

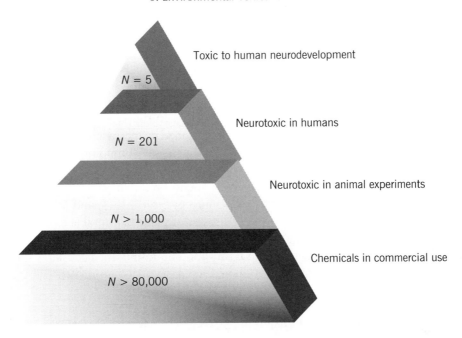

FIGURE 9.1. The current state of our knowledge of the neurotoxicity of environmental chemicals. Only a small fraction of substances in the commercial chemical universe have been shown to cause developmental neurotoxicity in humans. This reflects the absence of rigorous developmental neurotoxicity testing in laboratory animals, as well as the lack of human epidemiological studies of suspect compounds. The five compounds known to be toxic to human neurodevelopment are arsenic, lead, methylmercury, toluene, and the polychlorinated biphenyls (PCBs). Adapted from Grandjean and Landrigan (2006). Copyright 2006 by Elsevier. Adapted by permission.

In addition, children have different ecological niches in which they live and breathe. They play closer to the ground, where they are often in intimate contact with interior dust, exterior soil, and vegetation. This can result in exposure to toxicants through oral, dermal, and respiratory routes. The nature of children's behavior increases their exposure to environmental toxicants as well. Infants and preschoolers crawl on the floor and ground, and explore their environment by placing their hands and objects in their mouths. As a result of these normative early behaviors, they expose themselves to toxicant residues in the home as well as outdoors. Children also have immature metabolic pathways and thus handle chemical toxicants differently. There are important differences in absorption, activation, detoxification, distribution, and elimination of xenobiotics that increase the probability of harm. For example, children will absorb about 50% of ingested lead, whereas adults will absorb only about 10–15%. Finally, infants and children are uniquely vulnerable to environmental chemical exposure, because important physiological systems are still differentiating and growing.

The special vulnerability of fetuses and children was brought to light in the 1960s with the discovery of thalidomide's devastating effects (Lenz, 1988). Environmental disasters where industrial chemicals found their way into the bodies of pregnant women and children also highlighted this vulnerability, especially with respect to the developing central nervous system (CNS). Over 100 years ago, an epidemic of lead poisoning was described among Australian children who ingested leaded house paint (Gibson, 1904). These children presented with anemia, encephalopathy, peripheral neuropathies, paralysis, and blindness. Two other notable examples—one involving methylmercury poisoning in Minamata Bay, Japan, in the 1950s, and the other involving contamination of cooking oil by PCBs and related compounds in Japan and Taiwan in the 1960s and 1970s—have been described earlier (Dietrich, 2000) and are also discussed below. In the 1950s, residents of a Japanese fishing village on Minamata Bay were severely poisoned by methylmercury as a result of the ingestion of fish and mollusca contaminated by the massive dumping of industrial effluent into the sea (Harada, 1995). Children exposed *in utero* developed cerebral palsy, sensory handicaps, emotional disturbances, and severe mental retardation, even while their birth mothers were sometimes asymptomatic (see Smith & Smith, 1975, and Mishima, 1992, for vivid pictorial essays of this environmental disaster). In another notable case, rice bran oils contaminated with polychlorinated biphenyls (PCBs) and related compounds were consumed by pregnant women in Japan and Taiwan. The results included fetal wasting and mental and motor deficits in offspring (Chen, Guo, Hsu, & Rogan, 1992).

ANIMAL EXPERIMENTS AND HUMAN STUDIES

Most of the chemicals discussed in this review have been extensively studied in experimental animals. Animal experiments, in which dose and timing of exposure can be manipulated (and other environmental factors strictly controlled), afford firmer causal inferences than human studies do. Much of what is known regarding the biological mechanisms involved in environmental chemical damage to the brain has been derived from controlled experiments with animals (usually rodents, such as laboratory rats and mice). These studies have proven to be invaluable in advancing our understanding of how exposures to environmental chemicals affect behavior (Riley & Vorhees, 1986) and critical developmental processes in the brain (Rodier, 2004). Moreover, in the absence of human data, regulators depend heavily on experimental animal studies. Data from animal experiments are used to reveal any potential adverse health effects before human exposure can occur (e.g., premarket testing of a new compound).

However, animal models of human health effects are limited in terms of measuring the true risks of fetal and childhood exposure to developmental neurotoxicants in the environment. Sources of uncertainty that can arise from data derived solely from animal studies include (1) a short exposure period compared to that for humans; (2) testing limited to adult (nonpregnant) animals; (3) frequent use of genetically homogeneous animals (and thus the inability to detect sensitive individuals in genetically diverse subpopulations); (4) use of high test doses of a chemical (doses several orders of magnitude higher than typically observed in fetuses and children); (5) small numbers of test animals; and (6) the need to extrapolate across species to humans (Wigle & Lanphear, 2005). The last limitation is particularly germane when it comes to assessing the functional outcomes of chemically mediated damage to the developing brain. With the exception of some studies of nonhuman primates (e.g., Rice, 1999), most animal-testing paradigms of human developmental neurotoxicity cannot reflect the critical cognitive processes involved in human learning and behavior. Moreover, in some cases animals are not nearly as sensitive as humans to developmentally toxic drugs and environmental chemicals. In the case of thalidomide, for example, humans and other higher primates are vulnerable during embryogenesis, whereas most other animals (including rats) are resistant to thalidomide teratogenesis (Wilson, 1973). Furthermore, neurobehavioral effects of prenatal and early postnatal exposure to methylmercury, lead, and polychlorinated biphenyls (PCBs) occur in humans at doses at least three orders of magnitude lower than those predicted from rodent data alone (Rice, 1996).

Therefore, this chapter focuses primarily on human epidemiological studies of pregnant women, fetuses, and children. These studies have a number of limitations as well. It is clearly unethical to administer toxic substances experimentally to fetuses and children; thus biomarkers must be assessed as surrogates for dose to the target organ. The concentrations of toxicants and/or their metabolites are often measured as exposure biomarkers in body fluids, such as blood, breast milk, and urine. Cumulative exposure to toxicants can be assessed in body tissues that serve as long-term depositories, such as teeth, bone, fingernails, and hair. The concentration of bone-seeking substances like lead is measured in shed deciduous teeth (Needleman, Tuncay, & Shapiro, 1972) and in the skeleton *in vivo* by X-ray fluorescence (Chettle, 2005). Methylmercury can be measured in human hair (Clarkson, 1983), and approximately 80% of the mercury in hair is methylmercury (Phelps, Clarkson, Kershaw, & Wheatley, 1980). Since the hair shaft grows at a known rate during pregnancy (1 cm/month), segmental analyses of maternal hair at delivery can recapitulate fetal exposure throughout the course of gestation. These indirect indices of exposure and absorption are then correlated with the neurodevelopmental endpoints of interest. A limitation of these biomarkers is that they do not directly measure doses to the brain. With the exception of manganese, which can be assessed in regions of interest in the brain via magnetic resonance imaging (MRI) (Kim, 2004), there are no methods currently available to measure *in vivo* the concentration of environmental toxicants in tissues of the CNS. Nevertheless, the consistency with which these biomarkers are associated with neurobehavioral deficits in exposed fetuses and children suggests that they are valid indices of doses to the developing brain. In the case of methylmercury, for example, concentrations in maternal hair during pregnancy correlate closely with concentrations in the brains of deceased newborn infants at autopsy (Cernichiari et al., 1995).

A further problem with epidemiological studies arises from the fact that exposure to environmental chemicals is not random. Environmental chemical exposure occurs in the context of numerous exogenous factors that can influence child development. Recognizing this fact, investigators attempt to determine how a compound induces developmental neurotoxicity by identifying its distinct contribution from other influences within a child's total environment. In essence, these investigations statistically strip away the contributions of these other environmental factors (often referred to as *confounders* and/or *covariates*) to neurodevelopment. This is typically accomplished by application of various multivariable regression techniques. In the final step, the investigator determines whether the neurotoxicant of interest accounts for a significant portion of the residual variance in the outcome variable. This analytical strategy is specifically designed to achieve the aim of reducing Type I error (attributing to the chemical variance in outcome that should "belong" to other environmental or organismic cofactors). However, a potential risk of such a conservative analytical strategy is the inflation of Type II error by assuming that all of the variance belongs first to the model's set of covariates and confounders (Weiss & Bellinger, 2006). In this regard, studies of lead exposure and child development are instructive. Much of the debate surrounding the relationship between developmental lead exposure and intellectual attainment has focused on the ability of epidemiological studies to distinguish the contribution of lead from such potential confounders as parental IQ, socioeconomic status (SES), maternal drug use, caregiving quality, and other aspects of a child's sociohereditary milieu (Bellinger, 1995a). The problem of confounding and balancing Type I and Type II error in studies of lead and other neurotoxicants has been a dominant subject of debate in this field (Bellinger, 2004).

Complications can also arise when mediating variables are included in regression models as bona fide confounders. Jacobson and Jacobson (1996a) provide an interesting example. Birthweight is a robust predictor of neurodevelopmental delays and school-age disabilities (Avchen, Scott, & Mason, 2001). Maternal cocaine use during pregnancy is associated with low birthweight, owing to its action as an appetite depressant and vasoconstrictor. Thus the effect of prenatal exposure on neurobehavioral outcome could be mediated by reduced birth size. Including the mediating variable of birthweight as a confounder in multivariable regression models could spuriously reduce the estimate for cocaine's effect on neurodevelopment to nonsignificance (a Type II error). My colleagues and I (Dietrich et al., 1987) were the first environmental health researchers to utilize structural equation modeling (Joreskog, 1979) to address this problem in our Cincinnati birth cohort. Prenatal lead exposure in the Cincinnati cohort and others has been linked with lower birthweight and decreased gestational maturity (Andrews, Savitz, & Hertz-Picciotto, 1994). Rather than treating birthweight and gestational age as confounders of the blood lead–behavior relationship in multiple-regression analyses, we modeled these variables statistically as mediators of developmental delays in the first year of life. Specifically, we used structural equation analyses to test the hypothesis that lead-related deficits in infant neurodevelopmental status at 3, 6, and 12 months of age were due in part to lead-related lower birthweight and shortened gestational age. Results of these analyses showed that prenatal (maternal) blood lead concentrations were associated with lower Bayley Scales of Infant Development Mental and Motor Index scores, both directly and through lead-associated reductions in birthweight and gestational maturity. Although potential confounders should be included routinely in all analyses, biologically plausible mediators should not. At the very least, investigators should conduct multivariable statistical analyses with and without potential mediating variables, to evaluate their impact on the regression estimates (Jacobson & Jacobson, 1996a).

Epidemiological studies must also consider the possibility that a toxicant may interact with other presenting environmental and organismic factors. The magnitude of harm done by neurotoxicants may depend upon other operative factors in the population of interest. Epidemiologists refer to this as *effect modification*. Effect modification occurs when the estimate for the association between exposure and disease differs in different strata of the moderator variable. For example, several studies of the effect of lead exposure on IQ have found dose-related deficits to be greatest among children of lower SES (Bellinger, 2000). In a cohort study from the Netherlands, the effects of prenatal PCB exposure on IQ scores were greater among formula-fed children and those from educationally disadvantaged homes (Patandin et al., 1999; Vreugdenhil, Lanting, Mulder, Boersma, & Weisglas-Kuperus, 2002). In a study of fetal alcohol effects, dose-related deficits on a measure of early mental and motor development were found only among offspring of women over 30 years of age, suggesting that vulnerability to this neuroteratogen may depend on physiological changes in the mother associated with a history of heavy drinking (Jacobson et al., 1993).

Researchers are just beginning to study the interactions between human genetic differences and environmental chemical exposures. A heretofore unexplored area has been the interaction between toxicant dose and genetic polymorphisms involving neurotransmitter metabolism. For example, a recent study found interactive effects between lead and the dopamine receptor D4 (DRD4) gene. The effect of lead on rule learning and reversal (executive functions) in children was evident predominately among those lacking the DRD4 seven-repeat allele (Froehlich et al., 2007). Pearce (1989; cited in Weiss & Bellinger, 2006, p. 1479) has stated that "every effect estimate . . . reflects numerous unknown or unmeasured modifying factors." In essence, every main effect can be conceived of as an interaction that is incompletely characterized. The examination of differential vulnerabilities in these epidemiological studies is critical, because the ultimate goal is to understand the relationship between toxicant dose and disease among the most vulnerable groups in the population.

Another complication with epidemiological studies arises when the population under investigation is subject to multiple environmental chemical exposures. Unfortunately, most studies in this area measure only one environmental toxicant, or analyze the impact of multiple toxicants on neurodevelopment independently. For example, populations that consume fish and sea mammals are at risk of simultaneous exposure to methylmercury, PCBs, and persistent organochlorine pesticides (Muckle, Ayotte, Dewailly, Jacobson, & Jacobson, 2001). Some children living in older inner-city housing are exposed to a combination of lead paint and pesticide residues (Landrigan et al., 1999). Children exposed to lead are also more likely to be exposed to higher levels of environmental tobacco smoke (Mannino, Albalak, Grosse, & Repace, 2003). No study to date has reported on the additive or synergistic effects of simultaneous exposure to these CNS poisons, although some efforts in this area are underway (Fenske, Bradman, Whyatt, Wolf, & Barr, 2005). In fact, no studies have been fully successful in characterizing the complex mixture of environmental chemicals that fetuses and children are exposed to. The National Children's Study, a planned prospective investigation of 100,000 American children, has the potential to address the complex issues raised by exposure to chemical mixtures during early development (Landrigan et al., 2006).

NEUROTOXICANTS AND THE DEVELOPING HUMAN BRAIN

The developing human brain is inherently more susceptible to injury caused by neurotoxic agents than is the brain of a fully mature adult. Studies of the effects of environmental exposures on fetuses and children have repeatedly demonstrated that the developing brain is among the most sensitive human organs to damage. This extraordinary sensitivity to chemical influences stems from the fact that the human brain develops from a small strip of cells along the dorsal ectoderm of the embryo into an intricate organ consisting of approximately 100 billion neurons and many more functionally supportive neuroglial cells. Over the course of normal development, these neurons migrate to distinct positions in the brain, and establish abundant interconnections and specialized functions. The maturation of the CNS involves a more complex sequence of developmental processes than any other structure, making this organ uniquely vulnerable to environmental chemical exposures (Rodier, 2004).

Humans become potentially vulnerable to developmental neurotoxicants at least as early as conception (the germ cells may also be involved through mutagenic influences). Chemicals with low molecular weight, lipid affinity, nonpolarity, and low protein-binding properties cross the placenta with ease (Slikker & Miller, 1994). Most drugs and environmental chemicals possess one or more of these properties, cross the placenta, and enter the fetal circulation (Beckman & Brent, 1999). The immature blood–brain barrier of the fetus and young infant is more permeable to toxicants, and the fetus lacks drug-metabolizing and detoxification capacities present postnatally. However, there is no bright line between the prenatal and postnatal periods of CNS maturation (Figure 9.2). Processes such as cell proliferation and growth, and especially cortical cellular migration, myelination, dendritic arborization, synaptogensis, and programmed apoptosis, continue for a considerable period of time after birth. Unlike other organs, the human brain achieves its mature form only until approximately 21 years after conception (Rodier, 1995).

CHEMICALS IDENTIFIED
AS HUMAN DEVELOPMENTAL NEUROTOXICANTS

As illustrated in Figure 9.1, only a handful of environmental chemicals have been identified as neuroteratogenic in humans. Grandjean and Landrigan (2006) list five: arsenic and arsenical compounds, lead and lead compounds, methylmercury, toluene, and PCBs. Brent (2001), preferring a more severe definition and test of causal proof, lists only three: methylmercury, toluene, and the PCBs. An overview of all candidate human developmental

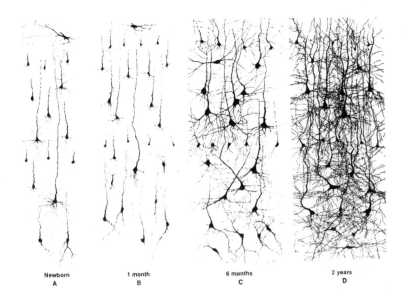

FIGURE 9.2. Golgi-stained section of human cerebral cortex taken from equivalent areas of the anterior portion of the middle frontal gyrus at different ages. The human brain has a protracted period of development and vulnerability to environmental toxicants. At maturity, the human cerebral cortex will consist of 30 billion neurons interconnected by 100,000 km of axons and dendrites. From Conel (1959), reprinted in Nolte (1993). Copyright 1959 by Harvard University Press. Reprinted by permission.

neurotoxicants is beyond the scope of this chapter. Instead, the principal focus is on those that are widely recognized for their neuroteratogenic potential (e.g., mercury and lead), as well as a few that have not been adequately studied in children, but are emerging as strong candidates (e.g., pesticides and environmental tobacco smoke).

MERCURY

Mercury's symbol on the periodic table (Hg) descends from the Greek term meaning "water silver." This unique metal and its compounds have been prescribed for centuries as antiseptics, antiparasitics, dental reconstructions, and a myriad of other allopathic medical applications, and incorporated into cultural rituals and folk remedies for relief from disease or other misfortunes. Mercury is still used commercially in thermometers, batteries, and switches, as well as in electrodes in the electrolytic production of chlorine and sodium hydroxide from saline (Agency for Toxic Substances and Disease Registry [ATSDR], 1999). Mercury is also in the new high-efficiency compact fluorescent light bulbs that, by law, will be the only domestic consumer option for light bulbs in the United States by 2012; this requirement has raised concerns among some about its implications for the contamination of lands and waterways (Lavelle, 2007).

Inorganic Mercury

Mercury is a natural constituent of the earth's crust, but anthropogenic sources (e.g., coal burning, incineration of contaminated waste, mining, and other industrial emissions) increase its discharge into the atmosphere, soil, and waterways. Mercury is present in the environment in a number of forms that vary in their developmental neurotoxicity. It exists as elemental or metallic metal (Hg), inorganic salt (Hg^{2+}), and organic forms such as methylmercury (CH_3Hg). In its fluid form (quicksilver), mercury is attractive to children who may encounter abandoned flasks of the substance at closed industrial sites.

Metallic mercury is highly volatile, even at ambient temperatures. In vapor form (Hg^0), metallic mercury is almost completely absorbed in the lungs and is extremely toxic to the CNS. Intoxication produces a complex of symptoms, including weakness, anorexia, fatigue, and *erethism* (an agitated depressive state characterized by shyness, irritability, memory loss, and insomnia). In the early part of the 20th century, mercurous mercury salt compounds such as calomel were prescribed by physicians and pharmacists in the United Kingdom, Australia, and the southern United States to treat a wide variety of unconnected childhood illnesses. The result was a sometimes fatal disorder of the sympathetic nervous system called *acrodynia* ("painful extremities") that afflicted hypersensitive children (Warkany, 1966). Acrodynia is characterized by the protean clinical signs and symptoms of irritability, paresthesias, insomnia, depression, cognitive deterioration, anorexia, excessive sweating, leg cramps, painful pink to red fingers, hands and feet, and peeling skin (Yeates & Mortensen, 1994). Although it is rare, acrodynia is not an extinct disease, as new cases are still documented from time to time (Goldman & Shannon, 2001).

A more common contemporary source of inorganic mercury exposure is dental restoration work. Dental amalgams consist of approximately 50% mercury combined with silver and copper. The process of chewing releases mercury vapor into the oral cavity, where it is inhaled and subsequently absorbed (Kingman, Albertini, & Brown, 1998). Although urinary mercury concentrations in people with amalgams are well below those associated with occupational exposure, significant concern has been raised about the hazards of long-term low-level exposure. This concern has been directed toward children as well, because pediatric urinary mercury concentrations are highly correlated with both number of amalgam fillings and the time since placement (Woods et al., 2007). Two recently reported clinical trials have addressed this question directly. In a study of 534 New England children 6–10 years of age, Bellinger et al. (2006) found that while children randomly assigned to the amalgam group had higher mean mercury levels than those in the resin-based composite group, there were no statistically significant differences between treatment arms in terms of 5-year change in IQ, 4-year change in a general memory index, or a visual–motor score. DeRouen et al. (2006) reported a similar clinical trial conducted on 507 children ages 8–10 from Lisbon, Portugal. At a 7-year follow-up, children in the amalgam group had higher urinary mercury concentrations, but there were no statistically significant differences between the treatment arms on assessments of memory, attention/concentration, visual–motor performance, and nerve conduction velocities. Both of these investigations support the view that amalgam dental restorations are safe for children, but some have argued that further studies are needed to establish this firmly (Needleman, 2006).

Organic Mercury

The form of mercury most toxic to the developing CNS is methylmercury. The first published report of methylmercury poisoning in humans was by Hunter and Russell (1954). They described the health problems of four men who were poisoned by inhaling methylmercury compounds in a London factory where fungicides were being applied to seeds being prepared and packaged for agriculture. This classic description of the sequential neurological manifestations of the disease later helped to identify methylmercury as the causative agent in several subsequent mass poisonings (including Minamata). The Hunter–Russell syndrome, as it came to be called, begins with paraesthesia, deterioration in fine motor coordination, and restriction of the visual fields, and proceeds to gross ataxia, dementia, and death. On autopsy, Hunter and Russell found marked destruction of neurons and cerebral atrophy in both hemispheres.

The methylation process is the key to understanding why methylmercury is viewed as a widespread and serious threat to human health. Sediments in both fresh and marine waters, through the action of microorganisms, convert inorganic mercury into methylmercury. Following conversion, methylmercury begins to ascend the aquatic food chain, attaining its highest concentrations in larger, predatory species of fish (e.g., pike, snapper, swordfish, tuna, and shark). Shellfish living in contaminated waters can also accumulate high concentrations of methylmercury. Seafood is by far the most significant source of human exposure to methylmercury (National Research Council [NRC], 2000). Methylmercury is rapidly absorbed in the human gastrointestinal tract, with about 95% of an ingested dose turned over to the bloodstream and with a half-life of approximately 2 months (Miettinen, 1973).

Methylmercury readily crosses the placenta and blood–brain barrier, is poorly excreted by the fetus, and interferes with a number of critical neurodevelopmental processes (Clarkson, Magos, & Myers, 2003). It is highly lipophilic and therefore capable of diffusing through cell membranes without the assistance of any specific carrier system. Unfortunately, methylmercury also gains access to brain tissues through a kind of molecular mimicry. In blood, methylmercury is bound to proteins and low-molecular-weight sulfhydryl compounds like cysteine. This methylmercury–cysteine complex acts as an amino acid analogue of methionine (an essential amino acid). The methylmercury–cysteine compound is actively transported into the endothelial cells in the blood–brain barrier on the methionine carrier, and ultimately into the brain on a glutathione carrier (Kerper, Ballatori, & Clarkson, 1992; Zheng, Aschner, & Ghersi-Egea, 2003).

Two epidemics of methylmercury poisoning in Japan in the 1950s and 1960s, and another in Iraq in the early 1970s, are among the classic geographic isolates in the annals of environmental neuroepidemiology. They are also signal events in the evolving understanding that the womb is not fully protected from exogenous environmental influences (Harada, 1995; Marsh, Clarkson, Cox, & Myers, 1987). Vivid historical and sociological reports of these human-made human health disasters have been written (Mishima, 1992; Smith & Smith, 1975).

In adults, methylmercury assaults specific areas of the CNS—the calcarine, temporal, precentral, and postcentral cortices, as well as the dorsal root spinal ganglia (Takeuchi, 1968). The primary clinical signs of poisoning are paraesthesia, concentric constriction of the visual fields, cortical hearing loss, dysarthria, intention tremor, and ataxia. These signs may be accompanied by disturbances in gustation and olfaction. Women exposed to high levels of methylmercury during their pregnancy produce offspring with a progressive cortical degenerative disease that manifests itself as a cerebral palsy accompanied by mental retardation, severe sensory deficits, microcephaly, and limb malformations (Harada, 1986). Neuropathological findings in these fetal cases are much more widespread than in adults or children, including atrophy and hypoplasia of the cerebral cortex and corpus callosum, abnormal cytoarchitecture, and dysmyelination of the pyramidal tract (Takeuchi, 1977). Incident cases of congenital and infant methylmercury poisoning are unknown today, although many survivors of these earlier tragedies continue to live in various states of disability (Eto, 1997, 2000). Furthermore, in the Japanese outbreak it was clear that the impact of chronic lower-level methylmercury poisoning within the Kumamoto Prefecture was underestimated. In 1970, investigators observed a rate of mental retardation of over 29% in children who were born in the most heavily contaminated areas between 1955 and 1958; 21% presented with sensory disturbances, and 12% with speech deficits (Harada, 1995). Children in Minamata with mental deficits of unknown etiology evinced methylmercury concentrations in preserved umbilical cord tissue that were significantly higher than in healthy controls, but lower than children certified as having congenital Minamata disease (Akagi, Grandjean, Takizawa, & Weihe, 1998). Thus methylmercury poisoning should not be regarded as a clinical entity that appears with all of its elements or none at all (Grandjean & White, 2001).

Mechanisms of Developmental Neurotoxicity

Many of the neurodevelopmental effects of methylmercury arise from the ability of this compound to depolymerize microtubules. Tubulin proteins are rich in sulfhydryl groups that readily bind to methylmercury. Methylmercury blocks the assembly process while disassembly proceeds, leading to the depolymerization of the tubule (Clarkson, Hursh, Sager, & Syversen, 1988). The result is inhibition of cell division and migration, leading to fewer brain cells and ectopic neurons. The molecular underpinnings of methylmercury's neuro-toxicity involve a number of overlapping toxic mechanisms, including inhibition of protein and macromolecular synthesis, mitochondrial dysfunction, defective calcium and ion flux (abnormal neurotransmitter homeostasis), initiation of oxidative stress (cell injury and death), and microtubular disaggregation (Verity, 1997).

Epidemiological Studies

After more than three decades since the last widespread outbreak of Minamata disease, researchers and regulators have turned their attention to the neurodevelopmental risks of chronic lower-level exposure to methylmercury (U.S. Environmental Protection Agency [U.S. EPA], 1997). Results of recent prospective studies in this area have generated considerable controversy regarding the risks and benefits of seafood, or what some have characterized as the "mercury-in-fish" debate (Gochfeld & Berger, 2005). Evidence of a lack of consensus on this issue can be found in the different recommendations adopted by various regulatory agencies with respect to the consumption of potentially contaminated fish. In the United States, the EPA has set a reference dose (RfD) for methylmercury of 0.1 μg/kg/day; Health Canada and the World Health Organization (WHO) have set current RfDs at approximately 0.5 μg/kg/day. Sports and subsistence harvesters of contaminated marine life can greatly exceed these limits (Wheatley & Pradis, 1998), and high-end consumers of commercially available predatory fish (10 or more meals per week) have been found to have blood and/or hair mercury concentrations in the range associated with clinical poisoning (Gochfeld, 2003; Hightower & Moore, 2003).

Prospective studies conducted in New Zealand, the Seychelle Islands, and the Faroe Islands have been especially influential in the ongoing debate regarding the neurodevelopmental effects of lower-level, chronic methylmercury exposure. These cohort studies were selected for review by an expert committee impaneled by the National Academy of Sciences (NAS) to determine whether the U.S. EPA's current RfD is scientifically defensible (NRC, 2000). Consistent with the concept that the developing CNS is especially vulnerable, NAS's panel of expert consultants concluded that an RFD could be calculated most reliably if based on neurobehavioral outcomes in children. All three cohort studies examined populations with a high intake of seafood with various levels of methylmercury contamination. These studies and their strengths and limitations are reviewed below.

The New Zealand cohort study examined children with varying degrees of prenatal exposure to methylmercury by virtue of maternal consumption of fish (mostly shark) served as a popular fast-food dish (fish and chips) in the northern island of the country. Out of an original birth cohort of more than 10,000 children, a small fraction of the original sample was targeted for assessment on the basis of maternal hair mercury concentrations at delivery (Kjellstrom, Kennedy, Wallis, & Mantell, 1986). At 6–7 years of age, 237 children divided into four exposure groups were assessed with a neuropsychological battery that included measures of achievement, language, neuromotor coordination, psychometric intelligence, and social adjustment (Crump, Kjellstrom, Shipp, Silvers, & Stewart, 1998; Kjellstrom et al., 1989). Mean maternal hair mercury concentrations were 8.3 parts per million (ppm) in the highest group and 2.0 ppm in the lowest. Following covariate adjustment, higher prenatal exposure as reflected by maternal hair mercury levels greater than 6 ppm were significantly associated with lower scores on the Speaking Language Quotient of the Test of Language Development, Full Scale IQ on the original edition of the Wechsler Intelligence Scale for Children (WISC), and the McCarthy Scales of Children's Abilities Perceptual–Performance subscale.

A more powerful approach to analysis of the New Zealand data was undertaken by Crump et al. (1998), who treated average mercury concentration in maternal hair as a continuous variable. This analysis also included parents' education as a covariate and discarded one outlying hair mercury concentration of 86 ppm, which was more than four times higher than the next highest level of 20 ppm. Without this extreme outlying value and with the control for parents' education, methylmercury was significantly associated only with the Perceptual–Performance subscale of the McCarthy Scales. However, negative trends above conventional levels of statistical significance ($p < .10$) were observed on other standardized measures, including the Clay Reading Test (letters and concepts), the McCarthy General Cognitive Index (GCI), and the Test of Language Development (grammar completion and grammar understanding).

An adequate appraisal of the New Zealand study is complicated by the fact that the primary reports do not provide sufficient information with respect to study procedures or data quality control. The study is limited by small sample size and lack of control for important sociohereditary factors such as parental IQ. Also, the primary analyses have never been published in the peer-reviewed scientific literature. Nevertheless, NAS experts gave considerable weight to this study in their deliberations and final report (NRC, 2000).

A second prospective study was conducted in the Seychelle Islands (Marsh et al., 1995), an archipelago located in the western part of the Indian Ocean. This island republic (with 80,000 residents of diverse ethnicity) is known mainly for fishing and tourism. Various species of finfish are the population's primary source of dietary protein. Residents of the Seychelles consume fish at almost every meal, and the mercury in seafood harvested from Seychelles waters is similar to levels found in fish in oceans around the world.

The Seychelles study represents a major advance in methylmercury neuroepidemiology. It is notable for its careful piloting of study procedures, large sample size (>700), prospective birth cohort design, serial evaluation of subjects utilizing a well-validated battery of standardized tests, an excellent rate of follow-up, and attention to the potential confounding factors (including parental intelligence and quality of caretaking in the home). There was also minimal exposure to other developmental toxicants, such as tobacco, alcohol, organochlorines (e.g., PCBs), or lead (Davidson et al., 1998). The index of prenatal exposure was total mercury in maternal hair, which ranged from 0.5 to 26.7 ppm (median = 5.9 ppm).

Seychelles children born of uncomplicated pregnancies and in good health were evaluated at 6, 19, 29, 66, and 107 months. At 6 months, infants were administered the Denver Developmental Screening Test—Revised (DDST-R) and the Fagan Test of Infant Intelligence (a measure of visual recognition memory) (Fagan & Shephard, 1987). A standard neurological examination was also performed (Myers et al., 1995). In addition to the sample's being developmentally robust (only 3 out of 737 infants received abnormal scores on the DDST-R), methylmercury was unrelated to any neurodevelopmental parameters, before or after adjustment for covariates. At 19 and 29 months, infants were administered the 1969 edition of the Bayley Scales of Infant Development (Davidson et al., 1995). Prior to and after adjustment for covariates, no statistically significant associations with methylmercury were observed, except for a rating of activity level from the Bayley Infant Behavior Record: In males, activity level decreased as maternal hair methylmercury concentrations increased.

As children reached 5½ years of age, the study was able to recall 91% of the original cohort (Davidson et al., 1998). At this wave, the test battery consisted of the GCI of the McCarthy Scales of Children's Abilities; the Preschool Language Scale; the Letter and Word Recognition (reading) and Applied Problems (math) subtests of the Woodcock–Johnson Tests of Academic Achievement; the Bender–Gestalt Forms Reproduction Test (visual–spatial abilities); and the Achenbach Child Behavior Checklist (CBCL), an inventory of behavioral problems completed by the primary caregiver. In addition to prenatal exposure, postnatal exposure to methylmercury was assessed by measuring total hair mercury (from a 1-cm segment of each child's hair nearest to the scalp) at the time of testing. Performance of Seychelles subjects on these standardized tests was similar to what would be expected in healthy U.S. children. No significant effects of prenatal or postnatal exposure to methylmercury were found before or after covariate adjustment. Indeed, for four of the six measures, slightly better performance was observed at higher exposures.

The Seychellois cohort was examined again at approximately 9 years of age (Myers et al., 2003). At this time, 643 subjects were administered the WISC-III and a comprehensive battery of domain-specific memory, attentional, motor, language, and scholastic achievement tests. Psychosocial adjustment was again assessed with the CBCL. Out of a very large number of outcomes, only performance on the grooved pegboard with the nondominant hand was inversely associated with methylmercury exposure. Using these same data, Davidson et al. (2006) employed a longitudinal multiple-regression approach focusing on outcomes that were repeatedly measured at different ages, including global cognition, reading and mathematics scholastic achievement, social behavior, and memory. No significant associations were found between prenatal methylmercury exposure and changes over time on any of these repeatedly measured neurodevelopmental endpoints.

A third major prospective study was conducted in the Faroe Islands. The Faroes (an autonomous province of Denmark) are located in the North Atlantic between the Shetland Islands and Iceland. The population of about 45,000 is mostly of Scandinavian descent. The principal industries are fishing, fish and sheep farming, and tourism. In 1986 a study of exposure to neurodevelopmental toxicants in seafood and potential effects on child development was initiated (Grandjean et al., 1992). This study shares all of the advanced methodological features of the Seychelles investigation. A cohort of over 1,000 singleton births was recruited during a 21-month period (Grandjean & Weihe, 1993). The residents of the Faroe Islands consume finfish with relatively low levels of methylmercury, as well as pilot whale meat with higher concentrations of methylmercury and pilot whale blubber with elevated concentrations of PCBs. Mercury concentrations were measured in maternal hair samples at delivery, in umbilical cord blood, and in children's hair at various points in time.

The most comprehensive neurobehavioral studies on the Faroese cohort were conducted when subjects reached 7 years of age (Grandjean et al., 1997). Neurophysiological and neuropsychological tests were administered to 917 children, or 90.3% of the original birth cohort. Rather than relying on global assessments of intellectual attainment, the Faroes investigators focused on measures of specific abilities that have been associated with early exposure to neurodevelopmental toxicants in past studies. Their battery assessed motor, attentional, visual–spatial, mnemonic, and language skills (White, Debes, Dahl, & Grandjean, 1994). Neurophysiological tests included pattern reversal evoked potentials, brainstem auditory evoked potentials, computerized posturography, and electrocardiography as a measure of autonomic nervous system function. The primary measure of prenatal exposure was the concentration of methylmercury in cord blood. In addition, hair was obtained from each child at the time of the examination to assess total mercury. Prenatal exposure to PCBs was assessed in umbilical cord tissue in 436 stored samples. Covariates were assessed as potential confounders, including use of alcohol and tobacco during pregnancy, sociodemographics, and parental intelligence.

The geometric mean methylmercury concentration was 22.9 µg/L in cord blood and 3.0 ppm in subjects' hair. Neurological test results were unrelated to exposure. Effects of prenatal methylmercury exposure on electrophysiological measures were found only for the auditory evoked potentials. Delays for peaks III and V were significantly associated with elevated cord blood methylmercury concentrations. Results of neuropsychological evaluations revealed a number of significant associations with cord blood methylmercury. Following covariate adjustment, higher cord blood methylmercury concentrations were associated with performance deficits in motor skills (finger tapping, reaction time), memory (Digit Span from the WISC-R, and short- and long-term reproduction of time-delayed word lists from the California Verbal Learning Test), and language (cued and noncued responses on the Boston Naming Test). In a further analysis of these data, the investigators segregated the subjects scoring below the 25th percentile on representative measures of motor, attentional, visual–spatial, language, and memory abilities. Faroese subjects were also grouped by their cord blood methylmercury concentrations from <15 to >50 µg/L. As illustrated in Figure 9.3, the dose–response relationship was statistically significant for the domains of attention (reaction time on a continuous-performance test) language (Boston Naming Test, cued condition), and memory (California Verbal Learning Test, long-delay recall). In general, maternal and child hair mercury concentrations were not as predictive of neuropsychological performance.

The Faroese cohort was examined a final time when subjects were 14 years of age (Debes, Budtz-Jorgensen, Weihe, White, & Grandjean, 2006). A domain-specific battery similar to the one administered at 7 years was employed. The previously observed associations were diminished in number and strength. However, significant relationships were observed between cord blood methylmercury and finger tapping speed and the Boston Naming Test cued correct score. Interestingly, higher cord blood and maternal hair methylmercury concentrations were associated with significantly better scores on the Wechsler Memory Scale–III Spatial Span subtest. The latter finding is particularly noteworthy, as seafood diets are high in long-chain omega-3 fatty acids, which are important for optimal development of the visual cortex and other parts of the CNS.

The conflicting findings of the Seychellois and Faroese studies have fueled a vigorous debate about the hazards of low-level exposure to methylmercury from seafood, as well as the relative virtues of the two prospective studies (Davidson, Myers, & Weiss, 2004; Grandjean, White, Weihe, & Jorgensen, 2003). For reasons that did not appear to be related to the scientific merits of the two studies, the experts impaneled by the NAS gave greater weight to the Faroese study's positive findings in their calculations of the neurodevelopmental hazards of methylmercury exposure (NRC, 2000). This has resulted in a backlash among some industry-sponsored consumer interest groups, which argue that the results of

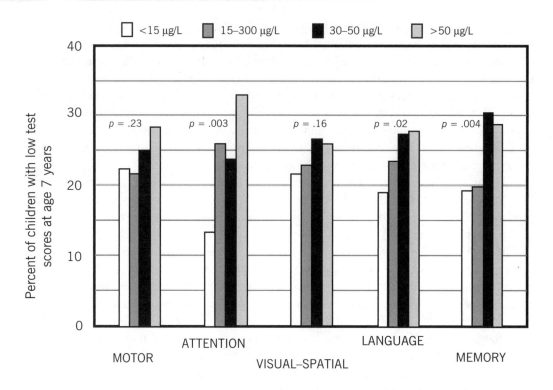

FIGURE 9.3. Effects of low-dose prenatal exposure to methylmercury among Faroese subjects at 7 years of age. The figure shows cord blood methylmercury concentrations of children with scores in the lowest quartile for each of the five neurocognitive domains assessed in the study. One neuropsychological test for each domain was selected for analysis: motor, finger tapping with preferred hand; attention, reaction time on continuous-performance test; visual–spatial, Bender Visual–Motor Gestalt Test error score; language, Boston Naming Test score after cues; memory, California Verbal Learning Test long-delay recall. From Grandjean et al. (1997). Copyright 1997 by Elsevier. Reprinted by permission.

these studies are too equivocal to be used as a basis for restrictions on seafood consumption (Center for Consumer Freedom, 2007). Scientific critics have also pointed out that the major source of methylmercury exposure in the Faroes is pilot whale meat, and that the ocean finfish diet of residents in the Seychelles is a closer approximation to the seafood consumed in the United States (Davidson et al., 2004). Whales have much higher levels of methylmercury in their edible tissues than most ocean fish, as well as other neurotoxicants, such as PCBs in the blubber (which is a popular snack food in the Faroes). Therefore, in terms of exposure to seafood toxicants, residents of the Faroes are more like natives in the Arctic regions—for example, the Inuit of Quebec and Greenland (Muckle et al., 2001). The average PCB concentration in pilot whale blubber in the Faroes is approximately 30 ppm (the current U.S. Food and Drug Administration tolerance level is 2 ppm). Not surprisingly, PCB concentration in collected umbilical cord tissue was significantly correlated with cord blood methylmercury ($r = .41$ for wet-weight PCB) (Weihe, Grandjean, Debes, & White, 1996). It has been shown in animal models that methylmercury and PCBs interact (Bemis & Seegal, 2000). For example, methylmercury potentiates the neurotoxic effects of PCBs on dopamine activity *in vitro* (Bemis & Seegal, 1999). Some analyses of the Faroes data suggest that methylmercury toxicity may be potentiated by PCBs (Budtz-Jorgensen, Keiding, Grandjean, White, & Weihe, 1999; Grandjean et al., 2001). Furthermore, a recent U.S. study (discussed below) reported a stronger association between intrauterine methylmercury exposure and global intelligence among preschoolers with higher levels of prenatal PCB exposure (Stewart, Reihman, Lonky, Darvill, & Pagano, 2003b). It has also been speculated that the high, intermittent methylmercury dose afforded by sporadic whale meat meals may be more toxic to the developing CNS than constant, low-level exposure from finfish (Davidson et al., 2004).

Even in the midst of this controversy and uncertainty, a pediatric neuropsychologist can confidently advise client families (Adams & Schantz, 2006). The health benefits of a seafood diet are undisputed (Cohen et al., 2005; Institute of Medicine, 2007). Seafood is rich in essential long-chain omega-3 fatty acids, such as docosahexaenoic acid and eicosapentaenoic acid. Deficiencies in these nutrients can adversely affect neurodevelopment (Wainright, 2002). A study of an Inuit population in Arctic Quebec found that higher cord plasma docosahexaenoic acid concentration was associated with longer gestation, better visual acuity, and advanced mental development in infants at approximately 1 year of age (Jacobson et al., 2008). A recent study of nearly 9,000 mother–child pairs enrolled in the Avon Longitudinal Study of Parents and Children observed that, after covariate adjustment, higher maternal prenatal seafood consumption (≥340 g per week) was significantly associated with a lower risk for suboptimum social, motor, and language development (Hibbeln et al., 2007).

It is relatively easy to enjoy the benefits of a seafood diet and avoid undue exposure to methylmercury. Several accessible resources are available to assist families in choosing fish species low in methylmercury. The U.S. EPA (at *epa.gov/waterscience/fish/MethylmercuryBrochure.pdf*) offers a helpful pamphlet, and state-by-state fishing advisories are also available (at *epa.gov/waterscience/fish/states.htm*).

Although the principal source of human exposure to organic mercury is fish consumption, vaccinations are the most common secondary source. For over 60 years, vaccines such as pertussis, diptheria, tetanus, and influenza were preserved with thimerosal, an antimicrobial preparation composed of 49.6% ethylmercury. Before the year 2000, there was 25 μg of mercury in each 0.5-mL dose of diphtheria and tetanus toxoids and acellular pertussis vaccines, as well as some *Haemophilus influenzae* type b, influenza, meningococcal, and pneumococcal vaccines. If we assume that the toxicity of ethylmercury is similar to methylmercury, the exposure from a single vaccination would exceed federal guidelines for that day (0.1 μg/kg/day), and adherence to the usual pediatric vaccination schedule would deliver up to 187.5 μg by 6 months of age (Goldman & Shannon, 2001). As a precautionary measure, the U.S. Public Health Service ordered the removal of thimerosal from vaccines as quickly as possible (CDC, 2000a).

At the same time that thimerosal was being eliminated from vaccines in the United States, concerns were being raised about the role of thimerosal-containing vaccines in the rise in cases of ASD in the United States and elsewhere (Bernard, Enayati, Redwood, Roger, & Binstock, 2001). The relationship between incident cases of ASD and exposure to thimerosal-containing pediatric vaccines has been examined in several studies. A population-based cohort study of over 450,000 subjects in Denmark compared children vaccinated with thimerosal-containing vaccine to children vaccinated with a thimerosal-free formulation of the same vaccine (Hviid, Stellfeld, Wohlfahrt, & Melbye, 2003). No difference in the rate of ASD was found between the groups. A retrospective cohort study in the United Kingdom examined the relationship between the amount of thimerosal received by infants via diphtheria–tetanus–pertussis or diphtheria–tetanus vaccination and a large number of subsequent neurodevelopmental disorders, including ASD (Andrews et al., 2004). With the exception of tics, there was no evidence that thimerosal exposure causes neurodevelopmental disorders. Rigorous critical reviews of studies in this area have reached the same conclusion: There is simply no reliable empirical evidence linking ASD or other neurodevelopmental disorders with thimerosal-containing vaccines (Clements, 2004; Nelson & Bauman, 2003; Parker, Schwartz, Todd, & Pickering, 2004; Rutter, 2005).

Nevertheless, there continues to be interest among scientists and advocacy groups in the possible link between exposure to environmental chemicals and ASD (Lathe, 2006). This is reflected in a remarkable clinical trial initiated in 2006 under the sponsorship of the National Institute of Mental Health (NIMH). In this study, children between 4 and 10 years of age with ASD and detectable but subtoxic levels of mercury in blood are being administered succimer (a chelating agent for heavy metal poisoning) or placebo. These subjects are subsequently being followed with measures designed to assess improvement in social reciprocity (NIMH, 2006).

PCBS AND RELATED COMPOUNDS

PCBs are a family of 209 synthetic hydrocarbons (congeners) that were once used in a wide variety of industrial products and processes, including insulating oil, microscope immersion oil, hydraulic fluids, plasticizers, electrical capacitors, transformers, and even carbonless copy paper. Although PCBs were banned in the United States in the 1970s and somewhat later internationally, careless disposal practices have left PCB residues in air, water, soil, and sediment around the world, and such residues can be detected in biological tissues sampled from most residents in industrial countries (Jensen, 1989). These organochlorine compounds are fat-soluble and typically have half-lives in humans of approximately 5–10 years, although the more highly chlorinated species may have half-lives of up to 50 years or more (Shirai & Kissel, 1996). PCBs also cross the placenta and, owing to their lipophilic nature, can be present in high concentrations in human breast milk. Indeed, lactation is the single physiological condition in which substantial quantities of PCBs are excreted over a short period of time (Masuda et al., 1978).

PCBs were first identified as developmental neurotoxicants in 1968 when, in Japan, large quantities of PCBs and their even more toxic thermal degradation by-products (e.g., polychlorinated dibenzofurans) were accidentally mixed with cooking oil during the decolorization process (Kuratsune, 1989). This resulted in an outbreak of severe cystic acne among the residents of Kyusho. It was estimated that more than 1,500 adults were affected. A similar episode occurred in Taiwan in 1979, in which approximately 2,000 individuals were exposed and developed clinical symptoms. The ensuing infirmities following these exposures were referred to as *Yusho* and *Yu-cheng* ("oil disease") in Japan and Taiwan, respectively. Many of the neonates exposed *in utero* were born with low birthweights, microcephaly, dark pigmentation of the skin and nails, early eruption of teeth, swollen eyelids and gums, and an anceform rash (*chloracne*) (Yamashita & Hayashi, 1985). In some cases, intrauterine exposure resulted in neonatal fatalities (Hsu et al., 1985). Developmentally, survivors of intrauterine poisoning lagged behind their unexposed peers in sensory–motor and cognitive abilities (Harada, 1976; Rogan et al., 1988).

Although most residents of industrialized countries are exposed to low levels of PCBs and other halogenated organic compounds, no recent outbreaks of clinical symptoms have occurred in nonoccupationally exposed persons. The greatest concern is presently focused on fetal exposure and the possibility of subtle effects on the developing CNS at low doses (Schantz, Widholm, & Rice, 2003).

Because PCBs were manufactured in such large quantities and carelessly disposed of, members of the general community can be exposed in several ways. Old appliances can leak small quantities of PCBs into the air when they get hot during operation. Breathing the air or drinking well water near hazardous waste sites can be another source of exposure. PCBs can also be present in some meats and dairy products. However, the principal way in which most people in the United States and worldwide are exposed to PCBs is through the consumption of seafood. Because of PCBs' lipophilicity and biological stability, these compounds are transmitted through the food chain and can become highly concentrated in fatty, apical predatory fish and sea mammals (ATSDR, 2000a). Consumption of predatory fish harvested from contaminated waters is strongly associated with the concentration of PCBs and other persistent toxic substances in human serum (Humphrey et al., 2000).

Mechanisms of Developmental Neurotoxicity

Halogenated organic compounds such as PCBs interfere with normal hormonal function and can adversely affect growth and maturation. As a group, PCBs and related compounds are called *endocrine disruptors* (Bonefeld-Jorgensen, Andersen, Rasmussen, & Vinggaard, 2001). Hormonally active agents such as PCBs can be potent developmental neurotoxicants because of their potential to disrupt CNS morphoregulation. Thus, for example, some of the developmental neurotoxicity of PCBs may be related to the antiestrogenic characteristics of dioxin-like PCB congeners, which in turn can affect neurochemistry (e.g., dopaminergic functions) during development (Korach, Sarver, Chae, McLachlan, & McKinney, 1987). PCBs are also structurally similar to the thyroid hormones (Porterfield, 1994). Thyroid hormones are essential for normal CNS development; they increase the rate of neuronal proliferation, and help initiate the process of neuronal maturation and differentiation (Hambaugh, Mendoza, Burkhart, & Weil, 1971). Hydroxylated metabolites of PCBs and related compounds bind to human transthyretin, the only thyroid-hormone-binding protein synthesized in the brain. By binding to transthyretin, some hydroxylated PCBs may alter brain free thyroxine levels and interfere with CNS development (Cheek, Kow, Chen, & McLachlan, 1999; Seegal, 2000). A recent study suggests that PCBs up-regulate several thyroid-hormone-responsive genes that are expressed during critical periods of brain development (Gauger et al., 2004). In this regard, it is noteworthy that Haddow et al. (1999) reported that even mild, asymptomatic maternal hypothyroidism during pregnancy can lead to subtle intellectual impairments in children.

Epidemiological Studies

The effects of PCBs on human neurodevelopment have been less studied than those of other widespread environmental neurotoxicants (e.g., mercury or lead). The seminal studies of Joseph and Sandra Jacobson and colleagues at Wayne State University, and of Walter Rogan and colleagues at the National Institute of Environmental Health Sciences, were reviewed previously (Dietrich, 2000). These Michigan and North Carolina studies were initiated following the *Yu-cheng* incident in Taiwan to assess the potential neurodevelopmental effects of *in utero* and lactational exposure to lower levels of PCBs. Both studies contributed substantially to our understanding of the effects of PCBs and related chemicals on neuropsychological development (Gladen & Rogan, 1991; Jacobson & Jacobson, 1996b). However, these important pioneering efforts were somewhat limited by the chemical-analytic techniques of their day. Since the publication of these historical cohort studies, advances in the analytic techniques for quantification of PCBs in biological tissues have advanced in sensitivity. Also, newer techniques have allowed congener-specific analyses. The latter advance is potentially important, because PCB congeners vary in their toxicity and effects on living tissues (Giesy & Kannan, 1998).

Earlier (Dietrich, 2000), it was noted that a cohort study of PCB exposure among Great Lakes fish eaters was underway in Oswego, New York. This later study was able to employ these advanced chemical-analytic techniques. Another strength of this study was the measurement of other potential developmental neurotoxicants in biomarker tissues, including dichlorodiphenyltrichloroethane (DDE), a contaminant of the pesticide dichlorodiphenyl-dichloroethane (DDT), as well as methylmercury and lead (Stewart et al., 1999).

Oswego is located on the southeastern shore of Lake Ontario, where the residents harvest and consume relatively large quantities of sportsfish (Lonky, Reihman, Darvill, Mather, & Daly, 1996). The Oswego longitudinal study was initiated in 1991 and consisted of 309 mother–child pairs who were followed longitudinally. PCB biomarkers employed in this study included the concentration of 68 PCB congeners in umbilical cord blood, placenta, and breast milk from a subgroup of lactating mothers. The median concentration of total PCBs in cord blood and breast milk fat were 0.52 and 153 ng/g, respectively. Exposure to PCBs in the Oswego cohort appears to have been lower than in the earlier Michigan study, which reported a median cord serum total PCB level of 2.0 μg/g (Schwartz, Jacobson, Fein, Jacobson, & Price, 1983).

Stewart and colleagues have not performed congener-specific analyses on biomarker tissues as yet. However, they have grouped PCB congeners by their degree of chlorination. The most highly chlorinated compounds (PCBs with seven or more chlorine atoms per biphenyl nucleus) are more persistent (but not necessarily more toxic) and can be measured more reliably, as they are less susceptible to analytical interference from other chemical contaminants in the sample (Schantz et al., 2003). Tissue levels of the more highly chlorinated PCBs were also more strongly associated with fish consumption than were total PCBs (Stewart et al., 1999). In most reports from the Oswego study, the associations between exposure to the most highly chlorinated PCBs (heptachlorinated, octachlorinated, and nonachlorinated biphenyl homologues) and neurodevelopmental outcomes are presented.

Newborns were evaluated with the Brazelton Neonatal Behavioral Assessment Scale (NBAS) at 12–24 and 25–48 hours of age (Lonky et al., 1996; Stewart, Reihman, Lonky, Darvill, & Pagano, 2000). Change scores based on the two assessments were calculated as the primary outcome variables. Following covariate adjustment, the concentration of the most highly chlorinated PCBs in cord blood was negatively associated with the NBAS autonomic and habituation cluster scores. This is similar to NBAS findings reported from the Michigan and North Carolina studies (Jacobson, Jacobson, Fein, Schwartz, & Dowler,

1984; Rogan et al., 1986). Infants were tested again at 6 and 12 months of age with the Fagan Test of Infant Intelligence. Higher total PCB concentrations in cord blood were associated with lower novel stimulus fixation times on the Fagan Test at both 6 and 12 months. The highly chlorinated PCBs were similarly associated with fixation time at 6 but not 12 months. This finding is in accord with the Michigan PCB study, which also used the Fagan Test to assess infant cognition (Jacobson, Fein, Jacobson, Schwartz, & Dowler, 1985). No other environmental toxicants examined in the Oswego study were significantly associated with either NBAS or Fagan Test measurements.

The Oswego cohort was examined again at 38 and 54 months of age (Stewart et al., 2003b). The GCI from the McCarthy Scales of Children's Abilities was the primary outcome measure at both ages. Approximately 200 subjects were examined at each age. Following adjustment for covariates, including methylmercury and DDE, there was a significant inverse association between highly chlorinated cord blood PCB concentrations and GCI at 38 months. A significant association was also observed between prenatal maternal hair methylmercury concentrations and GCI, but only in those subjects where PCBs were high enough to be detectable in cord blood. As previously discussed, this suggests that methylmercury's developmental neurotoxicity may be potentiated by concomitant prenatal exposure to PCBs. At 54 months, no significant relationships were observed between PCB biomarkers and the McCarthy GCI or subscales. There was also some evidence that subjects with higher exposure to chlorinated PCBs had recovered from their earlier deficits. This result was at odds with earlier findings from the Michigan cohort, wherein PCB-associated deficits in global intellectual attainment, information processing, and attention were observed in elementary school children (Jacobson & Jacobson, 1996b; Jacobson, Jacobson, Padgett, Brumitt, & Billings, 1992). One reason for this difference may lie in the probability that the Oswego cohort was more lightly exposed to seafood-borne toxicants. Although different chemical-analytic techniques were used, the reported cord blood PCB concentrations in Oswego were 0.5 ppb, compared to 2.0 ppm in Michigan. This may be due to differences in the amount of contaminated fish consumption among Oswego and Michigan mothers during pregnancy, as well as the fact that the Oswego cohort was developing during an era of declining levels of PCBs in some portions of the Great Lakes watershed (Stewart et al., 2003b).

As is sometimes the case in environmental health research, adverse effects of exposure to developmental neurotoxicants may become evident only in the fullness of time (Jacobson & Jacobson, 1996a). When the Oswego subjects were 54 months of age, Stewart et al. (2003a) observed a dose-dependent association between cord blood PCBs and errors of commission on a continuous-performance task. Using MRI, Stewart et al. (2003a) also measured the splenium in the corpus callosum in a small subsample of their cohort. This represents a neuropathway implicated in response inhibition and ADHD (Hynd et al., 1991; Lyoo, Noam, Lee, Kennedy, & Renshaw, 1996). The results indicated that the smaller the splenium, the larger the association between PCBs and errors of commission on the continuous-performance task. Exposure to PCBs was unrelated to splenium size, but the results of these studies suggested that children with suboptimal development of the splenium may be particularly vulnerable to these effects.

This led the Oswego investigators to speculate that prenatal exposure to PCBs may lead to persistent deficits in response inhibition. Thus Stewart et al. (2006) examined response inhibition again (and more directly) in their subjects when they reached 9 years of age, using a paradigm from animal model studies. The Oswego cohort was given a behavioral learning task that employed differential reinforcement of low response rates. In this task, the subject must learn to withhold responses before termination of the delay interval. Therefore, the investigators were tapping into a form of response inhibition in their subjects—an ability that is typically lacking in children with ADHD (Barkley, 1997). Both total and highly chlorinated PCBs were associated with shorter interresponse times and fewer earned reinforcements. Similar independent associations were also observed for prenatal methylmercury exposure (maternal hair) and postnatal blood lead concentrations assessed in Oswego subjects between 2 and 4 years of age. Unlike findings reported for global intellectual attainment, there were no significant neurotoxicant interactions. Impaired response inhibition and excessive responding during the delayed-reinforcement task are consistent with toxicant-related alterations in the development of the prefrontal cortex.

The Oswego studies are significant in that they largely replicate findings from the Michigan cohort in infancy and early childhood, and they provide direct empirical support for the possibility that PCB exposure may augment the associations between cognitive functions and methylmercury. Later findings with respect to deficiencies in attention and response inhibition can also be viewed as evidence of the persistent effects of exposure to low levels of PCBs in utero.

Another recent study using sensitive and congener-specific chemical analyses of biomarker tissues recruited a Dutch cohort of more than 400 healthy pregnant women and their offspring. Half of the women had been residing in heavily industrialized areas in and around Rotterdam (Koopman-Esseboom et al., 1994). Neurodevelopmental deficits in relationship to prenatal PCB exposure (maternal and cord plasma) have been reported from the neonatal period through 9 years of age (Patandin et al., 1999; Vreugdenhil, Mulder, Emmen, & Weisglas-Kuperus, 2004). Results from a contemporaneous German cohort of 171 healthy mother–infant pairs were generally in accord with the Dutch findings (Walkowiak et al., 2001).

It is unlikely that a pediatric neuropsychologist will encounter patients with neurodevelopmental issues specifically linked to exposure to PCBs and related compounds. However, parents and prospective parents can be counseled in a manner similar to that described for methylmercury concerns. The principal route of prenatal exposure is maternal consumption of seafood before and during pregnancy. Women can easily avoid consuming species that are higher in fat, where PCB residues reside. As noted in regard to methylmercury, the U.S. EPA and state fisheries are excellent sources of information on species and waters that should be avoided. However, the manner of seafood preparation can make a difference in PCB consumption, unlike methylmercury consumption. For example, consumption of PCB residues can be substantially decreased by trimming the skin and fatty darker fish flesh on the back and underbelly, as well as avoiding consumption of heads and entrails. Thus a mother and fetus can secure the nutritional benefits of seafood while limiting exposure to PCBs.

The principal source of early postnatal exposure to PCBs is breast milk. However, lactational exposure to PCBs (i.e., as calculated by breast milk PCB concentration × duration of breast feeding) has not been consistently associated with neurodevelopmental deficits in children, despite the fact that much larger absolute quantities of PCBs are transferred to the infant by breast feeding than transplacentally to the fetus (Jacobson & Jacobson, 2001). The confounding factor appears to be that breast-feeding mothers provide a home environment that is more favorable to cognitive development, thus compensating for any adverse developmental effects of postnatal exposure to PCBs through breast milk (Jacobson, Jacobson, & Humphrey, 1990). Furthermore, breast milk nutrients may be protective against functional neurotoxicity (Rogan & Gladen, 1993). As with methylmercury, admonitions concerning the consumption of seafood containing low levels of PCBs must be tempered by an appreciation of the nutritional benefits of such a diet for the mother and fetus. Findings from PCB studies also support continued encouragement of breast feeding in exposed populations (Dietrich, 1999).

INORGANIC LEAD

Lead is the environmental contaminant that pediatric neuropsychologists are most likely to encounter in their practices. A history of lead poisoning is responsible for more child and adolescent neuropsychological referrals than is exposure to any other developmental neurotoxicant (Lidsky & Schneider, 2006). A pediatric neuropsychologist's attention to lead as a causal factor in neurobehavioral problems is particularly appropriate when a practice includes infants and children with a history of residence in older substandard housing. In addition to its historical use as an additive to paint and motor fuels, lead has been and continues to be applied in a wide variety of industrial applications, making the metal a ubiquitous environmental contaminant.

For the pregnant woman and fetus, major sources of exposure are occupational, since the levels of lead in the atmosphere and diet have decreased substantially due to past regulatory actions by the U.S. EPA and the Food and Drug Administration (Annest et al., 1983; Bolger, Carrington, Capar, & Adams, 1991). Lead crosses the placenta readily and accumulates in fetal organs over the period of gestation (Barltrop & Burland, 1969). The transplacental passage of lead is thought to take place by diffusion and is linearly related to the rate of umbilical blood flow (Goyer, 1990). With some exceptions, the clinical picture of low-level prenatal lead exposure appears to be one of mild growth retardation *in utero* and mild developmental delay up to ages 1–2 years, with recovery by school age (Dietrich, 1996). Thus greater concern today is focused on low-level postnatal exposure.

Blood lead concentrations in the general population of U.S. children have declined dramatically since the discontinuation of lead as a gasoline additive (Schwemberger et al., 2005). However, a serious hazard continues to exist for children living in older housing with lead paint (Jacobs et al., 2002). This hazard is exacerbated by the lack of adequate screening and follow-up of children at risk for lead poisoning in some major urban centers in the United States. For example, a recent Government Accountability Office document reports that although lead screening is required by law as part of the Early and Periodic Screening, Diagnosis and Treatment program for children receiving care under Medicaid, it is carried out on fewer than 20% of eligible children (CDC, 2000b). In a recent report out from Michigan, 46% of children who had blood lead levels indicative of toxicity did not receive adequate follow-up testing (Kemper, Cohn, Fant, Dombkowski, & Hudson, 2005).

Lead paint residue in older housing is by far the most common source of exposure for young children. While children may be directly exposed to lead by ingesting paint chips, they are more commonly exposed by swallowing house dust or soil contaminated by leaded paint. Over time, lead paint chalks off interior and exterior walls, or peeling flakes become ground into tiny particles. These particles are often invisible to the naked eye and become constituents of the dust and soil in and around homes. Leaded paint particles can also be liberated during destruction, remodeling, paint removal, or preparation of painted surfaces for repainting. Other potential sources of undue exposure to lead include traditional home health remedies such as *azarcon* and *greta* (used for digestive maladies in the Hispanic community); imported candies; imported toys and toy jewelry; imported cosmetics, pottery, and ceramics; and drinking water contaminated by lead leaching from lead pipes, solder, brass fixtures, or valves (CDC, 2002).

The concentration of lead in blood is the exposure biomarker most often employed to define toxicity. The half-life of lead in the bloodstream is about 35 days; however, circulating levels of lead in blood reflect not only recent exposure, but ongoing mobilization of lead from soft tissues and long-term physiological depots such as bone (Rabinowitz, 1991). Clinical symptoms become visible in children when blood lead concentrations exceed 60–80 µg/dL. Common but nonspecific early symptoms include abdominal pain and arthralgia. Without immediate treatment, a progressive encephalopathy can develop, characterized by lethargy, anorexia, irritability, ataxia, and loss of mental developmental milestones. Presentations in the final stages include gasping respirations, reduced consciousness, seizures, coma, and death. Autopsy studies of nonsurvivors have shown severe cerebral edema attributable to injury to the capillaries, as well as a direct effect on neurons, including neuronal death in areas where neuronal cells are concentrated (such as gray matter and basal ganglia). Although symptomatic lead poisoning is now rare in the United States, cases still occasionally appear (Dietrich, Berger, & Bhattacharya, 2000). The pioneering work of Byers and Lord (1943) documented that children who recover from clinical encephalopathy are likely to have severe and irreversible cognitive and behavioral impairments.

The criterion for undue lead absorption or an elevated blood lead concentration has been revised downward several times over the preceding decades as a result of an accumulation of evidence from epidemiological studies. These investigations, reviewed below, have reported effects of lead on IQ, learning, and behavior at lower and lower levels of exposure. The blood lead "action level" or "level of concern" in infants and children as established by expert consensus has been gradually reduced: 60 µg/dL (1960–1970), 40 µg/dL (1970–1975), 30 µg/dL (1975–1985), 25 µg/dL (1985–1991), and 10 µg/dL (1991–present). Now the 10-µg/dL criterion has been challenged by several recent epidemiological studies of children with blood lead concentrations below the current action level (Gilbert & Weiss, 2006).

Mechanisms of Developmental Neurotoxicity

Lead has the potential to affect a large number of neurodevelopmental processes in the fetus and child. Although lead's toxic effects cannot be tied together by a single unifying mechanism, the metal's ability to mimic calcium is a factor common to many of its toxic actions (Goyer, 1995). For example, lead's ability to pass through the blood–brain barrier is largely due to its capacity to substitute for calcium ions (Kerper & Hinkle, 1997). Lead's long-recognized tendency to follow the calcium stream metabolically also appears to be at the foundation of these actions on the developing brain. The effects of lead on the brain are numerous and complex. Table 9.1 presents these effects and their putative mechanisms, as extensively reviewed by Lidsky and Schneider (2003). Ellen Silbergeld (1992) has condensed many of these effects and mechanisms into two distinct forms of lead neurotoxicity. She states:

TABLE 9.1. Mechanisms and Effects of Lead Toxicity

Mechanisms

Competition with and substitution for calcium
Disruption of calcium homeostasis
Stimulation of release of calcium from mitochondria
Opening of mitochondrial transition pore
Direct damage to mitochondria and mitochondrial membranes
Inhibition of antioxidative enzymes
Alteration of lipid metabolism
Substitution for zinc in zinc-mediated processes
Accumulation in the brain by astrocytes
Sequestration and mobilization of lead from bone stores
Long half-life in brain (2 years) and slow release from sites of accumulation

Effects

Apoptosis
Excitotoxicity
Decreased cellular energy metabolism
Impaired heme biosynthesis and anemia
Oxidative stress
Lipid peroxidation
Altered activity of second-messenger systems
Altered neurotransmitter release
Altered neurotransmitter receptor density
Impaired development and function of oligodendrocytes
Abnormal myelin formation
Abnormal neurotrophic factor expression
Abnormal dendritic branching patterns
Disruption of blood–brain barrier
Disruption of thyroid hormone transport into the brain
Altered regulation of gene transcription
Impaired neuropsychological functioning

Note. Adapted from Lidsky and Schneider (2003). Copyright 2003 by Oxford University Press. Adapted by permission.

. . . I propose that lead exerts neurotoxic effects in the following distinct ways: first, as a neurodevelopmental toxicant, interfering with the hard wiring and differentiation of the CNS [cell development, migration, and synaptogenesis]; second, as a neuropharmacological toxicant, interfering with ionic mechanisms of neurotransmission [cell-to-cell biochemical interactions and neurotransmitter metabolism]. (Silbergeld, 1992, p. 3202)

These generally recognized effects of lead on the development of the CNS establish the basis for the cognitive and motor impairments observed in lead-exposed children in the studies reviewed below.

Epidemiological Studies

The modern era of lead research on pediatric low-dose exposure began with a study by Herbert Needleman and his colleagues of school children in Chelsea and Somerville, Massachusetts (Needleman et al., 1979). This landmark study addressed many of the methodological problems of past investigations by assessment of historical or cumulative exposure to lead (through measurement of lead in deciduous teeth), assessment of potential confounding factors, and the use of multivariate statistical procedures. The authors reported a covariate-adjusted difference in child IQ of approximately 4.5 points between groups "high" and "low" in tooth lead. Teacher ratings of children's behavior in the classroom also suggested more behavioral problems and academic difficulties among children with higher concentrations of lead in shed teeth. Most of the cross-sectional studies that immediately followed the Needleman et al. report were attempts to replicate these findings. The question of low-level lead effects raised by the Chelsea and Somerville research also spawned a number of prospective studies of lead and child development in the United States, Europe, and Australia (Bellinger & Dietrich, 1994). The results of the Needleman et al. (1979) study ultimately provoked a bitter debate, which pitted the interests of children's health against the economic interests of the lead industry and their spokespersons in the academies (e.g., see Needleman, 1992).

Most of the major studies that followed the Needleman et al. (1979) report were reviewed in the first edition of this chapter (Dietrich, 2000), and only the more recent and relevant findings of the prospective investigations and cross-sectional studies are discussed here. An exhaustive review of studies conducted after those discussed in 2000 is beyond the scope of the present chapter. I wrote a detailed description of these investigations and their findings as part of the U.S. EPA's 2006 revised *Air Quality Criteria for Lead* document (USEPA, 2006, Chapter 6.2). However, several recent studies reviewed here have advanced our understanding of lead's effects on neurodevelopment in a number of areas. These include (1) relationships between lead exposure and global intellectual attainment in the international prospective studies (pooled data analysis); (2) assessments of specific cognitive abilities; (3) disturbances in behavior, mood, and social conduct; (4) neuroradiological studies of brain anatomical development and function; (5) reversibility of lead-related neurodevelopmental deficits; and (6) effects of environmental lead exposure within the lower blood lead range (i.e., <10 μg/dL).

Pooled Analysis of Prospective Longitudinal Cohort Studies

There continues to be some debate regarding the impact of lower-level lead exposure on global intellectual attainment. Critics sometimes point to perceived discrepancies in the results among various studies. In response, several meta-analyses have established that lead is robustly associated with dose-related declines in IQ (Needleman & Gatsonis, 1990; Schwartz, 1994; Pocock, Smith, & Baghurst, 1994).

An even more powerful approach toward addressing this question involves pooling the data from high-quality epidemiological studies to examine the dose–response relationships in a large sample of children with diverse sociodemographic backgrounds and levels of exposure. Lanphear et al. (2005a) conducted a pooled analysis of seven prospective studies that were initiated prior to 1995. The analysis involved 1,333 children with complete data on confounding factors used in the multivariable analyses. The participating sites included Boston, Massachusetts; Cincinnati and Cleveland, Ohio; Rochester, New York; Mexico City, Mexico; Port Pirie, Australia; and Kosovo (then part of Yugoslavia). The primary outcome measure was Full Scale IQ assessed in school-age children with the Wechsler scales; mean age of testing was 7 (range = 5–10) years. Four measures of lead exposure were examined: concurrent blood lead (blood lead concentration at the time of IQ testing), maximum blood lead concentration (peak blood lead level at any time prior to the IQ test), average lifetime blood lead (mean blood lead concentration from 6 months to the concurrent blood lead test), and early childhood blood lead (defined as the mean blood lead from 6 to 24 months).

The median lifetime average blood lead concentration was 12.4 μg/dL (5th–95th percentile = 4.1–34.8 μg/dL). The mean IQ of all children was 93.2 (SD = 19.2), but this varied greatly between studies. All four measures of postnatal lead exposure were highly correlated. However, the concurrent blood lead level exhibited the strongest relationship with IQ as assessed by R^2. Nevertheless, the results of regression analyses for all blood lead measures were very similar. Multivariable regression analysis resulted in a six-term model, including the log of concurrent blood lead, study site, maternal IQ, score on the HOME inventory (a measure of caretaking quality), birthweight, and maternal education.

Lanphear et al. (2005a) examined the fit of various models, including the linear model, the cubic spline function, the log-linear model, and the piecewise linear model. The shape of the dose–response curve was determined to be nonlinear; thus the log-linear model was found to be the best fit for the data. Using the log-linear model, the authors estimated a decrement of 1.9 points (95% confidence interval [CI] = 1.2, 2.6) in Full Scale IQ for a doubling of concurrent blood lead. However, the IQ point decrements associated with an increase in blood lead from 1 to 10 μg/dL versus 10 to 20 μg/dL were 6.2 points (95% CI = 3.8, 8.6) versus 1.9 points (95% CI = 1.2, 2.6). The individual effect estimates for the seven studies used in the Lanphear et al. pooled analysis also generally indicated steeper slopes in studies with lower blood lead levels. The issue of greater effects observed at lower blood lead concentrations is discussed later.

Assessments of Specific Cognitive Abilities

Earlier studies of lead and child development focused heavily on dose-related associations with psychometric intelligence. However, specific cognitive abilities in the domains of attention and other executive functions, language, memory and learning, and visual–spatial processing have been examined in greater detail by recent studies. Two areas of performance that appear to be affected in particular are the domains of attention/executive functions and visual–spatial skills.

In the aggregate, studies have suggested that lead exposure impairs a child's ability to engage several related higher-order cognitive processes that neuropsychologists have labeled *executive functions*. These include strategic planning, control of impulses, organized searching, flexibility of thought and action, and self-monitoring of one's own behavior—activities that help the subject maintain an appropriate mental set in order to achieve an immediate or future goal (Spreen, Risser, & Edgell, 1995). In some earlier studies, increased lead exposure was found to be associated with a higher frequency of negative ratings by teachers and/or parents on such behaviors as inattentiveness, impulsivity, distractibility, and less persistence in assigned tasks, as well as slow psychomotor responses and more errors on simple, serial, and choice reaction time tasks (e.g., Hatzakis et al., 1989; Needleman et al., 1979; Winneke, Brockhaus, Ewers, Kramer, & Neuf, 1990). The concept that lead exposure may affect executive functions in particular is biologically plausible. The prefrontal cortex is highly innervated by projections of neurons from the midbrain and has the highest concentration of dopamine of all cortical areas. Dopamine plays a key role in cognitive abilities mediated by the prefrontal cortex. Studies of rodents and nonhuman primates have indicated for some time that the dopamine system is particularly sensitive to lead (Cory-Slechta, 1995). Several epidemiological studies reviewed here have confirmed this.

Bellinger, Hu, Titlebaum, and Needleman (1994) examined a portion of the original Chelsea and Somerville cohorts at 19–20 years of age with a battery of attentional measures assembled by Mirsky (1987). Higher tooth lead concentrations were significantly associated with poorer scores on the Focus–Execute and Shift factors of the battery, leading to the conclusion that early lead exposure is associated with poorer executive/regulatory functions thought to depend on frontal or prefrontal regions of the brain. In studies of their Boston cohort at 10 years, Stiles and Bellinger (1993) found that higher blood lead concentrations at 2 years were significantly associated with lower scores on the Freedom from Distractibility factor of the Wechsler scales and an increase in the percentage of perseverative errors on the Wisconsin Card Sorting Test and the California Verbal Learning Test. Levels of lead exposure in the Boston cohort were low, since at 2 years 90% of the subjects had blood lead concentrations under 13 μg/dL.

Canfield and colleagues (Canfield et al., 2003a; Canfield, Kreher, Cornwell, & Henderson, 2003b; Canfield, Gendle, & Cory-Slechta, 2004) evaluated executive functioning and learning in their Rochester Lead Study cohort at 4 and 5 years of age. The mean blood lead level at 48 months was 6.5 μg/dL (range = 2–21), with 80% of the children below 10 μg/dL. The Shape School Task (Espy, 1997) was administered at 4 years. Although this task only requires the knowledge of simple shapes and primary colors, embedded in the tasks are protocols requiring inhibition and attention-switching mental sets. Following covariate adjustment, blood lead concentration at 48 months was negatively associated with children's focused attention, naming efficiency, and inhibition of automatic responding. Children with higher blood lead levels also completed fewer phases of the task and knew fewer color and shape names. At 6 years, the Working Memory and Planning protocols from the Cambridge Automated Neuropsychological Test Battery were administered to assess mnemonic and executive functions. Following covariate adjustment, children with higher blood lead concentrations showed impaired performance on tests of spatial working memory, spatial memory span, cognitive flexibility, and planning, as indexed by tests of intradimensional and extradimensional shifts and an analogue of the Tower of London task.

An extensive neuropsychological battery was administered to Cincinnati Lead Study subjects at 16 years of age (Ris, Dietrich, Succop, Berger, & Bornschein, 2004). Childhood blood lead levels in the Cincinnati cohort were high by contemporary standards, with 30% of the cohort having at least one blood lead concentration in excess of 25 μg/dL during the first 5 years of life. After covariate adjustment, the strongest association between lead exposure and cognitive performance was found for Attention factor scores derived from a principal-components analysis. This relationship was more prominent among male subjects.

Visual–spatial skills have also been explored in depth by some investigators (Baghurst, McMichael, Tong, Wigg, Vimpani, & Robertson, 1995). When studies of lead-exposed children have used global measures of IQ (e.g., Wechsler Full Scale IQ) and conducted subscale analyses, it has been observed that Performance IQ or subtests contributing to Performance IQ (e.g., Block Design) are frequently among the most strongly associated with biomarkers of lead exposure (Baghurst et al., 1992; Chiodo, Jacobson, & Jacobson, 2004; Dietrich, Berger, Succop, Hammond, & Bornschein, 1993b; Dietrich, Succop, Berger, Hammond, & Bornschein, 1991; Dietrich, Succop, Berger, & Keith, 1992; McMichael et al., 1988;

Wasserman et al., 1994). In addition, studies employing specific measures of visual–motor integration skills, such as the Developmental Test of Visual–Motor Integration (VMI), the Bender Visual–Motor Gestalt Test, and others, have found them to be among the most consistently associated with early lead exposure (Al-Saleh et al., 2001; Baghurst et al., 1995; Dietrich, Succop, & Berger, 1993a; Wasserman et al., 2000; Winneke et al., 1990). Ris et al. (2004) observed a significant association between prenatal maternal blood lead levels and deficits in visual–spatial and constructional skills as indexed by Visual-Constructional factor scores for Cincinnati Lead Study subjects at 16 years. Variables with high loadings on this factor included scores on the WISC-III Block Design subtest and selected variables from the Rey–Osterrieth Complex Figure task.

It remains unclear whether the domains of attention/executive functions or visual–spatial skills per se are specifically sensitive to developmental lead exposure. This is primarily because there is rarely a one-to-one correspondence between performance on a focused neuropsychological test and an underlying neuropsychological process (Bellinger, 1995b). For instance, a low score on the VMI may reflect singular or multiple neurobehavioral deficits, including difficulties with graphomotor control, visual perception, self-monitoring (impulsivity), or planning (executive functions).

Disturbances in Behavior and Social Conduct

As previously noted, cognitive functioning as assessed by IQ tests or specialized measures of performance has been the principal focus of pediatric lead studies. However, deficits in cognition may not be among the most important and persistent effects of early exposure (May, 2000). Needleman (2004) has pointed out that disturbances in behavior and social conduct are prototypical sequelae among victims of lead poisoning. Parents frequently report that following recovery from an episode of acute poisoning, their child's behavior changed dramatically and became restless, impulsive, inattentive, and aggressive. This is an old observation in the clinical literature; in 1943, Byers and Lord reported attentional problems and aggression in their patients who survived acute lead encephalopathy.

Low levels of lead in blood and/or teeth were associated with teacher ratings of hyperactivity, inattention, and behavioral problems in a number of earlier studies (e.g., Fergusson, Fergusson, Horwood, & Kinzett, 1988; Hatzakis et al., 1985; Needleman et al., 1979; Silva, Hughes, Williams, & Faed, 1988; Thomson, Raab, Hepburn, Fulton, & Laxen, 1989; Yule, Urbanowicz, Lansdown, & Millar, 1984). Although attentional deficits and hyperactivity are frequently cited as common problems among lead-poisoned children, until recently there has been a lack of compelling evidence that directly links lead exposure with most or all of the features of ADHD, including distractibility, poor organization, lack of persistence in completing tasks, and daydreaming (Bellinger & Rappaport, 2002). Previous studies that have examined the association of a medical diagnosis of ADHD with lead exposure have been limited by small sample size, ascertainment bias, and the possibility of residual confounding (David, Clark, & Voeller, 1972; Gittelman & Eskenazi, 1983).

A recent investigation utilized (1999–2002) data from the National Health and Nutrition Examination Survey (NHANES) to explore this question (Braun, Kahn, Froehlich, Auinger, & Lanphear, 2006). Blood lead concentrations were available for 4,704 subjects 4–15 years of age, 4.2% of whom were reported to have ADHD and to use stimulant medications. Following covariate adjustment, higher blood lead concentrations were significantly associated with ADHD. Subjects in the fifth quintile for blood lead (>2 µg/dL vs. <0.8 µg/dL) were four times more likely to have a diagnosis of ADHD and to be on stimulant medication. The authors calculated that on a national level, lead exposure accounts for 290,000 excess cases of ADHD in U.S. children.

Children with ADHD are at increased risk for disorders of conduct and behavior (Costello, Mustillo, Erkanli, Keeler, & Angold, 2003). Two prospective studies have examined the relationship between early exposure to lead and behavioral problems with the Achenbach CBCL. In the Kosovo prospective study, concurrent postnatal blood lead levels were significantly associated with parent ratings on the Destructive Behaviors subscale in 3-year-olds following covariate adjustment (Wasserman, Staghezza-Jaramillo, Shrout, Popovac, & Graziano, 1998). In the Port Pirie, Australia study, children's average lifetime blood lead concentrations were significantly associated with higher scores on the CBCL Externalizing Problems composite at 11–13 years of age. This relationship was strongest among male subjects.

Previous studies linking attention deficits, aggressive and disruptive behaviors, and poor self-regulation with lead absorption have raised the prospect that early exposure may result in an increased likelihood of engaging in antisocial behaviors in later life (Needleman, 2004). In an analysis of data from the Collaborative Perinatal Project, Denno (1990) found that a history of lead poisoning was among the most significant predictors of juvenile delinquency and adult criminality among male subjects. The relationship between lead exposure and several measures of behavioral disturbance and delinquent behavior was examined in the Pittsburgh Youth Study (Needleman, Riess, Tobin, Biesecker, & Greenhouse, 1996). Parents of subjects with higher lead levels in bone reported significantly more delinquent and aggressive behaviors, and higher Internalizing and Externalizing Problems scores, on the CBCL. Teachers reported significant lead-associated increases in CBCL scores tapping anxiety, social problems, attention problems, and delinquent and aggressive behavior. Significantly more subjects with high bone lead had CBCL scores in the clinical range on subscales assessing attention, aggression, and delinquency.

In the Cincinnati Lead Study, prenatal (maternal) blood lead levels were significantly associated with a covariate-adjusted increase in the frequency of parent-reported delinquent and antisocial acts, whereas prenatal and postnatal blood lead concentrations were significantly associated with a covariate-adjusted increase in the frequency of self-reported delinquent and antisocial acts (Dietrich, Ris, Succop, Berger, & Bornschein, 2001). In a case–control study of 240 delinquent and nondelinquent Pittsburgh-area youth, tibial bone lead concentrations were significantly higher in delinquent subjects after adjustment for covariates. Bone lead was the second strongest factor in the logistic regression models, exceeded only by race (Needleman, McFarland, Ness, Fienberg, & Tobin, 2002). In the Cincinnati Lead Study, prenatal and postnatal lead exposure was significantly associated with the number of officially documented criminal arrests in 250 young adults (age 22). These covariate-adjusted associations were particularly strong for arrests involving physically violent offenses (Wright et al., 2008). In consideration of these findings, it is noteworthy that a number of recent ecological investigations correlating leaded gasoline sales or atmospheric lead levels with crime rates also support an association between lead exposure and criminal behavior (Nevin, 2000, 2007; Stretesky & Lynch, 2001). This has led to speculation that one reason for the recent decline in crime rates in the general U.S. population is decreased exposure to lead.

The extension of lead effects into delinquent and criminal behavior is significant for both the individual and society as a whole. The specific biological mechanisms that may underlie lead effects on aggression, impulsivity, and poor self-regulation are not clearly understood. Lead affects a large number of sites and processes in the brain involved in impulse control (Lidsky & Schneider, 2003). Needleman et al. (2002) have proposed that in addition to direct impacts on brain development and neuronal function, impaired cognitive abilities and subsequent academic failure in lead-exposed children may increase risk. Students who have difficulties in school and fail to achieve academic goals are more likely to become lawbreakers.

Neuroradiological Studies of Brain Anatomical Development and Function

Advances in MRI technologies have provided a powerful tool for studying the effects of environmental chemicals and drugs on neurodevelopment. Trope and colleagues were the first to apply MRI and magnetic resonance spectroscopy (MRS) to the evaluation of lead-exposed subjects (Trope, Lopez-Villegas, Cecil, & Lenkinski, 2001; Trope, Lopez-Villegas, & Lenkinski, 1998). Trope et al. (2001) performed MRI and MRS studies on a sample of 16 subjects with a history of elevated blood lead levels (23–65 µg/dL) prior to 5 years of age. The average time of evaluation was 8 years. Compared to age-matched controls composed of siblings or cousins without a history of undue lead exposure (i.e., ≤10 µg/dL), lead-exposed subjects exhibited a significant reduction in ratios of N-acetylaspartate to creatine and phosphocreatine. N-acetylaspartate is a metabolite shown to decrease in processes that involve decreased neurononal densities and neuronal loss. The results of Trope et al. have recently been replicated in a similar study in China (Meng, Zhu, Ruan, She, & Luo, 2005).

Using functional MRI, Yuan et al. (2006) examined the influence of childhood lead exposure on language function in a subsample of 48 young adults from the Cincinnati Lead Study. Subjects performed an integrated verb-generating/finger-tapping paradigm. Higher childhood average blood lead levels were significantly associated with reduced activation in Broca's area, a recognized region of speech production in the left hemisphere. Higher blood lead levels were also associated with increased activation in the right temporal lobe, the homologue of Wernicke's area that is associated with speech perception. These associations were statistically significant following adjustment for covariates that were also predictive. These included the subject's own IQ score, birthweight, and marijuana consumption as assessed by a positive urine screen. The results of this study suggest that elevated childhood blood lead levels influence neural substrates of semantic language function, with concomitant recruitment of contralateral regions resulting in a striking, dose-dependent atypical reorganization of language function.

Using volumetric MRI, Cecil et al. (2008) also examined a subset of the Cincinnati Lead Study cohort. In studies of 157 subjects between the ages of 19 and 24 years, analyses of whole-brain MRI revealed significant decreases in brain volume associated with childhood blood lead concentrations. Following adjustment for other significant predictors, including age at time of imaging and birthweight, the most affected regions were within the frontal gray matter—specifically, the anterior cingulate cortex and ventrolateral prefrontal cortex, which are areas associated with executive functions (including mood regulation, decision making, and interpretation of sensory inputs). Areas of lead-associated gray matter volume loss were larger for males.

Reversibility of Lead-Related Neurodevelopmental Deficits

A unique aspect of lead poisoning relative to other environmental diseases of childhood is that it can be commonly treated with various chelating drugs that help the body to excrete the toxicant. Elemental mercury poisoning is also treated with chelating agents (Yeates & Mortensen, 1994), but these treatments are uncommon, given the relatively low number of incident cases per year.

The current standard of care calls for pharmacological intervention when blood lead concentrations exceed 44 µg/dL. In the past, these interventions have usually meant hospital treatment with parenteral administration of calcium disodium ethylenediaminetetraacetic acid (EDTA). At higher blood lead concentrations, treatment with EDTA may be accompanied by intramuscular injection of dimercaprol (British Antilewisite, or BAL). Today, pharmacotherapy is increasingly conducted on an outpatient basis with an orally administered drug—dimercaptosuccinic acid (succimer), a congener of BAL. In addition to drug treatment, it is absolutely essential to identify the sources of lead exposure and to eliminate any further contact with them. The availability of drugs that can reduce body burden of lead has permitted clinical studies aimed at reducing neurodevelopmental morbidity secondary to exposure.

Initial optimism that such interventions might be effective was raised by a study conducted in New York (Ruff, Bijur, Markowitz, Ma, & Rosen, 1993). Ruff et al. observed that among children 1–7 years of age (with blood lead levels of 25–55 µg/dL) who were given chelation with EDTA and/or therapeutic iron, those with the greatest decline in blood lead over a 6-month period showed the most improvement in cognitive test scores over baseline test results. This finding was independent of whether the subjects received iron alone or in combination with EDTA.

In 1991, the U.S. Food and Drug Administration approved succimer (Chemet) as the first oral chelating drug for the treatment of lead poisoning in children with blood lead concentrations in excess of 44 µg/dL (Nightingale, 1991). Soon afterward, the National Institute of Environmental Health Sciences launched the Treatment of Lead Exposed Children (TLC) clinical trial (Rogan, 1998). TLC was originally designed to test the hypothesis that children with "moderate" blood lead levels (20–44 µg/dL) who were given an oral chelating drug (succimer) would have better scores than children given placebo on a wide range of tests measuring cognition, neuropsychological functions, and behavior at a 36-month follow-up. In this study, 780 children, 12–33 months of age, from four clinical sites were enrolled in a randomized, placebo-controlled, double-blind trial of up to three 26-day courses of treatment with succimer or placebo. Most TLC subjects lived in deteriorating inner-city housing, with 77% of the subjects being African American. Although succimer was effective in lowering the blood lead levels of subjects on the active drug, no statistically significant differences were observed between treatment arms on a variety of outcomes, including standardized measures of intelligence, attention, language, sensory–motor skills, visual–spatial abilities, memory, and behavioral problems (Rogan et al., 2001).

Although results for the first wave of TLC follow-up were consistently negative for drug effects on cognition and behavior, they were not considered conclusive, since the benefits of therapy may be more clearly evident as the cohort ages. Therefore, subjects were followed into the first years of elementary education. A comprehensive battery of tests was administered to TLC subjects between 7 and 8 years of age. The battery included standardized measures of cognition, learning, memory, global intelligence, attention/executive functions, psychiatric status, behavioral and academic conduct, neurological functioning, and motor speed. Unfortunately, treatment resulted in no neuropsychological benefits (Dietrich et al., 2004). Indeed, children treated with succimer fared worse than children in the placebo group in several areas, including linear growth and neuropsychological deficits as assessed by the Attention and Executive Functions core domain from the NEPSY scales. Although the TLC results were negative, they highlight the apparent irreversibility of lead-associated cognitive deficits (Rosen & Mushak, 2001).

In an attempt to confirm the findings of Ruff et al. (1993), other investigators have examined the relationship between the rate of decline in blood lead concentrations during childhood and improvements in neurobehavioral performance. As in the Ruff et al. study, these investigations attempted to determine whether children recover from lead-associated neurodevelopmental deficits as blood lead levels decline, as they normally do during the later preschool years. Initial optimism raised by Ruff et al. about the reversibility of lead-induced cognitive impairments was tempered somewhat by a later report of an Australian study with longer follow-up. That study found small and inconsistent improvement in the IQs of children whose blood lead concentrations fell the most (Tong, Baghurst, Sawyer, Burns, & McMichael, 1998). Because of the lack of any salutary effects in the intent-to-treat analyses, TLC data were used to determine whether cognitive scores improved in subjects with the most rapidly declining blood lead concentrations (Liu et al., 2002). In analyses of the entire TLC cohort, there was no significant improvement in cognitive test scores in relationship to the rate of decline in blood lead over the first 36 months of follow-up. When the groups were divided into treatment and placebo arms, there was a small but statistically significant improvement in the placebo group only. Because of this inconsistency, the authors concluded that the results did not indicate that lead-induced cognitive defects are reversible. In general, these studies have not provided supportive evidence that lead-induced cognitive impairments are reversible as blood lead levels decline over time, or in response to nutritional interventions designed to limit lead absorption and/or increase excretion (Kordas, Stoltzfus, Lopez, Rico, & Rosado, 2005; Rico et al., 2006).

It remains unclear why these studies failed to firmly replicate the findings of Ruff et al (1993). The New York sample studied by Ruff and colleagues was very similar to the TLC cohort in terms of blood lead concentrations and other factors such as social disadvantage. Furthermore, the tests used to assess cognitive development in TLC and other studies reviewed here were similar to those used by the New York investigators (e.g., the Bayley and Wechsler scales). Unfortunately, at this point, the balance of the evidence indicates that pharmacological and nutritional interventions are relatively ineffective in improving the neuropsychological functioning of lead-exposed children.

Effects of Environmental Lead Exposure within the Lower Blood Lead Range

Over the past three decades, epidemiological studies of lead and child development have demonstrated inverse associations between blood lead concentrations and other biomarkers at successively lower lead exposure levels. In response to these data, agencies such as the CDC (1991) and the WHO (1995) have repeatedly lowered the definition of an elevated blood lead concentration. When these policies were put into place, there were few studies of children with blood lead concentrations consistently under 10 µg/dL on which to base a scientific consensus about effects within the lower blood lead range. Since the removal of lead from gasoline, the median blood lead concentration has dropped dramatically in U.S. children, permitting more studies of this nature in recent years. Also, the use of meta-analysis and pooled analysis has enabled investigators to get a clearer picture of effects below 10 µg/dL.

The Rochester Prospective Study (Canfield et al., 2003a) extended the relationship between deficits in IQ and blood lead concentrations to levels well below 10 µg/dL. Over half of the children in this study did not have a recorded blood lead concentration above 10 µg/dL. In the results of analyses using only children with peak blood lead levels less than 10 µg/dL, each 1-µg/dL increase in concurrent blood lead levels was associated with a statistically significant, covariate-adjusted –1.8-point decline in IQ at 5 years of age. Nonlinear semiparametric smoothing revealed a covariate-adjusted decline of more than –7 IQ points up to 10 µg/dL of childhood average blood lead, whereas a more gradual decline of –2.5 points was associated with an increase in blood lead from 10 to 20 µg/dL. The Rochester findings have been replicated in several other studies of children with blood lead levels below 10 µg/dL (Al-Saleh et al., 2001; Bellinger & Needleman, 2003; Chiodo et al., 2004; Kordas et al., 2006; Tellez-Rojo et al., 2006).

The most compelling evidence for effects at blood lead levels below 10 µg/dL comes from the international pooled analysis of seven prospective cohort studies (N = 1,333) by Lanphear et al. (2005a), described earlier. Although exposures in some cohorts were high, a substantial number (n = 244) of children with blood lead concentrations that never exceeded 10 µg/dL were included in the analysis when data from these diverse studies were pooled. As observed in Canfield et al. (2003a) and other studies mentioned above, the slope for lead effects on IQ was steeper at lower blood lead levels, as indicated by both cubic spline function and the log-linear model. As illustrated in Figures 9.4a and 9.4b, the shape of the log-linear model and the spline function indicated that the steepest declines in IQ were at blood lead concentrations below 10 µg/dL. The spline function results agreed quite closely with those of the parametric log-linear model. To further investigate whether the lead-associated decrement in IQ was greater at lower blood lead concentrations, Lanphear et al. divided the data at two cutoff points a priori—a maximal blood lead of 7.5 and 10 µg/dL. The blood lead coefficient for the 103 children with maximal blood lead levels below 7.5 µg/dL was significantly greater than the coefficient for the 1,230 children with a maximal blood lead greater than 7.5 µg/dL (–2.94 points [95% CI = –5.16, –0.71] per 1-µg/dL increase in blood lead vs. –0.16 points [95% CI = –0.24, –0.08]).

A nonlinear dose–response relationship appears to be a common observation in studies of low lead levels. At first this may seem at odds with fundamental toxicological concepts. However, nonlinear or supralinear dose–effect relationships are not uncommon in toxicology. It is conceivable that the initial neurodevelopmental lesions at lower lead levels may be disrupting very different biological mechanisms from those disrupted by the more severe lesions at high exposures, which result in symptomatic poisoning or frank mental retardation (Dietrich et al., 2001). As Kordas et al. (2006) state, this might help explain why, within the range of exposures not producing overt clinical symptoms, an increase in blood lead beyond a certain concentration might cause less additional impairment in children's cognitive functions. It is clear, however, that these studies strongly argue for a reevaluation of the current "action level" of 10 µg/dL by the CDC and other responsible national and international agencies.

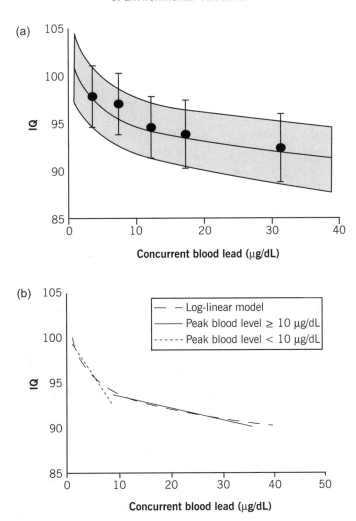

FIGURE 9.4. (a) Log-linear model (95% CI shaded) for concurrent blood lead concentration adjusted for HOME score, maternal education, maternal IQ, and birthweight. The mean IQ (95% CI) for the intervals 5, 5–110, 10–15, and ≥20 μg/dL are shown. (b) Log-linear model for concurrent blood lead concentration along with linear models for concurrent blood lead levels among children with peak blood lead levels above and below 10 μg/dL. Reprinted from Lanphear et al. (2005a) with permission from Environmental Health Perspectives.

The effects of lead on the neuropsychological functioning of children have been reported with remarkable consistency across numerous studies with various designs, populations studied, and developmental assessment protocols. The negative effects of lead on IQ and other neurobehavioral outcomes persist in most recent studies after adjustment for numerous confounding factors. Some of the effects attributed to lead, such as an increase in antisocial and criminal behaviors, can have devastating consequences for the individual and for society as a whole. These effects are not reversible through pharmacological or nutritional interventions. Therefore, the only certain way to prevent lead-associated neurodevelopmental morbidity is to prevent exposure in the first place; primary prevention is the only reasonable course of action (Rosen & Mushak, 2001). However, public health and housing agencies lack the resources needed to protect children fully from lead poisoning (Lanphear, 2005). Furthermore, current screening and treatment strategies often fall short (Kemper et al., 2005). Thus pediatric neuropsychologists will probably continue to encounter lead-poisoned patients in their clinics for some time to come. Sound strategies for the neuropsychological evaluation and follow-up of these children have been outlined by Bellinger and Rappaport (2002). Pediatric neuropsychologists with such children in their practices should study these recommendations carefully. Among other suggestions, the authors recommend long-term developmental surveillance and referral to early environmental enrichment programs.

The possibility that lead-exposed children from more disadvantaged circumstances may be particularly vulnerable to the metal's neurotoxicity has been raised by several studies. Indirectly, the significant interaction between lead exposure and various measures of SES suggests that differences among SES strata in the richness and variety of opportunities for environmental stimulation may be important (e.g., Tong, McMichael, & Baghurst, 2000). The potential importance of environmental stimulation as a prophylactic factor or treatment has also gained support from animal model studies demonstrating that environmental enrichment provides some protection from and can even reverse some of the cognitive and molecular deficits induced by developmental lead exposure (Guilarte, Toscano, McGlothan, & Weaver, 2003; Schneider, Lee, Anderson, Zuck, & Lidsky, 2001). Bellinger and Rappaport (2002) also recommend that in the developmental surveillance of children with elevated blood lead levels, neuropsychologists should watch for emerging difficulties at critical transition points in childhood (e.g., first, fourth, and sixth–seventh grades) and monitor the children for behaviors that interfere with learning, such as inattention and distractibility.

OTHER DEVELOPMENTAL NEUROTOXICANTS

Documentation of developmental effects in humans for compounds other than those reviewed above is relatively meager. However, four emerging and noteworthy environmental toxicants are reviewed below.

Pesticides

Research on the neurodevelopmental effects of pesticides in children is currently underway in prospective studies sponsored by the National Centers for Children's Environmental Health and for Disease Prevention Research (Fenske et al., 2006). There is a great deal of interest in pesticides because they are manufactured specifically as poisons, and although they are designed to act on the nervous systems of undesirable species, they also act on human nervous systems (Weiss, 1997). More than 4 billion pounds of pesticide chemicals are applied annually in the United States, and more than 75 million pounds are applied annually in U.S. households (Aspelin & Grube, 1999). Pesticide residues are found everywhere in the environment, and trace elements are commonly detected in food (including breast milk), in water, and on environmental surfaces in homes and yards.

The majority of pesticide-poisoning victims in the United States are preschool children (Litovitz et al., 2002). The neurotoxic potential of these compounds has been recognized for years, and some have even been exploited for chemical warfare. The two major classes of pesticides are the chlorinated hydrocarbons and the organophosphorus esters (OPs). Most pesticides now in commerce are OPs, as the organochlorine pesticides have been largely banned, owing to their long persistence in the environment and effects on the reproductive functions of wildlife. OPs exert their neurotoxic effects by inhibiting the activity of acetylcholinesterase, resulting in an excess of the neurotransmitter acetylcholine and a depolarizing blockade of neural transmissions (Weiss, 2004).

Although pesticides have been subjected to extensive testing in animal models, the neurodevelopmental toxicity of these compounds in humans is just beginning to be examined. The developmental neurotoxicity of pesticides was indicated by a unique anthropological study in Mexico (Guillette, Meza, Aquilar, Soto, & Garcia, 1998). Children in a lowland agricultural community that commonly used mixed pesticides in agriculture (including organochlorinated compounds and OPs), were compared to matched controls living in the foothills, where the use of these compounds is traditionally avoided. Compared to their less exposed peers in the foothills, lowland children displayed substantial deficits in memory, fine motor coordination, visual–spatial skills, and physical stamina. More studies are needed, but recent investigations have reported dose-related effects of prenatal exposure on intrauterine growth and neurodevelopment (Berkowitz et al., 2004; Rauh et al., 2006; Ruckart, Kakolewski, Bove, & Kaye, 2004; Young et al., 2005).

In most instances, a pediatric neuropsychologist will not be presented with cases of acute pesticide poisoning. These are more within the purview of a primary care or emergency room physician. However, clinicians can encourage parents to be careful when using pesticides in the home and other environments to which children have access. A recent prospective investigation has also shown that switching to organically grown vegetables and avoiding nondomestically grown produce can substantially reduce children's exposure to prevalent OPs such as malathion and chlorpyrifos (Lu, Barr, Pearson, & Waller, 2008). The U.S. EPA is another good source of information for clinicians and families on pesticides and child safety (*www.epa.gov/pesticides/factsheets/childsaf.htm*).

Manganese

Manganese (Mn) is an essential mineral element in mammals, yet it is neurotoxic in excess. The typical route of exposure is inhalation, through which it can gain direct access to tissues of the CNS. High-level exposures are usually occupational in origin and can produce a parkinsonian-like syndrome called *manganism*. This is largely due to the toxic effect of manganese on the dopaminergic neurons of the basal ganglia. Manganism is characterized by extrapyramidal and psychiatric symptoms that persist long after cessation of exposure (Olanow, 2004). Industrial and environmental exposures to manganese have been associated with other adverse neurobehavioral outcomes, including deficits in motor function, cognition, and affect (Ingren, 1999; Levy & Nassetta, 2003; Pal, Samili, & Caine, 1999).

The neurodevelopmental effects of this toxicant are largely unknown. Concerns about this metal have emerged in recent years, because the organic manganese compound methylcyclopentadienyl manganese tricarbonyl (MMT) has been added to gasoline as an octane-boosting agent in Mexico, Canada, and Australia, and plans to add MMT to fuels marketed in the United States are still in place. Manganese can cross the placenta as well as the blood–brain barrier (Aschner & Aschner, 1990; Wilson, Tubman, Halliday, & McMaster, 1992). In addition to inhalation, another major route of exposure is drinking water. Ecological studies of children exposed prenatally and postnatally via drinking water have observed neurobehavioral impairments (Zhang, Liu, & He, 1995; Wasserman et al., 2006). In a French birth cohort, cord blood manganese concentrations were inversely associated with selected subscales of the McCarthy Scales of Children's Abilities tapping, attention, nonverbal abilities, and eye–hand coordination (Tasker, Mergler, Hellier, Sahuquillo, & Huel, 2003). Fetuses and children in the United States can be exposed to manganese from a variety of sources, including well water, toxic waste sites, and point sources of industrial pollution.

Arsenic

Arsenic (As) is a ubiquitous heavy metal in the environment at low background levels. However, significant contamination can occur around mining and smelting operations, in agriculture as a herbicide or pesticide, and in the semiconductor industry. Pediatric cases of symptomatic arsenic poisoning in the United States are rare but not unheard of (Lai, Boyer, Kleinman, Rodig, & Ewald, 2005). The developmental neurotoxicity of arsenic has not been extensively examined, even though the toxicant has long been recognized to cause peripheral neuropathies in adults (ATSDR, 2000b). The health consequences of pediatric arsenic exposure first came to world attention in 1955, when infants in western Japan were exposed to arsenic-contaminated powdered milk manufactured by the Morinaga Milk Company (WHO, 1981). It is estimated that more than 12,000 infants were poisoned, 130 of whom died. Case–control follow-up studies observed substantially higher rates of sensory deficits and mental retardation in adolescent survivors of the Morinaga poisonings (Dakeishi, Murata, & Grandjean, 2006).

Arsenic is present in groundwater sources worldwide and in some hazardous waste sites in the United States. Concerns have been raised about the metal's developmental neurotoxicity at lower levels of exposure. In an ecological study, Wasserman et al. (2004) examined the relationship between arsenic concentrations in deep water wells in Araihazar, Bangladesh, and children's performance on the Wechsler scales at 10 years of age. Water arsenic was associated with reduced intellectual function in a dose-dependent manner on Performance and Full Scale weighted raw scores. A study of 32 children residing near a hazardous waste site in Oklahoma found a significant relationship between hair arsenic concentrations and IQ as measured by the Wechsler Abbreviated Scales of Intelligence after covariate adjustment. This relationship was particularly strong for Verbal IQ. An interaction between arsenic and manganese was also noted, with the lowest scores found among children who had hair arsenic and manganese concentrations above the median values in the sample (Wright, Amarasiriwardena, Woolf, Jim, & Bellinger, 2005). Although the data on arsenic's developmental neurotoxicity are currently meager, these studies suggest that lower-level exposures may be harmful.

Environmental Tobacco Smoke

The effects of prenatal exposure to tobacco smoke have been extensively examined. It has been well documented that prenatal maternal tobacco use is associated with a number of adverse reproductive outcomes and correlated neurodevelopmental morbidities (U.S.

Department of Health and Human Services, 2004). It has been estimated that approximately 40% of U.S. children are exposed postnatally to environmental tobacco smoke (ETS) in their homes (Pirkle et al., 1996). Remarkably, the NHANES 1999–2002 data showed that serum cotinine (a metabolite of nicotine) was highest in the youngest age range examined, 3–11 years (Needham, Calafat, & Barr, 2008).

Exposure to ETS has been linked with a number of adverse health effects, including middle-ear disease, colic, sudden infant death, asthma, and other respiratory difficulties (Cook & Strachan, 1999). ETS exposure has also been associated with a variety of adverse behavioral and cognitive outcomes in children (e.g., Eskanazi & Castorina, 1999; Johnson, Swank, Baldwin, & McCormick, 1999).

However, various methodological limitations of prior studies contribute to the lack of clarity in the findings. These limitations include small sample size, reliance on parental reports of child exposure, and the inability to distinguish prenatal and postnatal tobacco smoke exposure. We (Yolton, Dietrich, Auinger, Lanphear, & Hornung, 2005) have addressed a number of these limitations by using data from the third NHANES to examine the relationship between ETS exposure and cognitive abilities among U.S. children and adolescents 6–16 years of age. Serum cotinine, a metabolite of nicotine, was quantified and used as the biomarker of exposure. Children were only included in the analyses if their serum cotinine levels were ≤15 ng/mL, a level consistent with ETS exposure and not active use of tobacco products. Cognitive and academic abilities were assessed with the Reading and Math subtests of the Wide Range Achievement Test—Revised and with the Block Design and Digit Span subtests of the WISC-III. Following covariate adjustments that included control for prenatal tobacco exposure, there was a significant relationship between serum cotinine and scores on the Reading and Math achievement subtests and the WISC-III Block Design subtest. Dose-related deficits were evident even at the lowest levels of serum cotinine. Indeed, in a log-linear analysis, it was evident that ETS-associated decrements in cognitive test scores were greater at lower cotinine levels.

In addition to the documented effects of ETS on pediatric pulmonary health, there is mounting evidence that neurodevelopment is affected as well. In order to reduce or eliminate this avoidable risk, pediatric neuropsychologists should advise client families of the hazards to normal health and development that ETS presents.

CONCLUSIONS

The effects of environmental chemicals on child development have become a topic of considerable interest to behavioral scientists and clinicians. As in many areas of epidemiological research, controversies persist, and investigators have come to disparate conclusions. However, few credible clinicians or scientists today would argue that exposures to moderate or high levels of mercury or PCBs are inconsequential in terms of neurodevelopment. The adverse effects of lead at low doses have also come into focus, and some are now calling for a reevaluation of the current definition of toxicity by the CDC and other responsible agencies. Knowledge of the developmental hazards of other developmental neurotoxicants, such as pesticides and ETS, is also growing; studies that are now underway will provide much-needed information on these and other environmental chemical exposures.

As in the first edition of this chapter (Dietrich, 2000), the reader is again reminded that not all nonpharmaceutical chemical exposures suffered by fetuses are accidental or involuntary. For example, because of its anesthetic properties, toluene has been abused by sniffing or "huffing" the substance in readily available products (e.g., paint in aerosol spray cans). Cases where this abuse has affected fetuses have been documented by clinicians and researchers who described features in surviving newborns that bear some similarity to fetal alcohol syndrome (Hersch, Podruch, Rogers, & Weisskopf, 1985; Pearson, Hoyme, Seaver, & Rimsza, 1994). A recent study by the Substance Abuse and Mental Health Services Administration reported that over 1 million U.S. adolescents abused inhalants between 2002 and 2005, and that the numbers are increasing, particularly among teenage girls (Office of Applied Studies, 2006).

Whenever appropriate, this chapter has emphasized what the pediatric neuropsychologist can do to help clients and their families avoid the consequences of environmental chemical exposures. With respect to patient care, a network of health care providers with pediatric environmental health expertise is now regionally distributed across the United States. Funded by the U.S. EPA and ATSDR, 10 Pediatric Environmental Health Subspecialty Units (*www.atsdr.cdc.gov/HEC/natorg/pehsu.html*) serve the pediatric environmental health needs in their respective regions. Experts in these centers are available to answer questions from both health care providers and families regarding the prevention and treatment of pediatric environmental disease.

Pediatric neuropsychologists should continue to keep abreast of new developments in this field. Very few of the environmental chemical pollutants to which fetuses and children are exposed have been characterized in terms of their neurodevelopmental toxicity. As previously noted (Dietrich, 2000), a working knowledge of this area will not only enhance pediatric neuropsychologists' clinical and scientific acumen but may eventually help to identify as yet undiscovered environmental risks to normal CNS development. Clinicians, after all, were the first to identify some of the best-known environmental and pharmaceutical chemical risks to neurodevelopment. In commenting on the first edition of this chapter, Byron Rourke (2000) concluded, " As in so many areas of neuropsychological endeavor, good science and good practice go hand in hand" (p. 463).

ACKNOWLEDGMENTS

This work was supported by grants from the National Institute of Environmental Health Sciences and the U.S. Environmental Protection Agency.

REFERENCES

Adams, J., Barone, S., LaMantia, A., Philen, R., Rice, D. C., Spear, L., et al. (2000). Workshop to identify critical windows of exposure for children's health: Neurobehavioral Workforce Group summary. *Environmental Health Perspectives*, 108(Suppl. 3), 535–544.

Adams, J., & Schantz, S. L. (2006). Editors' note: Methylmercury 2006. *Neurotoxicology and Teratology*, 28, 527–528.

Agency for Toxic Substances and Disease Registry (ATSDR). (1999). *Toxicological profile for mercury*. Atlanta, GA: U.S. Department of Health and Human Services.

Agency for Toxic Substances and Disease Registry (ATSDR). (2000a). *Toxicological profile for polychlorinated biphenyls (PCBs)*. Atlanta, GA: U.S. Department of Health and Human Services.

Agency for Toxic Substances and Disease Registry (ATSDR). (2000b). *Toxicological profile for arsenic*. Atlanta, GA: U.S. Department of Health and Human Services.

Akagi, H., Grandjean, P., Takizawa, Y., & Weihe, P. (1998). Methylmercury dose estimation from umbilical cord concentrations in patients with Minamata disease. *Environmental Research, 77*, 98–103.

Al-Saleh, I., Nester, M., DeVol, E., Shinwari, N., Munchari, L., & Al-Sahria, A. S. (2001). Relationships between blood lead concentrations, intelligence, and academic achievement of Saudi Arabian schoolgirls. *International Journal of Hygiene and Environmental Health, 204*, 165–174.

American Academy of Pediatrics. (2003). *Pediatric environmental health* (2nd ed.). Elk Grove, IL: Author.

Andrews, K. W., Savitz, D. A., & Hertz-Picciotto, I. (1994). Prenatal lead exposure in relation to gestational age and birth weight: A review of epidemiologic studies. *American Journal of Industrial Medicine, 26*, 13–32.

Andrews, N., Miller, E., Grant, A., Stowe, J., Oxborne, V., & Taylor, B. (2004). Thimerosal exposure in infants and developmental disorders: A retrospective cohort study in the United Kingdom does not support a causal association. *Pediatrics, 114*, 584–591.

Annest, J. L., Pirkle, J. L., Makuc, D., Neese, J. W., Bayse, D. D., & Kovar, M. G. (1983). Chronological trends in blood lead levels between 1976 and 1980. *New England Journal of Medicine, 323*, 1096–1101.

Aschner, M., & Aschner, J. L. (1990). Manganese transport across the blood–brain barrier: Relationship to iron homeostasis. *Brain Research Bulletin, 24*, 857–860.

Aspelin, A. L., & Grube, A. H. (1999). *Pesticides industry sales and usage: 1996 and 1997 market estimates*. Washington, DC: Office of Pesticide Programs, U.S. Environmental Protection Agency.

Avchen, R. N., Scott, K. G., & Mason, C. A. (2001). Birth weight and school-age disabilities: A population-based study. *American Journal of Epidemiology, 154*, 895–901.

Baghurst, P. A., McMichael, A. J., Tong, S., Wigg, N. R., Vimpani, G. V., & Robertson, E. F. (1995). Exposure to environmental lead and visual–motor integration at age 7 years: The Port Pirie cohort study. *Epidemiology, 6*, 104–109.

Baghurst, P. A., McMichael, A. J., Wigg, N. R., Vimpani, G. V., Robertson, E. F., Roberts, R. J., et al. (1992). Environmental exposure to lead and children's intelligence at the age of seven years: The Port Pirie cohort study. *New England Journal of Medicine, 327*, 1279–1284.

Barkley, R. A. (1997). Behavioral inhibition, sustained attention, and executive functions: Constructing a unifying theory of ADHD. *Psychological Bulletin, 1212*, 65–94.

Barltrop, D., & Burland, W. L. (1969). *Mineral metabolism in pediatrics*. Philadelphia: Davis.

Beckman, D. A., & Brent, R. L. (1999). Basic principles of developmental toxicology. In E. A. Reece & J. C. Hobbins (Eds.), *Medicine of the fetus and the mother* (pp. 281–288). Philadelphia, PA: Lippincott-Raven.

Bellinger, D. C. (1995a). Interpreting the literature on lead and child development: The neglected role of the experimental system. *Neurotoxicology and Teratology, 17*, 201–212.

Bellinger, D. C. (1995b). Neuropsychological function in children exposed to environmental lead. *Epidemiology, 6*, 101–103.

Bellinger, D. C. (2000). Effect modification in epidemiologic studies of low-level neurotoxicant exposure and health outcomes. *Neurotoxicology and Teratology, 22*, 133–140.

Bellinger, D. C. (2004). Assessing environmental neurotoxicant exposures and child neurobehavior: Confounded by confounding. *Epidemiology, 15*, 383–384.

Bellinger, D. C., & Dietrich, K. N. (1994). Low-level lead exposure and cognitive function in children. *Pediatric Annals, 23*, 600–605.

Bellinger, D. C., Hu, H., Titlebaum, L., & Needleman, H. L. (1994). Attentional correlates of dentin and bone lead levels in adolescents. *Archives of Environmental Health, 49*, 98–105.

Bellinger, D. C., & Rappaport, L. (2002). Developmental assessment and interventions. In B. Harvey (Ed.), *Managing elevated blood lead levels among young children: Recommendations from the Advisory*

Committee on Childhood Lead Poisoning prevention (pp. 79–95). Atlanta, GA: Centers for Disease Control and Prevention.

Bellinger, D. C., Trachtenberg, F., Barregard, L., Tavares, M., Cernichiari, E., Daniel, D., et al. (2006). Neuropsychological and renal effects of dental amalgam in children: A randomized clinical trial. *Journal of the American Medical Association, 295,* 1775–1783.

Bemis, J., & Seegal, R. (1999). Polychlorinated biphenyls and methylmercury act synergistically to reduce rat brain dopamine content *in vitro. Environmental Health Perspectives, 107,* 879–885.

Bemis, J., & Seegal, R. (2000). Polychlorinated biphenyls and methylmercury alter intracellular calcium concentrations in rat cerebellar granule cells. *Neurotoxicology, 21,* 1123–1134.

Berkowitz, G. S., Wetmur, J. G., Birman-Deych, E., Obel, J., Lapinski, R. H., Godbold, J. H., et al. (2004). *In utero* pesticide exposure, maternal paraoxonase activity, and head circumference. *Environmental Health Perspectives, 112,* 388–391.

Bernard, S., Enayati, A., Redwood, L., Roger, H., & Binstock, T. (2001). Autism: A novel form of mercury poisoning. *Medical Hypotheses, 56,* 462–471.

Bolger, P. M., Carrington, C. D., Capar, S. G., & Adams, M. A. (1991). Reductions in dietary lead exposure in the United States. *Chemical Speciation and Bioavailability, 3,* 31–36.

Bonefeld-Jorgensen, E. C., Andersen, H. R., Rasmussen, T. H., & Vinggaard, A. M. (2001). Effect of highly bioaccumulated polychlorinated biphenyl congeners on estrogen and androgen receptor activity. *Toxicology, 158,* 141–153.

Braun, J. M., Kahn, R. S., Froehlich, T., Auinger, P., & Lanphear, B. P. (2006). Exposure to environmental toxicants and attention deficit hyperactivity disorder in U.S. children. *Environmental Health Perspectives, 114,* 1904–1909.

Brent, R. L. (2001). Addressing environmentally caused human birth defects. *Pediatrics in Review, 22,* 153–165.

Budtz-Jorgensen, E., Keiding, N., Grandjean, P., White, R. F., & Weihe, P. (1999). Methylmercury neurotoxicity independent of PCB exposure. *Environmental Health Perspectives, 107,* 236–237.

Byers, R. K., & Lord, E. E. (1943). Late effects of lead poisoning on mental development. *American Journal of Diseases of Children, 66,* 471–494.

Byrd, R. (2002). The epidemiology of autism in California. Retrieved from *www.dds.ca.gov/Autism/MindReport.cfm*

Canfield, R. L., Gendle, M. H., & Cory-Slechta, D. A. (2004). Impaired neuropsychological functioning in lead-exposed children. *Developmental Neuropsychology, 9,* 35–53.

Canfield, R. L., Henderson, C. R., Cory-Slechta, D. A., Cox, C., Jusko, T. Q., & Lanphear, B. P. (2003a). Intellectual impairment in children with blood lead concentrations below 10 micrograms per deciliter. *New England Journal of Medicine, 348,* 1517–1526.

Canfield, R. L., Kreher, D. A., Cornwell, C., & Henderson, C. R. (2003b). Low-level lead exposure, executive functioning, and learning in early childhood. *Child Neuropsychology, 9,* 35–43.

Cecil, K. M., Brubaker, C. J., Adler, C. M., Dietrich, K. N., Altaye, M., Egelhoff, J. C., et al. (2008). Decreased brain volume in adults with childhood lead exposure. *PLoS Medicine, 5,* 741–750.

Center for Consumer Freedom. (2007). Fishy mercury scare based on study of whale-heavy diets, says ad in *U.S. News & World Report.* Retrieved from *www.consumerfreedom.com*

Centers for Disease Control and Prevention (CDC). (1991). *Preventing lead poisoning in young children—October 1991.* Atlanta, GA: Author.

Centers for Disease Control and Prevention (CDC). (2000a). Summary of the joint statement on thimerosal in vaccines: American Academy of Family Physicians, American Academy of Pediatrics, Advisory Committee on Immunization Practices, Public Health Service. *Morbidity and Mortality Weekly Report, 49,* 622–631.

Centers for Disease Control and Prevention (CDC). (2000b). *Recommendations for blood lead screening of young children enrolled in Medicaid: Targeting a group at-risk.* Atlanta, GA: Author.

Centers for Disease Control and Prevention (CDC). (2002). *Managing elevated blood lead levels among young children: Recommendations from the Advisory Committee on Childhood Lead Poisoning Prevention.* Atlanta, GA: Author.

Centers for Disease Control and Prevention (CDC). (2005). *Third national report on human exposure to environmental chemicals*. Atlanta, GA: Author.

Cernichiari, E., Brewer, R., Myers, G. J., Marsh, D. O., Lapham, L. W., et al. (1995). Monitoring methylmercury during pregnancy: Maternal hair predicts prenatal brain exposure. *Neurotoxicology, 16,* 705–709.

Cheek, A. O., Kow, K., Chen, J., & McLachlan, J. A. (1999). Potential mechanisms of thyroid disruption in humans: Interaction of organochlorine compounds with thyroid receptor, transthyretin, and thyroid-binding globulin. *Environmental Health Perspectives, 107,* 273–278.

Chen, Y. C. J., Guo, Y. L., Hsu, C. D., & Rogan, W. J. (1992). Cognitive development of Yu-Cheng ("oil disease") children prentally exposed to heat-degraded PCBs. *Journal of the American Medical Association, 268,* 3213–3218.

Chettle, D. R. (2005). Three decades of *in vivo* X-ray fluorescence of lead in bone. *X-Ray Spectrometry, 34,* 446–450.

Chiodo, L. M., Jacobson, S. W., & Jacobson, J. L. (2004). Neurodevelopmental effects of postnatal lead exposure at very low levels. *Neurotoxicology and Teratology, 26,* 359–371.

Clarkson, T. W. (1983). Mercury. *Annual Review of Public Health, 4,* 375–380.

Clarkson, T. W., Hursh, J. B., Sager, P. R., & Syversen, T. L. M. (1988). Mercury. In T. W. Clarkson, L. Friberg, G. F. Nordberg, & P. R. Sager (Eds.), *Biological monitoring of heavy metals* (pp. 199–246). New York: Plenum Press.

Clarkson, T. W., Magos, L., & Myers, G. J. (2003). The toxicology of mercury: Current exposures and clinical manifestations. *New England Journal of Medicine, 349,* 1731–1737.

Clements, J. C. (2004). The evidence for the safety of thimerosal in newborn and infant vaccines. *Vaccine, 22,* 1854–1861.

Cohen, J. T., Bellinger, D. C., Conner, W. E., Kris-Etherton, P. M., Lawrence, R. S., Savitz, D. A., et al. (2005). A quantitative risk–benefit analysis of changes in population fish consumption. *American Journal of Preventive Medicine, 29,* 325–334.

Conel, J. L. (1939). *The postnatal development of the human cerebral cortex*. Cambridge, MA: Harvard University Press.

Cook, D. G., & Strachan, D. P. (1999). Health effects of passive smoking: 10. Summary of effects of parental smoking on the respiratory health of children and implications for research. *Thorax, 54,* 357–366.

Cory-Slechta, D. A. (1996). Bridging human and experimental animal studies of lead neurotoxicity: Moving beyond IQ. *Neurotoxicology and Teratology, 17,* 219–221.

Costello, E. J., Mustillo, S., Erkanli, A., Keeler, G., & Angold, A. (2003). Prevalence and development of psychiatric disorders in childhood and adolescence. *Archives of General Psychiatry, 60,* 837–844.

Crump, K. S., Kjellstrom, T., Shipp, A. M., Silvers, A., & Stewart, A. (1998). Influence of prenatal mercury exposure upon scholastic and psychological test performance: Benchmark analysis of a New Zealand cohort. *Risk Analysis, 18,* 701–713.

Dakeishi, M., Murata, K., & Grandjean, P. (2006). Long-term consequences of arsenic poisoning during infancy due to contaminated milk powder. *Environmental Health: A Global Access Science Source, 5:*31 doi:10.1186/1476-069X-5-31.

David, O. J., Clark, J., & Voeller, K. (1972). Lead and hyperactivity. *Lancet, ii,* 900–903.

Davidson, P. W., Myers, G. J., Cox, C., Axtell, C., Shamlaye, C., Sloane-Reeves, J., et al. (1998). Effects of prenatal and postnatal methylmercury exposure from fish consumption on neurodevelopment: Outcomes at 66 months of age in the Seychelles Child Development Study. *Journal of the American Medical Association, 280,* 701–707.

Davidson, P. W., Myers, G. J., Cox, C., Shamlaye, C. F., Marsh, D. O., Tanner, M. A., et al. (1995). Longitudinal neurodevelopmental study of Seychellois children following *in utero* exposure to methylmercury from maternal fish ingestion: Outcomes at 19 and 29 months. *Neurotoxicology, 16,* 677–688.

Davidson, P. W., Myers, G. J., Cox, C., Wilding, G. E., Shamlaye, C. F., Huang, L., et al. (2006). Methylmercury and neurodevelopment: Longitudinal analysis of the Seychelles Child Development cohort. *Neurotoxicology and Teratology, 28,* 529–535.

Davidson, P. W., Myers, G. J., & Weiss, B. (2004). Mercury exposure and child development outcomes. *Pediatrics, 113,* 1023–1029.

Debes, F., Budtz-Jorgensen, E., Weihe, P., White, R. F., & Grandjean, P. (2006). Impact of prenatal methylmercury exposure on neurobehavioral function at age 14 years. *Neurotoxicology and Teratology, 28,* 363–375.

Denno, D. (1990). *Biology and violence: From birth to adulthood.* New York: Cambridge University Press.

DeRouen, T. A., Martin, M. D., Leroux, B. G., Townes, B. D., Woods, J. S., Leitao, J., et al. (2006). Neurobehavioral effects of dental amalgam in children: A randomized clinical trial. *Journal of the American Medical Association, 295,* 1784–1792.

Dietrich, K. N. (1996). Low-level lead exposure during pregnancy and its consequences for fetal and child development. In S. M. Pueschel, J. G. Linakis, & A. C. Anderson (Eds.), *Lead poisoning in childhood* (pp. 117–139). Baltimore: Brookes.

Dietrich, K. N. (1999). Environmental chemicals and child development. *Journal of Pediatrics, 134,* 7–9.

Dietrich, K. N. (2000). Environmental neurotoxicants and psychological development. In K. O. Yeates, M. D. Ris, & H. G. Taylor (Eds.), *Pediatric neuropsychology: Research, theory, and practice* (pp. 206–234). New York: Guilford Press.

Dietrich, K. N., Berger, O. G., & Bhattacharya, A. (2000). Symptomatic lead poisoning in infancy: A prospective case analysis. *Journal of Pediatrics, 137,* 568–571.

Dietrich, K. N., Berger, O. G., & Succop, P. A. (1993b). Lead exposure and the motor developmental status of urban six-year-old children in the Cincinnati prospective study. *Pediatrics, 91,* 301–307

Dietrich, K. N., Berger, O. G., Succop, P. A., Hammond, P. B., & Bornschein, R. L. (1993a). The developmental consequences of low to moderate prenatal and postnatal lead exposure: Intellectual attainment in the Cincinnati Lead Study cohort following school entry. *Neurotoxicology and Teratology, 15,* 301–307.

Dietrich, K. N., Eskanazi, B., Schantz, S., Yolton, K., Rauh, V. A., Johnson, C. B., et al. (2005). Principles and practices of neurodevelopmental assessment in children: Lessons learned from the Centers for Children's Environmental Health and Disease Prevention Research. *Environmental Health Perspectives, 113,* 1437–1446.

Dietrich, K. N., Krafft, K. M., Bornschein, R. L., Hammond, P. B., Berger, O., Succop, P. A., et al. (1987). Low-level fetal lead exposure effect on neurobehavioral development in early infancy. *Pediatrics, 80,* 721–730.

Dietrich, K. N., Ris, M. D., Succop, P. A., Berger, O. G., & Bornschein, R. L. (2001). Early exposure to lead and juvenile delinquency. *Neurotoxicology and Teratology, 23,* 511–518.

Dietrich, K. N., Succop, P. A., Berger, O. G., Hammond, P. B., & Bornschein, R. L. (1991). Lead exposure and the cognitive development of urban preschool children: The Cincinnati Lead Study cohort at age 4 years. *Neurotoxicology and Teratology, 13,* 203–211.

Dietrich, K. N., Succop, P. A., Berger, O. G., & Keith, R. W. (1992). Lead exposure and the central auditory processing abilities and cognitive development of urban children: The Cincinnati Lead Study cohort at age 5 years. *Neurotoxicology and Teratology, 15,* 37–44.

Dietrich, K. N., Ware, J. H., Salganik, M., Radcliffe, J., Rogan, W. J., Rhoads, G. G., et al. (2004). Effect of chelation therapy on the neuropsychological and behavioral development of lead-exposed children after school entry. *Pediatrics, 114,* 19–26.

Eskanazi, B., & Castorina, R. (1999). Association of prenatal maternal or postnatal child environmental tobacco smoke exposure and neurodevelopmental and behavioral problems in children. *Environmental Health Perspectives, 107,* 991–1000.

Espy, K. E. (1997). The Shape School: Assessing executive function in preschool children. *Developmental Neuropsychology, 13,* 495–499.

Eto, K. (1997). Pathology of Minamata disease. *Toxicologic Pathology, 25,* 614–623.

Eto, K. (2000). Minamata disease. *Neuropathology, 20,* 14–19.

Fagan, J. F., & Shephard, P. A. (1987). *The Fagan Test of Infant Intelligence.* Cleveland, OH: Infantest.

Fenske, R. A., Bradman, A., Whyatt, R. M., Wolff, M. S., & Barr, D. B. (2005). Lessons learned for the assessment of children's pesticide exposure: Critical sampling and analytical issues for future studies. *Environmental Health Perspectives, 113*, 1455–1462.

Fergusson, D. M., Fergusson, J. E., Horwood, L. J., & Kinzett, N. G. (1988). A longitudinal study of dentine lead levels, intelligence, school performance and behaviour: Part III. Dentine lead levels and attention/activity. *Journal of Child Psychology and Psychiatry, 29*, 811–824.

Froehlich, T. E., Lanphear, B. P., Dietrich, K. N., Cory-Slechta, D. A., Wang, N., & Kahn, R. S. (2007). Interactive effects of DRD4 polymorphism, lead, and sex on executive functions in children. *Biological Psychiatry, 62*, 243–249.

Gauger, K. J., Kato, Y., Haraguchi, K., Lehmler, H-J., Robertson, L. W., Bansal, R., et al. (2004). Polychlorinated biphenyls (PCBs) exert thyroid hormone-like effects in the fetal rat brain but do not bind to thyroid hormone receptors. *Environmental Health Perspectives, 112*, 516–523.

Gibson, J. L. (1904). A plea for painted railings and painted walls of rooms as the source of lead poisoning among Queensland children. *Australian Medical Gazette, 23*, 149–153.

Giesy, J. P., & Kannan, K. (1998). Dioxin-like and non-dioxin-like toxic effects of polychlorinated biphenyls (PCBs): Implications for risk assessment. *Critical Reviews in Toxicology, 28*, 511–569.

Gilbert, S. G., & Weiss, B. (2006). A rationale for lowering the blood lead action level from 10 to 2 ug/dL. *Neurotoxicology, 27*, 693–701.

Gittelman, R., & Eskenazi, B. (1983). Lead hyperactivity revisited: An investigation of nondisadvantaged children. *Archives of General Psychiatry, 40*, 827–833.

Gladen, B. C., & Rogan, W. J. (1991). Effects of perinatal polychlorinated biphenyls and dichlorodiphenyl dichloroethane on later development. *Journal of Pediatrics, 119*, 58–63.

Gochfeld, M. (2003). Cases of mercury exposure, bioavailability, and absorption. *Ecotoxicology and Environmental Safety, 56*, 174–179.

Gochfeld, M., & Burger, J. (2005). Good fish/bad fish: A composite benefit–risk by dose curve. *Neurotoxicology, 26*, 511–520.

Goldman, L. R., & Shannon, M. W. (2001). Technical report: Mercury in the environment: Implications for pediatricians. *Pediatrics, 108*, 197–205.

Goyer, R. A. (1990). Transplacental transfer of lead. *Environmental Health Perspectives, 89*, 101–105.

Goyer, R. A. (1995). Nutrition and metal toxicity. *American Journal of Clinical Nutrition, 61*(Suppl.), 646S–650S.

Grandjean, P., & Landrigan, P. J. (2006). Developmental neurotoxicity of industrial chemicals. *Lancet, 368*, 2167–2178.

Grandjean, P., & Weihe, P. (1993). Neurobehavioral effects of intrauterine mercury exposure: Potential source of bias. *Environmental Research, 61*, 176–183.

Grandjean, P., Weihe, P., Burse, V. W., Needham, L. L., Storr-Hansen, E., Heinzow, B., et al. (2001). Neurobehavioral deficits associated with PCB in 7-year-old children prenatally exposed to seafood neurotoxicants. *Neurotoxicology and Teratology, 23*, 305–317.

Grandjean, P., Weihe, P., Jorgensen, P. J., Clarkson, T., Cernichiari, E., & Videro, T. (1992). Impact of a maternal seafood diet on fetal exposure to mercury, selenium, and lead. *Archives of Environmental Health, 47*, 185–195.

Grandjean, P., Weihe, P., White, R. F., Debes, F., Araki, S., Yokoyama, K., et al. (1997). Cognitive deficit in 7-year-old children with prenatal exposure to methylmercury. *Neurotoxicology and Teratology, 19*, 417–428.

Grandjean, P., & White, R. F. (2001). Neurobehavioral dysfunction as a possible sentinel of methylmercury exposure. *Human and Ecological Risk Assessment, 7*, 1079–1089.

Grandjean, P., White, R. F., Weihe, P., & Jorgensen, P. J. (2003). Neurotoxic risk caused by stable and variable exposure to methylmercury from seafood. *Ambulatory Pediatrics, 3*, 18–23.

Guilarte, T. R., Toscano, C. D., McGlothan, J. L., & Weaver, S. (2003). Environmental enrichment reverses cognitive and molecular deficits induced by developmental lead exposure. *Annals of Neurology, 53*, 50–56.

Guillette, E. A., Menza, M. M., Aquilar, M. G., Soto, A. D., & Garcia, I. D. (1998). An anthropological approach to the evaluation of preschool children exposed to pesticides in Mexico. *Environmental Health Perspectives, 106,* 347–353.

Haddow, J. E., Palomaki, G. E., Allan, W. C., Williams, J. R., Knight, G. J., Gagnon, J., et al. (1999). Maternal thyroid deficiency during pregnancy and subsequent neuropsychological development of the child. *New England Journal of Medicine, 341,* 549–555.

Hambaugh, M., Mendoza, L. A., Burkhart, J. F., & Weil, F. (1971). The thyroid as a time clock in the developing nervous system. In D. C. Pease (Ed.), *Cellular aspects of neuronal growth and differentiation* (pp. 321–328). Berkeley: University of California Press.

Harada, M. (1976). Intrauterine poisoning: Clinical and epidemiological studies of the problem. *Bulletin of the Institute of Constitutional Medicine of Kumamoto University, 25,* 1–60.

Harada, M. (1986). Congenital Minamata disease: Intrauterine methylmercury poisoning. In J. L. Brent & R. L. Brent (Eds.), *Teratogen update: Environmental birth defect risks* (pp. 123–126). New York: Liss.

Harada, M. (1995). Minamata disease: Methylmercury poisoning in Japan caused by environmental pollution. *Critical Reviews in Toxicology, 25,* 1–24.

Hatzakis, A, Salaminios, F., Kokevi, A., Katsouyanni, K., Maravelias, K., Kalandidi, A., et al. (1985). Blood lead and classroom behaviour of children in two communities with different degree of lead exposure: Evidence of a dose-related effect? In T. D. Lekkas (Ed.), *International conference: Heavy metals in the environment* (p. 47). Edinburgh, UK: CEP Consultants.

Hersch, J. H., Podruch, R. E., Rogers, G., & Weisskopf, P. (1985). Toluene embryopathy. *Journal of Pediatrics, 106,* 922–927.

Hibbeln, J. R., Davis, J. M., Steer, C., Emmett, P., Rogers, I., Williams, C., et al. (2007). Maternal seafood consumption in pregnancy and neurodevelopmental outcomes in childhood (ALSPAC study): An observational cohort study. *Lancet, 369,* 578–585.

Hightower, J. M., & Moore, D. (2003). Mercury levels in high-end consumers of fish. *Environmental Health Perspectives, 111,* 604–608.

Hsu, S. T., Ma, C. I., Hsu, S. K., Wu, S. S., Hsu, N. H., Yeh, C. C., et al. (1985). Discovery and epidemiology of PCB poisoning in Taiwan: A four year follow-up. *Environmental Health Perspectives, 59,* 5–10.

Humphrey, H. E. B., Gardiner, J. C., Pandya, J. R., Sweeney, A. M., Gasior, D. M., McCaffrey, R. J., et al. (2000). PCB congener profile in the serum of humans consuming Great Lakes Fish. *Environmental Health Perspectives, 108,* 167–172.

Hunter, D., & Russell, D. S. (1954). Focal cerebral and cerebellar atrophy in a human subject due to organic mercury compounds. *Journal of Neurology, Neurosurgery and Psychiatry, 17,* 235–241.

Hviid, A., Stellfeld, M., Wohlfarht, J., & Melbye, M. (2003). Association between thimerosal-containing vaccine and autism. *Journal of the American Medical Association, 290,* 1763–1766.

Hynd, G. W., Semrud-Clikeman, M., Lorys, A. R., Novey, E. S., Eliopulos, D., & Lyytinen, H. (1991). Corpus callosum morphology in attention deficit-hyperactivity disorder: Morphometric analysis of MRI. *Journal of Learning Disabilities, 24,* 141–146.

Ingren, A. (1999). Manganese neurotoxicity in industrial exposures: Proof of effects, critical exposure level, and sensitive tests. *Neurotoxicology, 20,* 315–323.

Institute of Medicine. (2007). *Seafood choices: Balancing benefits and risks* (M. C. Nesheim & A. L. Yaktine, Eds.). Washington, DC: National Academy Press.

Jacobs, D. E., Clickner, R. P., Zhou, J. Y., Viet, S. M., Marker, D. A., Roger, J. W., et al. (2002). The prevalence of lead-based paint hazards in U.S. housing. *Environmental Health Perspectives, 110,* A559–A606.

Jacobson, J. L., & Jacobson, S. W. (1996a). Prospective longitudinal assessment of developmental neurotoxicity. *Environmental Health Perspectives, 104*(Suppl. 2), 275–283.

Jacobson, J. L., & Jacobson, S. W. (1996b). Intellectual impairment in children exposed to polychlorinated biphenyls *in utero. New England Journal of Medicine, 335,* 783–789.

Jacobson, J. L., & Jacobson, S. W. (2001). Postnatal exposure to PCBs and childhood development. *Lancet, 358,* 1568–1569.

Jacobson, J. L., Jacobson, S. W., Fein, G. G., Schwartz, P. M., & Dowler, J. K. (1984). Prenatal exposure to an environmental toxin: A test of the multiple effects model. *Developmental Psychology, 20,* 523–532.

Jacobson, J. L., Jacobson, S. W., & Humphrey, H. E. (1990). Effects of *in utero* exposure to polyhclroinated biphenyls and related contaminants on cognitive functioning. *Journal of Pediatrics, 116,* 38–45.

Jacobson, J. L., Jacobson, S. W., Muckle, G., Kaplan-Estrin, M., Ayotte, P., & Dewailly, E. (2008). Beneficial effects of a polyunsaturated fatty acid on infant development: Evidence from the Inuit of Arctic Quebec. *Journal of Pediatrics, 152,* 356–354.

Jacobson, J. L., Jacobson, S. W., Padgett, R. J., Brumitt, G. A., & Billings, R. L. (1992). Effects of prenatal PCB exposure on cognitive processing efficiency and sustained attention. *Developmenal Psychology, 28,* 297–306.

Jacobson, J. L., Jacobson, S. W., Sokol, R. J., Martier, S. S., Ager, J. W., & Kaplan-Estrin, M. G. (1993). Teratogenic effects of alcohol on infant development. *Alcoholsim: Clinical and Experimental Research, 17,* 174–183.

Jacobson, S. W., Fein, G. G., Jacobson, J. L., Schwartz, P. M., & Dowler, J. K. (1985). The effect of PCB exposure on visual recognition memory. *Child Development, 56,* 853–860.

Jensen, A. A. (1989). Background levels in humans. In R. D. Kimbrough & A. A. Jensen (Eds.), *Topics in environmental health: Vol. 4. Halogenated biphenyls, napthalenes, dibenzodioxins, and related products* (pp. 385–390). Amsterdam: Elsevier.

Johnson, D. L., Swank, P. R., Baldwin, C. D., & McCormick, D. (1999). Adult smoking in the home environment and children's IQ. *Psychological Reports, 84,* 149–154.

Joreskog, K. G. (1979). Statistical estimation of structural models in longitudinal–developmental investigations. In J. R. Nesselroade & P. B. Baltes (Eds.), *Longitudinal research in the study of behavior and development* (pp. 303–374). New York: Academic Press.

Kelleher, K. J., McInerny, T. K., Gardner, W. P., Childs, G. E., & Wasserman, R. C. (2000). Increasing identification of psychosocial problems: 1979–1996. *Pediatrics, 105,* 1313–1321.

Kemper, A. R., Cohn, L. M., Fant, K. E., Dombkowski, K. J., & Hudson, S. R. (2005). Follow-up testing among children with elevated screening blood lead levels. *Journal of the American Medical Association, 293,* 2232–2237.

Kerper, L. E., Ballatori, N., & Clarkson, T. W. (1992). MeHg transport across the blood–brain barrier by an amino acid carrier. *American Journal of Physiology, 262,* 761–765.

Kerper, L. W., & Hinkle, P. M. (1997). Lead uptake in brain capillary endothelial cells: Activation by calcium store depletion. *Toxicology and Applied Pharmacology, 146,* 127–133.

Kim, Y. (2004). High signal intensities on T1-weighted MRI as a biomarker of exposure to manganese. *Industrial Health, 42,* 111–115.

Kingman, A., Albertini, T., & Brown, L. J. (1998). Mercury concentrations in urine and whole blood associated with amalgam exposure in a US military population. *Journal of Dental Research, 77,* 461–471.

Kjellstrom, T., Kennedy, P., Wallis, S., & Mantell, C. (1986). *Physical and mental development of children with prenatal exposure to mercury from fish: Stage 1. Preliminary tests at age 4* (Report No. 3080). Solna: National Swedish Environmental Protection Board.

Kjellstrom, T., Kennedy, P., Wallis, S., Stewart, A., Friberg, L., Lind, B., et al. (1989). *Physical and mental development of children with prenatal exposure to mercury from fish: Stage 2. Interviews and psychological tests at age 6* (Report No. 3642). Solna: National Swedish Environmental Protection Board.

Koopman-Esseboom, C., Morse, D. C., Weisglas-Kuperus, N., Lutkeschipholt, I. J., Van der Paauw, C. G., Tuinstra, L. G., et al. (1994). Effects of dioxins and polychlorinated biphenyls on thyroid hormone status of pregnant women and their infants. *Pediatric Research, 36,* 468–473.

Kordas, K., Stoltzfus, R. J., Lopez, P., Rico, J. A., & Rosado, J. L. (2005). Iron and zinc supplementation does not improve parent or teacher ratings of behavior in first grade Mexican children exposed to lead. *Journal of Pediatrics, 147,* 632–639.

Korach, K. S., Sarver, P., Chae, K., McLachlan, J. A., & McKinney, J. D. (1987). Estrogen receptor-binding activity of polychlorinated hydroxybiphenyls: Conformationally restricted structural probes. *Molecular Pharmacology, 33,* 120–126.

Kuratsune, M. (1989). Yusho with reference to Yu-cheng. In R. D. Kimbrough & A. A. Jensen (Eds.), *Topics in environmental health: Vol. 4. Halogenated biphenyls, terphenyls, napthalanes, dibenzodioxins, and related products* (pp. 381–400). Amsterdam: Elsevier.

Lai, M. W., Boyer, E. W., Kleinman, M. E., Rodig, N. M., & Ewald, M. B. (2005). Acute arsenic poisoning in two siblings. *Pediatrics, 116,* 249–257.

Landrigan, P. J., Claudio, L., Markowitz, S. B., Berkowitz, G. S., Brenner, B. L., Romero, H., et al. (1999). Pesticides and inner-city children: Exposures, risks, and prevention. *Environmental Health Perspectives, 107*(Suppl. 3), 431–437.

Landrigan, P. J., Trasande, L., Thorpe, L. E., Gwynn, C., Lioy, P. J., D'Alton, M. E., et al. (2006). The National Children's Study: A 21-year prospective study of 100,000 American children. *Pediatrics, 118,* 2173–2186.

Lanphear, B. P. (2005). Childhood lead poisoning prevention: Too little, too late. *Journal of the American Medical Association, 293,* 2274–2276.

Lanphear, B. P., Hornung, R., Khoury, J., Yolton, K., Baghurst, P., Bellinger, D. C., et al. (2005a). Low-level environmental lead exposure and children's intellectual function: An international pooled analysis. *Environmental Health Perspectives, 113,* 894–899.

Lanphear, B. P., Vorhees, C. V., & Bellinger, D. C. (2005b). Protecting children from environmental toxins. *PLoS Medicine, 2,* e61.

Lathe, R. (2006). *Autism, brain, and environment.* London: Kingsley.

Lavelle, M. (2007, December 19). The end of the light bulb as we know it. *U.S. News and World Report,* posted *www.usnews.com* accessed 6.23.2009.

Lenz, W. (1988). A short history of thalidomide embryopathy. *Teratology, 38,* 203–215.

Levy, B. S., & Nassetta, W. J. (2003). Neurologic effects of manganese in humans: A review. *International Journal of Occupational and Environmental Health, 9,* 153–163.

Lidsky, T. I., & Schneider, J. S. (2003). Lead neurotoxicity in children: Basic mechanisms and clinical correlates. *Brain, 126,* 5–19.

Lidsky, T. I., & Schneider, J. S. (2006). Adverse effects of childhood lead poisoning: The clinical neuropsychological perspective. *Environmental Research, 100,* 284–293.

Litovitz, T. L., Klein-Schwartz, W., Rodgers, G. C., Cobaugh, D., Youniss, J., Omslaer, J. C., et al. (2002). 2001 annual report of the American Association of Poison Centers toxic exposure surveillance system. *American Journal of Emergency Medicine, 20,* 391–452.

Liu, X., Dietrich, K. N., Radcliffe, J., Ragan, N. B., Rhoads, G. G., & Rogan, W. J. (2002). Do children with falling blood lead levels have improved cognition? *Pediatrics, 110,* 787–791.

Lonky, E., Reihman, J., Darvill, T., Mather, J., Sr., & Daly, H. (1996). Neonatal Behavioral Assessment Scale performance in humans influenced by maternal consumption of environmentally contaminated Lake Ontario fish. *Journal of Great Lakes Research, 22,* 198–212.

Lu, C., Barr, D. B., Pearson, M. A., & Waller, L. A. (2008). Dietary intake and its contribution to longitudinal organophosphorus pesticide exposure in urban/suburban children. *Environmental Health Perspectives, 116,* 537–542.

Lyoo, I. K., Noam, G. G., Lee, C. K., Kennedy, B. P., & Renshaw, P. F. (1996). The corpus callosum and lateral ventricles in children with attention deficit hyperactivity disorder: A magnetic resonance imaging study. *Biological Psychiatry, 40,* 1060–1063.

Mannino, D. M., Albalak, R., Grosse, S., & Repace, J. (2003). Second-hand smoke exposure and blood lead levels in U.S. children. *Epidemiology, 14,* 719–727.

Marsh, D. O., Clarkson, T. W., Cox, C., & Myers, G. J. (1987). Fetal methylmercury poisoning. *Archives of Neurology, 44,* 1017–1022.

Marsh, D. O., Clarkson, T. W., Myers, G. J., Davidson, P. W., Cox, C., Cernichiari, E., et al. (1995). The Seychelles study of fetal methylmercury exposure and child development: Introduction. *Neurotoxicology, 16,* 583–596.

Masuda, Y., Kagawa, R., Kuroki, H., Kuratsune, M., Yoshimura, T., Taki, I., et al. (1978). Transfer of polychlorinated biphenyls from mothers to fetuses and infants. *Food and Cosmetic Toxicology, 16,* 543–546.

May, M. (2000). Disturbing behavior: Neurotoxic effects in children. *Environmental Health Perspectives, 108,* A262–A267.

McMichael, A. J., Baghurst, P. A., Wigg, N. R. Vimpani, G. V., Robertson, E. F., & Roberts, R. J. (1988). Port Pirie cohort study: Environmental exposure to lead and children's abilities at the age of four years. *New England Journal of Medicine, 319,* 468–475.

Meng, X. M., Zhu, D. M., Ruan, D. Y., She, J. Q., & Luo, L. (2005). Effects of chronic lead exposure on H MRS of hippocampus and frontal lobes in children. *Neurology, 64,* 1644–1647.

Miettinen, J. K. (1973). Absorption and elimination of dietary Hg and methylmercury in man. In M. W. Miller & T. W. Clarkson (Eds.), *Mercury, mercurials, and mercaptans* (pp. 233–240). Springfield, IL: Thomas.

Mirsky, A. F. (1987). Behavioral and psychophysiological markers of disordered attention. *Environmental Health Perspectives, 74,* 191–199.

Mishima, A. (1992). *Bitter sea: The human cost of Minamata disease.* Tokyo: Kosei.

Muckle, G., Ayotte, P., Dewailly, E., Jacobson, S. W., & Jacobson, J. L. (2001). Prenatal exposure of the northern Quebec Inuit infants to environmental contaminants. *Environmental Health Perspectives, 109,* 1291–1299.

Myers, G. J., Davidson, P. W., Cox, C., Shamlaye, C. F., Palumbo, D., Cernichiari, E., et al. (2003). Prenatal methylmercury exposure from ocean fish consumption in the Seychelles Child Development Study. *Lancet, 361,* 1686–1692.

Myers, G. J., Marsh, D. O., Davidson, P. W., Cox, C., Shamlaye, C. F., Tanner, M., Cernichiari, E., et al. (1995). Main neurodevelopmental study of Seychellois children following *in utero* exposure to methylmercury from a maternal fish diet: Outcomes at six months. *Neurotoxicology, 16,* 653–664.

National Institute of Mental Health (NIMH). (2006). Mercury chelation to treat autism. Retrieved from *www.clinicaltrials.gov/ct/show/NCT00376194*

National Research Council (NRC). (2000). *Toxicological effects of methylmercury.* Washington, DC: National Academy Press.

Needham, L. L., Calafat, A. M., & Barr, D. B. (2008). Assessing developmental toxicant exposures via biomonitoring. *Basic and Clinical Pharmacology and Toxicology, 102,* 100–108.

Needleman, H. L. (1992). Salem comes to the National Institutes of Health: Notes from inside the crucible of scientific integrity. *Pediatrics, 90,* 977–981.

Needleman, H. L. (2004). Lead poisoning. *Annual Review of Medicine, 55,* 209–222.

Needleman, H. L. (2006). Mercury in dental amalgam: A neurotoxic risk? *Journal of the American Medical Association, 295,* 1835–1836.

Needleman, H. L., & Gatsonis, C. A. (1990). Low-level lead exposure and the IQ of children: A meta-analysis of modern studies. *Journal of the American Medical Association, 263,* 673–678.

Needleman, H. L., Gunnoe, C., Leviton, A., Reed, R., Peresie, H., Maer, C., et al. (1979). Deficits in psychologic and classroom performance of children with elevated dentine lead levels. *New England Journal of Medicine, 300,* 689–695.

Needleman, H. L., McFarland, C., Ness, R. B., Fienberg, S. E., & Tobin, M. J. (2002). Bone lead levels in adjudicated delinquents. A case–control study. *Neurotoxicology and Teratology, 24,* 711–717.

Needleman, H. L., Riess, J. A., Tobin, M. J., Biesecker, G. E., & Greenhouse, J. B. (1996). Bone lead levels and delinquent behavior. *Journal of the American Medical Association, 275,* 363–369.

Needleman, H. L., Tuncay, O. C., & Shapiro, I. M. (1972). Lead levels in deciduous teeth of urban and suburban American children. *Nature, 235,* 111–112.

Nelson, K. B., & Bauman, M. L. (2003). Thimerosal and autism? *Pediatrics, 111,* 674–678.

Nevin, R. (2000). How lead exposure relates to temporal changes in IQ, violent crime, and unwed pregnancy. *Environmental Research, 83,* 1–22.

Nevin, R. (2007). Understanding international crime trends: The legacy of preschool lead exposure. *Environmental Research, 104,* 315–336.

Nightingale, S. L. (1991). Succimer (DMSA) approved for severe lead poisoning. *Journal of the American Medical Association, 265,* 1802.

Nolte, J. (1993). *The human brain: An introduction to its functional neuroanatomy.* New York: Mosby–Year Book.

Office of Applied Studies. (2006). *Results from the National Survey on Drug Use and Health: National findings* (DHHS Publication No. SMA 06-4194, NSDUH Series No. H-30). Rockville, MD: Substance Abuse and Mental Health Services Administration.

Olanow, C. W. (2004). Manganese-induced parkinsonism and Parkinson's disease. *Annals of the New York Academy of Sciences, 1012,* 209–223.

Pal, P. K., Samili, A., & Caine, D. B. (1999). Manganese neurotoxicity: A review of clinical features, imaging and pathology. *Neurotoxicology, 20,* 227–238.

Parker, S. K., Schwartz, B., Todd, J., & Pickering, L. K. (2004). Thimerosal-containing vaccines and autism spectrum disorder: A critical review of published studies. *Pediatrics, 114,* 793–804.

Patandin, S., Lanting, C. J., Mulder, P. G. H., Boersma, E. R., Sauer, P. J. J., & Weisglas-Kuperus, N. (1999). Effects of environmental exposure to polychlorinated biphenyls and dioxins on cognitive abilities in Dutch children at 42 months of age. *Journal of Pediatrics, 134,* 33–41.

Pearce, N. (1989). Analytical implications of the epidemiological concept of interaction. *International Journal of Epidemiology, 18,* 976–980.

Pearson, M. A., Hoyme, E., Seaver, L. H., & Rimsza, M. A. (1994). Toluene embryopathy: Delineation of the phenotype and comparison with fetal alcohol syndrome. *Pediatrics, 93,* 211–215.

Phelps, R. W., Clarkson, T. W., Kershaw, T. G., & Wheatley, B. (1980). Interrelationships of blood and hair mercury concentrations in a North American population exposed to methylmercury. *Archives of Environmental Health, 35,* 161–168.

Pirkle, J. L., Flegal, K. M., Bernert, J. T., Brody, D. J., Etzel, R. A., & Maurer, K. R. (1996). Exposure of the US population to environmental tobacco smoke: The Third National Health and Nutrition Examination Survey, 1988–1991. *Journal of the American Medical Association, 275,* 1233–1240.

Plunkett, L. M. (2007). Developmental neurotoxicity of industrial chemicals (letter). *Lancet, 369,* 821.

Pocock, S. J., Smith, M., & Baghurst, P. (1994). Environmental lead and children's intelligence: A systematic review of the epidemiological evidence. *British Medical Journal, 309,* 1189–1197.

Porterfield, S. P. (1994). Vulnerability of the developing brain to thyroid abnormalities: Environmental insults to the thyroid system. *Environmental Health Perspectives, 102*(Suppl. 2), 125–130.

Rabinowitz, M. B. (1991). Toxicokinetics of bone lead. *Environmental Health Perspectives, 91,* 33–37.

Rauh, V. A., Garfinkel, R., Perera, F. P., Andrews, H. F., Hoepner, L., Barr, D. B., et al. (2006). Impact of prenatal chlorpyrofos exposure on neurodevelopment in the first 3 years of life among inner-city children. *Pediatrics, 118,* e1845–e1859.

Rice, D. C. (1996). Lessons for neurotoxicology from selected model compounds: SGOMSEC joint report. *Environmental Health Perspectives, 104*(Suppl. 2), S205–S215.

Rice, D. C. (1999). Behavioral impairment produced by low-level postnatal PCB exposure in monkeys. *Environmental Research, 80,* S113–S121.

Rico, J. A., Kordas, K., Lopez, P., Rosado, J. L., Vargas, G. G., Ronquillo, D., et al. (2006). Efficacy of iron and/or zinc supplementation on cognitive performance of lead-exposed Mexican schoolchildren: A randomized, placebo-controlled trial. *Pediatrics, 117*(3), e518–e527.

Riley, E. P., & Vorhees, C. V. (Eds.). (1986). *Handbook of behavioral teratology.* New York: Kluwer Academic.

Ris, M. D., Dietrich, K. N., Succop, P. A., Berger, O. G., & Bornschein, R. L. (2004). Early exposure to lead and neuropsychological outcome in adolescence. *Journal of the International Neuropsychological Society, 10,* 261–270.

Rodier, P. M. (1995). Developing brain as a target of toxicity. *Environmental Health Perspectives, 103*(Suppl. 6), 73–76.

Rodier, P. M. (2004). Environmental causes of central nervous system maldevelopment. *Pediatrics, 113,* 1076–1083.

Rogan, W. J. (1998). The Treatment of Lead Exposed Children (TLC) trial: Design and recruitment for a study of the effect of oral chelation on growth and development in toddlers. *Paediatric and Perinatal Epidemiology, 12*, 313–333.

Rogan, W. J., Dietrich, K. N., Ware, J. H., Dockery, D. W., Salganik, M., Radcliffe, J., et al. (2001). The effect of chelation therapy with succimer on neuropsychological development in children exposed to lead. *New England Journal of Medicine, 344*, 1421–1426.

Rogan, W. J., & Gladen, B. C. (1993). Breast-feeding and cognitive development. *Early Human Development, 31*, 181–193.

Rogan, W. J., Gladen, B. C., Hung, K., Koong, S., Shih, L., Taylor, J. S., et al. (1988). Congenital poisoning by polychlorinated biphenyls and their contaminants in Taiwan. *Science, 241*, 334–336.

Rogan, W. J., Gladen, B. C., McKinney, J. B., Carreras, N., Hardy, P., Thullen, J., et al. (1986). Neonatal effects of transplacental exposure to PCBs and DDE. *Journal of Pediatrics, 109*, 335–341.

Rosen, J. F., & Mushak, P. (2001). Primary prevention of childhood lead poisoning: The only solution. *New England Journal of Medicine, 344*, 1470–1471.

Rourke, B. P. (2000). Review and future directions. In K. O. Yeates, M. D. Ris, & H. G. Taylor (Eds.), *Pediatric neuropsychology: Research, theory, and practice* (pp. 459–469). New York: Guilford Press.

Ruckart, P. Z., Kakolewski, K., Bove, F. J., & Kay, W. E. (2004). Long-term neurobehavioral health effects of methyl parathion exposure in children in Mississippi and Ohio. *Environmental Health Perspectives, 112*, 45–51.

Ruff, H. A., Bijur, P. E., Markowitz, M. E., Ma, Y. C., & Rosen, J. F. (1993). Declining blood lead levels and cognitive changes in moderately lead-poisoned children. *Journal of the American Medical Association, 269*, 1641–1646.

Rutter, M. (2005). Incidence of autism spectrum disorders: Changes over time and their meaning. *Acta Paediatrica, 94*, 2–15.

Safer, D. J., Zito, J. M., & Fine, E. M. (1996). Increased methylphenidate usage for attention deficit disorder in the 1990s. *Pediatrics, 98*, 1084–1088.

Schantz, S. L., Widholm, J. J., & Rice, D. C. (2003). Effects of PCB exposure on neuropsychological function in children. *Environmental Health Perspectives, 111*, 357–376.

Schettler, T., Stein, J., Reich, F., & Valenti, M. (2000). *In harm's way: Toxic threats to child development.* Boston: Greater Boston Physicians for Social Responsibility.

Schneider, J. S., Lee, M. H., Anderson, D. W., Zuck, L., & Lidsky, T. I. (2001). Enriched environment during development is protective against lead-induced neurotoxicity. *Brain Research, 896*, 48–55.

Schwartz, J. (1994). Low-level lead exposure and children's IQ: A meta-analysis and search for a threshold. *Environmental Research, 65*, 42–55.

Schwartz, P. M., Jacobson, S. W., Fein, G. G., Jacobson, J. L., & Price, H. (1983). Lake Michigan fish consumption as a source of polychlorinated biphenyls in human cord serum, maternal serum, and milk. *Public Health Briefs, 73*, 293–296.

Schwemberger, J. G., Mosby, J. E., Jacobs, D. E., Ashley, P. J., Brody, D. J., Brown, M. J., et al. (2005). Blood lead levels—United States, 1999–2002. *Mortality and Morbidity Weekly Report, 54*, 513–516.

Seegal, R. F. (2000). The neurotoxicological consequences of developmental exposure to PCBs. *Toxicological Sciences, 57*, 1–3.

Shirai, J. H., & Kissel, J. C. (1996). Uncertainty in estimated half-lives of PCBs in humans: Impact on exposure assessment. *Science of the Total Environment, 187*, 199–210.

Silbergeld, E. K. (1992). Mechanism of lead neurotoxicity, or looking beyond the lamppost. *FASEB Journal, 6*, 3201–3206.

Silva, P. A., Hughes, P., Williams, S., & Faed, J. M. (1988). Blood lead, intelligence, reading attainment, and behaviour in eleven year old children in Dunedin, New Zealand. *Journal of Child Psychology and Psychiatry, 29*, 43–52.

Slikker, W., & Miller, R. K. (1994). Placental metabolism and transfer: Role in developmental toxicology. In C. A. Kimmel & J. Buelke-Sam (Eds.), *Developmental toxicology* (pp. 245–283). New York: Raven Press.

Smith, W. E., & Smith, A. W. (1975). *Minamata.* New York: Holt, Rinehart & Winston.

Spreen, O., Risser, A. T., & Edgell, D. (1995). *Developmental neuropsychology.* New York: Oxford University Press.

Stewart, P. W., Darvill, T., Lonky, E., Reihman, J., Pagano, J., & Bush, B. (1999). Assessment of prenatal exposure to PCBs from maternal consumption of Great Lakes fish: An analysis of PCB pattern and concentration. *Environmental Research, 80*(2, Pt. 2), S87–S96.

Stewart, P. W., Fitzgerald, S., Reihman, J., Gump, B., Lonky, E., Darvill, T., et al. (2003a). Prenatal PCB exposure, the corpus callosum, and response inhibition. *Environmental Health Perspectives, 111,* 1670–1677.

Stewart, P. W., Reihman, J., Lonky, E., Darvill, T., & Pagano, J. (2000). Prenatal PCB exposure and Neonatal Behavioral Assessment Scale (NBAS) performance. *Neurotoxicology and Teratology, 22,* 21–29.

Stewart, P. W., Reihman, J., Lonky, E. I., Darvill, T. S., & Pagano, J. (2003b). Cognitive development in preschool children prenatally exposed to PCBs and MeHg. *Neurotoxicology and Teratology, 25,* 11–22.

Stewart, P. W., Sargent, D. M., Reihman, J., Gump, B. B., Lonky, E., Darvill, T., et al. (2006). Response inhibition during differential reinforcement low rates (DRL) schedules may be sensitive to low-level polychlorinated biphenyl, methylmercury, and lead exposure. *Environmental Health Perspectives, 114,* 1923–1929.

Stiles, K. M., & Bellinger, D. C. (1993). Neuropsychological correlates of low-level lead exposure in school-age children: A prospective study. *Neurotoxicology and Teratology, 15,* 27–35.

Stretesky, P. B., & Lynch, M. J. (2001). The relationship between lead exposure and homicide. *Archives of Pediatrics and Adolescent Medicine, 155,* 579–582.

Takeuchi, T. (1968). Pathology of Minamata disease. In M. Kutsuma (Ed.), *Minamata disease* (pp. 141–228). Kumamoto, Japan: Kumamoto University, Study Group of Minamata Disease.

Takeuchi, T. (1977). Pathology of fetal Minamata disease. The effect of methylmercury on intrauterine life of human beings. *Pediatrician, 6,* 69–87.

Tasker, L., Mergler, D., Hellier, G., Sahuquillo, J., & Huel, G. (2003). Manganese, monoamine metabolite levels at birth, and child psychomotor development. *Neurotoxicology, 24,* 667–674.

Tellez-Rojo, M. M., Bellinger, D. C., Arroyo-Quiroz, C., Lamadrid-Figueroa, H., Mercado-Garcia, A., Schnaas-Arrieta, L., et al. (2006). Longitudinal associations between blood lead concentrations lower than 10 µg/dL and neurobehavioral development in environmentally exposed children in Mexico City. *Pediatrics, 118,* e323–e330.

Thomson, G. O. B., Raab, G. M., Hepburn, W. S., Fulton, M., & Laxen, D. P. H. (1989). Blood lead levels and children's behaviour: Results from the Edinburgh lead study. *Journal of Child Psychology and Psychiatry, 30,* 515–528.

Tong, S., Baghurst, P. A., Sawyer, M. G., Burns, J., & McMichael, A. J. (1998). Declining blood lead levels and changes in cognitive function during childhood: The Port Pirie cohort study. *Journal of the American Medical Association, 280,* 1915–1919.

Tong, S., McMichael, A. J., & Baghurst, P. A. (2000). Interactions between environmental lead exposure and sociodemographic factors on cognitive development. *Archives of Environmental Health, 55,* 330–335.

Trope, I., Lopez-Villegas, D., Cecil, K. M., & Lenkinski, R. E. (2001). Exposure to lead appears to selectively alter metabolism of cortical gray matter. *Pediatrics, 107,* 1437–1443.

Trope, I., Lopez-Villegas, D., & Lenkinski, R. E. (1998). Magnetic resonance imaging and spectroscopy of regional brain structure in a 10-year-old boy with elevated blood lead levels. *Pediatrics, 101,* e7.

U.S. Department of Health and Human Services. (2004). *The health consequences of smoking: A report of the Surgeon General—2004.* Atlanta, GA: Centers for Disease Control and Prevention.

U.S. Environmental Protection Agency (U.S. EPA). (1997). *Mercury study report to Congress.* Washington, DC: Author.

U.S. Environmental Protection Agency (U.S. EPA). (2006). *Air quality criteria for lead* (Chapter 6.2, Neurotoxic effects of lead in children). Research Triangle Park, NC: National Center for Environmental Assessment—RTP Division, U.S. Environmental Protection Agency.

Verity, M. A. (1997). Pathogenesis of methyl mercury neurotoxicity. In M. Yasui, M. J. Strong, K. Ota, & M. A. Verity (Eds.), *Mineral and metal neurotoxicology* (pp. 159–167). Boca Raton, FL: CRC Press.

Vreugdenhil, H. J., Lanting, C. I., Mulder, P. G., Boersma, E. R., & Weisglas-Kuperus, N. (2002). Effects of prenatal PCB and dioxin background exposure on cognitive and motor abilities of Dutch children at school age. *Journal of Pediatrics, 140,* 48–56.

Vreugdenhil, H. J. I., Mulder, P. G. H., Emmen, H. H., & Weisglas-Kuperus, N. (2004). Effects of perinatal PCBs on neuropsychological functions in the Rotterdam cohort at 9 years of age. *Neuropsychology, 18,* 185–193.

Wainright, P. E. (2002). Dietary essential fatty acids and brain function: A developmental perspective on mechanisms. *Proceedings of the Nutrition Society, 61,* 61–69.

Walkowiak, J., Wiener, J.-A, Fastabend, A., Heinzow, B., Kramer, U., Schmidt, E., et al. (2001). Environmental exposure to polychlorinated biphenyls and quality of the home environment: Effects on psychomotor development in early childhood. *Lancet, 358,* 1602–1607.

Wallis, C. (2007, January 12). Is the autism epidemic a myth? *Time,* posted January 12, 2007 *www.time.com* accessed June 23, 2009.

Warkany, J. (1966). Acrodynia: Postmortem of a disease. *American Journal of Diseases of Children, 112,* 147–156.

Wasserman, G. A., Graziano, J. H., Factor-Litvak, P., Popovac, D., Morina, N., Musabegovic, A., et al. (1994). Consequences of lead exposure and iron supplementation on childhood development at age 4 years. *Neurotoxicology and Teratology, 16,* 233–240.

Wasserman, G. A., Liu, X., Parvez, F. Ahsan, H., Factor-Litvak, P., van Geen, A., et al. (2004). Water arsenic exposure and children's intellectual function in Araihazar, Bangladesh. *Environmental Health Perspectives, 112,* 1329–1333.

Wasserman, G. A., Liu, X., Parvez, F., Ahsan, H., Levy, D., Factor-Litvak, P., et al. (2006). Water manganese exposure and children's intellectual function in Araihazar, Bangladesh. *Environmental Health Perspectives, 114,* 124–129.

Wasserman, G. A., Musabegovic, A., Liu, X., Kline, J., Factor-Litvak, P., & Graziano, J. H. (2000). Lead exposure and motor functioning in 4½-year-old children: The Yugoslavia prospective study. *Journal of Pediatrics, 137,* 555–561.

Wasserman, G. A., Staghezza-Jaramillo, B., Shrout, P., Popovac, D., & Graziano, J. (1998). The effect of lead exposure on behavior problems in preschool children. *American Journal of Public Health, 88,* 481–486.

Weihe, P., Grandjean, P., Debes, F., & White, R. (1996). Health implications for Faroe Islanders of heavy metals and PCBs from pilot whales. *Science of the Total Environment, 186,* 141–148.

Weiss, B. (1997). Pesticides as a source of developmental disabilities. *Mental Retardation and Developmental Disabilities Research Reviews, 3,* 246–256.

Weiss, B. (2004). Pesticides. *Pediatrics, 113,* 1030–1036.

Weiss, B., & Bellinger, D. C. (2006). Social ecology of children's vulnerability to environmental pollutants. *Environmental Health Perspectives, 114,* 1479–1485.

Weiss, B., & Landrigan, P. J. (2000). The developing brain and the environment: An introduction. *Environmental Health Perspectives, 107*(Suppl. 3), 373–374.

Wheatley, B., & Pradis, S. (1998). Northern exposure: Further analysis of the results of the Canadian aboriginal methylmercury program. *International Journal of Circumpolar Health, 57*(Suppl. 1), 586–590.

White, R. F., Debes, F., Dahl, R., & Grandjean, P. (1994). Development and field testing of a neuropsychological battery to assess the effects of methylmercury exposure in the Faroe Islands. In *Proceedings of the International Symposium on Assessment of Environmental Pollution and Health Effects of Methylmercury* (pp. 127–140). Kumamoto, Japan: Kumammoto University.

Wigle, D. T., & Lanphear, B. P. (2005). Human health risks from low-level environmental exposures: No apparent safety thresholds. *PLoS Medicine, 2,* 1232–1234.

Wilson, D. C., Tubman, T. R., Halliday, H. L., & McMaster, D. (1992). Plasma manganese levels in the very low birth weight infant are high in early life. *Biology of the Neonate, 61,* 42–46.

Wilson, J. G. (1973). *Environment and birth defects.* New York: Academic Press.

Winneke, G., Brockhaus, A., Ewers, U., Kramer, U., & Neuf, M. (1990). Results from the European multicenter study on lead neurotoxicity in children. *Neurotoxicology and Teratology, 12,* 553–559.

Woods, J. S., Martin, M. D., Leroux, B. G., DeRouen, T. A., Leitao, J. G., Bernardo, M. F., et al. (2007). The contribution of dental amalgam to urinary mercury excretion. *Environmental Health Perspectives, 115,* 1527–1531.

World Health Organization (WHO), International Programme on Chemical Safety. (1981). *Environmental health criteria 18: Arsenic.* Geneva: Author.

World Health Organization (WHO), International Programme on Chemical Safety. (1995). *Environmental health criteria 165: Inorganic lead.* Geneva: Author.

Wright, J. P., Dietrich, K. N., Ris, M. D., Hornung, R. W., Wessel, S. D., Lanphear, B. P., et al. (2008). Association of prenatal and childhood blood lead concentrations with criminal arrests in early adulthood. *PLoS Medicine, 5,* 732–740.

Wright, R. O., Amarasiriwardena, D., Woolf, A. D., Jim, R., & Bellinger, D. C. (2006). Neuropsychological correlates of hair arsenic, manganese, and cadmium levels in school-age children residing near a hazardous waste site. *Neurotoxicology, 27,* 210–216.

Yamashita, F., & Hayashi, M. (1985). Fetal PCB syndrome: Clinical features, intrauterine growth retardation and possible alteration in calcium metabolism. *Environmental Health Perspectives, 59,* 41–45.

Yeates, K. O., & Mortensen, M. E. (1994). Acute and chronic neuropsychological consequences of mercury vapor poisoning in two early adolescents. *Journal of Clinical and Experimental Neuropsychology, 16,* 209–222.

Yolton, K., Dietrich, K., Auinger, P., Lanphear, B. P., & Hornung, R. (2005). Exposure to environmental tobacco smoke and cognitive abilities among U.S. children and adolescents. *Environmental Health Perspectives, 113,* 98–113.

Young, J. G., Eskenazi, B., Gladstone, E. A., Bradman, A., Pedersen, L., Johnson, C., et al. (2005). Association between *in utero* oganophosphate pesticide exposure and abnormal reflexes in neonates. *Neurotoxicology, 26,* 199–209.

Yuan, W., Holland, S. K., Cecil, K. M., Dietrich, K. N., Wessel, S. D., Altaye, M., et al. (2006). The impact of early childhood lead exposure on brain organization: A functional magnetic resonance imaging study of language function. *Pediatrics, 118,* 971–977.

Yule, W., Urbanowicz, M. A., Lansdown, R., & Millar, I. B. (1984). Teachers' ratings of children's behavior in relation to blood lead levels. *British Journal of Developmental Psychology, 2,* 295–305.

Zhang, G., Liu, D., & He, P. (1995). Effects of manganese on learning abilities in school children. *Zhonghua Yu Fang Yi Xue Za Zhi, 29,* 156–158. (In Chinese)

Zheng, W., Aschner, M., & Ghersi-Egea, J.-F. (2003). Brain barrier systems: A new frontier in metal neurotoxicological research. *Toxicology and Applied Pharmacology, 192,* 1–11.

CHAPTER 10

Fetal Alcohol Spectrum Disorders

SARAH N. MATTSON
LINNEA VAURIO

HISTORICAL OVERVIEW AND DIAGNOSTIC CRITERIA

Although historical documentation suggests that the teratogenic effects of prenatal alcohol exposure have been known for centuries, fetal alcohol syndrome (FAS) was not recognized until 1973, when Kenneth Lyons Jones and David Smith described 11 children born to alcohol-abusing mothers (Jones, Smith, Ulleland, & Streissguth, 1973). Based on the examination of this small group of children, Jones and Smith (1973) delineated a pattern of malformation for FAS consisting of prenatal growth deficiency, developmental delay, craniofacial abnormality, and limb defects. Since the original description of FAS, diagnostic criteria have remained relatively consistent. According to the Centers for Disease Control and Prevention (CDC) and a recent clarification of the Institute of Medicine (IOM) guidelines (Bertrand, Floyd, & Weber, 2005; Hoyme et al., 2005; Stratton, Howe, & Battaglia, 1996), abnormalities in three domains are required for a diagnosis of FAS: prenatal or postnatal growth deficiency (growth ≤10th centile after adjustment for age, sex, gestational age, and race or ethnicity); specific pattern of facial dysmorphia (palpebral fissures ≤10th centile, smooth philtrum, and thin vermillion border); and evidence of central nervous system (CNS) dysfunction. These CNS deficits can vary from severe mental retardation to subtle nervous system dysfunction and can be structural, neurological, or functional. Structural deficits may be documented by neuroimaging or head circumference ≤10th centile, and functional deficits are defined as performance at or below the 3rd centile in global intelligence or in three or more specific functional domains (e.g., attention, motor functioning, or social skills). The criteria set forth by the CDC and the IOM vary slightly, with the CDC requiring all three facial features to be present, and the IOM requiring only two of three. However, the IOM guidelines as clarified by Hoyme et al. (2005) are more restrictive than those of the CDC in terms of the CNS abnormality (requiring either structural brain abnormalities as seen on neuroimaging or head circumference ≤10th centile), but do not include functional deficits as possible diagnostic criteria. Although the combination of the three criteria, including the facial features, is considered unique, several partial phenocopies (e.g., velocardiofacial, Williams, and de Lange syndromes) exist and should be ruled out prior to diagnosing FAS (Hoyme et al., 2005).

Early reports focused exclusively on children with FAS; however, converging and increasing evidence suggests that individuals exposed to large amounts of alcohol who do not have the physical markers seen in FAS have similar neurobehavioral deficits. Various terms have been used to describe individuals who are affected by the teratogenic effects of alcohol but who may not show all physical symptoms of FAS: *alcohol-related neurodevelopmental disorder, alcohol-related birth defects, fetal alcohol effects,* and *static encephalopathy.* The IOM guidelines (Hoyme et al., 2005; Stratton et al., 1996) provide criteria for the diagnosis of partial FAS, alcohol-related birth defects, and alcohol-related neurodevelopmental disorder, to facilitate identification of individuals with prenatal exposure to alcohol who may not meet all diagnostic criteria for FAS.

To acknowledge the continuum of deficits caused by prenatal alcohol exposure, the National Task Force on Fetal Alcohol Syndrome and Fetal Alcohol Effect adopted the term *fetal alcohol spectrum disorders* (FASD) (Bertrand et al., 2004), which was originally coined by the nonprofit organization NoFAS (*www.nofas.org*). FASD is not a diagnostic category, but an umbrella term used to emphasize the range of deleterious physical, mental, and behavioral outcomes that can occur with exposure to alcohol; FAS falls at the severe end of this spectrum of outcomes. In this chapter, we use the term FASD and focus on children with heavy prenatal alcohol exposure, including those with and without FAS. When we present results, the two groups are combined unless group differences have been found, in which case differences are made explicit.

EPIDEMIOLOGY

FAS and FASD are caused by maternal consumption of alcohol during pregnancy. Alcohol is recognized as toxic to the developing CNS (Stratton et al., 1996). Because alcohol freely crosses the placenta, a mother's blood alcohol content will be the same as that of the developing embryo or fetus, leading to CNS and other damage. Despite a proliferation of evidence demonstrating toxic effects of prenatal alcohol exposure, pregnant women continue to use alcohol. Approximately 10% of pregnant women in the United States report drinking alcohol during pregnancy, and 52.6% of women of childbearing age report drinking alcohol at risk levels, defined as consumption of five or more drinks on one occasion or seven or more drinks per week (CDC, 2004). Thus, although FASD is preventable, continued efforts are needed both to delineate effects and to develop intervention strategies suitable for children affected by prenatal alcohol exposure.

Estimates of the prevalence of FAS in the United States range between 0.5 and 2.0 cases per 1,000 live births, with current incidence estimates suggesting that 1,000–6,000 infants with FAS are born in the United States each year (Bertrand et al., 2005). However, as previously discussed, FAS is only one outcome along a spectrum of possible effects, and the variability in this spectrum makes estimating the prevalence and incidence of FASD more challenging. Prevalence estimates are as high as 1 per 100 live births (Sampson et al., 1997). A recent review estimated median adjusted annual expenditures for all individuals with FAS in the United States as $3.6 billion (Lupton, Burd, & Harwood, 2004). This estimate included costs associated with medical services, residential services, special education services, and lost productivity. Total lifetime cost per individual with FAS was estimated to be $2.9 million. No current estimates are available for costs associated with the full spectrum of outcomes of alcohol exposure. However, from the prevalence and incidence estimates given about, it can be assumed that expenditures increase dramatically when the full population with FASD is considered.

NEUROPATHOLOGY AND NEURAL SUBSTRATES

The brain is particularly sensitive to the teratogenic effects of alcohol exposure. In general, the patterns of brain size reduction and abnormality seen in imaging studies of individuals with FAS are also observed in individuals with nondysmorphic FASD, but with somewhat decreased severity (Riley, McGee, & Sowell, 2004; Roebuck, Mattson, & Riley, 1998a). See Table 10.1 for a summary of findings of brain changes noted in individuals with FASD.

Reduction in Total Brain Volume

One of the diagnostic features of FAS is head circumference ≤10th centile. Therefore, it is not surprising that consistent findings in neuroimaging investigations of FASD include reduced cranial vault and reduction of overall brain size (Archibald et al., 2001; Johnson, Swayze, Sato, & Andreasen, 1996; Mattson et al., 1994; Mattson et al., 1996c; Riikonen, Salonen, Partanen, & Verho, 1999; Swayze et al., 1997). As a result of overall reduction in brain size, examination of the specificity of alcohol's effects on CNS functioning is important. A pattern of diffuse and consistent overall reduction may indicate global effects of prenatal alcohol exposure, whereas a pattern of disproportionate reductions would indicate that certain areas are more sensitive to the teratogenic insult. By extension, behavioral and cognitive functions associated with areas of disproportionate reduction may be relatively more affected, and therefore may be domains of particular concern for neuropsychological investigation in this population. Although research in FASD using brain imaging is relatively sparse, a growing body of neuroimaging data suggests that certain brain regions and structures are differentially affected by prenatal alcohol exposure. Specifically, disproportionate size reductions and abnormalities have been found in the corpus callosum, basal ganglia, hippocampus, and cerebellum. Initial regional volumetric brain analyses have guided more focused investigations and have prompted investigation with additional imaging techniques, such as voxel-based morphometric (VBM) analyses, single-photon emission computerized tomography (SPECT), functional magnetic resonance imaging (fMRI), and diffusion tensor imaging (DTI). Research on the brains of individuals with FASD converges across neuroimaging modalities to suggest that certain brain regions are more vulnerable to the teratogenic effects of alcohol.

TABLE 10.1. Summary of Brain Changes Noted in Individuals with Fetal Alcohol Spectrum Disorders (FASD)

Brain region	Neuroimaging findings
Total brain	Overall reductions in brain size are found consistently in individuals with FASD (Archibald et al., 2001; Johnson et al., 1996; Mattson et al., 1994; Mattson et al., 1996c; Riikonen et al., 1999; Swayze et al., 1997).
Cortical regions	The parietal lobe is reduced in size (white matter more affected than gray matter) after whole-brain size is taken into account (Archibald et al., 2001). Abnormally increased gray matter and decreased white matter have also been seen in the left temporoparietal region (Sowell et al., 2001b). Thick cortex has been noted in bilateral temporal and parietal regions and the right frontal lobe (Sowell et al., 2008b). White matter microstructural abnormalities are seen in the right temporal lobe, bilateral medial parietal lobe (Sowell et al., 2008a), bilateral medial frontal lobe, and occipital lobe (Fryer et al., 2009).
Corpus callosum	Abnormalities in individuals with FASD can range from disproportionate reductions in size to total absence of the corpus callosum (Bhatara et al., 2002; Johnson et al., 1996; Riley et al., 1995; Swayze et al., 1997). Posterior regions (isthmus and splenium) are displaced and relatively reduced in size (Sowell et al., 2001a). Corpus callosum shape is more variable than in typically developing peers (Bookstein et al., 2002a). Microstructural abnormalities are found across several different regions of the corpus callosum (Fryer et al., 2009; Sowell et al., 2008a; Wozniak et al., 2006).
Subcortical regions	Individuals with FASD have reduced basal ganglia volume after brain size is taken into account, and these reductions are most pronounced in the caudate nucleus (Archibald et al., 2001; Mattson et al., 1992).
Hippocampus	Reductions in absolute hippocampal volume have been reported in some studies (Autti-Rämö et al., 2002; Bhatara et al., 2002), but in relation to overall brain reductions, the hippocampus appears to be relatively spared (Archibald et al., 2001).
Amygdala	Few studies have examined the amygdala in populations with FASD. Reductions that are noted appear to be proportional to overall brain reductions (Archibald et al., 2001; Mattson et al., 1992; Riikonen et al., 1999).
Cerebellum	Volumetric reductions in the cerebellum are greater than reductions seen in the cerebrum (Archibald et al., 2001; Mattson et al., 1992, 1994, 1996c). The anterior region of the cerebellar vermis appears to be more reduced than the posterior vermis (Autti-Rämö et al., 2002; O'Hare et al., 2005; Sowell et al., 1996).

Cortical Regions

In a study using whole-brain volumetric MRI analysis on a group of individuals with FASD, only the parietal lobe was relatively small in the alcohol-exposed group, while the temporal, frontal, and occipital lobes were reduced in proportion to brain size (Archibald et al., 2001). The reduction of parietal lobe volume was supported by findings of disproportionately reduced gray and white matter in this region (Archibald et al., 2001). VBM analyses have also been used to examine tissue constitution. This method allows for investigation of gray and white matter alterations and does not rely on predetermined regions of comparison, as are often used in traditional structural volumetric analyses. Therefore, abnormalities that occur in regions without clear structural boundaries can be detected. In one VBM study, increases in gray matter and decreases in white matter density occurred in the left posterior temporoparietal region of individuals with FAS (Sowell et al., 2001b). Nondysmorphic alcohol-exposed participants showed a similar pattern of tissue density in comparison with controls, but the differences were slightly less robust than those between controls and dysmorphic individuals with FAS.

DTI is a relatively new imaging technique used to investigate white matter integrity by examining tissue microstructure. An investigation using DTI to examine individuals with FASD found decreased fractional anisotropy (FA), indicative of compromised tissue integrity, in white matter in temporal and parietal lobes; decreased FA was also observed in the posterior cingulate, right internal capsule, and brainstem (Sowell et al., 2008a). Using VBM, this study found white matter in the right hemisphere to be relatively more pathological, which was inconsistent with previous investigations. Widespread microstructural abnormalities were observed in an additional whole-brain DTI study, with abnormalities observed in the parietal lobe and more prominently in the frontal and occipital lobes (Fryer et al., 2009).

In another study, brain surface anatomy and gray matter density were analyzed. Brain maps of alcohol-exposed participants and controls were matched along landmarks, and individual differences in spatial cortical patterns were investigated. Regional parietal abnormalities were confirmed; alcohol-exposed individuals had reduced brain growth in the inferior parietal (perisylvian) regions and ventral frontal lobes, with changes in the left hemisphere more pronounced than in the right (Sowell et al., 2002a). A separate study by the same authors found reduced asymmetry of the superior temporal and inferior parietal regions (Sowell et al., 2002b). A more recent investigation used novel techniques to analyze cortical thickness across the cortical surface and found increased thickness (indicative of less mature and less myelinated gray matter) in children with FASD in bilateral temporal, bilateral inferior parietal, and right frontal regions (Sowell et al., 2008b). Whereas abnormalities in the frontal region were associated with impaired verbal recall measures, alterations in left occipital regions were associated with poorer performance on visual–spatial measures in the group with FASD, suggesting that specific behavioral deficits observed in this population may be associated with particular brain anomalies.

From all these findings, it appears that prenatal alcohol exposure leads to alterations in size and structure in parietal, temporal, and frontal brain regions, although the perisylvian region of the left hemisphere appears to be especially affected. Examination of specific structures has further delineated the nature of abnormality in individuals with prenatal alcohol exposure.

Corpus Callosum

Dramatic abnormalities in the corpus callosum, the bundle of nerve fibers connecting the right and left hemispheres, were observed in early brain autopsies of children with FAS (Jones & Smith, 1975) and have been confirmed in more recent MRI investigations (Bhatara et al., 2002; Johnson et al., 1996; Riley et al., 1995; Swayze et al., 1997). Several studies have reported partial or full agenesis (absence) of the corpus callosum, leading to the suggestion that agenesis is found at a higher rate in FAS than in any other developmental disorder (Jeret & Serur, 1991). In an early imaging study, ranges of outcomes from dispro-portionate regional reductions to agenesis of the corpus callosum were found for individu-als with heavy prenatal alcohol exposure (Riley et al., 1995). Even among alcohol-exposed individuals, however, complete or partial agenesis is rare. Further investigations have delin-eated more specific structural displacements and shape abnormalities of the corpus callosum in individuals with FASD. For example, the isthmus and splenium, both posterior regions of the corpus callosum, are relatively more displaced in alcohol-exposed children than in controls, after adjustments for brain size and locations of other brain structures (Sowell et al., 2001a). These findings may relate to previously mentioned abnormalities in the parietal and temporal lobes, as the posterior corpus callosum regions contain fibers that connect perisylvian cortices (Hofer & Frahm, 2006). In addition to exhibiting spatial displacement, the splenium and isthmus were relatively reduced in size.

Several recent studies have used DTI to examine corpus callosum abnormalities in children (Fryer et al., 2009; Sowell et al., 2008a; Wozniak et al., 2006) and young adults with FASD (Ma et al., 2005). Results of these investigations showed that alcohol-exposed participants had altered diffusion in the corpus callosum, which is indicative of reduced fiber integrity, suggesting that this region is damaged at the microstructural level. The sub-regions of the corpus callosum that showed altered diffusion differed across these investiga-tions; thus microstructure abnormalities of the corpus callosum appear to be hypervariable in the population with FASD—a notion that has been suggested by other investigators (Bookstein, Sampson, Connor, & Streissguth, 2002a).

The nature of corpus callosum abnormality in individuals with heavy prenatal alco-hol exposure has been associated with specific neuropsychological deficits. In one study, affected participants with a relatively thick callosum had patterns of executive deficits, while a thin callosum was related to motor deficits (Bookstein, Streissguth, Sampson, Connor, & Barr, 2002b). Integrity of the corpus callosum is necessary for interhemispheric transfer of information, as it is the structural connection between the right and left hemispheres. In individuals with FASD, relations between reductions in callosal size and reduced inter-hemispheric transfer of somatosensory information (Roebuck, Mattson, & Riley, 2002) and between callosal displacement and verbal learning and memory (Sowell et al., 2001a) have been reported. These results suggest that the degree and nature of damage to the corpus callosum may be a predictor of functioning in some neurobehavioral domains.

Subcortical Regions

In addition to cortical changes, subcortical structures are affected by prenatal alcohol expo-sure. The basal ganglia appear to be particularly vulnerable to prenatal alcohol exposure. In one study, after microcephaly was controlled for, individuals with FAS and nondys-morphic FASD had reduced basal ganglia volume (Mattson et al., 1992). Further regional investigation of basal ganglia reductions demonstrated that the caudate nucleus accounted for most of the size reduction of the basal ganglia (Archibald et al., 2001; Mattson et al., 1992). Archibald et al. (2001) found evidence for reduction of the caudate for participants with nondysmorphic FASD in comparison to controls. In addition, those with nondysmor-phic FASD had caudate nuclei with marginally significant reductions when the caudate nucleus volume was compared to total subcortical gray volume (Archibald et al., 2001).

This finding supports general trends for individuals with nondysmorphic FASD to show brain abnormalities similar to, but less severe than, those of individuals with FAS. The caudate nucleus is extensively connected to prefrontal brain regions, and is associated with cognitive functions such as set shifting, appropriate inhibition, and spatial memory, all of which are impaired in alcohol-exposed individuals.

Hippocampus and Amygdala

Few imaging studies have reported alterations in the hippocampus. Significant findings from available studies have found gross abnormalities in the hippocampal region, but these studies have been based on small samples (Autti-Rämö et al., 2002; Bhatara et al., 2002), and it is not clear whether these reductions were relative to individual brain size or proportionate to overall brain reduction. One small study provided more specific results, finding that the hippocampus in alcohol-exposed individuals was relatively more reduced on the left than on the right side (Riikonen et al., 1999), although a subsequent report by the same authors did not support this effect (Riikonen et al., 2005). Investigations of the hippocampus that take overall brain size into consideration suggest that this region shows relative sparing; although reductions are apparent, they are proportional to those seen in overall brain size (Archibald et al., 2001). Similarly, the limited research on the amygdala shows relative sparing (Archibald et al., 2001; Mattson et al., 1992; Riikonen et al., 1999). The hippocampus and amygdala are thought to contribute to formation of long-term memories and emotions, respectively. Further analysis of these regions may elucidate whether these areas and associated functions are relatively spared in alcohol-exposed individuals.

Cerebellum

One region of the brain that is disproportionately affected by heavy prenatal alcohol exposure is the cerebellum, with several studies documenting greater reductions than those seen in the cerebrum (Archibald et al., 2001; Mattson et al., 1992, 1994, 1996c). Cerebellar volume reductions of approximately 15% have been reported in individuals with FAS, whereas reductions in individuals with nondysmorphic FASD are somewhat less dramatic (Archibald et al., 2001; Mattson et al., 1994). Investigations focused on the cerebellar vermis show that this structure is sensitive to alcohol exposure (Autti-Rämö et al., 2002; O'Hare et al., 2005; Sowell et al., 1996). More specifically, the anterior regions of the vermis are more affected than the posterior regions, and these alterations are related to verbal learning and memory deficits (O'Hare et al., 2005), suggesting that the size reductions in the vermis have behavioral relevance in this population.

Functional Brain Imaging Studies

Researchers have begun to use functional neuroimaging techniques to assess the neural substrates that contribute to cognitive dysfunction in FASD. One study used SPECT to examine regional alterations and found decreased cerebral blood flow in the left parieto-occipital region—a metabolic result that is consistent with the above-noted structural abnormality, and that the authors hypothesized to be related to arithmetic and speech difficulty in alcohol-exposed populations (Riikonen et al., 1999). In addition, controls had an expected pattern of asymmetric blood flow in the frontal lobe, while children with FAS had a pattern of abnormal functional symmetry, with similar blood flow in the right and left frontal lobes. A follow-up SPECT study examined serotonergic and dopaminergic neurotransmission in the striatal and frontal regions of alcohol-exposed participants, and found reduced serotonin in the medial frontal cortex and a significant but less robust increase in striatal dopamine transporter binding for individuals with FASD (Riikonen et al., 2005).

A positron emission tomography (PET) study of young adults showed that participants with FAS had subtle reductions in glucose metabolism in medial subcortical areas, including the caudate and thalamic nuclei (Clark, Li, Conry, Conry, & Loock, 2000). Additional investigations have used magnetic resonance spectroscopy (MRS) to examine individuals with FASD. An MRS study focusing on the caudate nucleus found abnormally elevated metabolites associated with pathological neuronal function in the left caudate nucleus of alcohol-exposed individuals (Cortese et al., 2006). A study examining cerebral metabolism of adolescents and young adults demonstrated altered metabolites in the frontal and parietal cortex, frontal white matter, corpus callosum, thalamus, and cerebellar dentate nucleus (Fagerlund et al., 2006), although altered metabolism was not observed in the caudate nucleus, as was previously reported. In addition, these widespread alterations were interpreted as stemming from glial cell abnormalities, rather than from neuronal alterations. Inconsistencies in findings of metabolic activity may relate to sample characteristics such as age. As indicated above, structural studies have previously identified abnormalities in each of these brain regions in alcohol-exposed populations; continued investigation providing specific information as seen on SPECT, PET, and MRS regarding neurotransmitter and glucose metabolism may be useful in further characterizing the nature and location of brain dysfunction contributing to impairments in cognitive abilities in alcohol-exposed populations.

Although early investigations using fMRI (Malisza et al., 2005) are difficult to interpret because of design flaws (Bookheimer & Sowell, 2005), more recent investigations have used fMRI effectively to examine hemodynamic response during neuropsychological tasks in alcohol-exposed children. An fMRI study focusing on response inhibition found that individuals with FASD had altered hemodynamic response during trials requiring inhibition of action, in comparison to controls (Fryer et al., 2007b). More specifically, the participants with FASD had increased areas of activation in left ventromedial and right dorsolateral prefrontal cortices, and decreased activation of the right caudate nucleus, despite comparable behavioral performance. These areas are consistent with frontal–striatal anatomical connections thought to be involved in response inhibition (Casey, Tottenham, & Fossella, 2002). Because task performance was comparable between the groups, the accompanying activation differences were probably task-specific; this suggests that the frontal–subcortical circuitry thought to mediate inhibitory control is sensitive to prenatal alcohol exposure. An additional investigation involving a verbal learning task found less activation in left medial and temporal regions, and increased activation in the left dorsal frontal cortex, in alcohol-exposed children versus controls. These differences remained after statistical controls for differences in task performance and were interpreted by the authors to reflect altered temporal lobe activity as an indicator of deficient processing of verbal information (Sowell et al., 2007). Increased frontal activation was hypothesized to reflect compensatory reliance on frontal systems for organization of verbally learned material; or, conversely, increased frontal activation may be indicative of less efficient systems' working to achieve the same level of frontally mediated performance as that of the controls.

Functional imaging techniques have been utilized rarely in alcohol-exposed populations, and increased use of measures that allow for examination of real-time brain responses may augment structural brain imaging and behavioral neuropsychological findings. Careful design and sufficient power in functional studies will assure that appropriate and applicable conclusions are reached. Over the past decade, brain imaging findings including abnormal brain surface morphology, anomalous patterns of gray matter, and (more recently) altered hemodynamics suggest that certain behavioral impairments seen in individuals with FASD may be associated with abnormalities of the cortex beyond size differences.

NEUROPSYCHOLOGICAL CONSEQUENCES

Like structural brain studies, neuropsychological studies are plagued by the question of relative sparing and impaired function. Delineation of a neuropsychological signature or profile has been the subject of much recent debate and investigation, and limited research has examined whether prenatal alcohol exposure results in general dysfunction or a more specific neurobehavioral profile of strengths and weaknesses. Although most research has focused on specific areas of deficit, with increasing neurobehavioral data and complementary brain findings, it appears that children with prenatal alcohol exposure have domains of functional vulnerability corresponding to differential brain involvement. In addition to generally diminished IQ, individuals with prenatal alcohol exposure have shown deficits in the domains of attention; learning and memory; speech and language; executive functioning (EF); motor functioning; visual–spatial ability; and social skills and secondary disabilities. See Table 10.2 for a summary of findings on neuropsychological deficits in individuals with FASD.

Global Deficits

When we consider the spectrum of outcomes in FASD, it is not surprising that estimates of general intellectual functioning vary. In studies of children with FAS, IQ scores range from 20 to 120, with an average between 65 and 72 (Mattson & Riley, 1998). Although FAS is thought to be the leading known cause of mental retardation in the United States (Pulsifer, 1996), most individuals with FAS do not have mental retardation (Streissguth, Barr, Kogan, & Bookstein, 1996). Nondysmorphic alcohol-exposed individuals tend to have slightly higher IQ scores than those of dysmorphic alcohol-exposed individuals, although still significantly lower than those of nonexposed peers (Mattson, Riley, Gramling, Delis, & Jones, 1997). Developmental delay, learning disability, and low academic achievement are outcomes related to decreased IQ in FASD (Bertrand et al., 2005). Although some reports indicate that children with FAS and FASD are relatively less impaired on nonverbal intelligence measures (as indicated by Performance IQ) than on verbal intelligence measures (Bertrand et al., 2005; Streissguth, Barr, Sampson, & Bookstein, 1994a), these findings are not consistent (Mattson & Riley, 1998).

TABLE 10.2. Summary of Neuropsychological Findings Noted in Individuals with FASD

Cognitive domain	Findings
Global deficits	IQ scores of individuals with FAS range from 20 to 120, with an average between 65 and 72 (Mattson & Riley, 1998). Alcohol-exposed individuals without facial dysmorphia tend to have slightly higher IQ scores than those of dysmorphic alcohol-exposed individuals, but still significantly lower IQs than those of nonexposed peers (Mattson et al., 1997).
Attention and hyperactivity	Visual sustained attention appears pervasively impaired. Deficits in auditory sustained attention may relate to task demands (Coles et al., 2002; Mattson et al., 2006b).
Verbal learning and memory	Children have impaired learning and memory of verbal material. However, retention of learned verbal information is spared when an implicit memory strategy is present (Mattson et al., 1996b, 1998).
Nonverbal learning and memory	Results are mixed. Some studies suggest that spatial recall is impaired (Hamilton et al., 2003; Mattson et al., 2006a; Uecker & Nadel, 1998); other studies indicate that spatial recall is intact (Kaemingk & Halverson, 2000). Some evidence suggests that object recall (Uecker & Nadel, 1998) and spatial retention (Mattson & Roebuck, 2002; Roebuck-Spencer & Mattson, 2004) may be spared in individuals with FASD.
Speech and language	There is some evidence suggesting speech production difficulties in children with FASD, possibly related to craniofacial abnormalities (Church et al., 1997). Children with FASD may be impaired in expressive and receptive language (Carney & Chermak, 1991), although these impairments may not be greater than expected from IQ (McGee et al., 2009).
Executive functioning (EF)	Deficits have been documented across several EF domains, including planning (Kodituwakku et al., 1995), utilization of feedback, cognitive flexibility, response inhibition, concept formation (Mattson et al., 1999), verbal fluency (poorer letter than category) (Kodituwakku et al., 1995, 2006; Mattson et al., 1999; Vaurio et al., 2008), and nonverbal fluency (Schonfeld et al., 2001).
Motor functioning	Both fine and gross motor abilities appear to be affected by prenatal alcohol exposure. Balance has been shown to be affected (Roebuck et al., 1998b), although this finding is possibly related to task demands (Adnams et al., 2001) and may not be evident in children with lower exposure (Richardson et al., 2002).
Visual–spatial ability	Only a few studies exist, but impairments have been documented in visual–motor tasks in individuals with alcohol exposure (Conry, 1990; Janzen et al., 1995; Mattson et al., 1998). These deficits may be related to impaired motor ability (Janzen et al., 1995). In addition, deficits are present in recalling local but not global features of hierarchical stimuli (Mattson et al., 1996a).
Social skills and secondary disabilities	Children with FASD are likely to be classified as hyperactive, disruptive, impulsive, or delinquent (Mattson & Riley, 2000; Roebuck et al., 1999), and to have elevated rates of comorbid disruptive behavior disorders and mood/anxiety disorders (Fryer et al., 2007a). Deficits in adaptive behavior are evident in childhood and adulthood (Streissguth et al., 1991a; Thomas et al., 1998), and are evident across socialization, communication, and daily living skills domains (Crocker, 2008).

Attention and Hyperactivity

A hallmark feature of prenatal alcohol exposure is attention deficit, and children with FASD frequently have a comorbid diagnosis of attention-deficit/hyperactivity disorder (ADHD) (Fryer, McGee, Matt, Riley, & Mattson, 2007a; Steinhausen & Spohr, 1998). Furthermore, attention deficits observed in heavily exposed children are worse than would be predicted by IQ scores (Mattson & Riley, 2000), and commonly used measures of attention and attention-related behavior can be used to discriminate alcohol-exposed children from controls with a high degree of accuracy even after overall IQ is controlled for (Lee, Mattson, & Riley, 2004). Thus attention deficits may be more sensitive than either intellectual deficits or facial dysmorphology in detecting prenatal alcohol exposure. In addition, it appears that attention deficits are not uniform in this population. Although visual sustained attention appears pervasively impaired, deficits in auditory sustained attention may relate to task demands (Coles, Platzman, Lynch, & Freides, 2002; Mattson, Calarco, & Lang, 2006b). Finally, although few studies comparing children with FASD to children with ADHD but no alcohol exposure exist, it appears that these two groups of children can be distinguished from each other on measures of vigilance, visual–spatial processing, EF, and adaptive behavior (Calarco, Mattson, Robertson, & Riley, 2003; Coles et al., 1997; Mattson, Lee, Hayden, & Riley, 2005; Vaurio, Riley, & Mattson, 2008). This is somewhat surprising, given the high rates of ADHD in the population with FASD, but it suggests that a single model of attention deficits may not be appropriate in classifying these two populations. Alcohol-related attention deficits are also apparent in prospective studies of individuals with low to moderate prenatal alcohol exposure (e.g., Burden, Jacobson, Sokol, & Jacobson, 2005; Streissguth et al., 1994a).

Learning and Memory

Multiple studies have addressed learning and memory in children with FASD. The general consensus is that deficits in this domain exist, but careful delineation of the nature and types of deficits is required and ongoing. As in other areas of function, it appears that some but not all types of learning and memory are affected in individuals with FASD. Most studies have focused on verbal learning and memory; a small number have addressed nonverbal learning and memory, and even fewer have made the distinction between learning and memory or retention and recall.

Verbal Learning and Memory

Several studies of FASD have used the California Verbal Learning Test—Children's Version (CVLT-C). This test allows for analysis of encoding, retrieval, and retention of a 15-word list. On this test, children with FASD learn fewer words initially and have more difficulty than controls in recalling words after a delay. However, children with FASD appear to benefit from repeated exposure to new material, although not as much as controls. Retention of learned verbal material is comparable between groups, suggesting that exposed children are able to retain verbal information that is encoded (Mattson, Riley, Delis, Stern, & Jones, 1996b; Mattson, Riley, Gramling, Delis, & Jones, 1998). A similar result was reported in a prospective study of children with lower levels of exposure; alcohol-related verbal memory deficits were apparent on the Children's Memory Scale, but were mediated by learning deficits, supporting a relative sparing in retention in the presence of impaired learning (Willford, Richardson, Leech, & Day, 2004). This spared retention may relate to differential explicit versus implicit memory abilities in this population. Although retention of learned material is intact on the CVLT-C, a task that involves an implicit learning strategy, alcohol-exposed individuals showed poor retention on the Wide Range Assessment of Memory Verbal Learning task, which involves no comparable implicit strategy (Mattson & Roebuck, 2002; Roebuck-Spencer & Mattson, 2004). In support of the possible role of task characteristics in accounting for these contrasting findings, one study demonstrated intact implicit memory but impaired explicit memory (recall) in the same group of children with FASD (Mattson & Riley, 1999).

Nonverbal Learning and Memory

Studies of nonverbal memory in children with FASD are sparse, and existing results are inconsistent. Some studies indicate that (as in the verbal domain) alcohol-exposed children benefit from repeated exposure, but demonstrate both encoding and retrieval deficits for nonverbal information (Mattson & Roebuck, 2002; Roebuck-Spencer & Mattson, 2004). However, other research demonstrates that alcohol-exposed children have a pattern of spared retention in visual learning measures similar to the pattern seen in the verbal domain (Kaemingk, Mulvaney, & Tanner Halverson, 2003). Furthermore, within the nonverbal memory domain, alcohol-exposed individuals may have specific strengths and weaknesses. For example, one study demonstrated intact object recall but impaired spatial location recall (Uecker & Nadel, 1996, 1998). Although these authors addressed recall, they did not analyze retention of learned material. However, examination of mean scores for the children with FAS and the control group suggests that despite impaired initial learning of spatial location, retention of spatial material may have been relatively less affected than retention of object material in the group with FAS. A separate study reported that when basic perceptual and verbal memory skills were taken into account, alcohol-exposed children performed similarly to controls on spatial recall tasks (Kaemingk & Halverson, 2000).

Although there are inconsistencies in the literature, a finding of spared spatial recall or retention may be due to task characteristics, as recent human (Hamilton, Kodituwakku, Sutherland, & Savage, 2003) and animal (Johnson & Goodlett, 2002) studies show convergent and specific place-learning deficits on a water maze task that has been shown to be sensitive to alcohol-related hippocampal damage. In one small study, participants with FAS demonstrated impaired performance on a virtual water maze task, which taps spatial memory. However, on a cued-navigation phase, which more directly tests visual–motor ability, the participants with FAS and the controls had comparable performance, suggesting a dissociable spatial recall deficit (Hamilton et al., 2003). Unfortunately, retention was not examined in this study. The spatial recall deficit was recently replicated in a large international study using the same virtual water maze task (Mattson, Autti-Rämö, May, Konovalova, & the CIFASD Consortium, 2006a). Thus evidence for spatial versus object memory deficits is limited and mixed, with some studies suggesting impaired spatial recall and intact object recall, and other studies indicating spared spatial recall or retention. Further investigation of retention of learned spatial and object information is necessary, as few studies have directly examined this relationship.

Speech and Language

A small number of studies have demonstrated both speech production and language-processing deficits in populations with heavy prenatal alcohol exposure (Church, Eldis, Blakley, & Bawle, 1997; Conry, 1990; Janzen, Nanson, & Block, 1995). Individuals with FASD demonstrate a range of speech production deficiencies, which can vary from less severe deficits in simple phonemic production to more marked deficits resulting in low intelligibility of speech. These speech production deficits are possibly related to the high proportion of craniofacial and dentofacial abnormalities in this population (Church et al., 1997). Individuals with FASD also may have impairments in grammatical components of expressive and receptive language ability. One study using the Test of Language Development showed that younger alcohol-exposed participants had global deficits in language, while older children had more specific syntactic deficits (Carney & Chermak, 1991). One investigation suggests that the receptive and expressive language deficits observed in children with heavy prenatal alcohol exposure may not be greater than would be predicted by IQ deficits (McGee, Bjorkquist, Riley, & Mattson, 2009). Although some research shows that prenatal alcohol exposure leads to speech and language deficits, as is evident, little information on this domain is available, and additional study in this area is needed.

Executive Functioning

EF is a complex set of abilities dependent on intact subprocessing, and is tapped by a variety of neuropsychological tasks. Examinations of various aspects of EF in individuals with FASD generally document impairments; however, the nature of these deficits is not yet conclusive. In a study assessing planning, self-regulatory behavior, and utilization of feedback in individuals with FASD, deficits were noted in some areas but not in others (Kodituwakku, Handmaker, Cutler, Weathersby, & Handmaker, 1995). Alcohol-exposed participants were significantly impaired on a task of planning. However, in the domain of self-regulatory behavior, alcohol-exposed participants had performance equal to that of controls. On tasks assessing utilization of feedback, alcohol-exposed participants were impaired on the Wisconsin Card Sorting Test (WCST), but had performance equal to that of controls on a go/no-go task. These results suggest that individuals with FASD have a specific pattern of EF deficits, rather than global deficits, dependent on underlying modality or task characteristics.

In another investigation, individuals with heavy alcohol exposure demonstrated deficits on tasks in the Delis–Kaplan Executive Functioning System (D-KEFS; Delis, Kaplan, & Kramer, 2001), which allows for a simultaneous hierarchical investigation of perceptual/lower-order and higher-order integrative abilities. Deficits were the same for dysmorphic and nondysmorphic individuals. Exposed children performed significantly worse on tests tapping cognitive flexibility, response inhibition, planning, and concept formation, even after lower-order processing was taken into account (Mattson, Goodman, Caine, Delis, & Riley, 1999). Deficits seen in children with prenatal alcohol exposure in the domains of concept formation and conceptual set shifting, as assessed by the D-KEFS California Card Sorting Test and the WCST, were confirmed in a recent investigation; however, although performance on these measures by alcohol-exposed children was better than expected from IQ estimates (McGee et al., 2009), suggesting that certain EF deficits may be relatively consistent with global functioning.

In examinations of verbal fluency ability in alcohol-exposed children, consistent impairment on letter fluency has been found, whereas category fluency performance appears to be diminished but less robustly affected (Kodituwakku et al., 1995, 2006; Mattson et al., 1999; Vaurio et al., 2008). This fluency deficit appears to be global, as children with FASD have shown similarly poor performance across verbal and nonverbal fluency tasks (Schonfeld, Mattson, Lang, Delis, & Riley, 2001). It may be related to the ability to switch cognitive set during fluency tasks (Hayden, 2005).

Performance on EF measures may serve to distinguish children with prenatal alcohol exposure from similar clinical groups, as a recent investigation demonstrated that children with FASD had a pattern of impairments different from that of nonexposed children with ADHD (Vaurio et al., 2008). EF deficits observed in children also appear to extend throughout the lifespan, as adults with FASD have similarly impaired performance on EF tasks (Connor, Sampson, Bookstein, Barr, & Streissguth, 2000).

Results are equivocal regarding the relationship of EF deficits and IQ, which are traditionally thought to be relatively independent. One study of adults found that EF deficits were worse than predicted from IQ, which implies that EF deficits are independent of diminished intellectual ability (Connor et al., 2000). Other studies find that EF ability in alcohol-exposed participants either is not significantly associated with IQ (Mattson et al., 1999) or is better than would be predicted from IQ (McGee et al., 2009; Vaurio et al., 2008) suggesting that at least some EF abilities may be relative strengths in this population.

One domain of EF that has been surprisingly understudied in individuals with heavy prenatal alcohol exposure is working memory. In one study using a delayed-matching-to-sample task and a self-ordered pointing task (two widely used working memory measures), no significant impairments were found in children with prenatal alcohol exposure (Kodituwakku et al., 1995). In a recent prospective study of children with low to moderate prenatal alcohol exposure, more moderately exposed children demonstrated worse performance on tasks thought to test working memory; a dose–response relationship was observed, with a 0.20 standard deviation decrease in working memory for each ounce of absolute alcohol consumed (Burden et al., 2005). However, a recent preliminary study found that when participants with lower-order processing deficits were excluded from analysis, performance of alcohol-exposed participants did not differ from that of controls (Vaurio, Repp, McGee, Riley, & Mattson, 2006). This suggests that deficits observed in working memory may be due to perceptual dysfunction, rather than specific higher-order deficits. Further systematic examination of working memory is required to determine whether it is indeed a central area of dysfunction in alcohol-exposed individuals.

Motor Functioning

Children with prenatal alcohol exposure demonstrate motor impairments. Tremors, weak grasp, and poor hand–eye coordination have been associated with FAS and FASD (Jones & Smith, 1973; Mattson & Riley, 1998). Both fine (e.g., grooved pegboard performance) and gross (e.g., balance) motor tasks appear to be affected in individuals with FASD. In one study, children with FASD showed impaired balance and were unable to compensate for body sway with their visual or vestibular systems when somatosensory and/or visual input was unreliable (Roebuck, Simmons, Mattson, & Riley, 1998b). To distinguish the source of these balance deficits, the authors conducted a follow-up study using electro-myographic data to measure short/medium-latency versus long-latency responses, which are thought to involve spinal pathways and transcortical pathways, respectively. Findings suggested that balance dysfunction was at least in part a central processing deficit rather than solely postsynaptic, as long-latency but not short- or medium-latency responses were significantly delayed in the alcohol-exposed participants (Roebuck, Simmons, Richardson, Mattson, & Riley, 1998c). In addition, it appears that motor deficits persist into adulthood for populations with heavy alcohol exposure (Connor, Sampson, Streissguth, Bookstein, & Barr, 2006).

However, some studies have not found motor impairments in this population. One study examined cognitive and motor ability in a South African sample, using several neu-robehavioral scales. A subscale measuring gross motor skills revealed no significant difference between the participants with FAS and the control group, although the authors suggest that their chosen measure may have not been sufficiently sensitive to detect motor deficits (Adnams et al., 2001). In addition, in a prospective study of children with low to moderate exposure, gross motor skills were not impaired at 3 years of age, and fine motor skills were not impaired at 10 years of age (Chandler, Richardson, Gallagher, & Day, 1996; Richardson, Ryan, Willford, Day, & Goldschmidt, 2002). As findings of motor impairments do occur in heavily exposed individuals, these negative findings may have been due to the lower levels of exposure in the sample.

Visual–Spatial Ability

In addition to exhibiting the spatial memory dysfunction mentioned above, children with prenatal alcohol exposure have shown deficits in visual–spatial construction. To examine this ability, most investigations have utilized a figure-copying test, the Beery–Buktenica Developmental Test of Visual–Motor Integration, and have found impairments in alcohol-exposed individuals (Conry, 1990; Janzen et al., 1995; Mattson et al., 1998). However, one study found no such impairment after motor drawing was controlled for, suggesting that visual–spatial abilities may be impaired due to motor rather than perceptual deficits (Janzen et al., 1995). To examine visual–spatial abilities more specifically, one study utilized a Global–Local Task (Mattson, Gramling, Delis, Jones, & Riley, 1996a), in which processing of hierarchical figures was tested. Deficits were found in recalling local but not global features of hierarchical stimuli, and these deficits were not due to the stimuli size or to memory performance. Previous research suggests that this type of performance may relate to a pattern of brain abnormality that involves the left hemisphere to a greater degree than the right hemisphere, and this suggestion is supported by brain imaging studies in this population (Sowell et al., 2001b). Although limited research has addressed the subprocesses that are involved in visual–spatial processing, preliminary data suggest that children with FASD are similarly impaired on measures of "what" processing (associated with the ventral visual processing stream) and "where" processing (associated with the dorsal processing stream) (Crocker, Wagner, Vaurio, & Mattson, 2009). Additional investigation is needed to determine if visual–spatial processing is affected in specific or global ways and to determine the contribution of lower order (perceptual, motor) deficits to visual–spatial processing.

Social Skills and Secondary Disabilities

In addition to perceptual and cognitive deficits, children with prenatal alcohol exposure demonstrate deficits in interpersonal domains. Parents are more likely to rate alcohol-exposed children as hyperactive, disruptive, impulsive, or delinquent (Mattson & Riley, 2000; Roebuck, Mattson, & Riley, 1999). In addition, significant deficits in adaptive behavior are notable throughout childhood and adulthood (Streissguth et al., 1991a; Thomas, Kelly, Mattson, & Riley, 1998). Domains of the Vineland Adaptive Behavior Scales may be useful in identifying alcohol-affected individuals. Two studies have documented relatively greater impairment on the Socialization domain (Streissguth et al., 1991; Thomas et al., 1998), even when Verbal IQ is controlled (Thomas et al., 1998). One study comparing children with FASD to children with ADHD indicated that the Socialization and Daily Living Skills domains were useful in distinguishing the groups (Crocker, 2008). Parent-reported deficits in social skills as measured by the Social Skills Rating System have been shown to be significantly correlated with parent-reported EF deficits, suggesting that higher-order cognitive deficits may contribute to interpersonal difficulty (Schonfeld, Paley, Frankel, & O'Connor, 2006).

Heavy prenatal alcohol exposure also relates to high levels of secondary disabilities and psychopathology. Secondary disabilities are important to consider, because individuals affected by prenatal alcohol exposure who do not have an IQ below 70 often are disabled but do not qualify for special services. High rates of inappropriate sexual behavior, disrupted school experience, trouble with the law, confinement, and drug and alcohol problems occur in children and adults with FASD (Streissguth et al., 1996). However, in a study of a predominantly African American sample with low socioeconomic status, no association was found between alcohol exposure and delinquency. Independent of alcohol exposure, delinquent acts were predicted by such factors as increased life stress, drug use, and decreased supervision (Lynch, Coles, Corley, & Falek, 2003). This finding highlights the importance of considering contextual factors when examining behavioral outcomes in alcohol-exposed individuals. In terms of psychopathology, elevated rates of ADHD, depressive disorders, oppositional defiant disorder, conduct disorder, and specific phobia have been documented (Famy, Streissguth, & Unis, 1998; Fryer et al., 2007a; Schonfeld, Mattson, & Riley, 2005; Steinhausen & Spohr, 1998). A recent prospective study of young adults with relatively low prenatal alcohol exposure documented elevations in substance abuse and personality disorders after confounding variables were controlled for (Barr et al., 2006). Although individuals with prenatal alcohol exposure may not always be identifiable on the basis of physical characteristics or intelligence scores, evidence of significant adaptive disability and risk for psychopathology and delinquency suggests that increased efforts to ameliorate negative outcomes are essential.

DEVELOPMENTAL CONSIDERATIONS

Although the initial brain insult caused by prenatal alcohol exposure will be expressed differently with advancing age, very few longitudinal studies have been conducted that can be used to describe developmental trends in FASD. Most relevant results have come from prospective studies of individuals with lower levels of exposure; this limited research suggests that disabilities seen in children with FASD persist into adulthood. One study of 40 individuals with FASD indicated that IQ deficits were stable and persistent over an average test–retest interval of 8 years (Streissguth, Randels, & Smith, 1991b). Similarly, separate studies of children and adults with FASD document the permanence of the neurobehavioral effects seen in this population. For example, such studies have indicated effects both in children and adults in the following domains: psychopathology (Famy et al., 1998; Fryer et al., 2007a); secondary disabilities (Streissguth et al., 1996); attention (Connor, Streissguth, Sampson, Bookstein, & Barr, 1999; Mattson et al., 2006b); motor performance (Connor et al., 2006; Roebuck et al., 1998b); verbal learning (Kerns, Don, Mateer, & Streissguth, 1997; Mattson, Riley, Delis, Stern, & Jones, 1996b); and EF (Kerns et al., 1997; Mattson et al., 1999). Longitudinal prospective studies that have followed cohorts of children into adulthood provide additional support for the long-term nature of alcohol's teratogenic effects (e.g., Richardson et al., 2002; Streissguth et al., 1994a).

PREDICTORS AND MODERATORS

Although prenatal alcohol exposure is a necessary precursor to development of FASD, it is not always sufficient, and not all children exposed to alcohol will develop the same outcome. Several factors related to alcohol consumption (e.g., dose, timing, pattern of exposure) may influence the effects seen in offspring, but few have been investigated in individuals with FASD. One recent study in a population of families in South Africa compared mothers of children with FAS to mothers without children with FAS; the former tended to have lower income, reported a lower level of education, were more likely to be employed on farms, and were more likely to cohabitate without marriage. In addition, a binge-drinking pattern was predictive of having a child with FAS, as were maternal anthropometric measures indicative of undernutrition and multigenerational prenatal alcohol exposure (May et al., 2005). A small number of studies have suggested that genetic factors are important in the expression of FAS or in alcohol's teratogenesis, and specifically that the ADH1B*3 allele may have a protective effect. The mechanism for this effect is unclear, however; it may relate to an effect on the efficiency by which alcohol is metabolized, or, more directly, to an effect on maternal alcohol-drinking behavior (Chambers & Jones, 2002; Warren & Li, 2005).

Most relevant results in this area come from prospective cohort studies. These studies have demonstrated a dose–response relationship: Increased alcohol consumption is associated with worse outcome in the domains of growth, head circumference, attention, memory, language, mathematical skills, and need for special education (Autti-Rämö, 2000; Day et al., 2002; Streissguth et al., 1994a). Although greater exposure is generally associated with worse outcomes, studies have demonstrated negative effects of prenatal alcohol exposure at doses as low as one to two drinks per day (Day et al., 2002; Streissguth, Barr, & Sampson, 1990). Studies using animal models of fetal alcohol exposure support these dose–response relationships, and indicate that timing and pattern of *in utero* alcohol exposure are additional moderators. Timing of exposure interacts with critical developmental periods to influence the nature of the deficits. Exposure in the first trimester interferes with migration of brain cells and facial development (Cook, Keiner, & Yen, 1990; Kotch & Sulik, 1992; Miller, 1993, 1996). Third-trimester exposure is related to malformations in the cerebellum, hippocampus, and prefrontal cortex (Coles et al., 1991; Livy, Miller, Maier, & West, 2003; Sutherland, McDonald, & Savage, 1997; West & Pierce, 1986). In addition, maternal drinking habits may relate to outcome. Some evidence suggests that maternal bingeing behavior may be more harmful than steady alcohol intake (e.g., Sampson, Streissguth, Barr, & Bookstein, 1989). Therefore, an exposed individual's deficits will relate not only to the amount but also to the timing and pattern of maternal alcohol consumption over the course of gestation. Because research has not identified a safe level of alcohol consumption during pregnancy, current guidelines from the American College of Obstetricians and Gynecologists (2000) recommend that pregnant women refrain from drinking alcohol.

A frequent confounding factor is comorbid use of other drugs by the mother during pregnancy. It is unlikely that abuse of one substance occurs in isolation. In one prospective longitudinal study examining the use of cocaine during pregnancy, women who used cocaine were more likely than controls to have used marijuana, alcohol, other amphetamines, and barbiturates prior to and during pregnancy (Richardson, Conroy, & Day, 1996). Substances such as cocaine and nicotine can have consequences for physical and behavioral outcomes (such as growth deficiency and attention deficits) that may be similar to the effects of prenatal alcohol exposure. This relationship can be complex, and it is difficult to isolate the effect of a substance in the presence of other prenatal exposures. One study found that prenatal exposure to alcohol, cocaine, and cigarettes each predicted low birthweight, whereas cocaine exposure was an independent predictor of short stature at age 7, and the effects of prenatal alcohol exposure on growth were moderated by maternal age (Covington, Nordstrom-Klee, Ager, Sokol, & Delaney-Black, 2002). Polysubstance use during pregnancy can also have complex effects on neurobehavioral outcomes (Streissguth et al., 1990). Although alcohol exposure has been associated with attention deficits and impulsivity, one study examining the effects of tobacco, marijuana, and alcohol exposures on a continuous-performance task found that both tobacco and marijuana exposure, but not alcohol exposure, were related to deficits (Richardson et al., 1996). Therefore, screening for exposure to other substances is essential in study designs, and determining a unique neurobehavioral profile resulting from prenatal alcohol exposure (rather than focusing on isolated deficits) may be the most useful approach.

Postbirth environmental factors have also been associated with outcome. Early diagnosis, a stable and enriched domestic environment, having basic needs met, and never experiencing violence were associated with improved outcomes in a heavily exposed population (Streissguth et al., 1996). Interestingly, having an FAS diagnosis, rather than a categorization of fetal alcohol effects, was associated with improved outcomes. The authors suggest that early and definitive FAS diagnosis may assist families in understanding expected disabilities, and also may allow the diagnosed individuals to qualify for special services (Streissguth et al., 1996). Conversely, living in a home with substance-abusing individuals and experiencing violence were associated with poor outcomes (Streissguth et al., 1996). Low paternal IQ and increased number of children present in the household have also been identified as risk factors (Streissguth et al., 1990). Children with prenatal alcohol exposure are at increased risk for exposure to abuse and neglect in their postnatal environments, and these comorbid risk factors are thought to contribute to relatively poorer cognitive outcomes, including language and communication deficits (Coggins, Timler, & Olswang, 2007). Identification of risk and protective environmental factors may indicate appropriate intervention strategies and improved outcomes.

CRITIQUE OF EXISTING RESEARCH

Certain characteristics of the population with FASD create significant obstacles to experimental investigation. As previously discussed, not every individual will exhibit quantifiable effects of prenatal alcohol exposure, and observed effects will vary among individuals. In addition, the influence of confounding variables is not yet known and is likely to differ among individuals. Furthermore, heavily exposed individuals tend to be oversampled to detect observable outcomes (Jacobson & Jacobson, 1996). Such oversampling may inflate the reported effects of prenatal alcohol exposure. An additional and important variable in studying neurotoxic effects of prenatal alcohol exposure is validation of maternal alcohol consumption. Accuracy of maternal report of prenatal alcohol consumption varies as a function of maternal anxiety, maternal age, maternal depression, amount of alcohol consumed, and timing of the report (concurrent vs. retrospective) (Alvik, Haldorsen, Groholt, & Lindemann, 2006). The nature of participant recruitment and confirmation of maternal alcohol consumption are two parameters that are addressed differently in prospective and retrospective investigations of FASD.

Most of the research discussed herein entailed retrospective study designs. Retrospective investigations of prenatal alcohol exposure involve identification of participants any time after birth. Recruitment of participants is typically based on known exposure or on clinical referral of children with identified difficulties, usually in behavior or learning. Because heavily exposed populations and participants with known deficits are likely to exhibit significant outcomes, larger effect sizes are seen in retrospectively recruited samples than in those recruited prospectively. Smaller sample sizes and overall lower costs are therefore possible with retrospective samples.

However, valuable information may be lost with the use of a retrospective design. Because of selective exclusion of those who have subtler or no deficits, most retrospective research focuses on heavily exposed individuals, and specific information on dose and timing of exposure is unavailable. In retrospective populations, birth mothers may be unavailable; valuable medical and demographic history, as well as data regarding dose and timing of alcohol consumption, are difficult to obtain in such cases. Retrospective designs are strengthened by selection of groups that are well matched on important confounders to help control for nonrandomization and the relatively remote reports of maternal alcohol consumption.

Recruitment for prospective studies involves identifying participants before behavioral outcomes are observed. Generally, this is accomplished by targeting women who are likely to drink during pregnancy or by identifying exposed infants at the time of birth. Although the diagnosis of FAS is based on an individual's physical characteristics and CNS function, obtaining accurate reports of maternal drinking during pregnancy is especially important in studies of FASD, given that physical markers of exposure are likely not to be apparent. An advantage of prospective studies is the observation of maternal drinking closer to the time of exposure, which may yield more accurate reports on timing and dosage of alcohol—two important parameters in research on teratogenic effects (Streissguth, Sampson, Barr, Bookstein, & Olson, 1994b). In addition, when the mother has been identified, more accurate information on demographic and environmental history is available. Another advantage of prospective studies is the possibility of adopting a longitudinal design. Initial brain damage resulting from prenatal alcohol exposure may not have consistent manifestations across different developmental periods, and repeated measures of an exposed individual's outcome can be helpful in detailing these changes over time.

Prospective designs also have drawbacks. One goal of teratogenic research is to delineate a dose–response relationship. However, prospectively identified participants typically are not heavily exposed, and therefore much larger samples are required to detect effects. Moreover, longitudinal prospective studies are costly and time-consuming, and therefore not always feasible. Nevertheless, public policy and funding are based at least in part on scientific investigation, and one consequence of not detecting teratogenic effects of alcohol is less allocation of resources to a disabled population (Vorhees, 1986).

SUGGESTIONS FOR FUTURE RESEARCH

Although over 30 years of research of the teratogenic effects of alcohol has yielded an impressive amount of information, some areas have been understudied, and current research will probably lead to new lines of investigation. Certain neuropsychological domains have not been adequately examined in populations with prenatal alcohol exposure. A critical goal in this field is to identify a well-defined neurobehavioral profile to assist in the identification of alcohol-exposed individuals. To do this, continued examination of specific but understudied domains (e.g., working memory, visual–spatial skills, speech and language, nonverbal memory, and specific aspects of attention) is required. Integration of these domains into the current literature, as well as comparisons with other clinical groups, will improve diagnostic specificity. In addition, increased use of longitudinal study designs will help in identifying the cognitive and behavioral manifestations of prenatal alcohol exposure over time, and may help demonstrate potential environmental moderators of the effect of the initial alcohol insult. Improved specification will also enable identification and diagnosis of alcohol-exposed individuals, leading to more appropriate and informed care.

A recent trend has been increasing attention to international research. Recent studies have demonstrated similarities in the manifestation of FAS, despite differing cultures and types of alcohol consumed (Strömland et al., 2005; Warren et al., 2001). Identification of high-risk populations in Russia and South Africa have led to the inclusion of these and other worldwide samples into current scientific examination. Because neurobehavioral profiles to identify children with prenatal alcohol exposure are still being developed, inclusion of more diverse samples will allow for better specification and an opportunity to assist underserved populations. Research including these regions may lead to valuable opportunities to intervene in a large underidentified population. In addition, an international strategy for identification of these children may allow for better diagnostic specificity; criteria that are both universal and useful worldwide may be delineated. This information may be applied specifically within the domain of international adoptions, as information on maternal drinking patterns is likely to be unavailable in such a population, and identification of effects of prenatal alcohol exposure in adopted individuals may allow for early intervention strategies to be applied.

Structural neuroimaging of individuals with FASD has increased awareness of brain areas particularly vulnerable to prenatal alcohol exposure. Increased use of functional brain imaging techniques may be helpful in elucidating brain–behavior correlates and abnormal patterns of brain activity. As with other clinical populations, and especially within a developmental context, researchers will need to give careful consideration to the experimental designs for these studies. It is necessary to assure that differential brain activity in alcohol-exposed populations is due to specific and attributable deficits rather than to differences in performance level. For future functional imaging studies, Bookheimer and Sowell (2005) suggest implementation of parametric designs and performance-matched comparisons to allow for contrast of hemodynamic patterns between alcohol-exposed and control participants, as well as studies of differential activation associated with increased effort/differential performance between the groups. If studies are limited to tasks on which alcohol-exposed subjects are proficient, abnormal patterns of brain activation related to impairments may be overlooked or may lead to nonrepresentative results. In addition, prenatal alcohol exposure leads to a spectrum of outcomes, and clinical populations tend to demonstrate variable performance (Bookheimer & Sowell, 2005). Therefore, large sample sizes and well-defined inclusion and exclusion criteria will help to assure sufficient power to detect differences in both brain structure and function.

Continued and increased use of multidisciplinary approaches will lead to well-informed scientific investigations. Prenatal alcohol exposure leads to significant negative outcomes in all spheres of functioning (e.g., health, neurocognitive, family, social, financial). Dissemination of current neurobehavioral and neuroimaging findings into medical and educational settings, and dialogue with health professionals and educators, will be essential in assuring that the questions asked and conclusions reached are ecologically valid for the population. Similarly, increased information on relative strengths and weaknesses in the population will aid in guiding intervention programs. Some promising research suggests that early identification and modification of environment may lead to better outcomes. Researchers have begun to develop school- and laboratory-based intervention programs, with some success (Adnams et al., 2007; Coles, Strickland, Padgett, & Bellmoff, 2007; Frankel, Paley, Marquardt, & O'Connor, 2006; Kable, Coles, & Taddeo, 2007). Along with continued efforts to identify individuals affected by FASD, developing avenues to assist with learning, attending, and understanding contingencies and consequences will be invaluable.

CONCLUSIONS

In utero exposure to alcohol can cause permanent brain damage and lifelong neurobehavioral deficits. Imaging research has revealed a general pattern of overall reduction in brain size for heavily exposed individuals, as well as areas of relative alteration, after overall brain size is taken into account. Size and cortical shape alterations have been found in parietal and frontal lobes. Specific structures of relative vulnerability include the corpus callosum, cerebellum, and caudate nucleus, which are reduced in size and altered in shape. Brain abnormalities are likely to be related to the cognitive deficits found in this population. Significant research efforts have begun to delineate a neurobehavioral profile for individuals with prenatal alcohol exposure. Determining strengths and weaknesses will allow for better diagnostic specificity and will guide interventions for the many adversely affected children in this large population. Findings thus far generally show that individuals with heavy prenatal alcohol exposure have reduced overall IQ, as well as specific deficits in visual–spatial, psychomotor, attention, learning, and EF domains. In addition, individuals with a history of alcohol exposure have impairments in socialization that are worse than expected from IQ, and they are at increased risk for negative life events (e.g., incarceration, substance abuse, and psychopathology). The effects of prenatal alcohol exposure on structure and function can vary among individuals, and some moderating factors have been identified, including timing and dose of maternal alcohol consumption, concurrent use of other substances by the mother, and other environmental factors.

Finally, the economic impact of FASD in the United States alone is staggering, as prevalence estimates of FASD suggest that as many as 1 in 100 individuals are affected by prenatal alcohol exposure. Recent inclusion of international samples has confirmed that alcohol consumption during pregnancy is a worldwide phenomenon, and that further investigation into diverse samples will provide a better representation of outcomes. Thus FASD is a widespread disorder with great public health and economic significance. Integration of new imaging techniques; continued delineation of neuropsychological profiles; and collaboration among medical, educational, and psychological disciplines are required to identify and assist this large and currently underidentified population.

ACKNOWLEDGMENTS

Preparation of this chapter was supported in part by National Institute on Alcohol Abuse and Alcoholism Grant Nos. R01 AA10820, R01 AA10417, U01 AA14834, and T32 AA13525. We gratefully acknowledge the assistance and support of the Center for Behavioral Teratology, San Diego State University.

REFERENCES

Adnams, C. M., Kodituwakku, P. W., Hay, A., Molteno, C. D., Viljoen, D., & May, P. A. (2001). Patterns of cognitive–motor development in children with fetal alcohol syndrome from a community in South Africa. *Alcoholism: Clinical and Experimental Research, 25,* 557–562.

Adnams, C. M., Sorour, P., Kalberg, W. O., Kodituwakku, P., Perold, M. D., Kotze, A., et al. (2007). Language and literacy outcomes from a pilot intervention study for children with fetal alcohol spectrum disorders in South Africa. *Alcohol, 41,* 403–414.

Alvik, A., Haldorsen, T., Groholt, B., & Lindemann, R. (2006). Alcohol consumption before and during pregnancy comparing concurrent and retrospective reports. *Alcoholism: Clinical and Experimental Research, 30,* 510–515.

American College of Obstetricians and Gynecologists. (2000). *Alcohol and pregnancy* (Education Pamphlet No. AP132). Washington, DC: Author.

Archibald, S. L., Fennema-Notestine, C., Gamst, A., Riley, E. P., Mattson, S. N., & Jernigan, T. L. (2001). Brain dysmorphology in individuals with severe prenatal alcohol exposure. *Developmental Medicine and Child Neurology, 43,* 148–154.

Autti-Rämö, I. (2000). Twelve-year follow-up of children exposed to alcohol *in utero. Developmental Medicine and Child Neurology, 42,* 406–411.

Autti-Rämö, I., Autti, T., Korkman, M., Kettunen, S., Salonen, O., & Valanne, L. (2002). MRI findings in children with school problems who had been exposed prenatally to alcohol. *Developmental Medicine and Child Neurology, 44,* 98–106.

Barr, H. M., Bookstein, F. L., O'Malley, K. D., Connor, P. D., Huggins, J. E., & Streissguth, A. P. (2006). Binge drinking during pregnancy as a predictor of psychiatric disorders on the Structured Clinical Interview for DSM-IV in young adult offspring. *American Journal of Psychiatry, 163,* 1061–1065.

Bertrand, J., Floyd, R. L., & Weber, M. K. (2005). Guidelines for identifying and referring persons with fetal alcohol syndrome. *Morbidity and Mortality Weekly Report Recommendations and Reports, 54,* 1–14.

Bertrand, J., Floyd, R. L., Weber, M. K., O'Connor, M., Riley, E. P., Johnson, K. A., et al. (2004). *National Task Force on FAS/FAE: Guidelines for referral and diagnosis.* Atlanta, GA: Centers for Disease Control and Prevention.

Bhatara, V. S., Lovrein, F., Kirkeby, J., Swayze, V., II, Unruh, E., & Johnson, V. (2002). Brain function in fetal alcohol syndrome assessed by single photon emission computed tomography. *South Dakota Journal of Medicine, 55,* 59–62.

Bookheimer, S. Y., & Sowell, E. R. (2005). Brain imaging in FAS: Commentary on the article by Malisza et al. *Pediatric Research, 58,* 1148–1149.

Bookstein, F. L., Sampson, P. D., Connor, P. D., & Streissguth, A. P. (2002a). Midline corpus callosum is a neuroanatomical focus of fetal alcohol damage. *Anatomical Record: Part B. New Anatomist, 269,* 162–174.

Bookstein, F. L., Streissguth, A. P., Sampson, P. D., Connor, P. D., & Barr, H. M. (2002b). Corpus callosum shape and neuropsychological deficits in adult males with heavy fetal alcohol exposure. *NeuroImage, 15,* 233–251.

Burden, M. J., Jacobson, S. W., Sokol, R. J., & Jacobson, J. L. (2005). Effects of prenatal alcohol exposure on attention and working memory at 7.5 years of age. *Alcoholism: Clinical and Experimental Research, 29,* 443–452.

Calarco, K. E., Mattson, S. N., Robertson, B., & Riley, E. P. (2003). Heavy prenatal alcohol exposure or ADHD?: Errors make the difference. *Journal of the International Neuropsychological Society, 9,* 152.

Carney, L. J., & Chermak, G. D. (1991). Performance of American Indian children with fetal alcohol syndrome on the test of language development. *Journal of Communication Disorders, 24,* 123–134.

Casey, B. J., Tottenham, N., & Fossella, J. (2002). Clinical, imaging, lesion, and genetic approaches toward a model of cognitive control. *Developmental Psychobiology, 40,* 237–254.

Centers for Disease Control and Prevention (CDC). (2004). Alcohol consumption among women who are pregnant or who might become pregnant—United States, 2002. *Morbidity and Mortality Weekly Report, 53,* 1178–1181.

Chambers, C. D., & Jones, K. L. (2002). Is genotype important in predicting the fetal alcohol syndrome? *Journal of Pediatrics, 141,* 751–752.

Chandler, L. S., Richardson, G. A., Gallagher, J. D., & Day, N. L. (1996). Prenatal exposure to alcohol and marijuana: Effects on motor development of preschool children. *Alcoholism: Clinical and Experimental Research, 20,* 455–461.

Church, M. W., Eldis, F., Blakley, B. W., & Bawle, E. V. (1997). Hearing, language, speech, vestibular, and dentofacial disorders in fetal alcohol syndrome. *Alcoholism: Clinical and Experimental Research, 21,* 227–237.

Clark, C. M., Li, D., Conry, J., Conry, R., & Loock, C. (2000). Structural and functional brain integrity of fetal alcohol syndrome in nonretarded cases. *Pediatrics, 105,* 1096–1099.

Coggins, T. E., Timler, G. R., & Olswang, L. B. (2007). A state of double jeopardy: Impact of prenatal alcohol exposure and adverse environments on the social communicative abilities of school-age children with fetal alcohol spectrum disorder. *Language, Speech, and Hearing Services in Schools, 38,* 117–127.

Coles, C. D., Brown, R. T., Smith, I. E., Platzman, K. A., Erickson, S., & Falek, A. (1991). Effects of prenatal alcohol exposure at school age: I. Physical and cognitive development. *Neurotoxicology and Teratology, 13,* 357–367.

Coles, C. D., Platzman, K. A., Lynch, M. E., & Freides, D. (2002). Auditory and visual sustained attention in adolescents prenatally exposed to alcohol. *Alcoholism: Clinical and Experimental Research, 26,* 263–271.

Coles, C. D., Platzman, K. A., Raskind-Hood, C. L., Brown, R. T., Falek, A., & Smith, I. E. (1997). A comparison of children affected by prenatal alcohol exposure and attention deficit, hyperactivity disorder. *Alcoholism: Clinical and Experimental Research, 21,* 150–161.

Coles, C. D., Strickland, D. C., Padgett, L., & Bellmoff, L. (2007). Games that "work": Using computer games to teach alcohol-affected children about fire and street safety. *Research in Developmental Disabilities, 28,* 518–530.

Connor, P. D., Sampson, P. D., Bookstein, F. L., Barr, H. M., & Streissguth, A. P. (2000). Direct and indirect effects of prenatal alcohol damage on executive function. *Developmental Neuropsychology, 18,* 331–354.

Connor, P. D., Sampson, P. D., Streissguth, A. P., Bookstein, F. L., & Barr, H. M. (2006). Effects of prenatal alcohol exposure on fine motor coordination and balance: A study of two adult samples. *Neuropsychologia, 44,* 744–751.

Connor, P. D., Streissguth, A. P., Sampson, P. D., Bookstein, F. L., & Barr, H. M. (1999). Individual differences in auditory and visual attention among fetal alcohol-affected adults. *Alcoholism: Clinical and Experimental Research, 23,* 1395–1402.

Conry, J. (1990). Neuropsychological deficits in fetal alcohol syndrome and fetal alcohol effects. *Alcoholism: Clinical and Experimental Research, 14,* 650–655.

Cook, R. T., Keiner, J. A., & Yen, A. (1990). Ethanol causes accelerated G1 arrest in differentiating HL-60 cells. *Alcoholism: Clinical and Experimental Research, 14,* 695–703.

Cortese, B. M., Moore, G. J., Bailey, B. A., Jacobson, S. W., Delaney-Black, V., & Hannigan, J. H. (2006). Magnetic resonance and spectroscopic imaging in prenatal alcohol-exposed children: Preliminary findings in the caudate nucleus. *Neurotoxicology and Teratology, 28,* 597–606.

Covington, C. Y., Nordstrom-Klee, B., Ager, J., Sokol, R., & Delaney-Black, V. (2002). Birth to age 7 growth of children prenatally exposed to drugs: A prospective cohort study. *Neurotoxicology and Teratology, 24,* 489–496.

Crocker, N., Wagner, A. E., Vaurio, L., & Mattson, S. N. (2009). Children with heavy prenatal alcohol exposure show what and where visuospatial deficits. *Journal of the International Neuropsychological Society, 15*(Suppl. S1). doi: 10.1017/S1355617709090420, Published online April 29, 2009, *heep:// journals.cambridge.org/action/displayIssue?jid=INS&volumeID=15&seriesID=0&issueID=S1.*

Crocker, N. A. (2008). *Comparison of adaptive behavior in children with fetal alcohol spectrum disorders and attention-deficit/hyperactivity disorder.* Unpublished master's thesis, San Diego State University.

Day, N. L., Leech, S. L., Richardson, G. A., Cornelius, M. D., Robles, N., & Larkby, C. (2002). Prenatal alcohol exposure predicts continued deficits in offspring size at 14 years of age. *Alcoholism: Clinical and Experimental Research, 26,* 1584–1591.

Delis, D. C., Kaplan, E., & Kramer, J. H. (2001). *Manual for the Delis–Kaplan Executive Function System.* San Antonio, TX: Psychological Corporation.

Fagerlund, Å., Heikkinen, S., Autti-Rämö, I., Korkman, M., Timonen, M., Kuusi, T., et al. (2006). Brain metabolic alterations in adolescents and young adults with fetal alcohol spectrum disorders. *Alcoholism: Clinical and Experimental Research, 30,* 2097–2104.

Famy, C., Streissguth, A. P., & Unis, A. S. (1998). Mental illness in adults with fetal alcohol syndrome or fetal alcohol effects. *American Journal of Psychiatry, 155,* 552–554.

Frankel, F., Paley, B., Marquardt, R., & O'Connor, M. (2006). Stimulants, neuroleptics, and children's friendship training for children with fetal alcohol spectrum disorders. *Journal of Child and Adolescent Psychopharmacology, 16,* 777–789.

Fryer, S. L., McGee, C. L., Matt, G. E., Riley, E. P., & Mattson, S. N. (2007a). Evaluation of psychopathological conditions in children with heavy prenatal alcohol exposure. *Pediatrics, 119,* e733–e741.

Fryer, S. L., Schweinsburg, B. C., Bjorkquist, O. A., Frank, L. R., Mattson, S. N., Spadoni, A. D., et al. (2009). Characterization of white matter microstructure in fetal alcohol spectrum disorders. *Alcoholism: Clinical and Experimental Research, 33*(3), 514–521.

Fryer, S. L., Tapert, S. F., Mattson, S. N., Paulus, M. P., Spadoni, A. D., & Riley, E. P. (2007b). Prenatal alcohol exposure affects frontal–striatal BOLD response during inhibitory control. *Alcoholism: Clinical and Experimental Research, 31,* 1415–1424.

Hamilton, D. A., Kodituwakku, P., Sutherland, R. J., & Savage, D. D. (2003). Children with fetal alcohol syndrome are impaired at place learning but not cued-navigation in a virtual Morris water task. *Behavioural Brain Research, 143,* 85–94.

Hayden, K. E. (2005). *Verbal fluency clustering and switching in children with heavy prenatal alcohol expo-sure.* Unpublished master's thesis, San Diego State University.

Hofer, S., & Frahm, J. (2006). Topography of the human corpus callosum revisited: Comprehensive fiber tractography using diffusion tensor magnetic resonance imaging. *NeuroImage, 32,* 989–994.

Hoyme, H. E., May, P. A., Kalberg, W. O., Kodituwakku, P., Gossage, J. P., Trujillo, P. M., et al. (2005). A practical clinical approach to diagnosis of fetal alcohol spectrum disorders: Clarification of the 1996 Institute of Medicine criteria. *Pediatrics, 115,* 39–47.

Jacobson, J. L., & Jacobson, S. W. (1996). Methodological considerations in behavioral toxicology in infants and children. *Developmental Psychology, 32,* 390–403.

Janzen, L. A., Nanson, J. L., & Block, G. W. (1995). Neuropsychological evaluation of preschoolers with fetal alcohol syndrome. *Neurotoxicology and Teratology, 17,* 273–279.

Jeret, J. S., & Serur, D. (1991). Fetal alcohol syndrome in adolescents and adults [Letter to the editor]. *Journal of the American Medical Association, 266,* 1077.

Johnson, T. B., & Goodlett, C. R. (2002). Selective and enduring deficits in spatial learning after limited neonatal binge alcohol exposure in male rats. *Alcoholism: Clinical and Experimental Research, 26,* 83–93.

Johnson, V. P., Swayze, V. W., II, Sato, Y., & Andreasen, N. C. (1996). Fetal alcohol syndrome: Craniofa-cial and central nervous system manifestations. *American Journal of Medical Genetics, 61,* 329–339.

Jones, K. L., & Smith, D. W. (1973). Recognition of the fetal alcohol syndrome in early infancy. *Lancet, ii*(7836), 999–1001.

Jones, K. L., & Smith, D. W. (1975). The fetal alcohol syndrome. *Teratology, 12,* 1–10.

Jones, K. L., Smith, D. W., Ulleland, C. N., & Streissguth, A. P. (1973). Pattern of malformation in off-spring of chronic alcoholic mothers. *Lancet, i*(7815), 1267–1271.

Kable, J. A., Coles, C. D., & Taddeo, E. (2007). Socio-cognitive habilitation using the math interactive learning experience program for alcohol-affected children. *Alcoholism: Clinical and Experimental Research, 31,* 1425–1434.

Kaemingk, K. L., & Halverson, P. T. (2000). Spatial memory following prenatal alcohol exposure: More than a material specific memory deficit. *Child Neuropsychology, 6,* 115–128.

Kaemingk, K. L., Mulvaney, S., & Tanner Halverson, P. (2003). Learning following prenatal alcohol exposure: Performance on verbal and visual multitrial tasks. *Archives of Clinical Neuropsychology, 18,* 33–47.

Kerns, K. A., Don, A., Mateer, C. A., & Streissguth, A. P. (1997). Cognitive deficits in nonretarded adults with fetal alcohol syndrome. *Journal of Learning Disabilities, 30,* 685–693.

Kodituwakku, P. W., Adnams, C. M., Hay, A., Kitching, A. E., Burger, E., Kalberg, W. O., et al. (2006). Letter and category fluency in children with fetal alcohol syndrome from a community in South Africa. *Journal of Studies on Alcohol, 67,* 502–509.

Kodituwakku, P. W., Handmaker, N. S., Cutler, S. K., Weathersby, E. K., & Handmaker, S. D. (1995). Specific impairments in self-regulation in children exposed to alcohol prenatally. *Alcoholism: Clini-cal and Experimental Research, 19,* 1558–1564.

Kotch, L. E., & Sulik, K. K. (1992). Experimental fetal alcohol syndrome: Proposed pathogenic basis for a variety of associated facial and brain anomalies. *American Journal of Medical Genetics, 44,* 168–176.

Lee, K. T., Mattson, S. N., & Riley, E. P. (2004). Classifying children with heavy prenatal alcohol expo-sure using measures of attention. *Journal of the International Neuropsychological Society, 10,* 271–277.

Livy, D. J., Miller, E. K., Maier, S. E., & West, J. R. (2003). Fetal alcohol exposure and temporal vulner-ability: Effects of binge-like alcohol exposure on the developing rat hippocampus. *Neurotoxicology and Teratology, 25,* 447–458.

Lupton, C., Burd, L., & Harwood, R. (2004). Cost of fetal alcohol spectrum disorders. *American Journal of Medical Genetics: Part C. Seminars in Medical Genetics, 127,* 42–50.

Lynch, M. E., Coles, C. D., Corley, T., & Falek, A. (2003). Examining delinquency in adolescents differentially prenatally exposed to alcohol: The role of proximal and distal risk factors. *Journal of Studies on Alcohol, 64,* 678–686.

Ma, X., Coles, C. D., Lynch, M. E., LaConte, S. M., Zurkiya, O., Wang, D., et al. (2005). Evaluation of corpus callosum anisotropy in young adults with fetal alcohol syndrome according to diffusion tensor imaging. *Alcoholism: Clinical and Experimental Research, 29,* 1214–1222.

Malisza, K. L., Allman, A.-A., Shiloff, D., Jakobson, L., Longstaffe, S., & Chudley, A. E. (2005). Evaluation of spatial working memory function in children and adults with fetal alcohol spectrum disorders: A functional magnetic resonance imaging study. *Pediatric Research, 58,* 1150–1157.

Mattson, S. N., Autti-Rämö, I., May, P. A., Konovalova, V., & the CIFASD Consortium. (2006a). Spatial learning and navigation deficits in an international sample of children with heavy prenatal alcohol exposure. *Alcoholism: Clinical and Experimental Research, 30*(9), 176A.

Mattson, S. N., Calarco, K. E., & Lang, A. R. (2006b). Focused and shifting attention in children with heavy prenatal alcohol exposure. *Neuropsychology, 20,* 361–369.

Mattson, S. N., Goodman, A. M., Caine, C., Delis, D. C., & Riley, E. P. (1999). Executive functioning in children with heavy prenatal alcohol exposure. *Alcoholism: Clinical and Experimental Research, 23,* 1808–1815.

Mattson, S. N., Gramling, L., Delis, D., Jones, K. L., & Riley, E. P. (1996a). Global–local processing in children prenatally exposed to alcohol. *Child Neuropsychology, 2,* 165–175.

Mattson, S. N., Lee, K. T., Hayden, K., & Riley, E. P. (2005). Comparison of adaptive behavior deficits in children with fetal alcohol spectrum disorders and/or ADHD. *Alcoholism: Clinical and Experimental Research, 29*(5), 46A.

Mattson, S. N., & Riley, E. P. (1998). A review of the neurobehavioral deficits in children with fetal alcohol syndrome or prenatal exposure to alcohol. *Alcoholism: Clinical and Experimental Research, 22,* 279–294.

Mattson, S. N., & Riley, E. P. (1999). Implicit and explicit memory functioning in children with heavy prenatal alcohol exposure. *Journal of the International Neuropsychological Society, 5,* 462–471.

Mattson, S. N., & Riley, E. P. (2000). Parent ratings of behavior in children with heavy prenatal alcohol exposure and IQ-matched controls. *Alcoholism: Clinical and Experimental Research, 24,* 226–231.

Mattson, S. N., Riley, E. P., Delis, D. C., Stern, C., & Jones, K. L. (1996b). Verbal learning and memory in children with fetal alcohol syndrome. *Alcoholism: Clinical and Experimental Research, 20,* 810–816.

Mattson, S. N., Riley, E. P., Gramling, L. J., Delis, D. C., & Jones, K. L. (1997). Heavy prenatal alcohol exposure with or without physical features of fetal alcohol syndrome leads to IQ deficits. *Journal of Pediatrics, 131,* 718–721.

Mattson, S. N., Riley, E. P., Gramling, L. J., Delis, D. C., & Jones, K. L. (1998). Neuropsychological comparison of alcohol-exposed children with or without physical features of fetal alcohol syndrome. *Neuropsychology, 12,* 146–153.

Mattson, S. N., Riley, E. P., Jernigan, T. L., Ehlers, C. L., Delis, D. C., Jones, K. L., et al. (1992). Fetal alcohol syndrome: A case report of neuropsychological, MRI and EEG assessment of two children. *Alcoholism: Clinical and Experimental Research, 16,* 1001–1003.

Mattson, S. N., Riley, E. P., Jernigan, T. L., Garcia, A., Kaneko, W. M., Ehlers, C. L., et al. (1994). A decrease in the size of the basal ganglia following prenatal alcohol exposure: A preliminary report. *Neurotoxicology and Teratology, 16,* 283–289.

Mattson, S. N., Riley, E. P., Sowell, E. R., Jernigan, T. L., Sobel, D. F., & Jones, K. L. (1996c). A decrease in the size of the basal ganglia in children with fetal alcohol syndrome. *Alcoholism: Clinical and Experimental Research, 20,* 1088–1093.

Mattson, S. N., & Roebuck, T. M. (2002). Acquisition and retention of verbal and nonverbal information in children with heavy prenatal alcohol exposure. *Alcoholism: Clinical and Experimental Research, 26,* 875–882.

May, P. A., Gossage, J. P., Brooke, L. E., Snell, C. L., Marais, A. S., Hendricks, L. S., et al. (2005). Maternal risk factors for fetal alcohol syndrome in the Western Cape Province of South Africa: A population-based study. *American Journal of Public Health, 95,* 1190–1199.

McGee, C. L., Bjorkquist, O. A., Riley, E. P., & Mattson, S. N. (2009). Impaired language performance in young children with heavy prenatal alcohol exposure. *Neurotoxicology and Teratology, 31*(2), 71–75.

Miller, M. W. (1993). Migration of cortical neurons is altered by gestational exposure to ethanol. *Alcoholism: Clinical and Experimental Research, 17,* 304–314.

Miller, M. W. (1996). Limited ethanol exposure selectively alters the proliferation of precursor cells in the cerebral cortex. *Alcoholism: Clinical and Experimental Research, 20,* 139–143.

O'Hare, E. D., Kan, E., Yoshii, J., Mattson, S. N., Riley, E. P., Thompson, P. M., et al. (2005). Mapping cerebellar vermal morphology and cognitive correlates in prenatal alcohol exposure. *NeuroReport, 16,* 1285–1290.

Pulsifer, M. B. (1996). The neuropsychology of mental retardation. *Journal of the International Neuropsychological Society, 2,* 159–176.

Richardson, G. A., Conroy, M. L., & Day, N. L. (1996). Prenatal cocaine exposure: Effects on the development of school-age children. *Neurotoxicology and Teratology, 18,* 627–634.

Richardson, G. A., Ryan, C., Willford, J., Day, N. L., & Goldschmidt, L. (2002). Prenatal alcohol and marijuana exposure: Effects on neuropsychological outcomes at 10 years. *Neurotoxicology and Teratology, 24,* 309–320.

Riikonen, R., Nokelainen, P., Valkonen, K., Kolehmainen, A. I., Kumpulainen, K. I., Kononen, M., et al. (2005). Deep serotonergic and dopaminergic structures in fetal alcoholic syndrome: A study with nor-ß-CIT-single-photon emission computed tomography and magnetic resonance imaging volumetry. *Biological Psychiatry, 57,* 1565–1572.

Riikonen, R., Salonen, I., Partanen, K., & Verho, S. (1999). Brain perfusion SPECT and MRI in fetal alcohol syndrome. *Developmental Medicine and Child Neurology, 41,* 652–659.

Riley, E. P., Mattson, S. N., Sowell, E. R., Jernigan, T. L., Sobel, D. F., & Jones, K. L. (1995). Abnormalities of the corpus callosum in children prenatally exposed to alcohol. *Alcoholism: Clinical and Experimental Research, 19,* 1198–1202.

Riley, E. P., McGee, C. L., & Sowell, E. R. (2004). Teratogenic effects of alcohol: A decade of brain imaging. *American Journal of Medical Genetics: Part C. Seminars in Medical Genetics, 127,* 35–41.

Roebuck, T. M., Mattson, S. N., & Riley, E. P. (1998a). A review of the neuroanatomical findings in children with fetal alcohol syndrome or prenatal exposure to alcohol. *Alcoholism: Clinical and Experimental Research, 22,* 339–344.

Roebuck, T. M., Mattson, S. N., & Riley, E. P. (1999). Behavioral and psychosocial profiles of alcohol-exposed children. *Alcoholism: Clinical and Experimental Research, 23,* 1070–1076.

Roebuck, T. M., Mattson, S. N., & Riley, E. P. (2002). Interhemispheric transfer in children with heavy prenatal alcohol exposure. *Alcoholism: Clinical and Experimental Research, 26,* 1863–1871.

Roebuck, T. M., Simmons, R. W., Mattson, S. N., & Riley, E. P. (1998b). Prenatal exposure to alcohol affects the ability to maintain postural balance. *Alcoholism: Clinical and Experimental Research, 22,* 252–258.

Roebuck, T. M., Simmons, R. W., Richardson, C., Mattson, S. N., & Riley, E. P. (1998c). Neuromuscular responses to disturbance of balance in children with prenatal exposure to alcohol. *Alcoholism: Clinical and Experimental Research, 22,* 1992–1997.

Roebuck-Spencer, T. M., & Mattson, S. N. (2004). Implicit strategy affects learning in children with heavy prenatal alcohol exposure. *Alcoholism: Clinical and Experimental Research, 28,* 1424–1431.

Sampson, P. D., Streissguth, A. P., Barr, H. M., & Bookstein, F. L. (1989). Neurobehavioral effects of prenatal alcohol: Part II. Partial least squares analysis. *Neurotoxicology and Teratology, 11,* 477–491.

Sampson, P. D., Streissguth, A. P., Bookstein, F. L., Little, R. E., Clarren, S. K., Dehaene, P., et al. (1997). Incidence of fetal alcohol syndrome and prevalence of alcohol-related neurodevelopmental disorder. *Teratology, 56,* 317–326.

Schonfeld, A. M., Mattson, S. N., Lang, A. R., Delis, D. C., & Riley, E. P. (2001). Verbal and nonverbal fluency in children with heavy prenatal alcohol exposure. *Journal of Studies on Alcohol, 62,* 239–246.

Schonfeld, A. M., Mattson, S. N., & Riley, E. P. (2005). Moral maturity and delinquency after prenatal alcohol exposure. *Journal of Studies on Alcohol, 66,* 545–555.

Schonfeld, A. M., Paley, B., Frankel, F., & O'Connor, M. J. (2006). Executive functioning predicts social skills following prenatal alcohol exposure. *Child Neuropsychology, 12,* 439–452.

Sowell, E. R., Jernigan, T. L., Mattson, S. N., Riley, E. P., Sobel, D. F., & Jones, K. L. (1996). Abnormal development of the cerebellar vermis in children prenatally exposed to alcohol: Size reduction in lobules I–V. *Alcoholism: Clinical and Experimental Research, 20,* 31–34.

Sowell, E. R., Johnson, A., Kan, E., Lu, L. H., Van Horn, J. D., Toga, A. W., et al. (2008a). Mapping white matter integrity and neurobehavioral correlates in children with fetal alcohol spectrum disorders. *Journal of Neuroscience, 28,* 1313–1319.

Sowell, E. R., Lu, L. H., O'Hare, E. D., McCourt, S. T., Mattson, S. N., O'Connor, M. J., et al. (2007). Functional magnetic resonance imaging of verbal learning in children with heavy prenatal alcohol exposure. *NeuroReport, 18,* 635–639.

Sowell, E. R., Mattson, S. N., Kan, E., Thompson, P. M., Riley, E. P., & Toga, A. W. (2008b). Abnormal cortical thickness and brain–behavior correlation patterns in individuals with heavy prenatal alcohol exposure. *Cerebral Cortex, 18,* 136–144.

Sowell, E. R., Mattson, S. N., Thompson, P. M., Jernigan, T. L., Riley, E. P., & Toga, A. W. (2001a). Mapping callosal morphology and cognitive correlates: Effects of heavy prenatal alcohol exposure. *Neurology, 57,* 235–244.

Sowell, E. R., Thompson, P. M., Mattson, S. N., Tessner, K. D., Jernigan, T. L., Riley, E. P., et al. (2001b). Voxel-based morphometric analyses of the brain in children and adolescents prenatally exposed to alcohol. *NeuroReport, 12,* 515–523.

Sowell, E. R., Thompson, P. M., Mattson, S. N., Tessner, K. D., Jernigan, T. L., Riley, E. P., et al. (2002a). Regional brain shape abnormalities persist into adolescence after heavy prenatal alcohol exposure. *Cerebral Cortex, 12,* 856–865.

Sowell, E. R., Thompson, P. M., Peterson, B. S., Mattson, S. N., Welcome, S. E., Henkenius, A. L., et al. (2002b). Mapping cortical gray matter asymmetry patterns in adolescents with heavy prenatal alcohol exposure. *NeuroImage, 17,* 1807–1819.

Steinhausen, H.-C., & Spohr, H.-L. (1998). Long-term outcome of children with fetal alcohol syndrome: Psychopathology, behavior and intelligence. *Alcoholism: Clinical and Experimental Research, 22,* 334–338.

Stratton, K., Howe, C., & Battaglia, F. (1996). *Fetal alcohol syndrome: Diagnosis, epidemiology, prevention, and treatment.* Washington, DC: National Academy Press.

Streissguth, A. P., Aase, J. M., Clarren, S. K., Randels, S. P., LaDue, R. A., & Smith, D. F. (1991a). Fetal alcohol syndrome in adolescents and adults. *Journal of the American Medical Association, 265,* 1961–1967.

Streissguth, A. P., Barr, H. M., Kogan, J., & Bookstein, F. L. (1996). *Final report: Understanding the occurrence of secondary disabilities in clients with fetal alcohol syndrome (FAS) and fetal alcohol effects (FAE).* Seattle: University of Washington Publication Services.

Streissguth, A. P., Barr, H. M., & Sampson, P. D. (1990). Moderate prenatal alcohol exposure: Effects on child IQ and learning problems at age 7 1/2 years. *Alcoholism: Clinical and Experimental Research, 14,* 662–669.

Streissguth, A. P., Barr, H. M., Sampson, P. D., & Bookstein, F. L. (1994a). Prenatal alcohol and offspring development: The first fourteen years. *Drug and Alcohol Dependence, 36,* 89–99.

Streissguth, A. P., Randels, S. P., & Smith, D. F. (1991b). A test–retest study of intelligence in patients with fetal alcohol syndrome: Implications for care. *Journal of the American Academy of Child and Adolescent Psychiatry, 30,* 584–587.

Streissguth, A. P., Sampson, P. D., Barr, H. M., Bookstein, F. L., & Olson, H. C. (1994b). The effects of prenatal exposure to alcohol and tobacco: Contributions from the Seattle longitudinal prospective study and implications for public policy. In H. L. Needleman & D. Bellinger (Eds.), *Prenatal exposure to toxicants: Developmental consequences* (pp. 148–183). Baltimore: Johns Hopkins University Press.

Strömland, K., Mattson, S. N., Adnams, C. M., Autti-Rämö, I., Riley, E. P., & Warren, K. R. (2005). Fetal alcohol spectrum disorders: An international prospective. *Alcoholism: Clinical and Experimental Research, 29,* 1121–1126.

Sutherland, R. J., McDonald, R. J., & Savage, D. D. (1997). Prenatal exposure to moderate levels of ethanol can have long-lasting effects on hippocampal synaptic plasticity in adult offspring. *Hippocampus, 7,* 232–238.

Swayze, V. W., II, Johnson, V. P., Hanson, J. W., Piven, J., Sato, Y., Giedd, J. N., et al. (1997). Magnetic resonance imaging of brain anomalies in fetal alcohol syndrome. *Pediatrics, 99,* 232–240.

Thomas, S. E., Kelly, S. J., Mattson, S. N., & Riley, E. P. (1998). Comparison of social abilities of children with fetal alcohol syndrome to those of children with similar IQ scores and normal controls. *Alcoholism: Clinical and Experimental Research, 22,* 528–533.

Uecker, A., & Nadel, L. (1996). Spatial locations gone awry: Object and spatial memory deficits in children with fetal alcohol syndrome. *Neuropsychologia, 34,* 209–223.

Uecker, A., & Nadel, L. (1998). Spatial but not object memory impairments in children with fetal alcohol syndrome. *American Journal of Mental Retardation, 103,* 12–18.

Vaurio, L., Repp, A., McGee, C. L., Riley, E. P., & Mattson, S. N. (2006). Visual working memory deficits in children with heavy prenatal alcohol exposure are secondary to lower-order deficits. *Alcoholism: Clinical and Experimental Research, 30*(9), 178A.

Vaurio, L., Riley, E. P., & Mattson, S. N. (2008). Differences in executive functioning in children with heavy prenatal alcohol exposure or attention-deficit/hyperactivity disorder. *Journal of the International Neuropsychological Society, 14,* 119–129.

Vorhees, C. V. (1986). Principles of behavioral teratology. In E. P. Riley & C. V. Vorhees (Eds.), *Handbook of behavioral teratology* (pp. 23–48). New York: Plenum Press.

Warren, K. R., Calhoun, F. J., May, P. A., Viljoen, D. L., Li, T.-K., Tanaka, H., et al. (2001). Fetal alcohol syndrome: An international perspective. *Alcoholism: Clinical and Experimental Research, 25,* 202S–206S.

Warren, K. R., & Li, T.-K. (2005). Genetic polymorphisms: Impact on the risk of fetal alcohol spectrum disorders. *Birth Defects Research: Part A. Clinical and Molecular Teratology, 73,* 195–203.

West, J. R., & Pierce, D. R. (1986). Perinatal alcohol exposure and neuronal damage. In J. R. West (Ed.), *Alcohol and brain development* (pp. 120–157). New York: Oxford University Press.

Willford, J. A., Richardson, G. A., Leech, S. L., & Day, N. L. (2004). Verbal and visuospatial learning and memory function in children with moderate prenatal alcohol exposure. *Alcoholism: Clinical and Experimental Research, 28,* 497–507.

Wozniak, J. R., Mueller, B. A., Chang, P.-N., Muetzel, R. L., Caros, L., & Lim, K. O. (2006). Diffusion tensor imaging in children with fetal alcohol spectrum disorders. *Alcoholism: Clinical and Experimental Research, 30,* 1799–1806.

PART II

NEURODEVELOPMENTAL DISORDERS

CHAPTER 11

Math Disabilities

MARCIA A. BARNES
LYNN S. FUCHS
LINDA EWING-COBBS

D isorders of mathematics have been identified and recognized in the neurological and neuropsychological literatures for as long as disorders of language such as aphasia and dyslexia have been, even though they have received much less study than language and reading (Kahn & Whitaker, 1991), and that disparity persists. For example, the ratio of reading studies to math studies over the last decade is 14:1 (Siegler, 2007), and reading intervention programs outnumber math programs by a factor of six (Ginsburg, Klein, & Starkey, 1998). For word-level reading disabilities (RDs), so much is known that there is a unifying theory that can explain both typical and atypical development of reading in relation to neurobiological and environmental factors, as well as the effects of intervention on both brain and behavior. In contrast, less is known about the typical development of math skills, math disabilities (MDs), math interventions, and neurobiological factors related to MDs. One possible reason for this imbalance is that RDs have traditionally been considered more costly to society in terms of school achievement as well as general health and employment (Fleishner, 1994); another is that, historically, less time has been spent on math than on reading both in and out of school in Western societies (Balfanz, 2000; Chen & Stevenson, 1995). Although literacy and numeracy are highly correlated in population-based samples, when numeracy is measured, it is found to be as important as literacy for predicting productivity, wages, and employment outcomes (Rivera-Batiz, 1992). Despite the fact that less is known about MDs than about RDs, strides have been made in recent years;

these reflect explicit attempts to increase understanding of MDs by considering evidence from research in cognitive development, cognitive neuroscience, developmental neuropsychology, education, and neurobiology. This chapter surveys the contributions from each of these areas to our current understanding of MDs. It focuses mainly on children with developmental MDs, but it includes some data relevant to children with genetic and acquired neurological disorders that place them at high risk of MDs. The last part of the chapter is devoted to a discussion of effective interventions for children with MDs, and highlights the essential ingredients of such interventions.

DEFINITIONAL ISSUES

Unlike many other disorders (e.g., as spina bifida, traumatic head injury, fragile X syndrome), which are defined by virtue of frank genetic or neurological markers, learning disabilities (LDs), although presumed to be neurobiological in origin, are defined behaviorally. When disorders are classified according to behavioral definitions, a lack of definitional clarity can result, and this has been very much the case for LDs. Because classification systems are fundamental to many areas of science and practice, scientific evaluation of their validity, reliability, and coverage is essential (Fletcher et al., 2002). Yet such scientific evidence was unavailable at the time LDs were first recognized as disabling disorders. Comprehensive reviews of the research on classification, definition, and identification of LDs can be found in Fletcher, Lyon, Fuchs, and Barnes (2007). The following briefly summarizes current knowledge on definitional issues with, particular reference to MDs.

Inherent in most of the classification systems described below is the idea that MDs are defined according to exclusionary criteria, as is the case for other LDs. These definitions include the finding of a discrepancy between IQ and math achievement, as well as deficits in mathematical function that are not due to a sensory or motor disability, mental retardation, emotional disturbance, or social, cultural, and economic factors (U.S. Office of Education, 1977; U.S. Department of Education, 1999). U.S. federal regulations governing special education make reference to two types of LDs in math—disabilities in *mathematics calculation* and *mathematics reasoning.* In Canada, education is under provincial, not federal, jurisdiction, although definitional issues such as the reliance on IQ–achievement discrepancy are similar to those in the United States. Many Canadian provinces include disorders in both computations and math reasoning/problem solving (Kozey & Siegel, 2008). The *Diagnostic and Statistical Manual of Mental Disorders,* fourth edition, text revision (American Psychiatric Association, 2000) classifies learning disorders into four categories, with *mathematics disorder* as one; the *International Classification of Diseases,* 10th revision (ICD-10; World Health Organization, 2007) includes *specific disorder of arithmetical skills,* as well as *mixed disorder of scholastic skills* for children with disorders of arithmetical skills as well as reading and/or spelling. Although some definitions (e.g., ICD-10) appear to focus on arithmetic or computation, most definitions are broad and refer to problems in arithmetic, word problem solving, and other abilities we might consider to be within the domain of mathematics. The term *specific MD* is often used to refer to a disability in math that is not accompanied by disabilities in other domains, such as reading (Rourke, 1993).

What is the evidence for these MD categories, the use of the IQ–achievement discrepancy for identifying those with MDs, and the assumption that we can define an MD separately from other disorders?

How Many Kinds of MDs Are There?

There is evidence for a disability in arithmetic or math computations, and this is the area of math that has received the most attention in cognitive, developmental, and neuropsychological studies. It is therefore the domain that we focus on in most of this chapter. There is little evidence at present for a disability in math reasoning and math concepts; *math reasoning* is not itself adequately defined (Lyon, Fletcher, & Barnes, 2003). From a scientific perspective, the purported distinction between math computations and math concepts/reasoning runs counter to developmental research, in which there is a reciprocal relationship between conceptual knowledge (e.g., understanding base 10) and procedural knowledge (e.g., regrouping in multidigit addition), and conceptual and procedural aspects of math are assumed to operate in most mathematical tasks (Rittle-Johnson, Siegler, & Alibali, 2001). More fundamentally, from a classification perspective, there is no widely agreed-upon set of core academic skills that can be said to represent markers for one or more types of MDs. By contrast, there is some consensus about component skills of reading (word recognition, reading fluency, and comprehension). This is not entirely surprising, given that math encompasses many domains, such as arithmetic, estimation, geometry, and topology—each of which may have different developmental trajectories, may be related to partially overlapping but also unique cognitive markers or correlates, and may have somewhat different neural signatures and genetic markers (Barnes & Fuchs, 2008). Furthermore, the applied aspects of math (word problem solving, measurement, etc.) would appear to draw on one or more of these mathematical domains as well as other aspects of cognition, such as language and general world knowledge.

Methods of Diagnosing MDs

As is the case for RDs, there is little validity for the use of an IQ–achievement discrepancy to diagnose and identify children with MDs (Fletcher, 2005; Mazzocco & Myers, 2003). For example, Fletcher (2005) compared children with MD (and no RD) who were identified by a significant IQ–achievement discrepancy (i.e., IQ much higher than achievement in arithmetic) to those who exhibited nondiscrepant low achievement. They were compared on a number of cognitive skills that have been variously related to math across a number of studies, including language skills, visual–spatial skills, concept formation skills, and attention. Not surprisingly, the group with IQ–achievement discrepancy had higher levels of ability on these other cognitive tasks; this is to be expected, because IQ was used to define the groups, and these various skills are moderately correlated with IQ. However, eliminating variability due to vocabulary (a proxy for IQ) eliminated most of the differences in level of performance between the groups, and the pattern or shape of the cognitive profiles did not differ between groups. Although there have been far fewer studies and meta-analyses of the validity of the discrepancy formula for identifying MDs than there have been for identifying RDs, the existing data suggest that this means of identifying

MDs has weak validity. Alternative methods of identifying children with MDs include response-to-intervention models (discussed in Fletcher et al., 2007; see also *www.student-progress.org*), in which children are screened for math difficulties at school entry, provided with evidence-based general education math instruction, monitored frequently for progress via brief fluency-based probes (e.g., curriculum-based measurement), and given more specialized or more intense intervention within the general education system before they are formally identified as having MDS.

Recently, some researchers (e.g., Geary, Hoard, Byrd-Craven, Nugent, & Numtee, 2007; Murphy, Mazzocco, Hanich, & Early, 2007) have suggested that the considerable definitional variability in research studies of MDs has contributed to a lack of clarity in the search for core deficits that are *causally* implicated in MDs. In research studies, children have been identified as having an MD if their scores on a standardized math test (typically computations) are as high as the 35th percentile; other studies use more stringent low achievement criteria or an IQ–achievement discrepancy. As well, math achievement is typically only assessed at one time point, although some have suggested that the persistence of math difficulties over time should contribute to the diagnosis of an MD (Geary et al., 2007; Murphy et al., 2007). Geary et al. (2007) have argued that a distinction should be made between children who are low achievers in math and those with actual MDs, using lenient and strict achievement cutoffs, respectively. The argument has been made that children with significant and persistent very low achievement in math may differ both quantitatively and qualitatively from those who are simply low-achieving. One hypothesis is that deficits in the central executive component of working memory characterize children with MDs and mediate their math performance. It is difficult at this point to say whether this alternate classification system will contribute to the search for the causal underpinnings of MDs. The same critiques would seem to apply to this classification method for MDs as those leveled against the use of cutoff scores for RDs: How does one apply nonarbitrary, scientifically valid cutoffs along what may be normally distributed abilities in an academic domain (Fletcher et al., 2007)?

Heterogeneity and Overlap with Other Disorders

Another important question about current definitions of LDs in general and of MDs in particular has to do with the heterogeneity of LDs. MDs co-occur with other academic and behavioral disorders with high frequency; they occurs in about 40–50% of children with RDs (Lewis, Hitch, & Walker, 1994; Shalev, Auerbach, Manor, & Gross-Tsur, 2000), and MDs and attention-deficit/hyperactivity disorder (ADHD) or other difficulties in attention also often co-occur (Fletcher, 2005; Marshall, Hynd, Handwerk, & Hall, 1997; Zentall, 1990). In most cases, comorbidity (e.g., RD + MD or MD + ADHD) is associated with greater impairment in academic domains than are independently occurring disorders (Fletcher et al., 2002). Certainly teachers' behavioral ratings of inattention are highly correlated with children's math difficulties (Fuchs et al., 2005) and with the types of errors they make in multidigit arithmetic (Raghubar et al., 2009), although the mechanisms behind such relations are not well understood. In any event, current classification systems do not take common comorbidities into account in terms of symptom severity; nor do they consider the overlap or differentiation of cognitive or neurobiological correlates when there is one LD (e.g., an MD) versus when there are two (e.g., RD + MD) or when there are co-occurring LDs and behavioral disorders (e.g., MD + ADHD).

EPIDEMIOLOGY

MDs are as common as word-level RDs (Shalev et al., 2000). In population studies, MDs are as prevalent as RDs when IQ–achievement discrepancy definitions are used (Badian & Ghublikian, 1983; Shalev et al., 2000). However, specific MD (i.e., MD without RD) is a little less than half as prevalent as MD + RD (Lewis et al., 1994), and is less common than specific RD. Of course, the prevalence of MDs varies with the way in which the MDs are defined—from a low of about 6% to a high of about 14%, depending on whether IQ–achievement discrepancy or low-achievement definitions are employed (Barbaresi, Katusic, Colligan, Weaver, & Jacobsen, 2005). Different approaches to identification yield different prevalence estimates, depending on decisions about cutoff points, the role of intervention in the definition (e.g., response-to-intervention methods of identification), and the type of math skill assessed (Fuchs et al., 2005).

Information on gender ratios in MDs is variable: Some studies show no gender differences in prevalence (Lewis et al., 1994); others show a higher prevalence in girls (Shalev et al., 2000); and yet others show a higher prevalence of MDs among males, depending on how MDs are identified (Barbaresi et al., 2005). This variability may be related to referral bias in some studies, differing definitions of MDs, and different ages at diagnosis (Shalev et al., 2000).

Similar to what has been found for RDs (e.g., Shaywitz et al., 1999), children move in and out of the MD category, depending on the cutoff points chosen for defining MDs (Gersten, Jordan, & Flojo, 2005; Mazzocco & Myers, 2003). For example, in one longitudinal study, Shalev and colleagues (Shalev, Manor, Auerbach, & Gross-Tsur, 1998; Shalev, Manor, & Gross-Tsur, 2005) showed that slightly fewer than half of children identified with an MD in grade 5 also met MD criteria in grade 8, and that only 40% met MD criteria in grade 11; in all grades, a stringent criterion of arithmetic scores at or below the 5th percentile was used. However, also consistent with studies of RDs, MDs tend to be persistent: Shalev et al. (2005) found that regardless of whether students diagnosed with an MD in grade 5 met strict criteria for diagnosis of an MD in grade 11, 95% of them were in the lowest 25% of students in math in grade 11.

NEUROBIOLOGICAL FACTORS

Genetic Studies

Risk of MDs in families of children with MDs appears to be about 10 times that expected in the general population (Gross-Tsur, Manor, & Shalev, 1996; Shalev et al., 2001). Twin and adoption studies on MDs have yielded heritability estimates between .20 and .90 (Alarcon, DeFries, Light, & Pennington, 1997; Thompson, Detterman, & Plomin, 1991). The contribution of genetic and shared environmental etiologies is similar in unselected samples and in samples that test these etiologies at the "extremes"—that is, in twin pairs where one or both twins have significant difficulties in math (Alarcon et al., 1997). Consistency between these different methodologies suggests that, as is the case for RDs, MDs may represent the tail end of a normally distributed skill spectrum (Petrill & Plomin, 2007).

A recent large study of 7-year-old twins (Kovas, Harlaar, Petrill, & Plomin, 2005) indicated substantial genetic influence as well as moderate environmental influence for math. The genetic correlations between mathematics and reading were high, which suggests that many of the genes predicting individual differences in one academic domain also predict individual differences in the other. Plomin and Kovas (2005) suggest a "generalist genes" theory of LDs. According to this view, the genes that affect learning in an academic skill such as reading are largely, though not completely, the same genes that affect learning in mathematics. In terms of genetic influences, Kovas et al. (2005) found that about a quarter of the variance in math was *not* shared with reading or general cognitive abilities. This theory is compatible with what is known about the substantial overlap between RDs and MDs. At present, only general math outcomes have been considered in these behavioral genetic studies, and no molecular genetic studies have been conducted on children with MD who do not also have genetic disorders such as fragile X syndrome (Petrill & Plomin, 2007). However, progress in understanding the cognitive phenotype of math abilities and MDs (e.g., similarities and differences in core cognitive correlates associated with MD only vs. RD + MD; potentially different types of MDs in different domains of mathematics) will be critical for informing behavioral genetic studies of mathematical skills.

Neuroimaging and Lesion Studies in Adults

Neuroimaging studies of math and math interventions in children with and without MDs are in their infancy. Different types of mathematical processing show clear dissociations in adults with brain lesions and in functional neuroimaging studies with normal adults (Dehaene, Spelke, Pinel, Stanescu, & Tsivkin, 1999). Some lesion studies have also shown dissociations between calculation and word reading (Dehaene & Cohen, 1997). In general, both adult lesion and imaging studies suggest that different neural circuits are involved in different types of mathematical processing. Dehaene and his colleagues (Dehaene et al., 1999; for a review, see Dehaene, Piaza, Pinel, & Cohen, 2005) propose that three circuits in the parietal lobe are implicated in mathematical function and dysfunction:

1. A bilateral intraparietal system for core quantitative processing, which is considered to be a domain-specific nonverbal analogue representational system for number or quantity. This system would be tapped by tasks such as approximate arithmetic or estimation, which are thought to draw on the so-called "mental number line."
2. A region of the left angular gyrus for verbal processing of numbers, such as multiplication facts and small-addition facts.
3. A posterior superior parietal system for aspects of mathematical processing such as number/quantity comparison, which is hypothesized not to be specific to number and which comes into play on numerical tasks that require spatial attention and visual–spatial working memory.

Consistent with aspects of the model are functional neuroimaging findings in adult women with Turner syndrome, who have high rates of MDs and do not show the typical modulation of intraparietal regions as a function of problem size (e.g., single-digit addition with sums under 10 vs. over 10) (Molko et al., 2003).

Neuroimaging Studies in Children

The model discussed above has been influential in guiding current neuroimaging studies of mathematical function. It is important to note, however, that even subtle changes in stimuli and processing requirements (e.g., task instructions, presentation rate, task complexity) can significantly alter activation patterns in math neuroimaging studies of skilled adults (reviewed in Simon & Rivera, 2007). There are also questions about the applicability of this model to typical and atypical development. First, studies of adult function are not the ideal model for determining whether any region of the brain is specific to or prewired for number processing (Simon & Rivera, 2007)—a question that is also at the heart of current domain-specific versus domain-general models of math abilities and MDs (discussed below). Second, it is questionable whether the model will provide a "good fit" for developmental data. Models derived from studies of acquired lesions in adults and neuroimaging findings from skilled adults are often incomplete and inaccurate in some of their causal inferences about the origins of skill impairments in developmental disorders, because they do not consider the process of change over development (Ansari & Karmiloff-Smith, 2002; Oliver, Johnson, Karmiloff-Smith, & Pennington, 2000).

Does the typically developing brain exhibit the same neural divisions identified in adult studies? What about the developing brain that is having difficulties in acquiring math skills? Only a few studies have begun to address these questions. Ansari and Dhital (2006) demonstrated that despite similar behavioral findings in adults and children on a test of magnitude comparison (e.g., indicating whether one side of a screen has more squares than the other), there were age-related differences in activation of the left intraparietal sulcus in relation to numerical distance on this task (e.g., a small distance of 3 dots vs. 4 dots, and a large distance of 3 dots vs. 9 dots). Rivera, Reiss, Eckert, and Menon (2005) have shown that even when younger and older children/youth are equally accurate on addition and subtraction calculations, they show somewhat different patterns of activation, with more activation in prefrontal cortex for younger children. Such findings, while preliminary, suggest developmental changes in the function of a brain area that has been consistently implicated in number processing in adults.

One study of adolescents born prematurely reported a correlation between gray matter in the left intraparietal sulcus and performance on a math achievement test (Isaacs, Edmonds, Lucas, & Gadian, 2001). A recent study comparing children with specific MD to typically developing controls (Kucian et al., 2006) showed similar activation patterns between the groups for approximate arithmetic (e.g., 2 + 5 is closer to 9 or 5?), exact calculation (e.g., 2 + 5 = 9 or 7?), and magnitude comparison (are there more objects on the left or right side of a screen?)—tasks that are thought to tap the three "systems" for mathematical processing proposed by Dehaene and colleagues (see above). The only group differences on some comparisons emerged for approximate arithmetic, where the group with specific MD showed weaker activation of the bilateral intraparietal region. It is unclear whether the findings reflect specific problems in accessing an analogue representational system for number, or differences between the groups in the strategies they brought to bear to solve approximate versus exact arithmetic problems (Simon & Rivera, 2007).

This seems particularly relevant, given the greater degree of interindividual performance variability in the group with specific MD (Kucian et al., 2006), and given that the strategies that children bring to bear to solve math problems change with age and skill level (Siegler, 1996).

Developmental models of mathematical skills—when they develop, what their cognitive precursors are, and which strategies individuals of different ages and skill levels bring to bear under different conditions—are likely to be critical for answering questions about the neural specificity and neural underpinnings of mathematical abilities and disabilities. To our knowledge, there are no neuroimaging studies in the literature that compare activation patterns in children with MDs prior to and following math interventions, such as the comparisons that have been made in reading intervention studies for children with RD; however such studies are currently underway.

THEORIES AND MODELS OF MDs: HISTORICAL AND CURRENT APPROACHES

Cognitive-Developmental and Neuropsychological Models

Neuropsychological studies were the first to discriminate between potentially different forms of MDs and the cognitive correlates associated with those MDs, depending on the presence or absence of a comorbid RD (reviewed in Rourke, 1993). These studies looked for group differences in such cognitive abilities as phonological skills and visual–spatial skills for children with MDs with and without co-occurring RDs. They focused on broad mathematical outcomes and were less concerned with analyzing typical and atypical growth in specific mathematical processes, such as understanding counting principles (e.g., understanding of one-to-one correspondence) or estimating quantities. These studies sought to understand individual differences, not normal developmental processes related to math. For example, several early studies suggested that children with disorders of both word recognition and mathematics have a different cognitive profile from that of children with a more restricted MD (Morrison & Siegel, 1991; Rourke, 1993). Children with both RD and MD have been found to have deficits in verbal and visual working memory (Siegel & Ryan, 1989) and phonological processing (Swanson & Sachse-Lee, 2001). In contrast, children with specific MD have been found to have deficits in visual memory, visual–spatial working memory, counting span (McLean & Hitch, 1999; Siegel & Ryan, 1989), and visual–spatial function (Rourke, 1993; Share, Moffitt, & Silva, 1988).

Earlier studies of MDs from educational research and a cognitive-developmental perspective typically did not subtype MDs, but focused on understanding the development and operation of the mathematical system itself (e.g., single-digit arithmetic and strategies children use to solve simple and more complex arithmetic problems; Russell & Ginsburg, 1984) and ways to remediate deficits in that system (Goldman, Pellegrino, & Mertz, 1988). As well, there were and continue to be many theoretically driven cognitive-developmental studies devoted to understanding the typical development of mathematical skills, such as conceptual understanding of counting principles (Gelman & Gallistel, 1978; LeFevre et al., 2006) and arithmetic problem solving (Rasmussen & Bisanz, 2005; Siegler & Shrager, 1984). Although such studies are potentially applicable to MDs, they are motivated by more general theories of cognitive development and mathematical development, rather than by models of individual differences in cognition per se. Some of the differences in these approaches are captured in Table 11.1.

More recent studies of MDs have proceeded from a cognitive-developmental approach, at the same time incorporating some of the theoretical and methodological aspects inherent in early neuropsychological models. Geary, in an influential 1993 paper (see also Geary, 2004), proposed a model of MDs based on an integrative review of the cognitive, developmental, neuropsychological, and neuroscience literatures on mathematical processing and MDs. Cognitive-developmental studies of arithmetic (e.g., Siegler & Shrager, 1984; Ashcraft, 1992) had shown that prior to formal schooling, children learn to solve simple everyday problems through the use of counting strategies (such as counting 1, 2, 3, 4 and 5, 6 either on fingers or verbally when adding four things to two things). Practice with computing typically leads to a more developmentally sophisticated strategy called the *min* or *counting up* strategy, in which the child counts up from the largest number (4, then 5, 6). Eventually the child comes to associate the problem with the answer in memory so that he or she "knows" that 4 and 2 is 6 (direct retrieval from memory), or uses sophisticated strategies such as *decomposition*, which involves knowledge of number combinations to solve larger or more complex problems (e.g., "For 5 + 8, I know that 5 + 5 = 10 and 3 more = 13"). Accurate and fluent single-digit arithmetic is thought to be important for freeing cognitive resources during the learning and application of more complex procedures such

TABLE 11.1. Differences between Cognitive-Developmental and Neuropsychological Studies of Math

Cognitive-developmental studies of math	Neuropsychological studies of math
Math is used to understand cognition more generally.	Math is used as an outcome.
Focus is on how math system operates in infants, preschoolers, children, adults.	Focus is on how neurocognitive skills such as spatial ability and working memory are related to math, and how these abilities differ in subtypes of children with MDs.
Complexity of math is acknowledged.	Computation is often studied, except in cognitive neuroscience studies where other aspects of math (estimation, magnitude comparison, etc.) may be investigated.
There is less focus on individual differences and disability.	There is an explicit focus on individual differences and disabilities, in both adult and child studies.
Earlier studies did not take reading into account.	Studies often took reading and RDs into account.
Developmental studies are concerned with capturing normative aspects of development of mathematical processes, such as changes in strategies for retrieving math facts.	Studies are not inherently developmental in nature.
There are few longitudinal studies from the preschool years into school age, or studies of developmental precursors of later-developing math skills.	There are few longitudinal studies or studies of deficits in suspected developmental precursors of later-developing math skills.

as carrying and borrowing, and fluency in math fact retrieval is strongly related to accurate performance in multidigit arithmetic (Barnes et al., 2006).

Geary (1993) combined these developmental data with the neuropsychological literature on MDs to suggest that MDs may take three forms. The first type is characterized by deficits in the accuracy, speed, and consistency of retrieving math facts or number combinations (e.g., 3 + 5 = 8) from semantic memory. Geary thought that this type might explain the relationship between RD and MD in many children with MD; that is, deficits in the phonological system may cause problems for both reading and math. He also suggested that this form of MD may represent a true cognitive deficit. The second type is characterized by difficulties in learning and implementing procedural aspects of math, such as delays in developing counting-up strategies in single digit arithmetic or in acquiring procedures for carrying in multidigit arithmetic. The relation to reading is not specified for this type, which Geary thought might reflect developmental delays rather than cognitive differences in acquiring math skills. The third type is related to difficulties in the understanding and manipulation of spatial aspects of number, which Geary thought might characterize the deficits of children with specific MD.

Several studies have tested aspects of the proposed model, including studies of children with developmental MD, as well as research on children with frank brain injury and those with genetic disorders associated with high rates of MDs. Recall that several of the early studies from the neuropsychological framework mentioned above suggested that children with disorders of both word recognition and mathematics have a different neurocognitive profile from that of children with a more restricted MD (Morrison & Siegel, 1991; Rourke, 1993). At first glance, these studies of the neurocognitive correlates (e.g., visual–spatial skill, phonological abilities) of MDs in children with specific MD and RD + MD would suggest that these correlates might affect the development of one type of MD versus another. However, the more recent studies of MDs that have tested Geary's model have suggested that children with MD and those with MD + RD look remarkably similar on most measures of mathematical processes (Barnes et al., 2006; Landerl, Bevan, & Butterworth, 2004; Jordan, Hanich, & Kaplan, 2003; Raghubar et al., 2008; Shalev et al., 1997), with a few exceptions such as math word problems (Fuchs & Fuchs, 2002; Hanich, Jordan, Kaplan, & Dick., 2001). The balance of the evidence suggests that the biggest difference between the two groups may be a quantitative rather than a qualitative one that affects the severity of the MD (Barnes et al., 2006; Shalev, Manor, & Gross-Tsur, 1997).

These studies have shown that regardless of whether there is a comorbid RD, or an acquired or congenital brain injury in childhood, children with MDs are characterized by difficulties in the accuracy and speed with which they can compute answers to single-digit problems (Ashcraft, Yamashita, & Aram, 1992; Barnes et al., 2006; Jordan et al., 2003). Given the evidence for deficits in math fact retrieval or number combinations in MDs, current research on the early identification of MDs is focusing on the developmental precursors of these characteristic deficits in math fact retrieval (e.g., Gersten et al., 2005).

To date, there is little evidence for the hypothesis that problems in visual–spatial processing directly affect learning or performance in the domain of mathematical computation. For example, the relationship of visual–spatial skill to either multidigit calculation or math fact performance is weak, even in populations where visual–spatial abilities are poorly developed (e.g., Barnes et al., 2006; Rovet, Szekely, & Hockenberry, 1994). Furthermore, children with visual–spatial deficits or those with specific MD do not make more visual–spatial errors in their calculations (Barnes et al., 2006; Raghubar et al., 2009), and differences in effect sizes for visual–spatial working memory between children with specific MD and those with RD + MD are small (Swanson & Jerman, 2006).

Although there is little evidence for a contribution of visual–spatial processing to arithmetic, visual–spatial skills do appear to be important for math in two ways. First, they are related to areas of math other than computation. Visual–spatial skills are related to algebra, word problem solving, trigonometry, and geometry in both typically developing and atypical populations (Barnes et al., 2002; Geary, 1996; Reuhkala, 2001). However, little is known about the cognitive correlates of and developmental pathways in these other math skills, or about why visual–spatial skills might be related to these areas of math. Second, visual–spatial abilities may show some developmentally limited relations with early informal aspects of math that are thought to provide some of the foundation for later math learning. For example, some early math skills in preschool children, such as quantity matching, adding to and taking away from small sets of objects, and an understanding of cardinality (i.e., the fact that the last count in a set represents the quantity of the set), are related to visual–spatial skills or visual–spatial memory (Ansari et al., 2003; Barnes, Smith-Chant, & Landry, 2005; Rasmussen & Bisanz, 2005). The idea that some math skills may be related to different cognitive processes at different points in development is one that has been suggested to operate in other cognitive domains as well, and it underlines the importance of a developmental perspective for pediatric neuropsychology (e.g., Oliver et al., 2000). As is the case for math fact retrieval, it is unclear whether the cognitive correlates of these other early math skills begin to change as a function of the strategies that individuals bring to bear in their problem solving. Longitudinal studies that track the development of mathematical knowledge—both conceptual and procedural—from the very early years into the school years are needed in order to answer some of these most fundamental questions about the developmental precursors of later-developing math abilities and disabilities in relation to different math skills.

Even though some of the specifics of Geary's original model have not held up in research studies, the finding that difficulties in learning and retrieving number combinations seem to characterize children with MDs (regardless of the presence of other disorders) has led to some reconceptualization of the hypothesized sources of MDs, the search for the developmental precursors of MDs, and the unique cognitive markers of MDs. Two main theoretical positions have been staked out: the *domain-specific* view, in which the origins of MDs are thought to reside in deficits in very basic aspects of number processing; and the *domain-general* view, in which the origins of MDs are thought to reside in deficits in more general cognitive systems, such as working memory and the central executive.

Domain-Specific and Domain-General Theories

In more recent research, the models and methods applied to the development of mathematical skills are the same models that are being applied to understand MDs. This research reflects the beginning of a theoretical and methodological convergence in the field of MDs, similar to that experienced earlier in the field of RDs. The two most prominent theoretical positions about MDs come from very different ways of explaining the origins of mathematical abilities and MDs. One position, the domain-specific view, proposes that MDs come about from deficits in the ability to recognize, represent, and manipulate quantities. The other proposes that MD comes about from deficits in more domain-general abilities, such as working memory, spatial cognition, and language. A third view is that the origin of MDs is confined to difficulties in accessing number information from the symbol systems for numbers (e.g., Arabic numerals), rather than from deficits in representing and understanding magnitudes per se or in domain-general abilities such as working memory (Rousselle & Noel, 2007).

The domain-specific view (e.g., Butterworth, 1999) comes from the hypothesis that, unlike reading (which is a relatively recent human achievement), an ability to understand magnitude or quantities and to compare numerosities is an ability that human and even nonhuman animals are born with, though domain specificity need not imply innateness (Karmiloff-Smith, Plunkett, Johnson, Elman, & Bates, 1998). There is debate over the interpretation of some of the infant research—that is, whether performance relies on an innate module for processing number or emerges from the operation of more basic cognitive systems in infancy, such as visual attention and visual preference (e.g., Cohen & Marks, 2002). However, very young infants are sensitive to differences in the numerosity of small sets (Starkey, Spelke, & Gelman, 1990). Five-months-olds also appear sensitive to changes in very small set sizes involving adding to and taking away (Wynn, 1992). Preschoolers can judge whether one set or number is bigger or smaller than another set or number (Ginsburg et al., 1998). Butterworth (1999) suggests that this sensitivity to number is the infant's "starter kit" for later mathematical development, and that deficits in these very basic mathematical abilities (which are not influenced by environment or schooling) underlie MDs. Proponents of this view do not argue that this is the only source of children's difficulty in mathematics. For example, mathematical tasks that require language (e.g., word problem solving) should be influenced by language skills, and inadequate teaching should lead to difficulties in learning a variety of mathematical skills in school.

In general, the proponents of this view tend to argue against the domain-general approach by citing evidence from both neuropsychological and developmental studies that are counter to what the domain-general view might predict. For example, the types of spatial acalculia that have been reported in adults with brain lesions (e.g., Hartje, 1987) are not found in children with MDs; variability in phonological memory is unrelated to math fact retrieval, the very mathematical skill that proponents of the domain-general view predict should be affected by poor phonological working memory (Temple & Sherwood, 2002); and studies that relate working memory to math abilities and MDs are inconsistent in their findings (e.g., McLean & Hitch, 1999; for a review, see Butterworth & Reigosa, 2007).

The evidence for the domain-specific view comes largely from two types of experimental or group studies. One type of study pits the ability to process non-numerical information (e.g., speed of physical judgments that do not involve number; letter naming) against the ability to process quantity-based information (e.g., speed of comparing which of two numbers is larger; naming digits or quantities) in children with MDs (Koontz & Berch, 1996; Landerl et al., 2004; van der Sluis, de Jong, & van der Leij, 2004). Another type of study tests for deficits in the "number module"—that is, in those number-related skills (e.g., subitizing) that are presumed to represent the operation of very basic number abilities present in young members of the species and sometimes across species (Landerl et al., 2004). The domain-specific view is considered to be compatible with neuroscience models that suggest some specificity for number processing in parietal lobes (Dehaene et al., 1999), though there is some controversy about whether any of the parietal systems implicated in number processing are actually specialized for number (Simon & Rivera, 2007).

In contrast, the domain-general view is that mathematical skills are built from other more basic or general cognitive systems, such as the language system (see discussion in Gelman & Butterworth, 2005), the visual–spatial system (Rourke, 1993), and the central executive or attentional and working memory systems (Swanson, 2007). Geary's more recent framework (Geary & Hoard, 2005) is the most comprehensive example of this view. In this framework, the skills that are important for the development of mathematical competence are the same ones proposed to be deficient in the development of MDs. According to this view, difficulties in math could arise in the language system; the visual–spatial system; the central executive, which sustains attention and inhibits irrelevant information; or any combination of these general cognitive systems. At present, there is some preliminary evidence for the framework (Geary & Hoard, 2005; Geary et al., 2007), but there is no coherent body of literature yet that would allow researchers to fully test the model or that pits this model against another MD model. For example, there is a considerable lack of precision in the measurement of cognitive processes within the domain of executive processes such as inhibition, switching, and updating, and there is a concomitant lack of precision over what aspects of mathematical function these executive skills are being used to predict (e.g., math fact retrieval, approximation, magnitude comparison). Swanson and Jerman (2006), in a meta-analysis of studies comparing children with MDs to those with average math achievement, found that the magnitude of effect sizes in overall functioning between the groups was related to deficits in verbal working memory after the effects of IQ and reading were partialed; this finding suggests that deficits in central executive processes may strongly characterize those with MDs. However, some studies have failed to show working memory differences in children with and without MD (McLean & Hitch, 1999; Temple & Sherwood, 2002). The real question in all of this work is whether a domain-general ability such as working memory is a primary *causal* factor in MDs.

A combination of the domain-general and domain-specific viewpoints can be found in another theoretical orientation from the developmental sciences. This suggests that infants are born with core knowledge systems, one of them akin to a number module (e.g., Spelke & Tviskin, 2001), and that the coordination of these core knowledge systems or modules (possibly via a domain-general ability such as language) extends and expands knowledge. The hypothesis is that this coordination drives skill development in math and in many other areas of cognition (see Spelke & Kinzler, 2007).

As well, a more recent and nuanced view of MDs takes into account the possibility that mathematical performance may be subserved by several representational systems that can be called upon to solve problems if one system is deficient (Bull, 2007). In her integrative review of studies of MDs in children with and without brain injuries or genetic disorders, Bull (2007) has suggested that mathematical performance may be achieved by different representational systems, depending on the integrity of the systems available to the child, and perhaps the age of the child as well (see also Ansari et al., 2003). For example, domain-general abilities such as visual–spatial skills or language may be related to MDs only when an alternative representational system for number cannot be accessed. Thus visual–spatial skills may be more closely related to MDs in individuals with fragile X syndrome (who have deficits in both language and space) than in those with Turner syndrome or spina bifida (who have spatial deficits, but whose language skills may be well developed).

MDs IN GENETIC AND NEURODEVELOPMENTAL DISORDERS

Some genetic, congenital and acquired neurodevelopmental disorders carry high risk for MDs even when reading develops relatively well. In some cases, the cognitive sources of MDs in these groups have been investigated via a combined cognitive-developmental and neuropsychological approach that provides information about the cognitive markers of the disability, sometimes in relation to the neurobiology of the disorder. For other disorders, there is information about math outcomes but less research at this time on the mathematical and neurocognitive processes implicated in the MDs.

Very low birthweight is associated with a host of LDs even when children have relatively spared cognitive and intellectual skills, and math may be particularly affected (Litt, Taylor, Klein, & Hack, 2005). Spina bifida (Ayr, Yeates, & Ernile, 2005; Barnes et al., 2006), hydrocephalus from several etiologies (Barnes et al., 2002), Turner syndrome (Mazzocco & McCloskey, 2005), fragile X syndrome (Mazzocco & McCloskey, 2005), and velocardiofacial syndrome (Simon, Bearden, McGinn, & Zackai (2005) are all associated with relatively high rates of MDs even when, in some of these neurodevelopmental disorders, word reading develops adequately. Traumatic brain injury is associated with difficulties in acquiring word-reading skills and math calculation skills, particularly for children who are injured in the preschool or very early school years (Ayr et al., 2005; Ewing-Cobbs et al., 2004). This relation of learning difficulties to an early age at injury is true for severe as well as mild to moderate injuries (Ewing-Cobbs et al., 2004). Standard academic achievement tests tend to underestimate the difficulties that children with traumatic brain injury have with academic skills in the classroom; these difficulties may reflect the influence of deficits in other cognitive systems, such as memory, attention, and executive functions that support learning (Barnes, Fletcher, & Ewing-Cobbs, 2007). Children with cancer (e.g., acute lymphoblastic leukemia) are also more affected by CNS treatment at younger ages of diagnosis. Difficulties have been found for such children in math as well as in reading, and the presentation of these LDs in the classroom may be exacerbated by accompanying deficits in information-processing speed, memory, attention, and visual–motor skills (reviewed in Armstrong & Briery, 2004).

Children with sickle cell disease are at high risk of LDs as well as other cognitive difficulties in domains (such as attention) known to be highly related to MDs; this is true not only of those with overt strokes, but also for children with silent strokes (see review in Bonner, Hardy, Ezell, & Ware, 2004). Furthermore, pain associated with the disease, medications to treat the pain, socioeconomic disadvantage, and behavioral issues may complicate how children with sickle cell disease function in the classroom, over and above the presence of LDs and other cognitive deficits. Indeed, any condition that results in frequent and/ or prolonged absence from school may be especially problematic for mathematics learning. This is the case because the development of math competence—possibly more so than that of early reading—is hierarchical, with skills building upon previous learned skills (Fuchs et al., 2006). This makes math more vulnerable not only to prolonged school absences, but also to the effects of poor instruction and variability in instructional quality.

INTERVENTIONS FOR MDs

Conceptual Approaches to Remediating LDs

Five conceptual approaches for treating the academic deficits of students with LDs have been most prominent in the past several years. The first three of these approaches have not been shown to be effective for improving outcomes of students with LDs in general or for those with MDs, in particular.

The *neuropsychological approach* incorporates concepts from medical and psychoeducational theories. In neuropsychological assessment, neurocognitive (e.g., visual–spatial cognition, memory) and behavioral skills are assessed; inferences about the effects of skill deficits on academic performance and social-emotional development are made; and neurocognitive strengths by which compensatory skills might be developed are identified. The interest is in determining what underlies a child's disabling condition, not just identifying the disability, with the goal of understanding how the underlying processing deficits might inform instruction. Unfortunately, at the present time, the value of this approach in terms of identifying the neurocognitive sources of MDs in groups of children or in individual children has not been proven (see Torgesen, 2002, for a discussion of this approach for LDs in general). Moreover, although neuropsychologically motivated intervention programs have proliferated in the last decade with advances in basic neuroscience, their importance for education has thus far not been demonstrated. That is, the practice has not been linked to improved outcomes (Lyon et al., 2003).

A related approach, also with limited efficacy data, focuses on *intraindividual differences in cognitive processes*. This approach focuses in greater depth on the cognitive profiles associated with LDs. Again, the hope is that the delineation of the cognitive profiles might inform treatment. For example, in designing an evaluation based on intraindividual differences in cognitive processes in the area of mathematics, one might assess language ability, which has been associated with deficits in math problem solving (Fuchs et al., 2008a), in the hope of deriving a cognitive profile associated with the predicted academic profile. This model also suffers from important weaknesses. For example, the focus is on test scores that describe cognitive performance in isolation from classroom performance and from academic skills. In addition, there is little empirical evidence to support its utility (Lyon et al., 2003).

The third model, *constructivism*, stresses teacher empowerment, child-centered instruction, and disavowal of explicit instruction. The view is that children are naturally predisposed to learning, and that educators should rely on unstructured activities from which learners will construct their own meaning (Hresko & Reid, 1981). In the past 20 years, math instruction has been strongly influenced by this discovery-oriented approach, which has been shown to promote learning and motivation for high- and average-achieving pupils (Woodward & Baxter, 1997). However, a meta-analysis of 58 math studies (Kroesbergen & Van Luit, 2003) reveals that students with MDs benefit more from explicit instruction than from discovery-oriented methods. Moreover, a 5-month randomized controlled field trial directly comparing the effects of constructivist versus explicit small-group math tutoring on 265 low-achieving 8- to 11-year-olds (Kroesbergen, Van Luit, & Maas, 2004) showed that explicit instruction was superior in enhancing automaticity, problem solving, strategy use, and motivation.

The remaining two approaches have proven more successful in remediating skill deficits in children with MDs. A *cognitive-behavioral approach* combines the methods of strategy instruction with behavioral principles (e.g., Fuchs et al., 2003). Typically, this approach is targeted at higher-level cognitive processes, such as reading comprehension and math problem solving. It also involves a strong focus on strategies underlying effective academic performance, such as having students develop reflective, self-regulated use of processes/ strategies and form positive attitudes about themselves and their academic capabilities. For example, some work has focused on the use of metacognitive planning and organization strategies for remediating word problem deficits. Montague and Bos (1986) assessed the effects of an eight-step metacognitive treatment that taught students to read problems, paraphrase the problems aloud, graphically display known and unknown information, state the known and unknown information, hypothesize solution methods, estimate answers, calculate answers, and check answers. Using a single-subject design, Montague and Bos found that this cognitive-behavioral strategy promoted word problem skill in adolescents with LDs.

The final approach, a *direct instruction model*, emphasizes the influence of environment while deemphasizing underlying causal mechanisms or thought processes. Such programs (e.g., Hallahan, Kauffman, & Lloyd, 1996; Rosenshine & Stevens, 1986) typically involve review of prerequisite learning; preview of goals; presentation of new concepts and material in small steps, with student practice after each step; provision of clear, explicit, detailed instructions and explanations; ongoing assessment of student understanding via teacher questioning; and systematic feedback and corrections. Direct instruction methods have been criticized, because they control the teaching process in ways that minimize professional discretion; however, the methods have been shown to be effective (e.g., Adams & Carnine, 2003; Gersten, White, Falco, & Carnine, 1982).

At the present time, the most persuasive evidence for promoting academic learning among students with LDs has been obtained for the cognitive-behavioral approach and for the direct instruction model. In a meta-analysis, Swanson, Hoskyn, and Lee (1999) found that direct instruction produced larger effect sizes than "other" interventions, as did strategy instruction. But combining direct instruction and strategy instruction yielded larger effect sizes than did either method alone, with moderate to large effects. Space limitations preclude a comprehensive review of mathematics programs within the direct instruction and cognitive-behavioral approaches. Instead, we illustrate the combined use of the direct instruction and strategy methods with two representative programs developed by Fuchs and colleagues, which have been evaluated based on random assignment, adequate description of interventions, sufficient intervention duration, and measurement of fidelity of implementation, with attention to external validity in regard to real classrooms (Lyon, Fletcher, Fuchs, & Chhabra, 2006). For examples of early intervention programs for very young children at risk of MDs, see the reviews by Griffin (2007) and Klein and Starkey (2004).

Remediating Number Combination Deficits

As discussed above, difficulties in accurately and fluently working with number combinations characterize children with MDs, regardless of the presence of coexisting academic and behavioral disorders or of frank brain injury. Number combination deficits are important to remediate not only because they form the foundational skills for more complex arithmetic, but also because they reflect a failure to develop basic conceptual skills related to understanding number. An intervention called Math Flash (Fuchs et al., 2008b), which remediates number combination deficits among third graders with MDs, is described.

Math Flash addresses 200 number combinations with addends and subtrahends from 0 to 9. It teaches these number combinations in a set sequence (e.g., facts of +1 and–1 are introduced first); does so by using manipulatives and the number line; and teaches the commutative property of addition (i.e., 4 + 1 = 1 + 4) while emphasizing that this property does not apply to subtraction. Each of the 48 Math Flash lessons (lasting 20–30 minutes each) comprises these activities: flash card warm-up, conceptual and strategic instruction, lesson-specific flash card practice, computerized practice with mastery assessment, and paper–pencil review. Some of these activities are highlighted below. In addition, a systematic reinforcement program is used to motivate good attention, hard work, and accurate work.

In flash card warm-up, tutors show flash cards representing the 200 combinations of numbers. At the end of 2 minutes, the number of cards answered correctly is counted, and each student enters this number on a graph, allowing the student to monitor his or her own progress over time. This promotes the use of self-regulation strategies—an effective instructional approach for children with MDs. During conceptual and strategic instruction, tutors introduce or review concepts and strategies. Throughout, tutors emphasize two strategies for deriving answers, "know it or count up"; they provide practice in counting up; and they require students to explain how to count up in addition and subtraction problems. As discussed earlier, typically developing children tend to "discover" strategies such as counting up to solve simple arithmetic problems; here, children with MD are explicitly taught this strategy to aid in accurate problem solving, but also to develop conceptual number knowledge. Computerized practice is used to build fluency with number combinations and to assess mastery with the day's set. A systematic reinforcement program using sticker charts that can be "cashed in" for a prize is also used as part of Math Flash, and it has proven to be helpful for increasing motivation in children with MDs.

Remediating Problem-Solving Deficits

In Pirate Math, 48 lessons are divided into four units. An introductory unit addresses skills foundational to word problems: the counting-up strategy for solving addition and subtraction number combinations; double-digit addition and subtraction; solving for *x* in any position in simple algebraic equations (i.e., $a + b = c$; $d–e = f$); and checking word problem work. The remaining units focus on solving word problems, and review the foundational skills taught in the introductory unit. Each unit introduces one type of word problem, while subsequent units provide systematic, mixed cumulative review. The problem types are *total* (two or more amounts being combined), *difference* (two amounts being compared), and *change* (initial amounts that increase or decrease). For each problem type, students are taught to identify and circle relevant information, mark missing information, construct an algebraic equation representing the underlying mathematical structure of the problem type, solve for the missing information, provide a word label for the answer, and check the reasonableness and accuracy of their work.

Similar to the lessons in Math Flash, Pirate Math daily lessons comprise these activities: flash card warm-up, conceptual and strategic instruction, flash card practice for each problem type, sorting word problems, and paper–pencil review. Flash card warm-up is identical to the flash card warm-up used in Math Flash. During conceptual and strategic instruction, tutors provide explicit instruction in solving the three types of word problems, along with instruction on identifying and integrating transfer features, using role playing, manipulatives, instructional posters, modeling, and guided practice. In each lesson, students solve three problems, as the tutor provides decreasing amounts of support (fading). Sorting word problems is used to promote transfer to new conceptually similar problems with different language and arithmetic content from the "learned" problems. The student listens to the problem and identifies the word problem type, but does not attempt to solve the problem. The Pirate Math reinforcement program is identical to the one used in Math Flash.

Fuchs et al. (2008b) randomly assigned 133 students who experienced substantial difficulty with calculations or word problems to receive Math Flash, to receive Pirate Math, or to continue in school without additional math tutoring (i.e., a control group). Half of the students in each intervention condition had MDs without RDs; the other half experienced concurrent difficulties with math and reading. On number combinations, both intervention conditions promoted improvement compared to the control group, and there were no significant differences between intervention conditions. Word problem performance improved significantly more for the Pirate Math group than for either the Math Flash group or the control group. So, interestingly, Math Flash enhances automatic retrieval of number combinations, whereas for a comparable amount of tutoring time, Pirate Math enhances word problem skill as well as fluency with number combinations. The findings applied across students with MDs, regardless of their reading skill.

How These Interventions Illustrate Key Principles of the Cognitive-Behavioral and Direct Approaches to Intervention

Math Flash and Pirate Math illustrate six principles of effective intervention for students with MDs. The first is *instructional explicitness*. Students who accrue serious mathematics deficits fail to profit from programs that rely on a constructivist, inductive instructional style (Kroesbergen & Van Luit, 2003). Therefore, effective intervention for students with MDs requires an explicit, didactic form of instruction, in which the teachers directly share the information the children need to learn.

Explicitness is not, however, sufficient. A second principle of effective mathematics intervention for students with MDs is *instructional design to minimize the learning challenge*. The goal is to anticipate and eliminate misunderstandings with precise explanations and with the use of carefully sequenced and integrated instruction, so that the achievement gap can be closed as quickly as possible. This may be especially important for mathematics, which involves many branches and strands, each with its own conceptual and procedural demands. Careful instructional design is illustrated in Math Flash in terms of sequencing, where number combination sets are introduced to capitalize on the knowledge a student brings to the table, while maximizing the student's rate of acquisition and sense of accomplishment. So +1/–1 facts are introduced first because they correspond well to a basic number line concept that is easy to teach, if not already achieved; because they ease counting demands; and because this results in a student's mastering 29 of the 200 number combinations in the first week of intervention. In Pirate Math, students recognize problem types similar to the kinds of problems found in the general education curriculum and in high-stakes tests. That way, novel story problems are not random events for students; they recognize novel problems as familiar and are able to use schemas for problem types the program teaches to apply appropriate solutions.

The third principle of effective mathematics intervention for students with MDs is providing a *strong conceptual basis* for procedures that are taught. Without a clear focus on the conceptual basis for each procedure, confusion, learning gaps, and a failure to maintain and integrate previously mastered content can result. Math Flash illustrates the need for conceptual instruction, as it relies strongly on manipulatives and number. *Drill and practice*, the fourth principle of effective intensive mathematics intervention, is also evident: in Math Flash, with the use of flash cards, computerized practice, and daily review; in Pirate Math, with practice in sorting problems into problem types, the mixing of problem types within the daily lesson, and daily review. This practice is rich in *cumulative review*, a fifth principle of effective mathematics intervention for students with MDs. This is reflected in Math Flash's flash card warm-up activity, computerized practice, and paper–pencil review, and in Pirate Math's continual reliance on the foundational skills taught in the introductory unit, the use of mixed problem types within conceptual instruction, sorting practice, and paper–pencil review.

Finally, intensive mathematics interventions need to incorporate *motivators* for students to regulate their attention and behavior and to work hard. Students with LDs often display attention, motivation, and self-regulation difficulties, which may adversely affect their behavior and learning (Fuchs et al., 2005, 2006; Montague, 2007). By the time students enter intensive intervention, they have experienced repeated failure, causing many to avoid the emotional stress associated with mathematics. For this reason, intensive intervention must incorporate systematic self-regulation and motivators, and for many students, tangible reinforcers are required. Math Flash illustrates this principle in the "beat your score" flash card activity, where goal-directed behavior is required; in having students graph the scores they achieve; and in the use of stars as rewards. Pirate Math incorporates similar activities.

CLINICAL IMPLICATIONS

At present, identification of children with MDs is hampered by the limited content of standardized assessments of math abilities. Particularly for children in grades 1–3, behavior sampling on calculation subtests at a given grade level is lean, with few items representing any given type of problem. This provides a poor basis for discriminating among children with different functional levels of competence. Fuchs et al. (2006) reported that the fluency of addition and subtraction fact retrieval in the early elementary years, predicted fluency in both double-digit algorithmic computation and solving word problems. In light of these findings, standardized assessments of fact retrieval accuracy and fluency may be critically important for identifying children in need of more intensive classroom-based or small-group instruction. In addition, developing standardized assessments of the strategies that children use to solve single-digit and more complex algorithmic computations may be helpful for identifying students who continue to use immature and inefficient strategies (such as finger counting), rather than making the transition to more efficient strategies (such as direct retrieval of math facts from memory). Using a response-to-intervention model that emphasizes more frequent curriculum-based progress-monitoring assessments, in conjunction with standardized measures of fact retrieval and strategy use, is likely to provide a basis for early identification and for monitoring the development of children with MDs. In later grades, more focused assessment of curriculum-based essential elements, such as performing operations involving multidigit division, proportions, or solving algebraic equations, may assist in identifying students who develop difficulties with more complex math concepts and procedures. In a related way, given work showing that difficulties with word problems may represent challenges with demands that differ from calculation skill, a great need exists for additional assessments of math problem-solving skills, to help practitioners identify students who require specific assistance in this subdomain of mathematics.

RDs and attention difficulties often co-occur with MDs. Moreover, the presence of these comorbidities appears to be associated with more severe academic difficulties (Fletcher et al., 2002). Therefore, assessment of learning competencies should be sufficiently broad to identify the presence of comorbidities indicating areas of weakness, as well as areas of strength that may serve as compensatory strategies. Assessment of learning competencies should include reading and language skills, as well as evaluation of the supporting cognitive competencies (e.g., attention, visual–spatial skills, nonverbal problem solving, and concept formation) that are related to performance on integrative math tasks such as solving word problems (Fuchs et al., 2006). As discussed in the preceding section, such knowledge may not determine the choice of intervention program, but may be useful in thinking about accommodations for specific children. For example, children with limitations in one area might use or be shown how to use different representational strategies to solve problems (e.g., visual strategies when language skills are weak or language-based strategies when visual–spatial skills are deficient; see Bull, 2007). Children with difficulties in attention and/or inhibitory control may require more explicit instruction in metacognitive strategies, such as identifying problem types, distinguishing relevant from irrelevant information, and evaluating the reasonableness of answers.

Affective variables also have a significant impact on math performance (Ashcraft, Krause, & Hopko, 2007). Provision of high-quality instruction in math—including instructional explicitness, teaching of metacognitive strategies, review and reteaching of concepts, and attention to motivational issues—will enhance mastery of mathematical concepts and be likely to reduce the development of negative affect, such as performance-based anxiety, that frequently impedes math achievement at higher grade levels. Moreover, for students with MDs, remedial programs must incorporate strong methods for encouraging on-task behavior, hard work, and accurate performance.

CONCLUDING COMMENTS

The active theoretical debates in the fields of mathematical development and disability, and the increasing focus on intervention studies for children with MDs that draw on the cognitive-developmental literature, as well as on the science of randomized controlled trials—should propel our knowledge of MDs forward over the next several years. However, several issues in research on MDs may require consensus or better instrumentation to help us make sense out of the increasingly large number of studies in this area and to guide future research. These issues include the following:

1. The varying cutoff scores and criteria used to define an MD.
2. The fact that different researchers use different tasks to measure both simple and more complex number skills. This seems particularly important given that even small changes in task variables—such as problem complexity and the use of Arabic numerals versus nonsymbolic representations of numbers (e.g., dots) as stimuli—may produce different results in both behavioral and neuroimaging studies.
3. The use of scores on standardized tests of calculation to define groups with MD, which may miss other types of MDs.
4. The reliance on adult lesion and neuroimaging studies for inferences about the neurobiological sources and neural signatures of MDs in childhood populations.
5. The lack of precision with which specific cognitive processes are defined in correlational studies relating such skills as working memory and math (see also Swanson, 2007).
6. The relative paucity of randomized controlled trials of math interventions for preschoolers and school-age children with MDs or at risk for MDs, including trials that take into account frequently co-occurring difficulties in reading and attention.

REFERENCES

Adams, G., & Carnine, D. (2003). Direct instruction. In H. K. Swanson, K. R Harris, & S. Graham (Eds.), *Handbook of learning disabilities* (pp. 403–416). New York: Guilford Press.

Alarcon, M., DeFries, J. C., Light, J. G., & Pennington, B. F. (1997). A twin study of mathematics disability. *Journal of Learning Disabilities, 30*(6), 617–623.

American Psychiatric Association. (2000). *Diagnostic and statistical manual of mental disorders* (4th ed., text rev.). Washington, DC: Author.

Ansari, D., & Dhital, B. (2006). Age-related changes in the activation of the intraparietal sulcus during nonsymbolic magnitude processing: An event-related functional magnetic resonance imaging study. *Journal of Cognitive Neuroscience, 18*(11), 1820–1828.

Ansari, D., Donlan, C., Thomas, M. S. C., Ewing, S. A., Peen, T., & Kamiloff-Smith, A. (2003). What makes counting count?: Verbal and visuo-spatial contributions to typical and atypical number development. *Journal of Experimental Child Psychology, 85*(1), 50–62.

Ansari, D., & Karmiloff-Smith, A. (2002). Atypical trajectories of number development: A neuroconstructivist perspective. *Trends in Cognitive Sciences, 6*(12), 511–516.

Armstrong, F. D., & Briery, B. G. (2004). Childhood cancer and the school. In R. T. Brown (Ed.), *Handbook of pediatric psychology in school settings* (pp. 263–281). Mahwah, NJ: Erlbaum.

Ashcraft, M. (1992). Cognitive arithmetic: A review of data and theory. *Cognition, 44*, 75–106.

Ashcraft, M. H., Krause, J. A., & Hopko, D. R. (2007). Is math anxiety a mathematical learning disability? In D. B. Berch & M. M. M. Mazzocco (Eds.), *Why is math so hard for some children?: The nature and origins of mathematical learning difficulties and disabilities* (pp. 329–348) Baltimore: Brookes.

Ashcraft, M. H., Yamashita, T. S., & Aram, D. M, (1992). Mathematics performance in left and right brain-lesioned children and adolescents. *Brain and Cognition, 19*(2), 208–252.

Ayr, L. K., Yeates, K. O., & Ernile, B. G. (2005). Arithmetic skills and their cognitive correlates in children with acquired and congenital brain disorder. *Journal of the International Neuropsychological Society, 11*(3), 249–262.

Badian, N., & Ghublikian, M. (1983). The personal–social characteristics of children with poor mathematical computation skills. *Journal of Learning Disabilities, 16*(3), 154–157.

Balfanz, R. (2000). Why do so many urban public school students demonstrate so little academic achievement? In M. G. Sanders (Ed.), *Schooling students placed at risk: Research, policy, and practice in the education of poor and minority adolescents* (pp. 37–62). Mahwah, NJ: Erlbaum.

Barbaresi, W. J., Katusic, S. K., Colligan, R. C., Weaver, A. L., & Jacobsen, S. J. (2005). Math learning disorder: Incidence in a population-based birth cohort, 1976–82, Rochester, Minn. *Ambulatory Pediatrics, 5*(5), 281–289.

Barnes, M. A., Fletcher, J. M., & Ewing-Cobbs, L. (2007). Mathematical disabilities in congenital and acquired neurodevelopmental disorders. In D. B. Berch & M. M. M. Mazzocco (Eds.), *Why is math so hard for some children?: The nature and origins of mathematical learning difficulties and disabilities* (pp. 195–217). Baltimore: Brookes.

Barnes, M. A., & Fuchs, L. (2008). Learning disabilities. In M. L. Wolraich, P. H. Dworkin, D. D. Drotar, & E. C. Perrin (Eds.), *Developmental–behavioral pediatrics: Evidence and practice.* Amsterdam: Elsevier.

Barnes, M. A., Pengelly, S., Dennis, M., Wilkinson, M., Rogers, T., & Faulkner, H. (2002). Mathematics skills in good readers with hydrocephalus. *Journal of the International Neuropsychological Society, 8*(1), 72–82.

Barnes, M. A., Smith-Chant, B., & Landry, S. (2005). Number processing in neurodevelopmental disorders: Spina bifida myelomeningocele. In J. I. D. Campbell (Ed.), *Handbook of mathematical cognition* (pp. 299–313). New York: Psychology Press.

Barnes, M. A., Wilkinson, M., Khemani, E., Boudesquie, A., Dennis, M., & Fletcher, J. M. (2006). Arithmetic processing in children with spina bifida: Calculation accuracy, strategy use, and fact retrieval fluency. *Journal of Learning Disabilities, 39*(2), 174–187.

Bonner, M. J., Hardy, K, K., Ezell, E., & Ware, R. (2004). Hematological disorders: Sickle cell disease and hemophilia. In R. T. Brown (Ed.), *Handbook of pediatric psychology in school settings* (pp. 241–261). Mahwah, NJ: Erlbaum.

Butterworth, B. (1999). *What counts: How every brain is hardwired for math.* New York: Free Press.

Butterworth, B., & Reigosa, V. (2007). Information processing deficits in dyscalculia. In D. B. Berch & M. M. M. Mazzocco (Eds.), *Why is math so hard for some children?: The nature and origins of mathematical learning difficulties and disabilities* (pp. 65–81). Baltimore: Brookes.

Bull, R. (2007). Commentary on Part II, Section III: Neuropsychological factors. In D. B. Berch & M. M. M. Mazzocco (Eds.), *Why is math so hard for some children?: The nature and origins of mathematical learning difficulties and disabilities* (pp. 265–278. Baltimore: Brookes.

Chen, C., & Stevenson, H. W. (1995). Motivation and mathematics achievement: A comparative study of Asian-American, Caucasian-American, and East Asian high school students. *Child Development, 66*(4), 1215–1234.

Cohen, L., & Marks, K. S. (2002). How infants process addition and subtraction events. *Developmental Science, 5*(2), 186–201.

Dehaene, S., & Cohen, L. (1997). Cerebral pathways for calculation: Double dissociation between rote verbal and quantitative knowledge of arithmetic. *Cortex, 33*(2), 219–250.

Dehaene, S., Piaza, M., Pinel, P., & Cohen, L. (2005). Three parietal circuits for number processing. In J. I. D. Campbell (Ed.), *Handbook of mathematical cognition* (pp. 433–453). New York: Psychology Press.

Dehaene, S., Spelke, E., Pinel, P., Stanescu, R., & Tsivkin, S. (1999). Sources of mathematical thinking: Behavioural and brain-imaging evidence. *Science, 284*(5416), 970–974.

Ewing-Cobbs, L., Barnes, M. A., Fletcher, J. M., Levin, H. S., Swank, P. R., & Song, J. (2004). Modeling of longitudinal academic achievement scores after pediatric traumatic brain injury. *Developmental Neuropsychology, 25*(1–2), 107–133.

Fleishner, J. E. (1994). Diagnosis and assessment of mathematics learning disabilities. In G. R. Lyon (Ed.), *Frames of reference for the assessment of learning disabilities: New views on measurement issues* (pp. 441–458). Baltimore: Brookes.

Fletcher, J. M. (2005). Predicting math outcomes: Reading predictors and comorbidity. *Journal of Learning Disabilities, 38*(4), 308–312.

Fletcher, J. M., Lyon, G. R., Barnes, M. A., Stuebing, K. K., Francis, D. J., Olson, R. K., et al. (2002). Classification of learning disabilities: An evidence-based evaluation. In R. Bradley, L. Danielson, & D. P. Hallahan (Eds.), *Identification of learning disabilities: Research to practice* (pp. 185–250). Mahwah, NJ: Erlbaum.

Fletcher, J. M., Lyon, G. R., Fuchs, L. S., & Barnes, M. A. (2007). *Learning disabilities: From identification to intervention.* New York: Guilford Press.

Fuchs, L. S., Compton, D. L., Fuchs, D., Paulsen, K., Bryant, J. D., & Hamlet, C. L. (2005). The prevention, identification, and cognitive determinants of math difficulty. *Journal of Educational Psychology, 97*(3), 493–513.

Fuchs, L. S., & Fuchs, D. (2002). Mathematical problem-solving profiles of students with mathematics disabilities with and without comorbid reading disabilities. *Journal of Learning Disabilities, 35*(6), 563–573.

Fuchs, L. S., Fuchs, D., Hamlet, C. L., Powell, S. R., Capizzi, A. M., & Seethaler, P. M. (2006). The effects of computer-assisted instruction on number combination skill in at-risk first graders. *Journal of Learning Disabilities, 39*(5), 467–475.

Fuchs, L. S., Fuchs, D., Prentice, K., Burch, M., Hamlett, C. L., Owen, R., et al. (2003). Enhancing third-grade students' mathematical problem solving with self-regulated learning strategies. *Journal of Educational Psychology, 95,* 306–315.

Fuchs, L. S., Fuchs, D., Stuebing, K., Fletcher, J. M., Hamlett, C. L., & Lambert, W. E. (2008a). Problem-solving and computation skills: Are they shared or distinct aspects of mathematical cognition? Journal of Educational Psychology, *100,* 30–47.

Fuchs, L. S., Seethaler, P. M., Powell, S. R., Fuchs, D., Hamlett, C. L., & Fletcher, J. M. (2008b). Effects of preventative tutoring on the mathematical problem solving of third-grade students with math and reading difficulties. *Exceptional Children, 74,* 155–173.

Geary, D. C. (1993). Mathematical disabilities: Cognitive, neuropsychological, and genetic components. *Psychological Bulletin, 114*(2), 345–362.

Geary, D. C. (1996). Sexual selection and sex differences in mathematical abilities. *Behavioral and Brain Sciences, 19,* 229–284.

Geary, D. C. (2004). Mathematics and learning disabilities. *Journal of Learning Disabilities, 37*(1), 4–15.

Geary, D. C., & Hoard, M. K. (2005). Learning disabilities in arithmetic and mathematics: Theoretical and empirical perspectives. In J. I. D. Campbell (Ed.), *Handbook of mathematical cognition* (pp. 253–267). New York: Psychology Press.

Geary, D. C., Hoard, M. K., Byrd-Craven, J., Nugent, L., & Numtee, C. (2007). Cognitive mechanisms underlying achievement deficits in children with mathematical learning disability. *Child Development, 78*(4), 1343–1359.

Gelman, R., & Butterworth, B. (2005). Number and language: How are they related? *Trends in Cognitive Sciences, 9*(1), 6–10.

Gelman, R., & Gallistel, C. R. (1978). *The child's understanding of number.* Cambridge, MA: Harvard University Press.

Gersten, R., Jordan, N. C., & Flojo, J. R. (2005). Early identification and interventions for students with mathematics difficulties. *Journal of Learning Disabilities, 38*(4), 293–304.

Gersten, R. M., White, W. A., Falco, R., & Carnine, D. (1982). Teaching basic discriminations to handicapped and non-handicapped individuals through a dynamic presentation of instructional stimuli. *Analysis and Intervention in Developmental Disabilities, 2*(4), 305–317.

Ginsburg, H. P., Klein, A., & Starkey, P. (1998). The development of children's mathematical thinking: Connecting research with practice. In W. Damon (Series Ed.) & I. E. Sigel & K. A. Renninger (Vol. Eds.), *Handbook of child psychology: Vol. 4. Child psychology in practice* (5th ed., pp. 401–476). New York: Wiley.

Goldman, S. R., Pellegrino, J. W., & Mertz, D. L. (1988). Extended practice of basic addition facts: Strategy changes in learning-disabled students. *Cognition and Instruction, 5*(3), 223–265.

Griffin, S. (2007). Early intervention for children at risk of developing mathematical learning difficulties. In D. B. Berch & M. M. M. Mazzocco (Eds.), *Why is math so hard for some children?: The nature and origins of mathematical learning difficulties and disabilities* (pp. 373–395). Baltimore: Brookes.

Gross-Tsur, V., Manor, O., & Shalev, R. S. (1996). Developmental dyscalculia: Prevalence and demographic features. *Developmental Medicine and Child Neurology, 38*(1), 25–33.

Hallahan, D. P., Kauffman, J., & Lloyd, J. (1996). *Introduction to learning disabilities*. Needham Heights, MA: Allyn & Bacon.

Hanich, L. B., Jordan, N. C., Kaplan, D., & Dick, J. (2001). Performance across different areas of mathematical cognition in children with learning difficulties. *Journal of Educational Psychology, 93*(3), 615–626.

Hartje, W. (1987). The effect of spatial disorders on arithmetical skills. In G. Deloche & X. Seron (Eds.), *Mathematical disabilities: A cognitive neuropsychological perspective* (pp. 121–135). Hillsdale, NJ: Erlbaum.

Hresko, W. P., & Reid, D. K. (1981). Five faces of cognition: Theoretical influences on approaches to learning disabilities. *Learning Disability Quarterly, 4*(3), 238–243.

Isaacs, E. B., Edmonds, C. J., Lucas, A., & Gadian, D. G. (2001). Calculation difficulties in children of very low birthweight: A neural correlate. *Brain, 124*(9), 1701–1707.

Jordan, N. C., Hanich, L. B., & Kaplan, D. (2003). A longitudinal study of mathematical competencies in children with specific mathematics difficulties versus children with comorbid mathematics and reading difficulties. *Child Development, 74*(3), 834–850.

Kahn, H. J., & Whitaker, H. A. (1991). Acalculia: An historical review of localization. *Brain and Cognition, 17*(2), 102–115.

Karmiloff-Smith, A., Plunkett, K., Johnson, M. H., Elman, J. L., & Bates, E. A. (1998). What does it mean to claim that something is innate?: A reply to Clark, Harris, Lightfoot & Samuels. *Mind and Language, 13*, 588–597.

Klein, A., & Starkey, P. (2004). Fostering preschool children's mathematical knowledge: Findings from the Berkeley math readiness project. In D. H. Clements, J. Sarama, & A. DiBiase (Eds.), *Engaging young children in mathematics: Standards for early childhood mathematics education* (pp. 343–360). Mahwah, NJ: Erlbaum.

Koontz, K. L., & Berch, D. B. (1996). Identifying simple numerical stimuli: Processing inefficiencies exhibited by arithmetic learning disabled children. *Mathematical Cognition, 2*(1), 1–23.

Kovas, Y. Harlaar, N., Petrill, S. A., & Plomin, R. (2005). 'Generalist genes' and mathematics in 7-year-old twins. *Intelligence, 33*(5), 473–489.

Kozey, M., & Siegel, L. S. (2008). Definitions of learning disabilities in Canadian provinces and territories. *Canadian Psychology, 49*(2), 162–171.

Kroesbergen, E. H., & Van Luit, J. E. H. (2003). Mathematics interventions for children with special education needs: A meta-analysis. *Remedial and Special Education, 24*(2), 97–114.

Kroesbergen, E. H., Van Luit, J. E. H., & Maas, C. J. M. (2004). Effectiveness of explicit and constructivist mathematics instruction for low-achieving students in The Netherlands. *Elementary School Journal, 104*(3), 244–251.

Kucian, K., Lonneker, T., Dietrich, T., Dosch, M., Martin, E., & von Aster, A. (2006). Impaired neural networks for approximate calculation in dyscalculic children: A functional MRI study. *Behavioural and Brain Functions, 2*(31).

Landerl, K., Bevan, A., & Butterworth, B. (2004). Developmental dyscalculia and basic numerical capacities: A study of 8–9-year-old students. *Cognition, 93*(2), 99–125.

LeFevre, J., Smith-Chant, B. L., Fast, L., Skwarchuk, S., Sargla, E., Arnup, J. S., et al. (2006). What counts as knowing?: The development of conceptual and procedural knowledge of counting from kindergarten through grade 2. *Journal of Experimental Child Psychology, 93*(4), 285–303.

Lewis, C., Hitch, G. J., & Walker, P. (1994). The prevalence of specific arithmetic difficulties and specific reading difficulties in 9- to 10-year old boys and girls. *Journal of Child Psychology and Psychiatry, 35*(2), 283–292.

Litt, J., Taylor, H. G., Klein, N., & Hack, M. (2005). Learning disabilities in children with very low birthweight: Prevalence, neuropsychological correlates, and educational interventions. *Journal of Learning Disabilities, 38*(2), 130–141.

Lyon, G. R., Fletcher, J. M., & Barnes, M. A. (2003). Learning disabilities. In E. J. Mash & R. A. Barkley (Eds.), *Child psychopathology* (2nd ed., pp. 520–586). New York: Guilford Press.

Lyon, G. R., Fletcher, J. M., Fuchs, L., & Chhabra, V. (2006). Treatment of learning disabilities. In E. J. Mash & R. A. Barkley (Eds.), *Treatment of childhood disorders* (3rd ed., pp. 512–592). New York: Guilford Press.

Marshall, R. M., Hynd, G. W., Handwerk, M. J., & Hall, J. (1997). Academic underachievement in ADHD subtypes. *Journal of Learning Disabilities, 30*(6), 635–642.

Mazzocco, M. M. M., & McCloskey, M. (2005). Math performance in girls with Turner or fragile X syndrome. In J. I. D. Campbell (Ed.), *Handbook of mathematical cognition* (pp. 269–297). New York: Psychology Press.

Mazzocco, M. M. M., & Myers, G. F. (2003). Complexities in identifying and defining mathematics learning disability in the primary school years. *Annals of Dyslexia, 53*, 218–253.

McLean, J. F., & Hitch, G. J. (1999). Working memory impairments in children with specific arithmetic learning difficulties. *Journal of Experimental Child Psychology, 74*(3), 240–260.

Molko, N., Cachia, A., Rivière, D., Mangin, J. F., Bruandet, M., Le Bihan, D., et al. (2003). Functional and structural alterations of the intraparietal sulcus in a developmental dyscalculia of genetic origin. *Neuron, 40*(4), 847–858.

Montague, M. (2007). Self-regulation and mathematics instruction. *Learning Disabilities Research and Practice, 22*(1), 75–83.

Montague, M., & Bos, C. S. (1986). The effect of cognitive strategy training on verbal math problem solving performance of learning disabled students. *Journal of Learning Disabilities, 19*, 26–33.

Morrison, S. R., & Siegel, L. S. (1991). Arithmetic disability: Theoretical considerations and empirical evidence for this subtype. In L. B. Feagans, E. J. Short, & L. J. Meltzer (Eds.), *Subtypes of learning disabilities: Theoretical perspectives and research* (pp. 189–208). Hillsdale, NJ: Erlbaum.

Murphy, M. M., Mazzocco, M. M. M., Hanich, L. B., & Early, M. C. (2007). Cognitive characteristics of children with mathematics learning disability (MLD) vary as a function of the cutoff criterion used to define MLD. *Journal of Learning Disabilities, 40*(5), 458–478.

Oliver, A., Johnson, M. H., Karmiloff-Smith, A., & Pennington, B. (2000). Deviations in the emergence of representations: A neuroconstructivist framework for analyzing developmental disorders. *Developmental Science, 3*(1), 1–23.

Petrill, S. A., & Plomin, R. (2007). Quantitative genetics and mathematical abilities/disabilities. In D. B. Berch & M. M. M. Mazzocco (Eds.), *Why is math so hard for some children?: The nature and origins of mathematical learning difficulties and disabilities* (pp. 307–322). Baltimore: Brookes.

Plomin, R., & Kovas, Y. (2005). Generalist genes and learning disabilities. *Psychological Bulletin, 131*(4), 592–617.

Raghubar, K. P., Cirino, P. T., Barnes, M. A., Ewing-Cobbs, L., Fletcher, J. M., & Fuchs, L. S. (2009). Errors in multi-digit arithmetic and behavioral inattention in children with math difficulties. *Journal of Learning Disabilities, 42*, 4, 356–371.

Rasmussen, C., & Bisanz, J. (2005). Representation and working memory in early arithmetic. *Journal of Experimental Child Psychology, 91*(2), 137–157.

Reuhkala, M. (2001). Mathematical skills in ninth-graders: Relationship with visuo-spatial abilities and working memory. Educational Psychology, 21(4), 387–399.

Rittle-Johnson, B., Siegler, R. S., & Alibali, M. W. (2001). Developing conceptual understanding and procedural skill in mathematics: An iterative process. *Journal of Educational Psychology, 93*(2), 346–362.

Rivera, S. M., Reiss, A. L., Eckert, M. A., & Menon, V. (2005). Developmental changes in mental arithmetic: Evidence for increased functional specialization in the left inferior parietal cortex. *Cerebral Cortex, 15*(11), 1779–1790.

Rivera-Batiz, F. L. (1992). Quantitative literacy and the likelihood of employment among young adults in the United States. *Journal of Human Resources, 27*(2), 313–328.

Rosenshine, B., & Stevens, R. (1986). Teaching functions. In M. C. Wittrock (Ed.), *Handbook of research on teaching* (3rd ed., pp. 376–391). New York: Macmillan.

Rourke, B. P. (1993). Arithmetic disabilities, specific and otherwise: A neuropsychological perspective. *Journal of Learning Disabilities, 26*(4), 214–226.

Rousselle, L., & Noël, M. (2007). Basic numerical skills in children with mathematics learning disabilities: A comparison of symbolic vs. non-symbolic number magnitude processing. *Cognition, 102*(3), 361–395.

Rovet, J., Szekely, C., & Hockenberry, M. (1994). Specific arithmetic calculation deficits in children with Turner syndrome. *Journal of Clinical and Experimental Neuropsychology, 16*(6), 820–839.

Russell, R. L., & Ginsburg, H. P. (1984). Cognitive analysis of children's mathematics difficulties. *Cognition and Instruction, 1*(2), 217–244.

Shalev, R. S., Auerbach, J., Manor, O., & Gross-Tsur, V. (2000). Developmental dyscalculia: Prevalence and prognosis. *European Child and Adolescent Psychiatry, 9*(Suppl. 2), 58–64.

Shalev, R. S., Manor, O., Auerbach, J., & Gross-Tsur, V. (1998). Persistence of developmental dyscalculia: What counts? Results from a 3-year prospective follow-up study. *Journal of Pediatrics, 133*(3), 358–362.

Shalev, R. S., Manor, O., & Gross-Tsur, V. (1997). Neuropsychological aspects of developmental dyscalculia. *Mathematical Cognition, 3*(2), 105–120.

Shalev, R. S., Manor, O., & Gross-Tsur, V. (2005). Developmental dyscalculia: A prospective six-year follow-up. *Developmental Medicine and Child Neurology, 47*(2), 121–125.

Shalev, R. S., Manor, O., Karem, B., Ayalia, M., Badichi, N., Friedlander, Y., et al. (2001). Developmental dyscalculia is a familial learning disability. *Journal of Learning Disabilities, 34*(1), 59–65.

Share, D. L., Moffitt, T. E., & Silva, P. A. (1988). Factors associated with arithmetic-and-reading disability and specific arithmetic disability. *Journal of Learning Disabilities, 21*(5), 313–320.

Shaywitz, S. E., Fletcher, J. M., Holahan, J. M., Shneider, A. E., Marchione, K. E., Stuebing, K. K., et al. (1999). Persistence of dyslexia: The Connecticut Longitudinal Study at adolescence. *Pediatrics, 10*(6), 1351–1359.

Siegel, L., & Ryan, E. B. (1989). Subtypes of developmental dyslexia: The influence of definitional variables. *Reading and Writing, 1*(3), 257–287.

Siegler, R. S. (1996). *Emerging minds: The process of change in children's thinking.* New York: Oxford University Press.

Siegler, R. S. (2007). Foreword: The birth of a new discipline. In D. B. Berch & M. M. M. Mazzocco (Eds.), *Why is math so hard for some children?: The nature and origins of mathematical learning difficulties and disabilities* (pp. xvii–xxii). Baltimore: Brookes.

Siegler, R. S., & Shrager, J. (1984). Strategy choice in addition and subtraction: How do children know what to do? In C. Sophian (Ed.), *Origins of cognitive skills* (pp. 229–293). Hillsdale, NJ: Erlbaum.

Simon, T. J., Bearden, C. E., McGinn, D. M., & Zackai, E. (2005). Visuospatial and numerical cognitive deficits in children with chromosome 22Q11.2 deletion syndrome. *Cortex, 41*(2), 145–155.

Simon, T. J., & Rivera, S. M. (2007). Neuroanatomical approaches to the study of mathematical ability and disability. In D. B. Berch & M. M. M. Mazzocco (Eds.), *Why is math so hard for some children?: The nature and origins of mathematical learning difficulties and disabilities* (pp. 283–305). Baltimore: Brookes.

Spelke, E. S., & Kinzler, K. D. (2007). Core knowledge. *Developmental Science, 10*(1), 89–96.

Spelke, E. S., & Tsivkin, S. (2001). Language and number: A bilingual training study. *Cognition, 78*(1), 45–88.

Starkey, P., Spelke, E. S., & Gelman, R. (1990). Numerical abstraction by human infants. *Cognition, 36*(2), 97–127.

Swanson, H. L. (2007). Commentary on Part I, Section II: Cognitive aspects of math disabilities. In D. B. Berch & M. M. M. Mazzocco (Eds.), *Why is math so hard for some children?: The nature and origins of mathematical learning difficulties and disabilities* (pp. 133–144). Baltimore: Brookes.

Swanson, H. L., Hoskyn, M., & Lee, C. (1999). *Interventions for students with learning disabilities: A meta-analysis of treatment outcomes.* New York: Guilford Press.

Swanson, H. L., & Jerman, O. (2006). Math disabilities: A selective meta-analysis of the literature. *Review of Educational Research, 76*(2), 249–274.

Swanson, H. K., & Sachse-Lee, C. (2001). Mathematical problem solving and working memory in children with learning disabilities: Both executive and phonological processes are important. *Journal of Experimental Child Psychology, 79*(3), 294–321.

Temple, C. M., & Sherwood, S. (2002). Representation and retrieval of arithmetical facts: Developmental difficulties. *Quarterly Journal of Experimental Psychology A: Human Experimental Psychology, 55A*(3), 733–752.

Thompson, L. A., Detterman, D. K., & Plomin, R. (1991). Associations between cognitive abilities and scholastic achievement: Genetic overlap but environmental differences. *Psychological Science, 2*(3), 158–165.

Torgesen, J. K. (2002). The prevention of reading difficulties. *Journal of School Psychology, 40*(1), 7–26.

U.S. Department of Education. (1999). 34 CFR Parts 300 and 303: Assistance to the states for the education of children with disabilities and the early intervention program for infants and toddlers with disabilities. Final regulations. *Federal Register, 64,* 12406–12672.

U.S. Office of Education. (1977). Assistance to states for education for handicapped children: Procedures for evaluating specific learning disabilities. *Federal Register, 42,* G1082–G1085.

Van der Sluis, S., de Jong, P. F., & van der Leij, A. (2004). Inhibition and shifting in children with learning deficits in arithmetic and reading. *Journal of Experimental Child Psychology, 87*(3), 239–266.

Woodward, J., & Baxter, J. (1997). The effects of an innovative approach to mathematics on academically low-achieving students in inclusive settings. *Exceptional Children, 63,* 373–388.

World Health Organization. (2007). *International classification of diseases* (10th rev., Version 2007). Geneva: Author.

Wynn, K. (1992). Addition and subtraction by human infants. *Nature, 358,* 749–750.

Zentall, S. S. (1990). Fact-retrieval automatization and math problem solving by learning disabled, attention-disordered, and normal adolescents. *Journal of Educational Psychology, 82*(4), 856–865.

CHAPTER 12

Reading Disability

ROBIN L. PETERSON
BRUCE F. PENNINGTON

HISTORY

Reading disability (RD), or *dyslexia*, is a learning disability in which children fail to make expected progress in learning to read. The disorder was first recognized in the late 19th century by Pringle-Morgan (1896), a British physician. He described Percy, a 14-year-old boy who could not read despite average intellect, good eyesight, and years of instruction. A number of similar reports were published soon afterward (Fisher, 1905; Hinshelwood, 1900, 1907; Kerr, 1897; Stephenson, 1907; Thomas, 1905). These authors noted the similarity to previously healthy adults who had lost the ability to read following stroke, a condition known as *word-blindness*, and called the new disorder *congenital word blindness*. The terms *developmental alexia* and *developmental dyslexia* were later used, and also implied a parallel to acquired forms of reading difficulty (Shaywitz, 2003).

Early theories of RD postulated a basic deficit in visual processing and focused on the reversal errors commonly made by individuals with RD, such as writing *b* for *d* or *was* for *saw*. Orton (1925, 1937) termed this deficit *strephosymoblia*—"twisted symbols"—and hypothesized that the visual problem arose because of a failure of hemispheric dominance, in which mirror images of visual stimuli were not inhibited, leading to reversal errors. Vellutino (1979) demonstrated that such reversal errors in RD were restricted to print in one's own language, and were thus really linguistic rather than visual in nature. Since then, a great deal of research has made clear that RD is a type of language disorder whose primary underlying deficit involves the development of phonological representations (for reviews, see Snowling, 2000; Vellutino, Fletcher, Snowling, & Scanlon, 2004). However, it is still possible that some sorts of visual processing problems are associated with RD.

DEFINITION

Children with RD have difficulties with accurate and/or fluent word recognition and spelling. Problems with reading comprehension are generally considered secondary (Lyon, Shaywitz, & Shaywitz, 2003). Definitions of RD exclude individuals whose reading problems arise from environmental deprivation, peripheral sensory impairment, or more severe developmental problems (e.g., intellectual disability). Research suggests that RD represents the lower end of a normal distribution of reading ability (e.g., Rodgers, 1983; Shaywitz, Escobar, Shaywitz, & Fletcher, 1992). Thus the diagnosis of RD requires setting a somewhat arbitrary cutoff on a continuous variable.

There has been debate as to whether the diagnostic threshold should be relative to the child's age or IQ. The logic of IQ–achievement discrepancy definitions is that low-IQ poor readers have a nonspecific learning problem and thus should not be grouped together with higher-IQ poor readers, whose reading problem presumably results from a different underlying deficit. There are several problems with this logic. First, IQ-referenced definitions ensure that many children whose reading problems cause significant impairment will not fit the definition of RD and will therefore not qualify for services. Second, although measures of IQ are moderately correlated with reading, we do not fully understand the causal basis of this correlation. IQ is likely to influence reading development, but there is also evidence that reading influences aspects of IQ, particularly vocabulary acquisition (Stanovich, 1986). In addition, a third variable, such as verbal short-term memory, could influence both reading and IQ test scores. IQ–achievement discrepancy definitions assume that the causal arrow is unidirectional—from IQ to reading. Third, the research literature does not support the external validity of the distinction between age- and IQ-referenced definitions in terms of either the underlying deficit (i.e., in phonological processing) or the kind of treatment that is helpful (Fletcher, Foorman, Shaywitz, & Shaywitz, 1999; Silva, McGee, & Williams, 1985; Stuebing et al., 2002). For clinical purposes, children who meet either an age- or an IQ-referenced definition should be identified and treated for RD.

EPIDEMIOLOGY

Prevalence estimates, of course, depend on definition. A cutoff for reading achievement set to 1.5 standard deviations below the mean for age necessarily identifies approximately 7% of the population as having RD. A similar IQ–achievement discrepancy definition (i.e., reading achievement at least 1.5 standard deviations below the score predicted by IQ) identifies a comparable proportion. For example, in an epidemiological sample of second and third graders, this definition identified approximately 9% of boys and 6% of girls as having RD (Shaywitz, Shaywitz, Fletcher, & Escobar, 1990). Of course, less extreme cutoffs will identify a larger proportion of children. However, some children will only meet the first definition (low ability, poor reading) and some will only meet the second (high ability, poorer-than-expected reading).

There has been some disagreement regarding whether RD is truly more common in boys than girls or whether apparent gender differences result from referral bias. A recent study of four epidemiological samples across two English-speaking countries found that in every case, there was a significant male predominance, with rates ranging from 1.4:1

to 3.3:1. Rates were similar for age- and IQ-referenced definitions, but there was a greater male predominance in New Zealand than in the United Kingdom (Rutter et al., 2004). Male predominance at the lower end of this range (i.e., 1.3–2:1) has been reported in epidemiological samples in the United States (Flannery, Liederman, Daly, & Schultz, 2000; Shaywitz et al., 1990; Smith, Gilger, & Pennington, 2001). However, the gender difference is even higher in referred samples, from about threefold to sixfold (Smith et al., 2001). The difference in gender ratios between epidemiological and referred samples means that girls with RD are less likely to be referred for services. The reason for this differential rate of referral appears to be higher rates of comorbid externalizing disorders—attention-deficit/ hyperactivity disorder (ADHD), oppositional defiant disorder (ODD), and conduct disorder (CD)—in boys with RD (Willcutt & Pennington, 2000).

RD is not diagnosed until after a child is exposed to formal reading instruction, but it is comorbid with several other developmental disorders that are apparent earlier and can therefore help indicate a child's risk for later reading problems. Work in our laboratory has tested the basis of these comorbidities. As mentioned above, RD is comorbid with externalizing problems, particularly in boys. Once the comorbidity between RD and ADHD is controlled for, the associations with ODD and CD become nonsignificant, so these appear to be secondary disorders or epiphenomenal comorbidities (Willcutt & Pennington, 2000). A longitudinal study showed that children with future RD had elevated rates of ADHD symptoms before kindergarten (Boetsch, 1996), consistent with other results indicating a shared genetic etiology between RD and ADHD (Willcutt, Pennington, & DeFries, 2000; Willcutt et al., 2002). So preschoolers who exhibit symptoms of ADHD are at increased risk for later RD.

RD is also comorbid with two other disorders of language development: specific language impairment (SLI) and speech sound disorder (SSD). SLI is defined as an unexpected difficulty with structural language acquisition, including the mastery of grammar (syntax) and vocabulary (semantics), while SSD (also called phonological disorder or articulation disorder) is an unexpected difficulty with accurately producing speech sounds. Both SLI and SSD can be apparent in the preschool years or earlier, and longitudinal studies have demonstrated that both predict later risk for RD, though the risk appears to be much greater for SLI (Bishop & Adams, 1990; Catts, Fey, Tomblin, & Zhang, 2002; Nathan, Stackhouse, Goulandris, & Snowling, 2004; Stothard, Snowling, Bishop, Chipchase, & Kaplan, 1998). In fact, the relationship between SSD and RD may arise largely because each is associated with SLI. Our laboratory and others (Smith, Pennington, Boada, & Shriberg, 2005; Stein et al., 2004) have found that genetic loci implicated in RD are also associated with SSD. To date, a different set of loci has been implicated in SLI (Bartlett et al., 2002; SLI Consortium, 2002, 2004). So there is a puzzle still to be resolved by the field, since the behavioral results indicate that the overlap between SSD and RD owes largely to the third variable of SLI, but the genetic results have told a different story. Practically speaking, preschool children who exhibit difficulties with speech *or* language development should be carefully monitored for later RD.

Although most of the research literature has investigated RD in English-speaking countries, there is mounting attention to reading difficulties in other languages (for reviews, see Caravolas, 2005; Goulandris, 2003). Written English is sometimes considered particularly difficult to learn, because the mapping between letters and sounds is less consistent than in many other alphabetic languages, such as Finnish, Italian, and Spanish (Seymour,

2005). In fact, children at the lower end of the reading distribution in languages with more consistent mappings do have less severe reading and spelling problems than their English-speaking counterparts, as least in terms of accuracy (Caravolas, Bruck, & Genesee, 2003; de Jong & van der Leij, 2003; Landerl, Wimmer, & Frith, 1997). Difficulties with reading fluency (i.e., speed of reading connected text) appear more comparable across languages (Caravolas, Volin, & Hulme, 2005; de Jong & van der Leij, 2003; Landerl et al., 1997). Furthermore, in many languages, children with RD exhibit phonological processing deficits (Caravolas et al., 2005; Landerl et al., 1997; Schneider, Roth, & Ennemoser, 2000). An influential neuroimaging study demonstrated that poor readers in English, French, and Italian all showed similar patterns of aberrant neural activation during a reading task (Paulesu et al., 2001). Consistent with other studies, the reading accuracy of the Italian participants (whose language has the most consistent letter–sound relations) was superior to that of the English and French participants. Furthermore, the Italian participants were least likely to have experienced clinically significant reading problems and to have been previously diagnosed with RD. These results suggest that for alphabetic languages, there is cross-cultural similarity in the neurocognitive underpinnings of poor reading, but that the same biological liability is more likely to cause significant impairment in some languages than in others (see Wydell & Butterworth, 1999, for a within-subject demonstration of this phenomenon).

A growing body of research is investigating RD in Chinese, a logographic language (e.g., Chan & Siegel, 2001; Shu & Anderson, 1997; Tzeng, Lin, Hung, & Lee, 1995). In contrast to alphabetic languages, in which letters represent phonemes (individual sounds), the smallest written units in Chinese are characters representing monosyllabic morphemes (units of language that convey meaning) (Hanley, 2005). Phonology is not irrelevant to reading in Chinese, however. Chinese characters have phonological elements (Hanley, 2005), and Chinese skilled readers show phonological effects on word recognition (Tan & Perfetti, 1998). Research supports the hypothesis that phonological deficits are associated with RD in Chinese, but may not be as critical as in alphabetic languages. For example, McBride-Chang et al. (2005) reported that both morphological and phonological tasks correlated with reading skill in Chinese and in two alphabetic orthographies (English and Korean). However, only the morphological tasks *uniquely* predicted reading ability in Chinese, while the opposite pattern held for the alphabetic orthographies. In a neuroimaging study, Siok, Perfetti, Jin, and Tan (2004) demonstrated that the pattern of aberrant neural activation in poor Chinese readers showed both similarities and differences to the pattern characterizing RD in alphabetic languages. More research is needed on this question, but it is possible that the etiologies and biological liabilities for reading difficulty in logographic versus alphabetic languages are partly independent. If so, RD across these languages would best be characterized as constituting overlapping, but not identical, disorders.

NEURAL SUBSTRATES

Anatomical Findings

Evidence for structural abnormalities in the brains of individuals with RD has primarily come from two sources: postmortem studies and magnetic resonance imaging (MRI). One group of postmortem findings relates to the planum temporale, a region of the superior temporal gyrus implicated in auditory and language processing. Most typically developing individuals show an asymmetry of this structure, with larger left-hemisphere than right-hemisphere volumes, while autopsies of several brains of individuals with RD showed symmetry (Galaburda, Sherman, Rosen, Aboitiz, & Geschwind, 1985; Humphreys, Kaufmann, & Galaburda, 1990). A second group of postmortem findings concerns histological anomalies, including abnormally sized cells, as well as ectopias and dysplasias presumed to result from failures of neural migration. Overall, these anomalies were more common in the brains of persons with RD than of controls. In particular, findings have been reported in the left hemisphere, particularly in perisylvian regions (Galaburda et al., 1985); in the medial and lateral geniculate nuclei (MGN and LGN) of the thalamus (Galaburda, Menard, & Rosen, 1994; Livingstone, Rosen, Drislane, & Galaburda, 1991); and in the cerebellum (Finch, Nicolson, & Fawcett, 2002).

Postmortem studies are inherently limited. Diagnosis must be retrospective, and the consequences of any abnormalities are unknown, since no behavioral measures are available. In addition, postmortem studies have used very small sample sizes and have not always carefully controlled for such factors as educational history or handedness. The advent of MRI has provided a powerful means of examining more brains of persons with RD *in vivo*. Furthermore, a number of exciting recent studies have combined behavioral methods with structural imaging techniques to examine the potential consequences of anatomical abnormalities more directly.

Many MRI studies followed up on the postmortem results by focusing on the planum temporale. Although early reports supported the absence of a normal leftward asymmetry in RD (Hynd, Semrud-Clikeman, Lorys, & Novey, 1990; Larsen, Hoien, Lundberg, & Odegaard, 1990), there have since been numerous failures to replicate this finding (Best & Demb, 1999; Eckert et al., 2003; Robichon, Levrier, Farnarier, & Habib, 2000; Rumsey et al., 1997a; Schultz, Cho, Staib, & Kier, 1994), and some reports of *greater* leftward asymmetry for individuals with RD than for controls (Leonard et al., 2001; Leonard, Voeller, Lombardino, & Morris, 1993). The initial association between RD and planum temporale symmetry may have resulted at least partly from subject characteristics that are not central to RD (e.g., left-handedness). In addition, meaningful variability within samples with RD could make it difficult to obtain positive results, especially since asymmetry measures require two volumes and are thus intrinsically less reliable than measurements of a single structure. A series of studies by Hugdahl and colleagues has shed some light on this issue (Heirvang et al., 2000; Hugdahl et al., 2003). The most recent study employed the largest sample size and reported no group differences (RD vs. control) for planum temporale asymmetry. However, asymmetry was correlated with ear preference in a dichotic listening task for the group with RD only, indicating within-group structural variability with functional consequences.

In general, there has been a heterogeneity of findings in structural MRI studies of RD (see Eckert, 2004, for a review). The inconsistency probably owes to multiple methodological factors and participant characteristics, including differing methods for identifying brain regions, small sample sizes, a range of statistical thresholds, different definitions of RD, and varying exclusionary criteria (e.g., comorbid diagnoses) (Filipek, 1996, 1999). Thus firm conclusions about brain structure in RD await greater methodological consistency and meta-analysis. Nonetheless, some intriguing findings have begun to emerge. Some of the findings to be replicated across samples and laboratories include reduced total cerebral volume and abnormalities of the cerebellum, temporal lobes, and a variety of perisylvian regions. We now briefly review this evidence.

A number of studies have reported reduced total cerebral volumes in participants with RD even after controlling for IQ (Casanova, Araque, Giedd, & Rumsey, 2004; Eckert et al., 2003; Phinney, Pennington, Olson, Filley, & Filipek, 2007), but other studies (Pennington et al., 1999; Vinckenbosch, Robichon, & Eliez, 2005) have obtained null results. The functional correlates of the group difference have yet to be investigated in detail. One of the few studies to examine the issue directly (Phinney et al., 2007) reported the surprising finding that after age, gender, and IQ were controlled, total cerebral volume was correlated with phonological skill for controls, but not for participants with RD. Reduced cerebral volume may be partly accounted for by disorders that are comorbid with RD. Leonard et al. (2001) reported that cerebral volume was not correlated with symptom measures considered central to RD (e.g., pseudoword reading), but was correlated with measures more commonly associated with SLI, including oral comprehension (see also Leonard et al., 2002).

Reductions in right cerebellar anterior lobe volume (Eckert et al., 2003; Leonard et al., 2001) and in total right cerebellar gray matter (Rae et al., 2002) have been reported in RD. Rae et al. demonstrated that relatively less gray matter in the right than left cerebellum (as indexed by a symmetry ratio) was correlated with slower pseudoword reading for participants with RD but not for controls. Eckert et al. reported correlations between right anterior cerebellar volume and multiple behavioral tasks that distinguished participants with RD from controls, including reading, phonological, and rapid naming tasks. The agreement across these two studies is particularly promising, since one included only adult males (Rae et al.), while the other included male and female children (Eckert et al.). Gray matter reductions in cerebellar posterior lobes have also been reported in RD. Brown et al. (2001) reported bilateral reductions in the similunar lobule, while Eckert et al. (2003) reported reductions in the left side of this structure.

Multiple studies have found temporal lobe anomalies in RD, though the more specific location of findings, including whether the differences were lateralized or bilateral, has varied (Brambati et al., 2004; Brown et al., 2001; Eliez et al., 2000; Hynd et al., 1990; Pennington et al., 1999; Vinckenbosch et al., 2005). Across these studies, volume reductions in the inferior, middle, and superior temporal gyri have been reported, as well as in the planum temporale and insula. When findings have been lateralized, reductions have typically been on the left. Vinckenbosch et al. (2005) reported that gray matter density within the middle temporal gyri bilaterally was correlated with performance on a visual rhyme judgment task that is sensitive to RD.

Perisylvian regions of the frontal and parietal lobes have also shown structural differences in RD. Brown et al. (2001) reported gray matter decreases in the left inferior frontal gyrus (IFG), and Eckert et al. (2003) found bilateral surface area reductions in this region. Another study reported that an abnormal rightward asymmetry of the IFG in RD was correlated with pseudoword-reading performance (Robichon et al., 2000). Gray matter reductions in the left supramarginal gyrus were found in a sample of children with RD (Eckert et al., 2005), while *increased* leftward asymmetry of the parietal operculum (Robichon et al., 2000) and planum parietal (Leonard et al., 2001) have both been reported in high-functioning adults with RD. Given the findings of structural abnormality in both anterior and posterior perisylvian regions, we might predict that the white matter tracts connecting these regions would also be damaged in RD. Klingberg et al. (2000) used diffusion tensor imaging (DTI) to compare adults with RD to controls, and found support for this hypothesis. They reported white matter disturbance in bilateral temporoparietal regions, with the axons predominantly oriented in the anterior–posterior direction. The integrity of white matter in the left (but not the right) temporoparietal region was correlated highly with measures of real-word and pseudoword reading ($r = .5$–$.7$). A very similar finding was subsequently reported in a sample of children (Deutsch et al., 2005).

In summary, the anatomical findings in RD implicate left-hemisphere networks involved in skilled reading and language (Sandak, Mencl, Frost, & Pugh, 2004), and differences also exist in the cerebellum and a number of other brain regions. As we will see, a similar story has emerged from studies of brain function.

Functional Findings

Numerous investigations have attempted to further elucidate the neural bases of RD by examining brain function during reading and language tasks, using positron emission tomography (PET) and functional MRI (fMRI). This literature has been marked by many of the same methodological concerns as the anatomical literature (e.g., different definitions of RD and of various brain regions). Interpretation of functional results is further limited in studies that use a case–control design but do not equate performance across the two groups (see Price & McCrory, 2005). In these cases, it is not clear whether the neural differences are a cause or a result of impaired performance.

Functional neuroimaging studies of reading and language tasks have identified aberrant activation patterns in participants with RD across a distributed set of left-hemisphere sites, including many of the same regions implicated in the anatomical literature. The most common findings have been reduced activation of left occipitotemporal (Brunswick, McCrory, Price, Frith, & Frith, 1999; Paulesu et al., 2001; Rumsey et al., 1997b; Shaywitz et al., 2003) and temporoparietal (Shaywitz et al., 2002; Shaywitz et al., 2003; Temple et al., 2001) regions. Findings in the region of the left IFG have been mixed, with several studies reporting increased activation in RD (Brunswick et al., 1999; Shaywitz et al., 1998; Temple et al., 2001) and others reporting decreased activation (Aylward et al., 2003; Corina et al., 2001; Georgiewa et al., 1999). Both task and participant characteristics have probably contributed to the difference in findings. Increased IFG activity in RD has most often emerged in the context of reading aloud (Price & McCrory, 2005). In silent reading or other language tasks, decreased activity in this region is more likely among the most impaired readers (Shaywitz et al., 2003). A common interpretation of the full pattern of results is that decreased occipitotemporal activity corresponds to deficits in word recognition processes, decreased temporoparietal activity corresponds to phonological processing difficulties, and increased IFG activity relates to compensatory processes. Notably, very few studies have equated performance across groups (RD vs. control). This limitation particularly complicates the interpretation of temporoparietal findings, which (to date) have emerged only in the context of group performance differences (Price & McCrory, 2005).

Some authors have argued that the left occipitotemporal region includes a "visual word form area" (McCandliss, Cohen, & Dehaene, 2003), which is specifically responsible for orthographic processing of words. A PET study (McCrory, Mechelli, Frith, & Price, 2005) tested whether aberrant activation of this region in RD was specific to word reading. The authors compared adults with RD and control participants on both a picture-naming task and a word-reading task. Behavioral performance was comparable across the two groups. The participants with RD exhibited reduced left occipitotemporal activation for both tasks; further, there was no group by task interaction. The authors concluded that the left occipitotemporal area is important in the integration of visual and phonological information, and that this process is impaired in RD. Given the relative recency of written language, it is unsurprising that the neural basis for reading in general, and impaired reading in particular, would relate to more general cognitive processes.

Consistent with the anatomical literature, some studies of RD have also reported activation differences in the cerebellum. For example, Brunswick et al. (1999) found that, compared to controls, adults with RD underactivated the cerebellum bilaterally during reading tasks. Another study by the same research group (McCrory, Frith, Brunswick, & Price, 2000) reported that participants with RD exhibited reduced activity in the left cerebellum during a word repetition task. These findings are unsurprising in light of the growing appreciation for the cerebellum's importance in a wide variety of cognitive processes, including language (e.g., Schmahmann & Caplan, 2006). However, the precise role of the cerebellum in RD, including the specific regions that are implicated, is not yet well understood.

Exciting new research is using fMRI to investigate the neural correlates of improved performance following treatment for RD (Aylward et al., 2003; Richards et al., 2006; Shaywitz et al., 2004; Temple et al., 2003). In general, these studies have reported that successful behavioral treatment is correlated with a normalization of brain activation patterns, such that participants with RD begin to resemble controls more closely. The Shaywitz et al. study particularly merits discussion because it had the largest sample size and longest follow-up time, and because in-scanner performance was comparable across groups. The study compared three groups of 6- to 9-year-old children: participants with RD receiving an intensive, year-long experimental treatment (Blachman, Schatschneider, Fletcher, & Clonan, 2003); participants with RD receiving standard community intervention; and controls. Experimental treatment provided 50 minutes of daily individual tutoring, including practice with letter–sound associations, phoneme analysis and blending, and timed reading of both single words and connected text. The treatment was significantly more effective than the community treatment in promoting reading fluency. Brain activation was measured during a letter identification task. Following treatment, the experimental group but not the community group demonstrated increased activation in a number of left-hemisphere sites, including the IFG and the posterior middle temporal gyrus. Importantly, the control group showed activation changes similar to those of the experimental group, and previous work demonstrated that left IFG activation is correlated positively with age in reading-related tasks (Shaywitz et al., 2002). Thus these results suggest that in the absence of successful treatment, the community group did not exhibit normal age-related changes in brain activity.

Summary

In summary, RD is associated with differences across multiple brain regions. The most consistent evidence points to aberrant structure and function of left-hemisphere networks important to reading and language. Furthermore, correlational and treatment studies indicate that these brain differences have meaningful behavioral consequences. However, these regions do not appear to tell the whole story in RD. The cerebellum is one structure likely to be fruitful for future research, since it has been implicated by histological, structural, and functional studies, but its role in RD is not yet well understood. Another important direction for future work will be to continue to investigate the connections among the brain regions involved in RD. The recent application of DTI to RD research (e.g., Deutsch et al., 2005; Klingberg et al., 2000) holds promise for addressing this question.

NEUROPSYCHOLOGY

There is a long and rich research history investigating the neuropsychology of RD. The goal of this research is to discover which aspects of the reading process go awry in RD, and then to identify the specific underlying cognitive deficits. Therefore, neuropsychological theories of RD have benefited greatly from cognitive models of skilled reading (e.g., Coltheart, Curtis, Atkins, & Haller, 1993; Coltheart, Rastle, Perry, Langdon, & Ziegler, 2001; Harm & Seidenberg, 1999, 2004; Seidenberg & McClelland, 1989).

The ultimate goal of reading is comprehension, which depends on many higher processes such as reasoning and memory. However, it turns out that a substantial proportion of the variation in reading comprehension can be accounted for by individual differences in the accuracy and speed of printed-word recognition, especially in children (Perfetti, 1985). According to the "simple view of reading" (Gough & Walsh, 1991), reading comprehension (hereafter abbreviated as RC) equals the product of single-word recognition (hereafter abbreviated as WR) and listening comprehension (LC). Empirical evidence has demonstrated that, in children, the product of WR and LC is correlated highly with RC (.84; Gough & Walsh, 1991). Since children begin school with much better-developed LC than WR, it makes sense that WR would be the main contributor to individual differences in RC in the early school years. One study found that, among second graders, the correlation between WR and RC was .78, whereas LC had a negligible contribution. By fifth grade, the balance between these two factors had shifted considerably; the correlation for WR was now .45, whereas LC had increased to .74 (Curtis, 1980). In other words, by fifth grade, most students had developed enough WR skill that individual LC differences emerged as the major factor limiting RC, but individual WR differences still played a substantial role. The external validity of defining RD as characterized by deficits in accurate and fluent WR derives partly from the relationship of WR to RC. Of course, some children may have RC difficulties despite good WR skills because of impairments in LC. There is now evidence that such a group of children exists. They have been called "poor comprehenders" and are considered to have a learning disability differing from RD (see Nation, 2005, for a review). By definition, poor comprehenders have good single-word-decoding skills relative to their RC ability—the opposite of a "pure" dyslexic profile. There is evidence that poor comprehenders and children with SLI overlap somewhat (Nation, Clarke, Marshall, & Durand, 2004), although most children with SLI have problems with both WR and LC.

Given that RD is characterized by deficits in WR, an important question concerns the cognitive mechanisms that underlie skilled WR. This has been a topic of ongoing debate in both the adult and developmental literatures (see Coltheart et al., 2001; Harm & Seidenberg, 1999; Jackson & Coltheart, 2001; Plaut, McClelland, Seidenberg, & Patterson, 1996). The influential dual-route theory of Coltheart and colleagues holds that skilled readers have two mechanisms for reading words: a direct look-up mechanism for words the reader knows well, and an indirect mechanism that converts letters into sounds and assembles the sounds into words. Only the direct mechanism can read exception words, such as *yacht*, that disobey the normal rules of letter–sound correspondence, whereas only the indirect mechanism can read pseudowords, such as *plim*, that the reader has never encountered before. Critical distinctions between the routes are that the indirect route, but not the direct route, relies on sublexical phonology, and that the indirect route is much slower. Dual-route theory was originally built on the strength of evidence from adult patients with brain damage; since then, support has come from computational models and behavioral data. An alternative approach holds that phonological processing is critical for skilled reading of even very familiar words (Van Orden & Kloos, 2005). Support for the alternative approach comes from behavioral evidence that phonological activation occurs very quickly in virtually every instance of WR (Frost, 1998; Van Orden, Pennington, & Stone, 1990), and from neuroimaging data indicating that all kinds of words and pseudowords appear to be handled by the same neural machinery (see Price & McCrory, 2005).

Although this debate is not covered in any detail here, our view is that the alternative approach better accounts for the developmental data, including both the development of skilled reading and RD. For example, in young, normal readers, the correlation between nonword and exception-word reading is high (.66–.90, Gough & Walsh, 1991)—not what we would predict if these two stimuli are handled by two distinct mechanisms. Similarly, as a group, children with RD are impaired at reading both exception words and pseudowords (Castles, Datta, Gayan, & Olson, 1999; Manis, Seidenberg, Doi, & McBride-Chang, 1996; Stanovich, Siegel, & Gottardo, 1997). The pseudoword-reading deficit is generally considered more central to RD, because of extensive research documenting that, on the whole, individuals with RD read pseudowords less accurately than even younger, normal readers matched on real-word reading accuracy do (see Rack, Snowling, & Olson, 1992, for a review). Although some researchers have argued that there are subtypes of RD resulting from a selective deficit to either the direct or indirect mechanism (Castles & Coltheart, 1993), pure cases, with normal performance at one process and impaired performance on the other, have been rare. Furthermore, a recent influential connectionist model (Harm & Seidenberg, 1999) simulated these two patterns of performance (worse exception-word reading than pseudoword reading, and vice versa) in a network that did not include discrete direct and indirect mechanisms. Overall, the current balance of evidence suggests that the great majority of children with RD have difficulties with word recognition that result largely from deficits in phonological coding (i.e., converting letter strings into their appropriate sound sequences).

A complete neuropsychological theory of RD must also specify the cognitive deficits that lead to phonological coding difficulties. As a group, individuals with RD have been shown to perform more poorly than controls on a wide variety of tasks, including tasks assessing auditory, visual, motor, and linguistic skill; working memory; and speed of processing (see discussion below). A challenge for the field has been to identify which of these deficits are causal in RD, as opposed to resulting from RD or merely correlated with RD because of some third variable. One family of tasks that has received particular attention measures *phoneme awareness*, an oral language skill that includes the ability to manipulate and attend to individual sounds in words. As an example of one kind of phoneme awareness task, the child is asked to say *fixed* without the /k/, with the correct answer being *fist* (Wagner, Torgesen, & Rashotte, 1999). Individuals with RD perform poorly on phoneme awareness tasks, relative to both age-matched controls and younger, typically developing readers (Bruck, 1992; Fawcett & Nicolson, 1995; Liberman, Shankweiler, Fischer, & Carter, 1974; Pennington, Van Orden, Smith, & Green, 1990; Wagner & Torgesen, 1987). Furthermore, these tasks are among the best predictors of later reading ability (e.g., Pennington & Lefly, 2001; Schatschneider, Fletcher, Francis, Carlson, & Foorman, 2004; Snowling, Gallagher, & Frith, 2003; see also Goswami & Bryant, 1990; Wagner & Torgesen, 1987), and phoneme awareness training positively influences later reading skill (Bradley & Bryant, 1983; Cunningham, 1990; Lundberg, Frost, & Petersen, 1988; Wise, Ring, & Olson, 1999). Taken together, the evidence suggests that phoneme awareness plays a causal role in RD (though see Castles & Coltheart, 2004). This relationship presumably arises because the ability to map individual sounds onto letters—the defining characteristic of phonological coding—relies on the ability to break spoken words apart into sounds and to attend to those sounds individually.

Despite agreement about the importance of phoneme awareness deficits in RD, there is disagreement about whether or not these difficulties are themselves caused by lower-level processing deficits. Phoneme awareness is a complex metalinguistic skill that clearly involves multiple components. One argument is that phoneme awareness deficits arise from impaired phonological representations (Fowler, 1991; Swan & Goswami, 1997a). Another argument postulates that the central deficit is not specific to language, but occurs at a lower level of auditory processing (Tallal, 1980). We believe the most parsimonious explanation for current data is that deficits in phonological representations lead to both phoneme awareness and phonological coding difficulties in RD. An important caveat is that the relationship between phoneme awareness and reading is bidirectional, so that over time, poor reading also causes poor phoneme awareness (Morais, Cary, Alegria, & Bertelson, 1979; Perfetti, Beck, Bell, & Hughes, 1987; Wagner, Torgesen, & Rashotte, 1994). Although some lower-level sensory problems are correlated with RD, there is not much evidence for a causal relationship. We now briefly review the evidence for this argument.

Phonological Representations

The hypothesis of impaired phonological representations is appealing because it helps explain why RD is associated not only with deficits in phoneme awareness, but also with impairments on a wide variety of phonological tasks, including phonological memory (Byrne & Shea, 1979; Shankweiler, Liberman, Mark, Fowler, & Fischer, 1979), confrontational naming (Fowler & Swainson, 2004; Swan & Goswami, 1997b), and rapid naming (Bowers & Wolf, 1993; Denckla & Rudel, 1976–though there is debate as to whether rapid naming tasks are best conceptualized as phonological; see Vellutino et al., 2004, for a discussion). It is important to note that these are all *oral* language tasks, buttressing the argument that RD is a language disorder. Researchers have proposed a number of ways in which phonological representations may be impaired. For example, the representations of individual phonemes may be somehow distorted (Harm & Seidenberg, 1999). An alternative proposal, the segmentation hypothesis (Bird & Bishop, 1992; Fowler, 1991; Metsala, 1997b), is concerned with the grain size of phonological representations. During language acquisition, typically developing children build increasingly fine-grained phonological representations, from the whole-word level to the level of the syllable and eventually the phoneme (Metsala, 1997a; Metsala & Walley, 1998; Walley, 1993). The segmentation hypothesis holds that RD results from a delay in this process. Because alphabetic languages require establishing mappings between phonemes and letters, phonological representations specified at the level of the demisyllable or the syllable would greatly complicate the task of learning to read.

Some evidence for impaired phonological representations in RD comes from studies of speech perception. In a typical experiment, synthetic speech sounds are manipulated along a continuum, with the ends of the continuum representing syllables beginning with two different consonants (e.g., *da* and *ga*). Research has demonstrated that although the acoustic properties vary continuously, human listeners perceive discrete categories—a phenomenon known as *categorical perception* (Cooper, Delattre, Liberman, Borst, & Gerstman, 1952; Liberman, Cooper, Shankweiler, & Studdert-Kennedy, 1967). Several studies have shown impaired categorical perception in RD, manifested as a shallower slope between categories and/or less accurate identification at the ends of the continuum (Godfrey, Syrdal-Lasky, Millay, & Knox, 1981; Manis, McBride-Chang, Seidenberg, & Keating, 1997; Reed, 1989; Werker & Tees, 1987). However, close inspection of data has suggested that the deficit is limited to individuals with severe RD and/or a comorbid language impairment (Joanisse, Manis, Keating, & Seidenberg, 2000). Thus there is not clear evidence that deficits in speech perception can account for all cases of RD. One possible explanation is a severity hypothesis, in which individuals with mild damage to phonological representations have RD, while individuals with more severe damage have both severe RD and speech perception deficits (Harm & Seidenberg, 1999). A second, not mutually exclusive, explanation derives from the segmentation hypothesis. Someone with poorly segmented phonological representations might nonetheless demonstrate good categorical perception for the syllabic stimuli typically used in speech perception experiments. Thus researchers have also used a different kind of task to investigate the underlying phonological impairment in RD.

A recent study in our laboratory (Boada & Pennington, 2006) compared 11- to 13-year old children with RD with both age-matched and reading-level controls on three tasks designed to be sensitive to the grain size of phonological representations. For example, a syllable similarity task provided a measure of whether children were more likely to confuse nonsense words that were similar in syllabic structure or that shared an initial phoneme. There is normal developmental change in this task; compared to adults, children, whose phonological representations are presumably less well segmented, are more likely to confuse words that share syllabic structure (Treiman & Breaux, 1982). Another task investigated whether participants' identification of a spoken word was aided by a very short prime that primarily carried initial phoneme information, versus a longer prime that carried more information about the whole first syllable. Across all three tasks, the performance of participants with RD was consistent with less well-segmented phonological representations. For example, in the priming task, the participants with RD benefited from the longer prime as much as controls, but did not benefit from the shorter prime. These performance differences were evident in comparisons to both age-matched and reading-level controls, suggesting that they did not result solely from reduced exposure to print. Furthermore, results did not vary as a function of whether the participants with RD had a history of speech or language impairments, so this kind of task may hold more promise than typical speech perception tasks for explaining all cases of RD.

Of course, language is a highly interconnected system (Bishop, 1997). Many children with phonological impairments might be expected to show difficulties with other aspects of language, such as semantics (word meanings) or syntax (grammar). In fact, on IQ tests, children with RD tend to underperform their typically developing counterparts not only on the most phonological tasks, such as digit span, but on all Verbal IQ subtests (D'Angiulli & Siegel, 2003). Some of this performance deficit is likely to have resulted from RD, since children with reading difficulties have impoverished opportunities to learn from print (e.g., Stanovich, 1986; but see Scarborough & Parker, 2003); however, some may well reflect subtle, wide-ranging language impairments. Nonverbal reasoning skills are relatively, but not absolutely, spared in RD. Children with RD tend to obtain lower nonverbal or Performance IQ scores than typically developing children, though the effect size is typically smaller than for Verbal IQ (D'Angiulli & Siegel, 2003; Snowling et al., 2003). This finding is unsurprising, given that in the population as a whole, Verbal and Performance IQ scores are highly correlated (Sattler & Dumont, 2004).

In summary, RD is associated with performance deficits on a wide variety of phonological tasks, including tasks that do not require metalinguistic awareness. Evidence suggests that many of the deficits result from poorly segmented phonological representations. More severe cases of RD may additionally be complicated by distortions within the representations. Future longitudinal studies should attempt to establish that poorly segmented phonological representations cause the phonological coding deficits that are central to RD. Although RD-related impairments are most striking on phonological tasks, linguistic difficulties also extend to verbal conceptual measures.

Auditory Processing

An influential theory (Tallal, 1980) holds that phonological impairments in RD arise from lower-level deficits in auditory processing that are not specific to language. This theory developed out of earlier work demonstrating auditory processing deficits in SLI (Tallal & Percy, 1973, 1975). Indeed, as a group, individuals with RD have demonstrated impaired performance on a variety of nonspeech auditory tasks (for reviews, see Farmer & Klein, 1995; Tallal, Miller, Jenkins, & Merzenich, 1997). Methodological concerns have been raised about this literature (Vellutino et al., 2004). Perhaps more importantly, the argument for causality is damaged by a case-by-case inspection of data, which has consistently revealed that many participants with RD do not have auditory deficits, while some control participants do (see Ramus, 2003, for a review). For example, Ramus et al. (2003) compared 16 participants with RD to 16 controls on an extensive battery of phonological, auditory, and other sensory–motor tasks. Although there was a mean group difference on the nonspeech auditory tasks, a minority of individual cases with RD (approximately 6, or 38%) showed evidence of a deficit. This result contrasted with the phonological tasks, on which 100% of the participants with RD (and only 6% of controls) were impaired.

The auditory processing hypothesis assumes that a low-level sensory deficit causes a higher-level linguistic deficit. However, it is also possible that linguistic deficits have top-down effects on audition. Longitudinal studies have generally failed to establish a connection between earlier auditory deficits and later reading problems (Heath & Hogben, 2004;

Share, Jorm, Maclean, & Matthews, 2002). Similarly, Boets, Wouters, van Wieringen, and Ghesquiere (2006) compared preschoolers at high and low familial risk for later RD on a variety of low-level auditory tasks and did not find group differences. Instead, consistent with earlier studies (Pennington & Lefly, 2001; Scarborough, 1998), the high- and low-risk groups were distinguished by measures of phonological skill and letter knowledge.

Anatomical results from animal models are more consistent with a top-down than a bottom-up relationship between cognitive and sensory processing in RD (see Ramus, 2004, for a discussion). Galaburda and colleagues (Rosen, Press, Sherman, & Galaburda, 1992) have developed a rat model of RD that depends on induction of the kinds of cortical anomalies found in postmortem studies (see discussion above). Although the rats obviously cannot demonstrate reading difficulties, they have shown evidence of learning deficits (Rosen, Waters, Galaburda, & Denenberg, 1995). Some of the rats with cortical damage later developed anomalies in the MGN of the thalamus, which in turn impaired auditory processing (Herman, Galaburda, Fitch, Carter, & Rosen, 1997; Peiffer, Rosen, & Fitch, 2002). Of course, much more research would be needed to establish whether a similar phenomenon is at play in humans. However, this work serves as a good reminder that while a bottom-up explanation often seems more intuitive, top-down processes are equally plausible.

Other Sensory–Motor Findings

There is a long history of theories positing a causal visual deficit in dyslexia (Hinshelwood, 1907; Orton, 1925, 1937; Pringle-Morgan, 1896). The most straightforward of these theories have long been discredited (Vellutino, 1979, 1987; Vellutino & Scanlon, 1982). However, participants with RD have shown reliable group deficits on certain low-level visual processing tasks, including motion perception and detection of low spatial frequencies (Badcock & Lovegrove, 1981; Eden et al., 1996; Martin & Lovegrove, 1984). Because such tasks specifically engage the magnocellular pathway of the visual system, these findings have led to a magnocellular theory of RD (Stein & Walsh, 1997). Further support for the theory comes from the autopsy findings discussed earlier, since thalamic abnormalities in brains of individuals with RD were found in magnocellular layers of the LGN. As a causal hypothesis, this theory has faced some of the same challenges as the auditory theory. Studies have generally found that many individual participants with RD do not have visual deficits, while some control participants do (Ramus et al., 2003; see Vellutino et al., 2004). Furthermore, this theory lacks surface validity to explain the WR deficit in RD. The magnocellular system is responsible for large-scale visual tasks, such as detection of motion and rapid changes in the visual field. In contrast, the parvocellular system is responsible for fine, high-frequency discriminations (Gazzaniga, Ivry, & Magnun, 2002). Although it is conceivable that a magnocellular deficit could negatively affect the reading of connected text, it is not clear how such a deficit could influence single word reading under central fixation (Hulme, 1988). And yet a deficit in reading single words is the defining symptom in RD!

Studies have also reported tactile (Laasonen, Service, & Virsu, 2001; Stoodley, Talcott, Carter, Witton, & Stein, 2000) and motor skill deficits (Fawcett, Nicolson, & Dean, 1996; Nicolson & Fawcett, 1990; Ramus et al., 2003) in some participants with RD. The magnocellular theory has been proposed as an overarching explanation for these diverse findings, since there are magnocellular pathways within every sensory modality, and because the cerebellum receives massive magnocellular input (Stein, 2001). As discussed above, such a theory cannot account for all cases of RD, and probably not even for the majority of cases. Thus one interpretation is that RD sometimes co-occurs with more general sensory–motor difficulties that are not the cause of the central phonological coding deficit (Hulslander et al., 2004; Ramus, 2003).

Given some of the brain findings discussed earlier (i.e., reduced cerebral volume, widespread neural differences), it is not surprising that RD might be associated with a variety of symptoms. On the basis of the rat model, Ramus (2004) has advanced a specific brain-based hypothesis for why a sensory–motor syndrome should sometimes, but not always, accompany RD. In rats, cortical disruption only sometimes leads to thalamic abnormalities, with the likelihood being moderated by the presence of fetal testosterone (Rosen, Herman, & Galaburda, 1999). Ramus has suggested that RD results from phonological impairments caused by cortical damage, and that under certain hormonal conditions, the cortical damage also leads to thalamic damage, which in turn causes the sensory–motor syndrome. This is an intriguing hypothesis that merits future research.

Psychosocial Outcomes

RD is associated with a variety of poor psychosocial outcomes, including both externalizing and internalizing problems (Hinshaw, 1992; McGee, Share, Moffitt, Williams, & Silva, 1988). As discussed earlier, there is evidence that externalizing problems precede reading failure, particularly in boys, and share a common genetic basis with RD. A different story has emerged for internalizing problems. For example, work in our lab found that RD was correlated with elevated rates of dysthymia, particularly in girls (Willcutt & Pennington, 2000). However, children with future dyslexia did not differ from controls on measures of dysthymia before kindergarten (Boetsch, 1996). This result suggests that dysthymia is secondary to RD, presumably in reaction to school failure. Two more recent studies have replicated the association between internalizing problems and RD in school-age children (Maughan, Rowe, Loeber, & Stouthamer-Loeber, 2003; Scarborough & Parker, 2003). In a longitudinal sample, Scarborough and Parker found that internalizing problems among children with RD remained stable from second grade to eighth grade; Maughan et al. reported a similar result in a cross-sectional sample. These findings indicate that the risk for developing dysthymia, depressed mood, or low self-esteem in response to reading failure may be highest early in the school years, between kindergarten and second grade.

Summary

In summary, there is evidence for both specificity and generality in the neuropsychology of RD. RD is associated with difficulties across a wide variety of domains, including low-level sensory processing, verbal and nonverbal reasoning, and social-emotional functioning. Some of these difficulties are likely to *result* from reading failure (i.e., reduced vocabulary development, dysthymia) whereas others are correlated with RD for reasons that are not yet well understood (i.e., sensory processing, nonverbal reasoning). Currently, the most viable causal hypothesis points to a relatively specific deficit in phonological representations. However, as we describe in the next section, studies of RD across the lifespan suggest that other aspects of language function interact with the phonological deficit to determine the severity and course of the disorder.

DEVELOPMENTAL CONSIDERATIONS

RD in Adulthood

There is both continuity and change in the developmental course of RD. Difficulties with reading fluency, phonological coding, spelling, and phoneme awareness are most likely to persist into adulthood (Bruck, 1990, 1992, 1993; Hatcher, Snowling, & Griffiths, 2002; Pennington et al., 1990). In contrast, a subset of dyslexic readers are able to compensate for problems with single-word reading accuracy and RC (Bruck, 1990; Hatcher et al., 2002; Lefly & Pennington, 1991; Shaywitz et al., 2003). These findings have theoretical implications, since one criterion for an underlying cognitive deficit is that the impairment be persistent. They also have practical implications, because they point to the kinds of tests that will be most useful for diagnosing RD in adults or older adolescents.

In a series of studies, Bruck (1990, 1992, 1993) investigated the reading, spelling, and phoneme awareness skills of adults with childhood histories of RD. She found that the group with RD performed more poorly on all tasks than chronological-age controls. The most interesting results emerged in comparison to a reading-level control group (elementary school children with reading skills at or above the 60th percentile for their age). Even compared with children more than 10 years younger, the adults with RD demonstrated great difficulty with phonological coding, as measured by pseudoword reading and pseudoword spelling. The single-word accuracy of the two groups was similar by definition, but the participants with RD read more slowly and spelled more poorly. Finally, the phoneme awareness skills of the group with RD were much weaker than those of the reading-level controls, especially on the most sensitive (i.e., difficult) tasks. Pennington et al. (1990) also found poor phoneme awareness in adults with RD and reported that the phonological deficit was relatively specific; it did not extend to articulatory speed, confrontational naming, or phoneme perception. Although there was some suggestion of a deficit in phonological memory, this finding was not consistent across different samples of adults with RD.

Bruck reported a different pattern of results for RC. On this measure, scores for the sample with RD as a whole were within the average range (though still below those of an age- and IQ-matched control group), with raw scores that did not differ from those of their reading-level controls. Bruck next compared two subgroups with RD: those with good RC (similar to that of controls), and those with poor RC. Surprisingly, the subgroups did not differ on word-reading accuracy. Instead, they were distinguished by measures of childhood IQ and adult receptive vocabulary. Bruck suggested that higher IQ provided a compensatory mechanism, allowing some adults with RD to understand text well despite deficits in decoding. This result is consistent with the simple view of reading, since LC correlates highly with Verbal IQ scores.

A more recent study (Shaywitz et al., 2003) also found suggestive evidence for the role of IQ as a compensatory mechanism. These authors used a longitudinal design to investigate outcomes for older adolescents who had met criteria for RD in elementary school. By 10th grade, a subgroup of participants no longer had deficits in single-word-reading accuracy and were termed the "accuracy-improved (AI)" readers. A second subgroup, the "persistently poor (PP)" readers, had ongoing difficulties with word-reading accuracy. Both subgroups had impaired reading fluency compared to controls, but only the PP group showed deficits in reading comprehension. The AI group had significantly higher IQ scores than the PP group, both as young children and as older adolescents, leading the authors to speculate that stronger cognitive abilities allowed the AI group to (partly) compensate for deficits in phonological processing. However, there was also a trend for the AI readers to have attended more advantaged schools, so it is possible that the group difference was largely driven by superior remedial instruction or other environmental factors. In either case, the results are consistent with Bruck's findings in demonstrating that a subgroup of adults with RD attain age-appropriate RC skills, despite continuing deficits with at least some components of decoding.

One research team (Hatcher et al., 2002) recently investigated which cognitive measures are most appropriate for diagnosing RD in university students. These authors compared undergraduate and graduate students with a previous diagnosis of RD to their typically developing peers. Consistent with earlier studies, many phonological and literacy measures differentiated the groups, with the largest effect sizes for spelling, phonological coding (speed and accuracy), and phoneme awareness. A discriminant-function analysis correctly classified 95% of individuals (96% sensitivity and 96% specificity), using spelling, pseudoword reading, and two tests from the Wechsler Adult Intelligence Scale—Digit Span and Digit Symbol. Of course, this study used a highly selected population, and the results may not apply to adults with RD who achieve lower levels of education. However, there is convergence across studies in suggesting that assessment of adult RD should include measures of spelling, phonological coding, and reading fluency. Tests of single-word-reading accuracy are less sensitive, especially in adults with higher IQ and/or a history of remediation. Although word-reading accuracy may be more sensitive in younger children, it is still advisable to include measures of spelling, reading fluency, phonological coding, and phoneme awareness in assessments for RD at any age.

Overall, studies of RD in adulthood have provided both support and challenge for the phonological representations hypothesis. The hypothesis predicts that the most persistent symptom of RD should be in phonological coding. Although this symptom is indeed persistent, it is no more so than are difficulties with spelling and reading fluency. One interpretation is that these symptoms are secondary. On this view, spelling impairments persist because spelling is a more difficult task than reading, requiring more detailed knowledge of letter–sound correspondences (Romani, Olson, & Di Betta, 2005). Similarly, poor reading fluency reflects the inefficient WR that results from failure to automatize knowledge of letter–sound relations. However, alternate explanations are also plausible. For example, something about the automaticity of WR, apart from phonological coding, may be central to RD. Such a hypothesis has been proposed, in varied forms, by a number of researchers who challenge a strict phonological hypothesis (e.g., Jackson & Coltheart, 2001; Nicolson, Fawcett, & Dean, 2001; Wolf & Bowers, 1999). To date, however, these arguments have been largely concerned with subtypes of RD, either explicitly (Jackson & Coltheart, 2001; Wolf & Bowers, 1999) or implicitly, by reference to correlated symptoms that are present in only a subset of individuals with RD (Nicolson et al., 2001). Thus a fuller understanding of the developmental relationship between phonological coding and reading fluency awaits future research. Cross-linguistic data will be relevant here, because of the finding (discussed earlier) that in regular orthographies, reading difficulties are more apparent for fluency than for accuracy. Treatment studies will also provide valuable data, because of the growing attention to fluency difficulties in RD and the burgeoning of programs to treat the problem (Shaywitz, 2003).

The study of underlying cognitive deficits in adult RD has also produced mixed results for the phonological representations hypothesis. In this case, the hypothesis predicts that adults should show persistent impairment on phoneme awareness tasks *and* other tasks requiring access to phonological representations. To date, only the first part of the prediction has received unequivocal support (Pennington et al., 1990). One explanation for why Pennington et al. failed to find group differences on other phonological tasks is that phoneme awareness measures were the most difficult, and therefore the most sensitive to group differences. However, group differences did emerge on other phonological measures between the older and younger control groups, suggesting that lack of sensitivity could not explain the null results. A second possibility is that because of their metalinguistic nature, phoneme awareness measures tap higher language abilities in addition to phonological skills. This argument suggests that a deficit in phonological representations by itself does not cause RD; broader linguistic difficulties must also be present. In fact, research at the other end of the developmental spectrum, in very young children, has provided some support for such a hypothesis. This research is reviewed below.

Precursors of RD

Researchers have capitalized on the familial nature of RD (Hallgren, 1950) to study its developmental precursors by identifying children who are at family risk for the disorder and following them from preschool (Pennington & Lefly, 2001; Snowling et al., 2003) or even earlier (Koster et al., 2005; Lyytinen et al., 2004; Scarborough, 1990). Among the most important findings to come out of this work are that (1) reading problems are foreshadowed by difficulties on a wide range of oral language measures, not just phonological ones; (2) the best predictor of later reading attainment depends partly on the age at which the predictor is measured; and (3) family risk for dyslexia is continuous, not categorical.

Scarborough (1990, 1991a, 1991b) identified a group of 2-year-old children who were at high family risk for RD and a comparison group matched on age and socioeconomic status (SES). At the end of second grade, 65% of the high-risk children had developed RD. She used retrospective analyses to investigate which oral language measures best predicted later literacy skills. The children who later developed RD were distinguished from their normally achieving peers (both controls and high-risk children who did not develop RD) by syntax and articulation at age 2.5–3 years; by syntax and vocabulary at age 3.5–4; and by vocabulary, phoneme awareness, and letter knowledge at age 4.5–5. Because the best predictors changed over time, these results point to the importance of using repeated measures in the search for underlying deficits in RD. And because difficulties with vocabulary and syntax were evident long before phoneme awareness impairments, the results pose a challenge for the view that a selective phonological deficit causes RD.

Later studies have also found that problems with literacy are preceded by a range of oral language difficulties (Frost, Madsbjerg, Niedersoe, Olofsson, & Sorensen, 2005; Koster et al., 2005; Snowling et al., 2003; van Alphen et al., 2004). For example, Lyytinen and colleagues have followed children at high family risk for dyslexia and their controls from birth (see Lyytinen et al., 2004, for a review). By age 6 months, the high- and low-risk groups showed differences in a categorical speech perception task, evidenced by both behavioral and electrophysiological responses. Measures of morphological and vocabulary development distinguished the high- and low-risk groups during the toddler and preschool years, and by age 3.5, group differences emerged on a simple phonological awareness task. Children at high and low risk showed no differences in early motor development or in Performance IQ scores. In general, the measures that discriminated the high- and low-risk groups also distinguished children who later developed RD from those who did not.

Another finding replicated across longitudinal studies is that family risk of dyslexia is continuous. Pennington and Lefly (2001) found that those children at high family risk who did not meet criteria for RD nevertheless showed subtle impairments on a wide range of phonological tasks, including phoneme awareness, phoneme perception, verbal short-term memory, and rapid naming. Furthermore, the reading and spelling skills of these children, though above the diagnostic threshold, were nevertheless poorer than those of controls matched on age, IQ, and SES. Similarly, Snowling et al. (2003) reported that members of a high-risk group who were not classified as having RD at age 8 still obtained scores on standardized literacy tests that were lower than those of appropriate controls. These results suggest that the etiology for RD is multifactorial. The high-risk children who did not develop RD probably carried some of the risk factors for the disorder, but not enough to push them over the diagnostic threshold.

Snowling et al. (2003) further reported a surprising finding: The high-risk children who did and did not develop RD at age 8 did not differ statistically on measures of phonological coding at age 6. This null result may have resulted partly from a lack of power and floor effects, especially for pseudoword reading. Even so, the high-risk, no-RD group showed larger-than-expected deficits on these tasks, given their later literacy attainment. In general, the earlier oral language development of this group had been good; at age 3, they had performed similarly to controls (and better than the high-risk group with RD) on measures of expressive and receptive vocabulary, as well as verbal short-term memory. The researchers suggested that strong oral language skills had allowed these children to compensate in part for their phonological difficulties. This result is similar to the adult studies (Bruck, 1990; Shaywitz et al., 2003) suggesting that outcome in RD may be moderated by Verbal IQ.

Summary

Taken together, the family risk and adult RD studies render the simplest causal story of RD—in which a single etiology causes a phonological deficit, which in turn impairs phonological coding and causes RD—implausible. Instead, it appears that a phonological deficit interacts with other factors, including broader language development, and probably also including environmental and educational factors, to determine an individual's literacy development. Despite this challenge to a strong phonological hypothesis, the developmental work provides convergent evidence for the importance of phonology in reading development. Beginning shortly before the start of formal literacy instruction, phonological tasks are the best oral language predictors of later reading skill; moreover, they are among the most persistent cognitive markers for RD, even in adults who have attained age-appropriate levels of RC. One interpretation of the full pattern of results is that an isolated phonological deficit may not be sufficient to cause RD. Individuals with enough protective factors, including strong broader language skills, can compensate for phonological deficits to a degree. However, this compensation is rarely, if ever, complete.

ETIOLOGY

Genetics

For the last century, clinicians have known that RD runs in families (Fisher, 1905; Hinshelwood, 1907; Stephenson, 1907; Thomas, 1905). Hallgren (1950) confirmed the familiality of the disorder with the first large-scale epidemiological investigation. In the last 25 years, the field has used behavioral and molecular genetics approaches to make significant progress in understanding the genetics of RD (see Pennington & Olson, 2005, for a more in-depth review). We now know that the disorder is heritable, and linkage studies have identified the approximate location of seven risk loci (see below). Specific candidate genes have recently been proposed within three of these regions (for reviews, see Fisher & Francks, 2006; McGrath, Smith, & Pennington, 2006). An important point to keep in mind is that since reading is a relatively recent cultural invention, none of these can be a gene "for reading" or "for RD." Instead, it appears that multiple genetic influences act on the evolved language and cognitive traits that are necessary for reading proficiency.

Twin studies confirmed the heritability of RD in the 1980s (DeFries, Fulker, & LaBuda, 1987). A more recent analysis of a large twin sample at the Colorado Learning Disabilities Research Center (CLDRC) indicated that just over half the group deficit in RD was due to heritable genetic influences (Wadsworth, Olson, Pennington, & DeFries, 2000). A large longitudinal twin sample from the United Kingdom (the Twins Early Development Study, or TEDS) obtained a remarkably similar result (Harlaar, Spinath, Dale, & Plomin, 2005). These estimates are group averages, and the balance of genetic and environmental influences on RD is likely to vary widely for individuals within a group. It is also important to remember that heritability estimates depend on the environmental range that is relevant to the target skill (in this case, reading). There is some evidence for a restricted environmental range in both the CLDRC and TEDS samples. The CLDRC primarily includes twins attending schools with average or above-average academic ratings, while the children in the TEDS sample were taught to read under a highly structured national curriculum (Harlaar et al., 2005). A smaller twin study whose population may have had a broader range of socioeconomic and educational backgrounds found a much lower estimate for the heritability of the group deficit in RD (Stevenson, 1991). So these results suggest that in environments that are generally supportive of learning to read, most of the variability in the group deficit for RD is due to genetic factors. Not surprisingly, as the environmental range expands, it plays an increasingly important role in determining individual differences.

Current evidence indicates that genetic influence may be stronger for RD with high IQ than for RD with low IQ (Knopik et al., 2002; Olson, Datta, Gayan, & DeFries, 1999; Wadsworth et al., 2000). This result suggests that there could be etiological subtypes of RD, with experiential or instructional factors playing a somewhat larger role for those with lower IQ. However, the results do not necessitate that such subgroups look different in terms of underlying cognitive skills (i.e., phonological coding, phoneme awareness) or in terms of the treatments that are helpful. In fact, as discussed previously, phonological deficits have been implicated in RD with both high and low IQ, and treatments targeting these deficits help both groups.

Behavioral genetic analyses have also been used to investigate the validity of neuropsychological theories of RD. If a component skill (e.g., phonological coding) is responsible for a heritable behavioral symptom (e.g., poor word recognition), then the component skill must also be heritable; furthermore, there should be a high genetic correlation between the two measures (which would indicate that common genetic influences are operating on both). In fact, Gayan and Olson (2001) established that both phonological coding and phoneme awareness deficits were heritable, and found a genetic correlation of .99 for group deficits in real-word reading and a measure of phonological coding. A substantial genetic correlation was also reported for phoneme awareness and word reading (r_g = .67). These results are consistent with the argument that poor phonological processing leads to a weakness in phonological coding, which in turn impairs word recognition. However, other findings from this research (Gayan & Olson, 2001) suggest that there are also genetically mediated influences on RD that are separate from phonological skill. A high genetic correlation (r_g = .81) was also found for group deficits in word reading and orthographic coding (recognition of specific word forms). The genetic correlation between orthographic coding and phoneme awareness deficits was much lower (r_g = .28), indicating that some of the genetic influences on deficits in these reading-related skills are independent.

Once behavioral genetic studies established that RD is partly heritable, the next logical question concerned the locations of the particular genes that cause the heritability. Genes that influence a continuous (as opposed to a categorical) trait are called *quantitative trait loci* (QTLs) (Eley & Craig, 2005). To date, linkage studies of RD have reported replicated regions for QTLs on seven chromosomes: 1p36–p34, 2p16–p15, 3p12–q13, 6p22.2, 15q21, 18p11.2, and Xq27.3 (see Fisher & Francks, 2006; McGrath et al., 2006). The discovery of multiple QTLs indicates that several different genes contribute to RD, consistent with the results from family risk studies suggesting a multifactorial etiology. The QTLs for RD are best conceptualized as susceptibility loci, whereby each confers a susceptibility to develop poor reading skills, but only in a probabilistic fashion. It is unlikely that any one QTL is either necessary or sufficient to cause RD.

Recently, four candidate genes within three of the replicated linkage regions have been proposed: DYX1C1 on 15q21 (Taipale et al., 2003), ROBO1 on 3p12–q13 (Hannula-Jouppi et al., 2005), and DCDC2 and KIAA0319 on 6p22 (Cope et al., 2005; Deffenbacher et al., 2004; Francks et al., 2004; Meng et al., 2005; Paracchini et al., 2006; Schumacher et al., 2006). Precise risk variants have yet to be identified in any of these genes, which will be an important next step in attempting to establish a causal relationship to RD. All four genes have been implicated in general brain development processes, including neural migration and axon guidance (Meng et al., 2005; Paracchini et al., 2006; Rosen et al., 2007; Seeger, Tear, Ferres-Marco, & Goodman, 1993; Threlkeld et al., 2007; Wang et al., 2006). Thus the known functions of these candidate genes for RD are consistent with some of the anatomical findings discussed earlier, including histological anomalies and white matter differences. However, a puzzle to be resolved by future research concerns how genes involved in global brain development cause the relatively specific phenotype of RD.

Environmental Factors

It goes without saying that literacy is dependent on environmental factors, since in cultures without written language, no one can read or write. Because the heritability of RD is not 100%, we also know that the environment contributes to individual differences in reading deficits within cultures. Two kinds of environmental risk factors for RD have received some attention in the literature: home literacy environment and instruction quality/type. Each of these is reviewed briefly below. It is also important to acknowledge that environmental events with more direct effects on biology (e.g., head injuries, lead poisoning) can have a significant influence on a child's ability to learn to read (Phillips & Lonigan, 2005).

Home literacy environment is an umbrella construct that includes such factors as joint parent–child reading, child's total exposure to print, and parent modeling of literate behavior (Rashid, Morris, & Sevcik, 2005). Studies of reading ability across the whole range have shown that joint parent–child reading predicts later literacy (see Phillips & Lonigan, 2005). Unfortunately, these studies have tended not to use genetically sensitive designs, so genetic explanations for the correlation cannot be ruled out. This limitation is avoided in treatment studies that use random assignment. In two such studies, Whitehurst and colleagues (Lonigan & Whitehurst, 1998; Whitehurst, Epstein, Angel, & Payne, 1994) found that training low-income parents in joint reading techniques produced gains in their preschoolers' expressive vocabulary lasting at least 6 months (a measure that, as discussed earlier, predicts later literacy skill). So there is suggestive, but not direct, evidence that joint parent–child reading has an impact on children's later literacy.

Studies of home literacy environment specific to RD have been rare. An exception is a study by Scarborough, Dobrich, and Hager (1991), who compared three groups: (1) children with RD whose parents also had RD; (2) typically achieving children of parents with RD; and (3) typically achieving children of typically achieving parents. As expected, parents with RD read less for pleasure themselves than parents who did not have RD. However, adult reading skill was not associated with frequency of joint parent–child reading. Children who later developed RD had indeed been read to somewhat less in preschool than children who did not develop RD. However, several results suggested that this finding was driven largely by child factors (e.g., interest in books). First, children who become poor readers had also spent less solitary time with books as preschoolers than either of the two eventual good-reader groups, who were similar to each other. Second, parents with RD whose children did not develop RD tended, if anything, to read to their children somewhat *more* than did typically achieving parents. Even if differences in print exposure were child-driven, they still may have had detrimental effects on later literacy. These results could be one example of a gene–environment correlation, in which children with a genetic liability for RD self-select environments that put them at even greater risk for reading failure.

The school environment has also been considered as a potential risk factor for RD. In the United States, there has been historical debate regarding whether or not reading instruction should include explicit teaching of phonics (letter–sound relationships) (e.g., Goodman, 1986). Given the association between poor phonological coding and RD, an instructional program that downplayed phonics could well increase many students' risk of reading failure. Brown and Felton (1990) identified kindergartners at risk for RD and assigned them to receive instruction that emphasized either phonics or the use of context. By the end of second grade, the phonics group attained superior scores on measures of both real-word and pseudoword reading. Therefore, among children beginning to experience reading failure, receiving phonics instruction reduced the risk of meeting standard diagnostic criteria for RD.

More recent intervention studies have been conducted by Vellutino and colleagues (Vellutino, Scanlon, Sipay, & Small, 1996; Vellutino, Scanlon, Small, & Fanuele, 2006). These researchers studied kindergarten and first-grade students exhibiting early signs of reading failure. Children received tutoring that included training in phoneme awareness, decoding, WR, and reading fluency. More than two-thirds of the poor readers attained average-range reading skill within 6 months, and most retained this level of achievement for at least 3 years. The authors' interpretation was that reading difficulties in many children are caused by instructional or experiential deficits. However, we think it is important to point out that the issue of etiology is in many ways orthogonal to ease of remediation. In this case, children were selected for intensive tutoring in the first place because their reading was falling behind that of other students in the same school, who presumably had a similar instructional background. Therefore, we believe these results may be better conceptualized as an example of a gene–environment interaction. Some children could have had a genetic liability that rendered them particularly vulnerable to a lack of specialized instruction. Indirect support for such an interpretation comes from a study by Hatcher, Hulme, and Snowling (2004). These researchers reported that children at risk for RD, but not typically developing children, responded differentially to type of reading instruction. Regardless of the etiology of children's difficulties, the results of these studies are extremely important in demonstrating that educational interventions can positively affect outcome in RD. Effective interventions are discussed further below.

TREATMENT

A number of empirically supported interventions have been developed for RD. The development of successful treatments has benefited from our understanding of the neuropsychology of RD, and the best interventions directly target phonological coding, phoneme awareness, and reading fluency. A review of specific commercially available programs is beyond the scope of this chapter; the reader is referred to Shaywitz (2003) for further information.

Several studies (Bradley & Bryant, 1983; Cunningham, 1990; Lundberg et al., 1988; Wise et al., 1999) have demonstrated that phoneme awareness training promotes later reading skill. However, when phoneme awareness training alone is compared to phoneme awareness plus direct reading instruction (e.g., letter–sound training, practice reading connected text), research has consistently found stronger effects for the integrated treatment (e.g., Bradley & Bryant, 1983; Cunningham, 1990; see also National Reading Panel, 2000). One carefully controlled study (Hatcher, Hulme, & Ellis, 1994) identified 7-year-old children experiencing early reading failure and randomly assigned them to one of four conditions: phonological training only (both rhyme and phoneme awareness); reading training only (including explicit phonics teaching); reading plus phonological training; and control. Immediately after training and at the 9-month follow-up, the group receiving reading plus phonological training showed the largest gains on all reading measures. In contrast, the group receiving phonological training only showed the greatest gains on the phoneme awareness measures themselves. So these results showed that extensive training in phoneme awareness promotes phoneme awareness, but that the effects transfer to reading better when intervention also includes direct reading instruction.

It is not terribly surprising that the best intervention for reading failure includes reading instruction. Hatcher et al. (1994) reported a second important finding: Phonological awareness training provided an additional boost over and above the benefits of reading instruction alone (see also Ball & Blachman, 1991; Byrne & Fielding-Barnsley, 1989;

National Reading Panel, 2000). A more recent study (Hatcher et al., 2004) demonstrated that the added effect of phoneme awareness training may be specific to children at risk for RD. These researchers implemented a highly structured, phonics-based reading program in 20 Reception classrooms (for children ages 4–5) in England. Some classes additionally received phoneme awareness instruction. Children who scored in the bottom third on pre-reading measures at study entry were considered at risk for reading failure. At-risk children showed differential effects of instruction, with the best effects for the program that included phoneme awareness training. In contrast, the typically developing children experienced no additional boost of phoneme awareness training over and above the phonics program. Presumably, the phoneme awareness training helped the at-risk children develop the skills they needed to benefit most from reading instruction, while the typically developing children may have been able to infer the necessary skills without explicit instruction. A separate but related phenomenon is that, compared to eventual good readers, young children who will later become RD have deficits not only in their absolute levels of phoneme awareness skill, but also in the rate at which they respond to phoneme awareness training (Byrne, Fielding-Barnsley, & Ashley, 2000). It is important to note that the added benefit of phoneme awareness training over and above direct reading instruction may not generalize to older struggling readers (Alexander & Slinger-Constant, 2004; Wise, Ring, & Olson, 2000).

A limitation of many early treatment studies is that the dependent measures included word-reading accuracy but not reading fluency. More recent studies have begun to investigate the impact of intervention on fluency (for reviews, see Alexander & Slinger-Constant, 2004; Torgesen, 2005). These studies have generally found that slow reading is more difficult to remediate than inaccurate reading. However, difficulties with reading fluency appear preventable when intervention is begun early enough. For example, Torgesen et al. (2001) administered a treatment integrating phoneme awareness, phonological coding, and reading connected text to children experiencing reading failure. The treatment remediated deficits in single-word-reading accuracy, word-reading accuracy in context, and RC, but not reading fluency. It is important to note that roughly half of instructional time was spent reading connected text, generally considered an appropriate intervention for fluency difficulties (Shaywitz, 2003). However, it is still possible that more attention to reading speed in particular would have produced a different pattern of results. This possibility is made somewhat less likely by the contrasting results of prevention studies (Torgesen, Rose, Lindamood, Conway, & Garvan, 1999; Torgesen, Wagner, Rashotte, & Herron, 2003). When a similar intervention was administered to kindergarten and first-grade children most at risk of reading failure, it effectively promoted both accuracy and fluency up to a year later. Torgesen (2005) suggested that once children have experienced several years of reading failure, they have accumulated dramatically less practice in reading than their typically developing peers have had (Cunningham & Stanovich, 1998). Even if their word-reading accuracy deficit is largely remediated, these long-standing differences in print exposure make it difficult or impossible for them to "close the gap" on their peers in reading fluency.

In summary, numerous studies have demonstrated that combined instruction in phoneme awareness training, phonological coding, and reading connected text is effective in treating word-reading accuracy difficulties in RD (National Reading Panel, 2000; Torgesen, 2005). Studies with children as young as 4 years old demonstrate that there is no need to wait for students to experience years of reading failure to begin intervention. On the contrary, some of the most promising results have been obtained in prevention studies. We speculate that such an approach should be effective not just in promoting reading accuracy and fluency, but also in preventing the correlated psychosocial problems secondary to school failure.

CONCLUSIONS AND FUTURE DIRECTIONS

The study of RD in many ways represents a great success story for developmental neuropsychology (Stanovich, 1991). In the last three decades, we have learned a tremendous amount about the disorder across levels of analysis. We now know that RD is genetically influenced. Multiple risk loci have been identified, and specific genes known to influence brain development have been proposed. At the level of the brain, structural and functional approaches have converged in implicating networks that are important for normal reading and language. And in terms of behavior, we have a neuropsychological theory built on the strength of correlational, treatment, family risk, and adult development studies. Despite these successes, it is clear that our understanding of RD is lacking in many ways. In particular, there is a growing acknowledgment that the phonological theory of RD, while not entirely incorrect, cannot be complete (Pennington, 2006; Ramus, 2004; Scarborough, 2005; Snowling et al., 2003).

One serious challenge to a strict phonological theory comes from the developmental work showing that a broad range of oral language measures are important predictors of later RD. To date, we have little understanding of the relationships among these measures at different time points. As Scarborough (2005) has pointed out, there are at least two ways in which various symptoms may be connected to each other. One possibility is a causal chain, in which (for example), early difficulties in morphology or syntax cause later problems with vocabulary, which in turn damage phonological development and impair reading. Alternately, all of the symptoms may be different manifestations of a common underlying problem. A deficit in phonological representations—in particular, the segmentation hypothesis—cannot yet be ruled out as a potential underlying problem. Early in development, more holistic phonological representations could logically affect the learning of morphology by making it difficult to identify commonalities below the level of the word or the syllable (e.g., in English, -ed or -s). Similarly, research suggests a relationship between vocabulary size and segmentation of phonological representations (Metsala, 1997a; Walley, 1993), but the nature of this relationship is not yet well understood. Learning of new vocabulary items may be impaired in an individual who has trouble discriminating between phonologically similar words as a consequence of more holistic representations. Tests of the segmentation hypothesis have not yet been integrated into longitudinal family risk studies to evaluate this possibility. Future studies should investigate this and other potential underlying deficits in order to understand the relationships among different oral language symptoms. Such studies would contribute greatly not only to our understanding of RD, but also to our knowledge of language development in general.

A second challenge to the phonological hypothesis, and one that our lab has investigated over many years, concerns the issue of comorbidity. If a phonological deficit is necessary and sufficient to cause RD, then it is not clear why RD is comorbid with other disorders that presumably result from different deficits. Our lab is currently examining the relationship of RD to ADHD, SSD, and SLI at the etiological and behavioral levels. Our current working hypothesis (Pennington, 2006) is that each comorbidity is caused by shared etiological risk factors that in turn lead to shared cognitive deficits. The overlap is not complete, because each disorder also has unique risk factors leading to unique deficits. In the case of RD and ADHD, we know that there is genetic overlap. At the cognitive level, we now have evidence that deficits in processing speed are common to both disorders (Shanahan et al., 2006). This study utilized multiple measures of processing speed (e.g., subtests from WISC-R, the baseline condition of the Stroop task, the Trail Making Test, Colorado Perceptual Speed), collapsed into a verbal and a nonverbal factor. Somewhat surprisingly, the groups with RD and with ADHD both showed deficits on both the verbal and nonverbal processing speed factors. Future work will attempt to establish a connection across these levels of analysis; in other words, do the shared genes in fact cause the slow processing speed, and if so, how? In the case of RD and SSD, there is accumulating evidence for a genetic overlap, and we know that each disorder is associated with phonological deficits. Currently, we are working to establish that a phonological deficit contributes to the overlap between the disorders. A full understanding of the relationship between RD and other disorders will also require neuroimaging work with attention to comorbidity. Because of sample size restrictions, many imaging studies either exclude individuals with comorbid disorders or analyze participants with and without comorbidities in a single group. Future studies should compare individuals with (for example) RD alone, ADHD alone, RD + ADHD, and no disorder (controls) to identify shared and unique brain differences.

A challenge that cuts across many areas of research in RD concerns the tension between specificity and generality. In terms of symptoms, a phonological deficit does the best job of accounting for all cases of RD, but problems across a wide variety of domains are associated with the disorder. At the etiological level, researchers have proposed four genes that are involved in global brain development; it is not yet clear how perturbations in these processes yield a phenotype with any specificity. Similarly, though some brain findings implicate a relatively restricted set of left-hemisphere regions, there is also evidence for much more widespread neural differences (e.g., reduced cerebral volume, subcortical and cerebellar anomalies). We do not yet understand the relationships among these brain differences; nor do we know which are causal in RD, which result from RD, and which are correlated because of some third variable. This question and others can only be answered with a combination of research methods. RD researchers have already begun to integrate neuroimaging into cross-cultural and longitudinal designs, and treatment studies into genetically sensitive designs, for example. Such approaches ensure that the next three decades will bring an even richer understanding of why some children struggle to learn to read.

REFERENCES

Alexander, A. W., & Slinger-Constant, A.-M. (2004). Current status of treatments for dyslexia: Critical review. *Journal of Child Neurology, 19*(10), 744–758.

Aylward, E. H., Richards, T. L., Berninger, V. W., Nagy, W. E., Field, K. M., Grimme, A. C., et al. (2003). Instructional treatment associated with changes in brain activation in children with dyslexia. *Neurology, 61*(2), 212–219.

Badcock, D., & Lovegrove, W. (1981). The effects of contrast, stimulus duration, and spatial frequency on visible persistence in normal and specifically disabled readers. *Journal of Experimental Psychology: Human Perception and Performance, 7*(3), 495–505.

Ball, E. W., & Blachman, B. A. (1991). Does phoneme awareness training in kindergarten make a difference in early word recognition and developmental spelling? *Reading Research Quarterly, 26*(1), 49–66.

Bartlett, C. W., Flax, J. F., Logue, M. W., Vieland, V. J., Bassett, A. S., Tallal, P., et al. (2002). A major susceptibility locus for specific language impairment is located on 13q21. *American Journal of Human Genetics, 71*(1), 45–55.

Best, M., & Demb, J. B. (1999). Normal planum temporale asymmetry in dyslexics with a magnocellular pathway deficit. *NeuroReport, 10*(3), 607–612.

Bird, J., & Bishop, D. (1992). Perception and awareness of phonemes in phonologically impaired children. *European Journal of Disorders of Communication, 27*(4), 289–311.

Bishop, D. V. M. (1997). *Uncommon understanding: Development and disorders of language comprehension in children.* Hove, UK: Psychology Press.

Bishop, D. V. M., & Adams, C. (1990). A prospective study of the relationship between specific language impairment, phonological disorders and reading retardation. *Journal of Child Psychology and Psychiatry, 31*(7), 1027–1050.

Blachman, B. A., Schatschneider, T., Fletcher, J. M., & Clonan, S. M. (2003). Early reading intervention: A classroom prevention study and a remediation study. In B. R. Foorman (Ed.), *Preventing and remediating reading difficulties: Bringing science to scale* (pp. 253–271). Timonium, MD: York Press.

Boada, R., & Pennington, B. F. (2006). Deficient implicit phonological representations in children with dyslexia. *Journal of Experimental Child Psychology, 95*, 153–193.

Boets, B., Wouters, J., van Wieringen, A., & Ghesquiere, P. (2006). Auditory temporal information processing in preschool children at family risk for dyslexia: Relations with phonological abilities and developing literacy skills. *Brain and Language, 97*(1), 64–79.

Boetsch, E. A. (1996). *A longitudinal study of the relationship between dyslexia and socioemotional functioning in young children.* Unpublished doctoral dissertation, University of Denver.

Bowers, P. G., & Wolf, M. (1993). Theoretical links among naming speed, precise timing mechanisms and orthographic skill in dyslexia. *Reading and Writing, 5*(1), 69–85.

Bradley, L., & Bryant, P. E. (1983). Categorizing sounds and learning to read: A causal connection. *Nature, 301*(5899), 419–421.

Brambati, S. M., Termine, C., Ruffino, M., Stella, G., Fazio, F., Cappa, S. F., et al. (2004). Regional reductions of gray matter volume in familial dyslexia. *Neurology, 63*(4), 742–745.

Brown, I. S., & Felton, R. H. (1990). Effects of instruction on beginning reading skills in children at risk for reading disability. *Reading and Writing, 2*(3), 223–241.

Brown, W. E., Eliez, S., Menon, V., Rumsey, J. M., White, C. D., & Reiss, A. L. (2001). Preliminary evidence of widespread morphological variations of the brain in dyslexia. *Neurology, 56*(6), 781–783.

Bruck, M. (1990). Word-recognition skills of adults with childhood diagnoses of dyslexia. *Developmental Psychology, 26*(3), 439–454.

Bruck, M. (1992). Persistence of dyslexics' phonological deficits. *Developmental Psychology, 28*(5), 874–886.

Bruck, M. (1993). Word recognition and component phonological processing skills of adults with childhood diagnosis of dyslexia. *Developmental Review, 13*(3), 258–268.

Brunswick, N., McCrory, E., Price, C. J., Frith, C. D., & Frith, U. (1999). Explicitly and implicit processing of words and pseudowords by adult developmental dyslexics. *Brain, 122*(10), 1901–1917.

Byrne, B., & Fielding-Barnsley, R. (1989). Phonemic awareness and letter knowledge in the child's acquisition of the alphabetic principle. *Journal of Educational Psychology, 81*(3), 313–321.

Byrne, B., Fielding-Barnsley, R., & Ashley, L. (2000). Effects of preschool phoneme identity training after six years: Outcome level distinguished from rate of response. *Journal of Educational Psychology, 92*(4), 659–667.

Byrne, B., & Shea, P. (1979). Semantic and phonetic memory codes in beginning readers. *Memory and Cognition, 7*(5), 333–338.

Caravolas, M. (2005). The nature and causes of dyslexia in different languages. In M. J. Snowling & C. Hulme (Eds.), *The science of reading: A handbook* (pp. 336–355). Oxford: Blackwell.

Caravolas, M., Bruck, M., & Genesee, F. (2003). Similarities and differences between English- and French-speaking poor spellers. In N. Goulandris (Ed.), *Dyslexia in different languages: Cross-linguistic comparisons* (pp. 157–180). London: Whurr.

Caravolas, M., Volin, J., & Hulme, C. (2005). Phoneme awareness is a key component of alphabetic literacy skills in consistent and inconsistent orthographies: Evidence from Czech and English children. *Journal of Experimental Child Psychology, 92*(2), 107–139.

Casanova, M. F., Araque, J., Giedd, J., & Rumsey, J. M. (2004). Reduced brain size and gyrification in the brains of dyslexic patients. *Journal of Child Neurology, 19*(4), 275–281.

Castles, A., & Coltheart, M. (1993). Varieties of developmental dyslexia. *Cognition, 47*(2), 149–180.

Castles, A., & Coltheart, M. (2004). Is there a causal link from phonological awareness to success in learning to read? *Cognition, 91*(1), 77–111.

Castles, A., Datta, H., Gayan, J., & Olson, R. K. (1999). Varieties of developmental reading disorder: Genetic and environmental influences. *Journal of Experimental Child Psychology, 72*(2), 73–94.

Catts, H. W., Fey, M. E., Tomblin, J. B., & Zhang, X. (2002). A longitudinal investigation of reading outcomes in children with language impairments. *Journal of Speech, Language, and Hearing Research, 45*(6), 1142–1157.

Chan, C. K. K., & Siegel, L. S. (2001). Phonological processing in reading Chinese among normally achieving and poor readers. *Journal of Experimental Child Psychology, 80*(1), 23–43.

Coltheart, M., Curtis, B., Atkins, P., & Haller, M. (1993). Models of reading aloud: Dual-route and parallel-distributed-processing approaches. *Psychological Review, 100*(4), 589–608.

Coltheart, M., Rastle, K., Perry, C., Langdon, R., & Ziegler, J. (2001). DRC: A dual route cascaded model of visual word recognition and reading aloud. *Psychological Review, 108*(1), 204–256.

Cooper, F. S., Delattre, P. C., Liberman, A. M., Borst, J. M., & Gerstman, L. J. (1952). Some experiments on the perception of synthetic speech sounds. *Journal of the Acoustical Society of America, 24,* 597–606.

Cope, N., Harold, D., Hill, G., Moskvina, V., Stevenson, J., Holmans, P., et al. (2005). Strong evidence that KIAA0319 on chromosome 6p is a susceptibility gene for developmental dyslexia. *American Journal of Human Genetics, 76*(4), 581–591.

Corina, D. P., Richards, T. L., Serafini, S., Richards, A. L., Steury, K., Abbott, R. D., et al. (2001). FMRI auditory language differences between dyslexic and able reading children. *NeuroReport, 12*(6), 1195–1201.

Cunningham, A. E. (1990). Explicit versus implicit instruction in phonemic awareness. *Journal of Experimental Child Psychology, 50*(3), 429–444.

Cunningham, A. E., & Stanovich, K. E. (1998). The impact of print exposure on word recognition. In J. L. Metsala & L. C. Ehri (Eds.), *Word recognition in beginning literacy* (pp. 235–262). Mahwah, NJ: Erlbaum.

Curtis, M. E. (1980). Development of components of reading skill. *Journal of Educational Psychology, 72*(5), 656–669.

D'Angiulli, A., & Siegel, L. S. (2003). Cognitive functioning as measured by the WISC-R: Do children with learning disabilities have distinctive patterns of performance? *Journal of Learning Disabilities, 36*(1), 48–58.

Deffenbacher, K. E., Kenyon, J. B., Hoover, D. M., Olson, R. K., Pennington, B. F., DeFries, J. C., et al. (2004). Refinement of the 6p21.3 quantitative trait locus influencing dyslexia: Linkage and association analyses. *Human Genetics, 115*(2), 128–138.

DeFries, J. C., Fulker, D. W., & LaBuda, M. C. (1987). Evidence for a genetic aetiology in reading disability of twins. *Nature, 329*(6139), 537–539.

de Jong, P. F., & van der Leij, A. (2003). Developmental changes in the manifestation of a phonological deficit in dyslexic children learning to read a regular orthography. *Journal of Educational Psychology,* 95(1), 22–40.

Denckla, M. B., & Rudel, R. G. (1976). Rapid 'automatized' naming (R.A.N.): Dyslexia differentiated from other learning disabilities. *Neuropsychologia,* 14(4), 471–479.

Deutsch, G. K., Dougherty, R. F., Bammer, R., Siok, W. T., Gabrieli, J. D. E., & Wandell, B. (2005). Children's reading performance is correlated with white matter structure measured by tensor imaging. *Cortex,* 41(3), 354–363.

Eckert, M. A. (2004). Neuroanatomical markers for dyslexia: A review of dyslexia structural imaging studies. *Neuroscientist,* 10(4), 362–371.

Eckert, M. A., Leonard, C. M., Richards, T. L., Aylward, E. H., Thomson, J., & Berninger, V. W. (2003). Anatomical correlates of dyslexia: Frontal and cerebellar findings. *Brain,* 126(2), 482–494.

Eckert, M. A., Leonard, C. M., Wilke, M., Eckert, M., Richards, T., Richards, A., et al. (2005). Anatomical signatures of dyslexia in children: Unique information from manual and voxel based morphometry brain measures. *Cortex,* 41(3), 304–315.

Eden, G. F., VanMeter, J. W., Rumsey, J. M., Maisog, J. M., Woods, R. P., & Zeffiro, T. A. (1996). Abnormal processing of visual motion in dyslexia revealed by functional brain imaging. *Nature,* 382(6586), 66–69.

Eley, E. C., & Craig, I. W. (2005). Introductory guide to the language of molecular genetics. *Journal of Child Psychology and Psychiatry,* 46, 1039–1041.

Eliez, S., Rumsey, J. M., Giedd, J. N., Schmitt, J. E., Patwardhan, A. J., & Reiss, A. L. (2000). Morphological alteration of temporal lobe gray matter in dyslexia: An MRI study. *Journal of Child Psychology and Psychiatry,* 41(5), 637–644.

Farmer, M. E., & Klein, R. M. (1995). The evidence for a temporal processing deficit linked to dyslexia: A review. *Psychonomic Bulletin and Review,* 2(4), 460–493.

Fawcett, A. J., & Nicolson, R. I. (1995). Persistence of phonological awareness deficits in older children with dyslexia. *Reading and Writing,* 7(4), 361–376.

Fawcett, A. J., Nicolson, R. I., & Dean, P. (1996). Impaired performance of children with dyslexia on a range of cerebellar tasks. *Annals of Dyslexia,* 46, 259–283.

Filipek, P. A. (1996). Structural variations in measures in the developmental disorders. In R. W. Thatcher, G. R. Lyon, J. Rumsey, & N. Krasnegor (Eds.), *Developmental neuroimaging: Mapping the development of brain and behavior* (pp. 169–186). San Diego, CA: Academic Press.

Filipek, P. A. (1999). Neuroimaging in the developmental disorders: The state of the science. *Journal of Child Psychology and Psychiatry,* 40(1), 113–128.

Finch, A. J., Nicolson, R. I., & Fawcett, A. J. (2002). Evidence for a neuroanatomical difference within the olivo-cerebellar pathway of adults with dyslexia. *Cortex,* 38(4), 529–539.

Fisher, J. H. (1905). Case of congenital word-blindness. *Ophthalmic Review,* 24, 315.

Fisher, S. E., & Francks, C. (2006). Genes, cognition and dyslexia: Learning to read the genome. *Trends in Cognitive Sciences,* 10(6), 250–257.

Flannery, K. A., Liederman, J., Daly, L., & Schultz, J. (2000). Male prevalence for reading disability is found in a large sample of black and white children free from ascertainment bias. *Journal of the International Neuropsychological Society,* 6(4), 433–442.

Fletcher, J. M., Foorman, B. R., Shaywitz, S. E., & Shaywitz, B. A. (1999). Conceptual and methodological issues in dyslexia research: A lesson for developmental disorders. In H. Tager-Flusberg (Ed.), *Neurodevelopmental disorders* (pp. 271–305). Cambridge, MA: MIT Press.

Fowler, A. E. (1991). How early phonological development might set the stage for phoneme awareness. In S. A. Brady & D. P. Shankweiler (Eds.), *Phonological processes in literacy: A tribute to Isabelle Y. Liberman* (pp. 97–117). Hillsdale, NJ: Erlbaum.

Fowler, A. E., & Swainson, B. (2004). Relationships of naming skills to reading, memory, and receptive vocabulary: Evidence for imprecise phonological representations of words by poor readers. *Annals of Dyslexia,* 54(2), 247–280.

Francks, C., Paracchini, S., Smith, S. D., Richardson, A. J., Scerri, T. S., Cardon, L. R., et al. (2004). A

77-kilobase region of chromosome 6p22.2 is associated with dyslexia in families from the United Kingdom and from the United States. *American Journal of Human Genetics, 75*(6), 1046–1058.

Frost, J., Madsbjerg, S., Niedersoe, J., Olofsson, A., & Sorensen, P. M. (2005). Semantic and phonological skills in predicting reading development: From 3–16 years of age. *Dyslexia, 11*(2), 79–92.

Frost, R. (1998). Toward a strong phonological theory of visual word recognition: True issues and false trails. *Psychological Bulletin, 123*(1), 71–99.

Galaburda, A. M., Menard, M. T., & Rosen, G. D. (1994). Evidence for aberrant auditory anatomy in developmental dyslexia. *Proceedings of the National Academy of Sciences USA, 91*(17), 8010–8013.

Galaburda, A. M., Sherman, G. F., Rosen, G. D., Aboitiz, F., & Geschwind, N. (1985). Developmental dyslexia: Four consecutive patients with cortical anomalies. *Annals of Neurology, 18*(2), 222–233.

Gayan, J., & Olson, R. K. (2001). Genetic and environmental influences on orthographic and phonological skills in children with reading disabilities. *Developmental Neuropsychology, 20*(2), 483–507.

Gazzaniga, M. S., Ivry, R. B., & Magnun, G. R. (2002). *Cognitive neuroscience: The biology of the mind* (2nd ed.). New York: Norton.

Georgiewa, P., Rzanny, R., Hopf, J.-M., Knab, R., Glauche, V., Kaiser, W.-A., et al. (1999). fMRI during word processing in dyslexic and normal reading children. *NeuroReport, 10*(16), 3459–3465.

Godfrey, J. J., Syrdal-Lasky, A. K., Millay, K. K., & Knox, C. M. (1981). Performance of dyslexic children on speech perception tests. *Journal of Experimental Child Psychology, 32*(3), 401–424.

Goodman, K. S. (1986). *What's whole in whole language: A parent–teacher guide.* Portsmouth, NH: Heinemann.

Goswami, U., & Bryant, P. (1990). *Phonological skills and learning to read.* Hillsdale, NJ: Erlbaum.

Gough, P. B., & Walsh, M. A. (1991). Chinese, Phoenicians, and the orthographic cipher of English. In S. A. Brady & D. P. Shankweiler (Eds.), *Phonological processes in literacy: A tribute to Isabelle Y. Liberman* (pp. 199–209): Hillsdale, NJ: Erlbaum.

Goulandris, N. (Ed.). (2003). *Dyslexia in different languages: Cross-linguistic comparisons.* London: Whurr.

Hallgren, B. (1950). Specific dyslexia (`congenital word-blindness'): A clinical and genetic study. *Acta Psychiatrica et Neurologica Supplement, 65*, 1–287.

Hanley, J. R. (2005). Learning to read in Chinese. In M. J. Snowling & C. Hulme (Eds.), *The science of reading: A handbook* (pp. 316–335). Oxford: Blackwell.

Hannula-Jouppi, K., Kaminen-Ahola, N., Taipale, M., Eklund, R., Nopola-Hemmi, J., Kaariainen, H., et al. (2005). The axon guidance receptor gene ROBO1 is a candidate gene for developmental dyslexia. *PLoS Genetics, 1*(4), e50.

Harlaar, N., Spinath, F. M., Dale, P. S., & Plomin, R. (2005). Genetic influences on early word recognition abilities and disabilities: A study of 7-year-old twins. *Journal of Child Psychology and Psychiatry, 46*(4), 373–384.

Harm, M. W., & Seidenberg, M. S. (1999). Phonology, reading acquisition, and dyslexia: Insights from connectionist models. *Psychological Review, 106*(3), 491–528.

Harm, M. W., & Seidenberg, M. S. (2004). Computing the meanings of words in reading: Cooperative division of labor between visual and phonological processes. *Psychological Review, 111*(3), 662–720.

Hatcher, J., Snowling, M. J., & Griffiths, Y. M. (2002). Cognitive assessment of dyslexic students in higher education. *British Journal of Educational Psychology, 72*(1), 119–133.

Hatcher, P. J., Hulme, C., & Ellis, A. W. (1994). Ameliorating early reading failure by integrating the teaching of reading and phonological skills: The phonological linkage hypothesis. *Child Development, 65*(1), 41–57.

Hatcher, P. J., Hulme, C., & Snowling, M. J. (2004). Explicit phoneme training combined with phonic reading instruction helps young children at risk of reading failure. *Journal of Child Psychology and Psychiatry, 45*(2), 338–358.

Heath, S. M., & Hogben, J. H. (2004). Cost-effective prediction of reading difficulties. *Journal of Speech, Language, and Hearing Research, 47*(4), 751–765.

Heirvang, E., Hugdahl, K., Steinmetz, H., Smievoll, A. I., Stevenson, J., Lund, A., et al. (2000). Planum temporale, planum parietale and dichotic listening in dyslexia. *Neuropsychologia, 38*(13), 1704–1713.

Herman, A. E., Galaburda, A. M., Fitch, R. H., Carter, A. R., & Rosen, G. D. (1997). Cerebral microgyria, thalamic cell size and auditory temporal processing in male and female rats. *Cerebral Cortex, 7*(5), 453–464.

Hinshaw, S. P. (1992). Academic underachievement, attention deficits, and aggression: Comorbidity and implications for intervention. *Journal of Consulting and Clinical Psychology, 60*(6), 893–903.

Hinshelwood, J. (1900). Congenital word-blindness. *Lancet, i*, 1506–1508.

Hinshelwood, J. (1907). Four cases of congenital word-blindness occurring in the same family. *British Medical Journal, 21*, 1229–1232.

Hugdahl, K., Heiervang, E., Ersland, L., Lundervold, A., Steinmetz, H., & Smievoll, A. I. (2003). Significant relation between MR measures of planum temporale area and dichotic processing of syllables in dyslexic children. *Neuropsychologia, 41*(6), 666–675.

Hulme, C. (1988). The implausibility of low-level visual deficits as a cause of children's reading difficulties. *Cognitive Neuropsychology, 5*(3), 369–374.

Hulslander, J., Talcott, J., Witton, C., DeFries, J., Pennington, B., Wadsworth, S., et al. (2004). Sensory processing, reading, IQ, and attention. *Journal of Experimental Child Psychology, 88*(3), 274–295.

Humphreys, P., Kaufmann, W. E., & Galaburda, A. M. (1990). Developmental dyslexia in women: Neuropathological findings in three patients. *Annals of Neurology, 28*(6), 727–738.

Hynd, G. W., Semrud-Clikeman, M., Lorys, A. R., & Novey, E. S. (1990). Brain morphology in developmental dyslexia and attention deficit disorder/hyperactivity. *Archives of Neurology, 47*(8), 919–926.

Jackson, N. E., & Coltheart, M. (2001). *Routes to reading success and failure: Toward an integrated cognitive psychology of atypical reading.* New York: Psychology Press.

Joanisse, M. F., Manis, F. R., Keating, P., & Seidenberg, M. S. (2000). Language deficits in dyslexic children: Speech perception, phonology, and morphology. *Journal of Experimental Child Psychology, 77*(1), 30–60.

Kerr, J. (1897). School hygiene, in its mental, moral, and physical aspects: Howard Medical Prize essay. *Journal of the Royal Statistical Society, 60*, 613–680.

Klingberg, T., Hedehus, M., Temple, E., Salz, T., Gabrieli, J. D., Moseley, M. E., et al. (2000). Microstructure of temporo-parietal white matter as a basis for reading ability: Evidence from diffusion tensor magnetic resonance imaging. *Neuron, 25*(2), 493–500.

Knopik, V. S., Smith, S. D., Cardon, L., Pennington, B., Gayan, J., Olson, R. K., et al. (2002). Differential genetic etiology of reading component processes as a function of IQ. *Behavioral Genetics, 32*(3), 181–198.

Koster, C., Been, P. H., Krikhaar, E. M., Zwarts, F., Diepstra, H. D., & Van Leeuwen, T. H. (2005). Differences at 17 months: Productive language patterns in infants at familial risk for dyslexia and typically developing infants. *Journal of Speech, Language, and Hearing Research, 48*(2), 426–438.

Laasonen, M., Service, E., & Virsu, V. (2001). Temporal order and processing acuity of visual, auditory, and tactile perception in developmentally dyslexic young adults. *Cognitive, Affective, and Behavioral Neuroscience, 1*(4), 394–410.

Landerl, K., Wimmer, H., & Frith, U. (1997). The impact of orthographic consistency on dyslexia: A German–English comparison. *Cognition, 63*(3), 315–334.

Larsen, J. P., Hoien, T., Lundberg, I., & Odegaard, H. (1990). MRI evaluation of the size and symmetry of the planum temporale in adolescents with developmental dyslexia. *Brain and Language, 39*(2), 289–310.

Lefly, D. L., & Pennington, B. F. (1991). Spelling errors and reading fluency in compensated adult dyslexics. *Annals of Dyslexia, 41*, 143–162.

Leonard, C. M., Eckert, M. A., Lombardino, L. J., Oakland, T., Kranzler, J., Mohr, C. M., et al. (2001). Anatomical risk factors for phonological dyslexia. *Cerebral Cortex, 11*(2), 148–157.

Leonard, C. M., Lombardino, L. J., Walsh, K., Eckert, M. A., Mockler, J. L., Rowe, L. A., et al. (2002). Anatomical risk factors that distinguish dyslexia from SLI predict reading skill in normal children. *Journal of Communication Disorders, 35*(6), 501–531.

Leonard, C. M., Voeller, K. K., Lombardino, L. J., & Morris, M. K. (1993). Anomalous cerebral structure in dyslexia revealed with magnetic resonance imaging. *Archives of Neurology, 50*(5), 461–469.

Liberman, A. M., Cooper, F. S., Shankweiler, D. P., & Studdert-Kennedy, M. (1967). Perception of the speech code. *Psychological Review, 74*(6), 431–461.

Liberman, I. Y., Shankweiler, D., Fischer, F. W., & Carter, B. (1974). Explicit syllable and phoneme segmentation in the young child. *Journal of Experimental Child Psychology, 18*(2), 201–212.

Livingstone, M. S., Rosen, G. D., Drislane, F. W., & Galaburda, A. M. (1991). Physiological and anatomical evidence for a magnocellular defect in developmental dyslexia. *Proceedings of the National Academy of Sciences USA, 88*(18), 7943–7947.

Lonigan, C. J., & Whitehurst, G. J. (1998). Relative efficacy of parent and teacher involvement in a shared-reading intervention for preschool children from low-income backgrounds. *Early Childhood Research Quarterly, 13*(2), 263–290.

Lundberg, I., Frost, J., & Petersen, O.-P. (1988). Effects of an extensive program for stimulating phonological awareness in preschool children. *Reading Research Quarterly, 23*(3), 263–284.

Lyon, G. R., Shaywitz, S. E., & Shaywitz, B. A. (2003). A definition of dyslexia. *Annals of Dyslexia, 53*, 1–14.

Lyytinen, H., Ahonen, T., Eklund, K., Guttorm, T., Kulju, P., Laakso, M. L., et al. (2004). Early development of children at familial risk for dyslexia: Follow-up from birth to school age. *Dyslexia, 10*(3), 146–178.

Manis, F. R., McBride-Chang, C., Seidenberg, M. S., & Keating, P. (1997). Are speech perception deficits associated with developmental dyslexia? *Journal of Experimental Child Psychology, 66*(2), 211–235.

Manis, F. R., Seidenberg, M. S., Doi, L. M., & McBride-Chang, C. (1996). On the bases of two subtypes of development dyslexia. *Cognition, 58*(2), 157–195.

Martin, F., & Lovegrove, W. (1984). The effects of field size and luminance on contrast sensitivity differences between specifically reading disabled and normal children. *Neuropsychologia, 22*(1), 73–77.

Maughan, B., Rowe, R., Loeber, R., & Stouthamer-Loeber, M. (2003). Reading problems and depressed mood. *Journal of Abnormal Child Psychology, 31*(2), 219–229.

McBride-Chang, C., Cho, J.-R., Liu, H., Wagner, R. K., Shu, H., Zhou, A., et al. (2005). Changing models across cultures: Associations of phonological awareness and morphological structure awareness with vocabulary and word recognition in second graders from Beijing, Hong Kong, Korea, and the United States. *Journal of Experimental Child Psychology, 92*(2), 140–160.

McCandliss, B. D., Cohen, L., & Dehaene, S. (2003). The visual word form area: Expertise for reading in the fusiform gyrus. *Trends in Cognitive Sciences, 7*(7), 293–299.

McCrory, E., Frith, U., Brunswick, N., & Price, C. (2000). Abnormal functional activation during a simple word repetition task: A PET study of adult dyslexics. *Journal of Cognitive Neuroscience, 12*(5), 753–762.

McCrory, E. J., Mechelli, A., Frith, U., & Price, C. J. (2005). More than words: A common neural basis for reading and naming deficits in developmental dyslexia? *Brain, 128*(2), 261–267.

McGee, R., Share, D., Moffitt, T. E., Williams, S., & Silva, P. A. (1988). Reading disability, behaviour problems and juvenile delinquency. In D. H. Saklofske & S. B. G. Eysenck (Eds.), *Individual differences in children and adolescents* (pp. 158–172). New Brunswick NJ: Transaction.

McGrath, L. M., Smith, S. D., & Pennington, B. F. (2006). Breakthroughs in the search for dyslexia candidate genes. *Trends in Molecular Medicine, 12*, 333–341.

Meng, H., Smith, S. D., Hager, K., Held, M., Liu, J., Olson, R. K., et al. (2005). DCDC2 is associated with reading disability and modulates neuronal development in the brain. *Proceedings of the National Academy of Sciences USA, 102*(47), 17053–17058.

Metsala, J. L. (1997a). An examination of word frequency and neighborhood density in the development of spoken-word recognition. *Memory and Cognition, 25*(1), 47–56.

Metsala, J. L. (1997b). Spoken word recognition in reading disabled children. *Journal of Educational Psychology, 89*(1), 159–169.

Metsala, J. L., & Walley, A. C. (1998). Spoken vocabulary growth and the segmental restructuring of lexical representations: Precursors to phonemic awareness and early reading ability. In J. L. Metsala & L. C. Ehri (Eds.), *Word recognition in beginning literacy* (pp. 89–120). Mahwah, NJ: Erlbaum.

Morais, J., Cary, L., Alegria, J., & Bertelson, P. (1979). Does awareness of speech as a sequence of phones arise spontaneously? *Cognition, 7*(4), 323–331.

Nathan, L., Stackhouse, J., Goulandris, N., & Snowling, M. J. (2004). The development of early literacy skills among children with speech difficulties: A test of the 'critical age hypothesis.' *Journal of Speech, Language, and Hearing Research, 47*(2), 377–391.

Nation, K. (2005). Children's reading comprehension difficulties. In M. J. Snowling & C. Hulme (Eds.), *The science of reading: A handbook* (pp. 248–265). Oxford: Blackwell.

Nation, K., Clarke, P., Marshall, C. M., & Durand, M. (2004). Hidden language impairments in children: Parallels between poor comprehension and specific language impairment? *Journal of Speech, Language, and Hearing Research, 47*, 199–211.

National Reading Panel. (2000). *Teaching children to read: An evidence-based assessment of the scientific research literature on reading and its implications for reading instruction.* Washington, DC: National Institute for Child Health and Human Development.

Nicolson, R. I., & Fawcett, A. J. (1990). Automaticity: A new framework for dyslexia research? *Cognition, 35*(2), 159–182.

Nicolson, R. I., Fawcett, A. J., & Dean, P. (2001). Developmental dyslexia: The cerebellar deficit hypothesis. *Trends in Neurosciences, 24*(9), 508–511.

Olson, R. K., Datta, H., Gayan, J., & DeFries, J. C. (1999). A behavioral-genetic analysis of reading disabilities and component processes. In R. M. Klein & P. A. McMullen (Eds.), *Converging methods for understanding reading and dyslexia* (pp. 133–151). Cambridge, MA: MIT Press.

Orton, S. T. (1925). 'Word-blindness' in school children. *Archives of Neurology and Psychiatry, 14*, 581–615.

Orton, S. T. (1937). *Reading, writing and speech problems in children.* New York: Norton.

Paracchini, S., Thomas, A., Castro, S., Lai, C., Paramasivam, M., Wang, Y., et al. (2006). The chromosome 6p22 haplotype associated with dyslexia reduces the expression of KIAA0319, a novel gene involved in neuronal migration. *Human Molecular Genetics, 15*(10), 1659–1666.

Paulesu, E., Demonet, J. F., Fazio, F., McCrory, E., Chanoine, V., Brunswick, N., et al. (2001). Dyslexia: Cultural diversity and biological unity. *Science, 291*(5511), 2165–2167.

Peiffer, A. M., Rosen, G. D., & Fitch, R. H. (2002). Rapid auditory processing and MGN morphology in microgyric rats reared in varied acoustic environments. *Developmental Brain Research, 138*(2), 187–193.

Pennington, B. F. (2006). From single to multiple deficit models of developmental disorders. *Cognition, 101*, 385–413.

Pennington, B. F., Filipek, P. A., Lefly, D., Churchwell, J., Kennedy, D. N., Simon, J. H., et al. (1999). Brain morphometry in reading-disabled twins. *Neurology, 53*(4), 723–729.

Pennington, B. F., & Lefly, D. L. (2001). Early reading development in children at family risk for dyslexia. *Child Development, 72*(3), 816–833.

Pennington, B. F., & Olson, R. K. (2005). Genetics of dyslexia. In M. J. Snowling & C. Hulme (Eds.), *The science of reading: A handbook* (pp. 453–472). Oxford: Blackwell.

Pennington, B. F., Van Orden, G. C., Smith, S. D., & Green, P. A. (1990). Phonological processing skills and deficits in adult dyslexics. *Child Development, 61*(6), 1753–1778.

Perfetti, C. A. (1985). *Reading ability.* Oxford: Oxford University Press.

Perfetti, C. A., Beck, I., Bell, L. C., & Hughes, C. (1987). Phonemic knowledge and learning to read are reciprocal: A longitudinal study of first grade children. *Merrill–Palmer Quarterly, 33*(3), 283–219.

Phillips, B. M., & Lonigan, C. J. (2005). Social Correlates of Emergent Literacy. In M. J. Snowling & C. Hulme (Eds.), *The science of reading: A handbook* (pp. 173–187). Oxford: Blackwell.

Phinney, E., Pennington, B. F., Olson, R., Filley, C. M., & Filipek, P. A. (2007). Brain structure correlates of component reading processes: Implications for reading disability. *Cortex, 43*, 777–791.

Plaut, D. C., McClelland, J. L., Seidenberg, M. S., & Patterson, K. (1996). Understanding normal and impaired word reading: Computational principles in quasi-regular domains. *Psychological Review*, *103*(1), 56–115.

Price, C. J., & McCrory, E. (2005). Functional brain imaging studies of skilled reading and developmental dyslexia. In M. J. Snowling & C. Hulme (Eds.), *The science of reading: A handbook* (pp. 473–496). Oxford: Blackwell.

Pringle-Morgan, W. (1896). A case of congenital word blindness. *British Medical Journal, ii*(1871), 1543–1544.

Rack, J. P., Snowling, M. J., & Olson, R. K. (1992). The nonword reading deficit in developmental dyslexia: A review. *Reading Research Quarterly, 27*(1), 28–53.

Rae, C., Harasty, J. A., Dzendrowskyj, T. E., Talcott, J. B., Simpson, J. M., Blamire, A. M., et al. (2002). Cerebellar morphology in developmental dyslexia. *Neuropsychologia, 40*(8), 1285–1292.

Ramus, F. (2003). Developmental dyslexia: Specific phonological deficit or general sensorimotor dysfunction? *Current Opinion in Neurobiology, 13*(2), 212–218.

Ramus, F. (2004). Neurobiology of dyslexia: A reinterpretation of the data. *Trends in Neurosciences, 27*(12), 720–726.

Ramus, F., Rosen, S., Dakin, S. C., Day, B. L., Castellote, J. M., White, S., et al. (2003). Theories of developmental dyslexia: Insights from a multiple case study of dyslexic adults. *Brain, 126*(4), 841–865.

Rashid, F. L., Morris, R. D., & Sevcik, R. A. (2005). Relationship between home literacy environment and reading achievement in children with reading disabilities. *Journal of Learning Disabilities, 38*(1), 2–11.

Reed, M. A. (1989). Speech perception and the discrimination of brief auditory cues in reading disabled children. *Journal of Experimental Child Psychology, 48*(2), 270–292.

Richards, T. L., Aylward, E. H., Berninger, V. W., Field, K. M., Grimme, A. C., Richards, A. L., et al. (2006). Individual fMRI activation in orthographic mapping and morpheme mapping after orthographic or morphological spelling treatment in child dyslexics. *Journal of Neurolinguistics, 19*(1), 56–86.

Robichon, F., Levrier, O., Farnarier, P., & Habib, M. (2000). Developmental dyslexia: Atypical cortical asymmetries and functional significance. *European Journal of Neurology, 7*(1), 35–46.

Rodgers, B. (1983). The identification and prevalence of specific reading retardation. *British Journal of Educational Psychology, 53*(3), 369–373.

Romani, C., Olson, A., & Di Betta, A. M. (2005). Spelling disorders. In M. J. Snowling & C. Hulme (Eds.), *The science of reading: A handbook* (pp. 431–447). Oxford: Blackwell.

Rosen, G. D., Bai, J., Wang, Y., Fiondella, C. G., Threlkeld, S. W., LoTurco, J. J., et al. (2007). Disruption of neuronal migration by RNAi of Dyx1c1 results in neocortical and hippocampal malformations. *Cerebral Cortex, 17*(11), 2562–2572.

Rosen, G. D., Herman, A. E., & Galaburda, A. M. (1999). Sex differences in the effects of early neocortical injury on neuronal size distribution of the medial geniculate nucleus in the rat are mediated by perinatal gonadal steroids. *Cerebral Cortex, 9*(1), 27–34.

Rosen, G. D., Press, D. M., Sherman, G. F., & Galaburda, A. M. (1992). The development of induced cerebrocortical microgyria in the rat. *Journal of Neuropathology and Experimental Neurology, 51*(6), 601–611.

Rosen, G. D., Waters, N. S., Galaburda, A. M., & Denenberg, V. H. (1995). Behavioral consequences of neonatal injury of the neocortex. *Brain Research, 681*(1), 177–189.

Rumsey, J. M., Donohue, B. C., Brady, D. R., Nace, K., Giedd, J. N., & Andreason, P. (1997a). A magnetic resonance imaging study of planum temporale asymmetry in men with developmental dyslexia. *Archives of Neurology, 54*(12), 1481–1489.

Rumsey, J. M., Nace, K., Donohue, B., Wise, D., Maisog, J. M., & Andreason, P. (1997b). A positron emission tomographic study of impaired word recognition and phonological processing in dyslexic men. *Archives of Neurology, 54*(5), 562–573.

Rutter, M., Caspi, A., Fergusson, D., Horwood, L. J., Goodman, R., Maughan, B., et al. (2004). Sex differences in developmental reading disability: New findings from 4 epidemiological studies. *Journal of the American Medical Association, 291*(16), 2007–2012.

Sandak, R., Mencl, W. E., Frost, S. J., & Pugh, K. R. (2004). The neurobiological basis of skilled and impaired reading: Recent findings and new directions. *Scientific Studies of Reading, 8*(3), 273–292.

Sattler, J. M., & Dumont, R. (2004). *Assessment of children: WISC-IV and WPPSI-III supplement*. San Diego, CA: Jerome M. Sattler.

Scarborough, H. S. (1990). Very early language deficits in dyslexic children. *Child Development, 61*(6), 1728–1743.

Scarborough, H. S. (1991a). Antecedents to reading disability: Preschool language development and literacy experiences of children from dyslexic families. *Reading and Writing, 3*(3), 219–233.

Scarborough, H. S. (1991b). Early syntactic development of dyslexic children. *Annals of Dyslexia, 41*, 207–220.

Scarborough, H. S. (1998). Early identification of children at risk for reading disabilities: Phonological awareness and some other promising predictors. In B. K. Shapiro, P. J. Accardo, & A. J. Capute (Eds.), *Specific reading disability: A view of the spectrum* (pp. 75–119). Timonium, MD: York Press.

Scarborough, H. S. (2005). Developmental relationships between language and reading: Reconciling a beautiful hypothesis with some ugly facts. In H. W. Catts & A. G. Kamhi (Eds.), *The connections between language and reading disabilities* (pp. 3–24). Mahwah, NJ: Erlbaum.

Scarborough, H. S., Dobrich, W., & Hager, M. (1991). Preschool literacy experience and later reading achievement. *Journal of Learning Disabilities, 24*(8), 508–511.

Scarborough, H. S., & Parker, J. D. (2003). Children's learning and teachers' expectations: Matthew effects in children with learning disabilities. Development of reading, IQ, and psychosocial problems from grade 2 to grade 8. *Annals of Dyslexia, 53*, 47–71.

Schatschneider, C., Fletcher, J. M., Francis, D. J., Carlson, C. D., & Foorman, B. R. (2004). Kindergarten prediction of reading skills: A longitudinal comparative analysis. *Journal of Educational Psychology, 96*(2), 265–282.

Schmahmann, J. D., & Caplan, D. (2006). Cognition, emotion and the cerebellum. *Brain, 129*(2), 290–292.

Schneider, W., Roth, E., & Ennemoser, M. (2000). Training phonological skills and letter knowledge in children at risk for dyslexia: A comparison of three kindergarten intervention programs. *Journal of Educational Psychology, 92*(2), 284–295.

Schultz, R. T., Cho, N. K., Staib, L. H., & Kier, L. E. (1994). Brain morphology in normal and dyslexic children: The influence of sex and age. *Annals of Neurology, 35*(6), 732–742.

Schumacher, J., Anthoni, H., Dahdouh, F., Konig, I. R., Hillmer, A. M., Kluck, N., et al. (2006). Strong genetic evidence of DCDC2 as a susceptibility gene for dyslexia. *American Journal of Human Genetics, 78*(1), 52–62.

Seeger, M., Tear, G., Ferres-Marco, D., & Goodman, C. S. (1993). Mutations affecting growth cone guidance in *Drosophila*: Genes necessary for guidance toward or away from the midline. *Neuron, 10*(3), 409–426.

Seidenberg, M. S., & McClelland, J. L. (1989). A distributed, developmental model of word recognition and naming. *Psychological Review, 96*(4), 523–568.

Seymour, P. H. K. (2005). Early reading development in European orthographies. In M. J. Snowling & C. Hulme (Eds.), *The science of reading: A handbook* (pp. 296–315). Oxford: Blackwell.

Shanahan, M. A., Pennington, B. F., Yerys, B. E., Scott, A., Boada, R., Willcutt, E. G., et al. (2006). Processing speed deficits in attention deficit/hyperactivity disorder and reading disability. *Journal of Abnormal Child Psychology, 34*, 585–602.

Shankweiler, D. P., Liberman, I. Y., Mark, L. S., Fowler, C. A., & Fischer, F. W. (1979). The speech code and learning to read. *Journal of Experimental Psychology: Human Learning and Memory, 5*, 531–545.

Share, D. L., Jorm, A. F., Maclean, R., & Matthews, R. (2002). Temporal processing and reading disability. *Reading and Writing, 15*(1), 151–178.

Shaywitz, B. A., Shaywitz, S. E., Blachman, B. A., Pugh, K. R., Fulbright, R. K., Skudlarski, P., et al.

(2004). Development of left occipitotemporal systems for skilled reading in children after a phonologically-based intervention. *Biological Psychiatry, 55*(9), 926–933.

Shaywitz, B. A., Shaywitz, S. E., Pugh, K. R., Mencl, W. E., Fulbright, R. K., Skudlarksi, P., et al. (2002). Disruption of posterior brain systems for reading in children with developmental dyslexia. *Biological Psychiatry, 52*(2), 101–110.

Shaywitz, S. E. (2003). *Overcoming dyslexia: A new and complete science-based program for reading problems at any level.* New York: Knopf.

Shaywitz, S. E., Escobar, M. D., Shaywitz, B. A., & Fletcher, J. M. (1992). Evidence that dyslexia may represent the lower tail of a normal distribution of reading ability. *New England Journal of Medicine, 326*(3), 145–150.

Shaywitz, S. E., Shaywitz, B. A., Fletcher, J. M., & Escobar, M. D. (1990). Prevalence of reading disability in boys and girls: Results of the Connecticut Longitudinal Study. *Journal of the American Medical Association, 264*(8), 998–1002.

Shaywitz, S. E., Shaywitz, B. A., Fulbright, R. K., Skudlarski, P., Mencl, W. E., Constable, R. T., et al. (2003). Neural systems for compensation and persistence: Young adult outcome of childhood reading disability. *Biological Psychiatry, 54*(1), 25–33.

Shaywitz, S. E., Shaywitz, B. A., Pugh, K. R., Fulbright, R. K., Constable, R. T., Mencl, W. E., et al. (1998). Functional disruption in the organization of the brain for reading in dyslexia. *Proceedings of the National Academy of Sciences USA, 95*(5), 2636–2641.

Shu, H., & Anderson, R. C. (1997). Role of radical awareness in the character and word acquisition of Chinese children. *Reading Research Quarterly, 32*(1), 78–89.

Silva, P. A., McGee, R., & Williams, S. (1985). Some characteristics of 9-year-old boys with general reading backwardness or specific reading retardation. *Journal of Child Psychology and Psychiatry, 26*(3), 407–421.

Siok, W. T., Perfetti, C. A., Jin, Z., & Tan, L. H. (2004). Biological abnormality of impaired reading is constrained by culture. *Nature, 431*(7004), 71–76.

SLI Consortium. (2002). A genomewide scan identifies two novel loci involved in specific language impairment. *American Journal of Human Genetics, 70*(2), 384–398.

SLI Consortium. (2004). Highly significant linkage to the SLI1 locus in an expanded sample of individuals affected by specific language impairment. *American Journal of Human Genetics, 74*(6), 1225–1238.

Smith, S. D., Gilger, J. W., & Pennington, B. F. (2001). Dyslexia and other specific learning disorders. In D. L. Rimoin, J. M. Conner, & R. E. Pyeritz (Eds.), *Emery and Rimoin's principles and practice of medical genetics* (4th ed.). New York: Churchill Livingstone.

Smith, S. D., Pennington, B. F., Boada, R., & Shriberg, L. D. (2005). Linkage of speech sound disorder to reading disability loci. *Journal of Child Psychology and Psychiatry, 46*(10), 1057–1066.

Snowling, M. J. (2000). *Dyslexia* (2nd ed.). Oxford: Blackwell.

Snowling, M. J., Gallagher, A., & Frith, U. (2003). Family risk of dyslexia is continuous: Individual differences in the precursors of reading skill. *Child Development, 74*(2), 358–373.

Stanovich, K. E. (1986). Matthew effects in reading: Some consequences of individual differences in the acquisition of literacy. *Reading Research Quarterly, 21*(4), 360–406.

Stanovich, K. E. (1991). Cognitive science meets beginning reading. *Psychological Science, 2*, 70–81.

Stanovich, K. E., Siegel, L. S., & Gottardo, A. (1997). Converging evidence for phonological and surface subtypes of reading disability. *Journal of Educational Psychology, 89*(1), 114–127.

Stein, C. M., Schick, J. H., Gerry Taylor, H., Shriberg, L. D., Millard, C., Kundtz-Kluge, A., et al. (2004). Pleiotropic effects of a chromosome 3 locus on speech-sound disorder and reading. *American Journal of Human Genetics, 74*(2), 283–297.

Stein, J. (2001). The sensory basis of reading problems. *Developmental Neuropsychology, 20*(2), 509–534.

Stein, J., & Walsh, V. (1997). To see but not to read: The magnocellular theory of dyslexia. *Trends in Neurosciences, 20*(4), 147–152.

Stephenson, S. (1907). Six cases of congential word-blindness affecting three generations of one family. *Ophthalmoscope, 5,* 482–484.

Stevenson, J. (1991). Which aspects of processing text mediate genetic effects? *Reading and Writing, 3*(3), 249–269.

Stoodley, C. J., Talcott, J. B., Carter, E. L., Witton, C., & Stein, J. F. (2000). Selective deficits of vibrotactile sensitivity in dyslexic readers. *Neuroscience Letters, 295*(1–2), 13–16.

Stothard, S. E., Snowling, M. J., Bishop, D. V. M., Chipchase, B. B., & Kaplan, C. A. (1998). Language-impaired preschoolers: A follow-up into adolescence. *Journal of Speech, Language, and Hearing Research, 41*(2), 407–418.

Stuebing, K. K., Fletcher, J. M., LeDoux, J. M., Lyon, G. R., Shaywitz, S. E., & Shaywitz, B. A. (2002). Validity of IQ-discrepancy classifications of reading disabilities: A meta-analysis. *American Educational Research Journal, 39*(2), 469–518.

Swan, D., & Goswami, U. (1997a). Phonological awareness deficits in developmental dyslexia and the phonological representations hypothesis. *Journal of Experimental Child Psychology, 66*(1), 18–41.

Swan, D., & Goswami, U. (1997b). Picture naming deficits in developmental dyslexia: The phonological representations hypothesis. *Brain and Language, 56*(3), 334–353.

Taipale, M., Kaminen, N., Nopola-Hemmi, J., Haltia, T., Myllyluoma, B., Lyytinen, H., et al. (2003). A candidate gene for developmental dyslexia encodes a nuclear tetratricopeptide repeat domain protein dynamically regulated in brain. *Proceedings of the National Academy of Sciences USA, 100*(20), 11553–11558.

Tallal, P. (1980). Auditory temporal perception, phonics, and reading disabilities in children. *Brain and Language, 9*(2), 182–198.

Tallal, P., Miller, S. L., Jenkins, W. M., & Merzenich, M. M. (1997). The role of temporal processing in developmental language-based learning disorders: Research and clinical implications. In B. A. Blachman (Ed.), *Foundations of reading acquisition and dyslexia: Implications for early intervention* (pp. 49–66). Mahwah, NJ: Erlbaum.

Tallal, P., & Percy, M. (1973). Developmental aphasia: Impaired rate of nonverbal processing as a function of sensory modality. *Neuropsychologia, 11,* 389–398.

Tallal, P., & Percy, M. (1975). Developmental aphasia: The perception of brief vowels and extended stop consonants. *Neuropsychologia, 13,* 69–74.

Tan, L.-H., & Perfetti, C. A. (1998). Phonological codes as early sources of constraint in Chinese word identification: A review of current discoveries and theoretical accounts. *Reading and Writing, 10*(3), 165–200.

Temple, E., Deutsch, G. K., Poldrack, R. A., Miller, S. L., Tallal, P., Merzenich, M. M., et al. (2003). Neural deficits in children with dyslexia ameliorated by behavioral remediation: Evidence from functional MRI. *Proceedings of the National Academy of Sciences USA, 100*(5), 2860–2865.

Temple, E., Poldrack, R. A., Salidis, J., Deutsch, G. K., Tallal, P., Merzenich, M. M., et al. (2001). Disrupted neural responses to phonological and orthographic processing in dyslexic children: An fMRI study. *NeuroReport, 12*(2), 299–307.

Thomas, C. J. (1905). Congenital word-blindness and its treatment. *Ophthalmoscope, 3,* 380–385.

Threlkeld, S. W., McClure, M. M., Bai, J., Wang, Y., LoTurco, J. J., Rosen, G. D., et al. (2007). Developmental disruptions and behavioral impairments in rats following *in utero* RNAi of Dyx1c1. *Brain Research Bulletin, 71,* 508–514.

Torgesen, J. K. (2005). Recent discoveries on remedial interventions for children with dyslexia. In M. J. Snowling & C. Hulme (Eds.), *The science of reading: A handbook* (pp. 521–537). Oxford: Blackwell.

Torgesen, J. K., Alexander, A. W., Wagner, R. K., Rashotte, C. A., Voeller, K. K. S., & Conway, T. (2001). Intensive remedial instruction for children with severe reading disabilities: Immediate and long-term outcomes from two instructional approaches. *Journal of Learning Disabilities, 34,* 33–58.

Torgesen, J. K., Rose, E., Lindamood, P., Conway, T., & Garvan, C. (1999). Preventing reading failure in young children with phonological processing disabilities: Group and individual responses to instruction. *Journal of Educational Psychology, 91,* 579–594.

Torgesen, J. K., Wagner, R. K., Rashotte, C. A., & Herron, J. (2003). *Summary of outcomes from first grade study with Read, Write, Type and Auditory Discrimination in Depth instruction and software with at-risk children* (Technical Report No. 3). Tallahassee: Florida Center for Reading Research.

Treiman, R., & Breaux, A. M. (1982). Common phoneme and overall similarity relations among spoken syllables: Their use by children and adults. *Journal of Psycholinguistic Research, 11*(6), 569–598.

Tzeng, O. J. L., Lin, Z. H., Hung, D. L., & Lee, W. L. (1995). Learning to be a conspirator: A tale of becoming a good Chinese reader. In B. de Gelder & J. Morais (Eds.), *Speech and reading: A comparative approach* (pp. 227–246). Hove, UK: Taylor & Francis.

van Alphen, P., de Bree, E., Gerrits, E., de Jong, J., Wilsenach, C., & Wijnen, F. (2004). Early language development in children with a genetic risk of dyslexia. *Dyslexia, 10*(4), 265–288.

Van Orden, G. C., & Kloos, H. (2005). The question of phonology and reading. In M. J. Snowling & C. Hulme (Eds.), *The science of reading: A handbook* (pp. 61–78). Oxford: Blackwell.

Van Orden, G. C., Pennington, B. F., & Stone, G. O. (1990). Word identification in reading and the promise of subsymbolic psycholinguistics. *Psychological Review, 97*(4), 488–522.

Vellutino, F. R. (1979). The validity of perceptual deficit explanations of reading disability: A reply to Fletcher and Satz. *Journal of Learning Disabilities, 12*(3), 160–167.

Vellutino, F. R. (1987). Dyslexia. *Scientific American, 256*(3), 34–41.

Vellutino, F. R., Fletcher, J. M., Snowling, M. J., & Scanlon, D. M. (2004). Specific reading disability (dyslexia): What have we learned in the past four decades? *Journal of Child Psychology and Psychiatry, 45*(1), 2–40.

Vellutino, F. R., & Scanlon, D. M. (1982). Verbal processing in poor and normal readers. In C. J. Brainerd & M. Pressley (Eds.), *Verbal processes in children* (pp. 189–264). New York: Springer-Verlag.

Vellutino, F. R., Scanlon, D. M., Sipay, E. R., & Small, S. G. (1996). Cognitive profiles of difficult-to-remediate and readily remediated poor readers: Early intervention as a vehicle for distinguishing between cognitive and experiential deficits as basic causes of specific reading disability. *Journal of Educational Psychology, 88*(4), 601–638.

Vellutino, F. R., Scanlon, D. M., Small, S., & Fanuele, D. P. (2006). Response to intervention as a vehicle for distinguishing between children with and without reading disabilities: Evidence for the role of kindergarten and first-grade interventions. *Journal of Learning Disabilities, 39*(2), 157–169.

Vinckenbosch, E., Robichon, F., & Eliez, S. (2005). Gray matter alteration in dyslexia: Converging evidence from volumetric and voxel-by-voxel MRI analyses. *Neuropsychologia, 43*(3), 324–331.

Wadsworth, S. J., Olson, R. K., Pennington, B. F., & DeFries, J. C. (2000). Differential genetic etiology of reading disability as a function of IQ. *Journal of Learning Disabilities, 33*(2), 192–199.

Wagner, R. K., & Torgesen, J. K. (1987). The nature of phonological processing and its causal role in the acquisition of reading skills. *Psychological Bulletin, 101*(2), 192–212.

Wagner, R. K., Torgesen, J. K., & Rashotte, C. A. (1994). Development of reading-related phonological processing abilities: New evidence of bidirectional causality from a latent variable longitudinal study. *Developmental Psychology, 30*(1), 73–87.

Wagner, R. K., Torgesen, J. K., & Rashotte, C. A. (1999). *Comprehensive Test of Phonological Processing.* Austin, TX: PRO-ED.

Walley, A. C. (1993). The role of vocabulary development in children's spoken word recognition and segmentation ability. *Developmental Review, 13*(3), 286–350.

Wang, Y., Paramasivam, M., Thomas, A., Bai, J., Kaminen-Ahola, N., Kere, J., et al. (2006). DYX1C1 functions in neuronal migration in developing neocortex. *Neuroscience, 143*(2), 515–522.

Werker, J. F., & Tees, R. C. (1987). Speech perception in severely disabled and average reading children. *Canadian Journal of Psychology, 41*(1), 48–61.

Whitehurst, G. J., Epstein, J. N., Angel, A. L., & Payne, A. C. (1994). Outcomes of an emergent literacy intervention in Head Start. *Journal of Educational Psychology, 86*(4), 542–555.

Willcutt, E. G., & Pennington, B. F. (2000). Psychiatric comorbidity in children and adolescents with reading disability. *Journal of Child Psychology and Psychiatry, 41*(8), 1039–1048.

Willcutt, E. G., Pennington, B. F., & DeFries, J. C. (2000). Etiology of inattention and hyperactivity/

impulsivity in a community sample of twins with learning difficulties. *Journal of Abnormal Child Psychology, 28*(2), 149–159.

Willcutt, E. G., Pennington, B. F., Smith, S. D., Cardon, L. R., Gayan, J., Knopik, V. S., et al. (2002). Quantitative trait locus for reading disability on chromosome 6p is pleiotropic for attention-deficit/hyperactivity disorder. *American Journal of Medical Genetics, 114*(3), 260–268.

Wise, B. W., Ring, J., & Olson, R. K. (1999). Training phonological awareness with and without explicit attention to articulation. *Journal of Experimental Child Psychology, 72*(4), 271–304.

Wise, B. W., Ring, J., & Olson, R. K. (2000). Individual differences in gains from computer-assisted remedial reading. *Journal of Experimental Child Psychology, 77*(3), 197–235.

Wolf, M., & Bowers, P. G. (1999). The double-deficit hypothesis for the developmental dyslexias. *Journal of Educational Psychology, 91*(3), 415–438.

Wydell, T. N., & Butterworth, B. (1999). A case study of an English–Japanese bilingual with monolingual dyslexia. *Cognition, 70*(3), 273–305.

CHAPTER 13

Specific Language Impairment

MARGARET J. SNOWLING
MARIANNA E. HAYIOU-THOMAS

Specific language impairment (SLI) is a neurodevelopmental disorder characterized by delayed or disordered language development in the absence of general cognitive deficits, hearing impairments, psychiatric problems, or frank neurological damage. Children with SLI have been studied by professionals from a wide range of disciplines, including neurology, speech pathology, psychology, and linguistics. A number of different terms have been used to describe the condition, including *developmental dysphasia*, *specific developmental language disorder*, and *language-learning impairment*, and there have been attempts to delineate qualitatively distinct subtypes.

The *Diagnostic and Statistical Manual of Mental Disorders*, fourth edition, text revision (DSM-IV-TR; American Psychiatric Association, 2000) uses the diagnostic category of *communication disorders* to classify children described clinically as having SLI—that is, children whose scores obtained on individually administered measures of language development are below expectation, given their nonverbal intellectual capacity. The term can also be applied if a child has suffered an accompanying sensory deficit, learning difficulties, or environmental deprivation, provided that the language difficulties exceed those usually associated with these problems. DSM-IV-TR goes on to distinguish several types of communication disorders, including expressive language disorder (primarily affecting language production), mixed receptive–expressive language disorder (affecting both language comprehension and production), and phonological disorder (affecting the use of speech sounds to signal meaning). In a similar vein, the 10th revision of the *International Classification of Diseases* (ICD-10; World Health Organization, 1993) lays out criteria for expressive language disorder, receptive language disorder, and specific speech articulation disorder. Both classification schemes also exclude children with pervasive developmental disorders (e.g., autism) from receiving diagnoses of communication disorders (DSM-IV-TR) or specific developmental disorders of speech and language (ICD-10).

Clinicians can screen for SLI by taking a developmental and school history, using behavioral observations during the evaluation, and administering standardized tests (Pennington, 2009a). A scale in wide use in the United Kingdom is the Children's Communication Checklist (Bishop, 2003), which is completed by parents or professionals to rate the nature of a child's speech, language, and communication difficulties. As discussed later, children with SLI will have an early history of delayed language milestones, particularly in expressive language (e.g., word-finding problems) and verb acquisition. Parents may have noticed that a child's grammar sounds immature because of problems with verb tense (e.g., *walk* for *walked*), pronouns, and word order. In school, the child will almost invariably have trouble across the curriculum, in subjects that require reading comprehension and writing. During the evaluation, children with SLI will typically say rather little compared with other children their age, and they may exhibit problems with word finding and grammar. On standardized tests, a child with SLI will almost invariably have a depressed Verbal IQ and poor reading comprehension scores, and will perform poorly on measures of verbal working memory. Arguably the most widely used standardized test battery for assessing receptive and expressive language skills is the Clinical Evaluation of Language Fundamentals (Semel, Wiig, & Secord, 2006), which comprises subtests tapping aspects of grammatical and semantic processing as well as verbal working memory. Since reading difficulties (affecting decoding, comprehension, or both) are so common in SLI, clinical assessment should also include evaluations of these skills.

A contentious issue is the extent to which SLI can truly be considered a *specific* disorder of language development. Although is it possible to find children with seemingly circumscribed language delays and difficulties, it is more often the case that the language impairment is accompanied by lower-than-average levels of nonverbal ability (Bishop, North, & Donlan, 1995), so it is not clear that the diagnostic requirement of a significant discrepancy between language development and nonverbal IQ is warranted. A complicating factor is that nonverbal IQ may fall with age among individuals with SLI (Botting, 2005; Stothard, Snowling, Bishop, Chipchase, & Kaplan, 1998). Such findings suggest that language difficulties can have a downstream effect on general cognitive ability. Moreover, SLI very often co-occurs with other learning and behavioral disorders and sensory impairments. In particular, there is a high degree of comorbidity between language impairments and reading disorders (Bishop & Snowling, 2004; Pennington, 2009b), developmental coordination disorder (Hill, 2001), and attention-deficit/hyperactivity disorder (ADHD) (Cohen, Davine, Horodezky, Lipsett, & Isaacson, 1993).

The present chapter aims to provide an overview of current knowledge concerning the nature of SLI; its behavioral manifestations across the lifespan; and variations in these manifestations, depending on the language a child speaks. There are several different theoretical approaches to SLI, and hence the research literature is both varied and complex. At the biological level, investigations have explored the genetic and neurobiological bases of the condition; we touch on these studies, but our main focus is on cognitive and linguistic explanations for the disorder. Broadly speaking, the linguistic approaches have focused on the language behaviors observed in SLI and have tended to test specific rather than alternative hypotheses. On the other hand, cognitive approaches have attempted to explain the underlying proximal causes of the disorder; to some extent, these approaches are guided by the language behaviors that are observed (see Morton & Frith, 1995, for a discussion of different levels of explanation for developmental disorders). Following a brief review of what is known about the neurobiology of SLI, we discuss the main theoretical approaches. We first review work following from a Chomskyean perspective, which has focused on grammatical aspects of SLI (particularly the use of inflections, passives, and complex syntax), and then proceed to discuss the primary cognitive explanations: SLI as a speed-of-processing impairment, an auditory processing impairment, and a phonological memory impairment. We also review a number of "hybrid" accounts that have tried to unite cognitive and linguistic theories before we consider the etiology of SLI and possible treatments. We close by discussing hypotheses that hold promise for integrating a diverse set of findings, and argue that future progress will require framing research within a developmental model of language development and disorder.

NATURE AND PREVALENCE

Depending on the precise criteria used for diagnosing SLI, different numbers of children will be identified, and the characteristics they show will vary. Prevalence estimates range from 3% to 6%, but are complicated by the fact that SLI is not a static condition (Bishop & Edmundson, 1987; Tomblin et al., 1997). As with many other developmental disorders, more males than females are affected with SLI (between 3:1 and 4:1), although the epidemiological study of Tomblin et al. (1997) reported a more even male–female ratio of 1.33:1.

Children with SLI constitute a heterogeneous group with a wide range of language difficulties. As noted above, There have been several attempts to specify subtypes of SLI, some based on clinical judgments and others on statistical approaches. Conti-Ramsden, Crutchley, and Botting (1997) used cluster analysis to identify five unique profiles of difficulty in a large sample of children attending language units in U.K. schools. Children with severe *expressive and receptive impairments* constituted the largest group of children and performed poorly on all language tests administered and in word reading. A group with *complex multiword deficits* had difficulties with word reading, grammar, and narrative skills, but relatively good phonology, and expressive vocabulary. A group with *expressive–phonological impairments* had adequate expressive vocabulary and comprehension, but poor word reading, phonology and narrative skills. The fourth group had poor expressive vocabulary but was otherwise similar to the group with expressive–phonological impairments. Finally, some children with adequate phonology, expressive vocabulary, comprehension of grammar, and word reading were considered by their teachers to have difficulties with the social use of language. This group was referred to as having *pragmatic language impairments* (PLI). Using a similar procedure, van Weerdenburg, Verhoeven, and van Balkom (2006) identified four clusters of Dutch-speaking children with SLI according to their performance on tasks tapping lexical–semantic abilities (including morphology), verbal sequential memory, speech production phonology, and auditory conceptualization.

Although there are synergies between the clusters of difficulties described by different researchers, it is difficult to draw parallels between studies—particularly if they include children speaking different languages, for whom the linguistic manifestations of SLI may change with age. For present purposes, we note that contemporary practice is to consider the problems of children with pure speech impairments (sometimes described as *speech sound disorder*) as experiencing a different form of disorder from those with language impairments (Bird, Bishop, & Freeman, 1995; Nathan, Stackhouse, Goulandris, & Snowling, 2004; Raitano, Pennington, Tunick, Boada, & Shriberg, 2004), and to differentiate children with classic impairments in the form and structure of language (SLI) from those who have deficits that are relatively restricted to its use for the purposes of communication (Bishop, 1997; Bishop & Norbury, 2002), now referred to as PLI (see above). Since children with PLI display some characteristics usually associated with autism, and since the region of overlap between autism and PLI is the subject of an increasing amount of research, we restrict our review to the more classic form of SLI.

NEUROBIOLOGY

Children with SLI do not typically show any detectable abnormality on gross inspection of the brain, which is puzzling. Given what is known about brain plasticity, any change in brain development in SLI is likely to be early and widespread, but of a nature that differentially affects language development and does not produce global cognitive dysfunction (i.e., intellectual disability). We currently lack a neurobiological model of SLI that adequately addresses this issue. The extant research findings suggest that subtle neurodevelopmental abnormalities primarily affecting left-hemisphere language systems may be implicated; unfortunately, however, progress in this field has been hampered by a lack of agreement surrounding diagnostic criteria and by the possible inclusion of individuals with comorbid disorders in study samples. In addition, it needs to be borne in mind that few studies have conducted comprehensive analyses, and frontal and temporal regions have attracted the most scrutiny (Leonard, Eckert, & Bishop, 2005).

There are now some studies that have used brain imaging or electrophysiological techniques to reveal converging evidence of abnormalities in brain structure and function in individuals with SLI. Abnormalities of structure have primarily been reported in frontal and perisylvian language regions of the cortex, most often on the left but sometimes bilaterally distributed. Fewer studies have investigated the basal ganglia, but here too damage or reduction in volume has been noted, as have changes bilaterally in the structure of the cerebellum. The smaller number of functional imaging studies tend to confirm patterns of under- or overactivation of these same areas during language-processing tasks (Ullman & Pierpont, 2005; Webster & Shevell, 2004).

Two sets of recent investigations deserve discussion because they have used more comprehensive methods of analysis. Studies of an extended family in which many members are affected by SLI with severe speech difficulties (the KE family) have compared affected and nonaffected family members (Belton, Salmond, Watkins, Vargha-Khadem, & Gadian, 2002; Vargha-Khadem et al., 1998; Watkins et al., 2002). In initial studies, Vargha-Khadem and colleagues reported reduced gray matter in Broca's left area; increased gray matter in left anterior insular and right sensory–motor cortex; changes in volume in regions of the basal ganglia and thalamus; and bilaterally increased gray matter in posterior temporal cortex and angular gyrus. Subsequent studies have broadly replicated this pattern of abnormalities, although detailed analyses reveal variability in the quantities of gray matter in different regions. One problem in generalizing from studies of the KE family is that it may not be representative of the population with SLI. The frequency of oral–motor impairments among family members is high, and their speech dyspraxia is more severe than is typically the case.

Leonard et al. (2002) compared brain structure in children with SLI to that of children with dyslexia. This research strategy is useful because it controls for the comorbidity of language and reading impairments. Building on earlier work that had identified four anatomical "risk factors" that distinguished people with dyslexia from controls (rightward cerebral asymmetry; leftward asymmetry of the anterior lobe of the cerebellum; combined leftward asymmetry of the planum and posterior ascending ramus of the sylvian fissure; and a large duplication of Heschl's gyrus on the left), Leonard et al. (2002) reported that the two groups did not differ on these factors, but that the children with SLI had a smaller surface area of Heschl's gyrus on the left, and that the planum temporale in these children tended to be symmetric.

The neuroscientific study of language impairment is still in its infancy; the findings to date suggest that brain development is atypical in SLI (though it should be noted that anatomical risk is sometimes seen in control brains). Moreover, a significant interpretive issue is the extent to which differences in brain structure and function are causes of language impairment. Although there are strong indications that differences in brain structure in SLI may be under genetic control, patterns of brain organization are likely to change over time as a function of language processing (Karmiloff-Smith, 1998; Mills & Neville, 1997). In particular, increases in brain volume and in brain activity in specific regions may reflect compensatory processes that children with SLI bring to bear in the attempt to overcome their communication impairment.

LANGUAGE DEVELOPMENT IN CHILDREN

Perhaps the most striking characteristic of the language of children with SLI is its delayed onset and slow rate of development. Whereas the majority of typically developing children produce their first words by about 11 months of age, the average age at which these emerge among those with language impairment is about 2 years, with multiword combinations occurring much later. In general, the lexical abilities of children with SLI are the least affected of their language skills, while their sentence grammar is the most impaired (Leonard, 1998). In addition, most children with SLI have some difficulties with phonology, although these difficulties are frequently resolved by school age.

The most common manifestation of the lexical problems that children with SLI have is a word-finding difficulty. The other lexical difficulty they exhibit is with the acquisition of verbs. Experimental studies have shown that new word learning takes longer for children with SLI than for typically developing controls (Rice, Oetting, Marquis, Bode, & Pae, 1994), and that verb acquisition is particularly problematic. It is possible that the problem with verbs is a consequence of syntactic difficulties, since their meaning is only apparent within a sentence frame, and it has been suggested that parsing sentences to learn new verbs may exceed the processing capacity of children with SLI (Leonard, 1998). Verb morphology also appears to present more difficulty than noun morphology, and the difficulty continues into the school years (Conti-Ramsden, Botting, & Faragher, 2001).

THEORETICAL APPROACHES

Research on SLI has primarily emanated from psychology and linguistics; the two disciplines have tended to focus on different features of the disorder and offer different theoretical explanations. At the outset, it is important to note that there are many competing theories of SLI, each positing a deficit in a single factor, and that so far none of these theories has proven to be adequate. This situation is not dissimilar to that for other developmental disorders reviewed in this book, notably autism and ADHD. Some experts in the field of SLI are starting to espouse a multiple-deficit approach to understanding SLI, as we discuss later.

One of the main theoretical accounts of SLI starts from the assumption that the mental representation of language is modular (Fodor, 1983) and operates independently of other cognitive functions. Within this view, SLI represents a deficit in linguistic (i.e., grammatical) knowledge. The alternative approach views language as an inherent aspect of cognition. Within this view, a grammatical deficit is likely to be the outcome of a deficit in the cognitive processes that underpin language (Ullman & Pierpont, 2005). Such cognitive deficit approaches can be broadly subdivided into "general" and "specific" processing accounts. The former invokes the notion of a general resource underlying all cognitive processing (Kail & Salthouse, 1994). Language is a complex operation that requires analysis of rapidly incoming signals; encoding and storage of large amounts of multilayered information (phonological, lexical, semantic, syntactic, pragmatic); and retrieval and automatic production of this same information. It is precisely the kind of task that should suffer in the face of limited processing capacity. At the same time, any other task that makes similarly complex demands should also suffer, and the presence in SLI of deficits in demanding motor or memory tasks, for example, is crucial to the arguments leveled by those espousing the concept of a general processing deficit.

The concept of a specific processing deficit, on the other hand, suggests a deficit in specific resources or processes that are necessary to language learning and functioning. For instance, impaired phonological memory could interfere with the consolidation of new lexical knowledge. Similarly, a deficit in auditory processing could affect speech perception, which in turn would have an impact on word acquisition and the development of sentence comprehension (Bishop, 1997).

Linguistic Arguments

Although the manifestations of SLI are variable, it is generally accepted that *morphosyntax* (the use of morphemes and word order to signal meaning) is an area of particular weakness for many of these children. English-speaking children with SLI use grammatical morphemes when they are obligatory much less frequently than younger typically developing children whose language is at a similar level in terms of mean length of utterance (MLU). The morphemes they find difficult include inflections that signal noun plural (-s), third-person singular (-s), and regular past tense (-ed), as well as forms of the verb *to be*, such as *am*, *is*, and *are* (Leonard, Bortolini, Caselli, McGregor, & Sabbadini, 1992; Rice, Wexler, & Cleave, 1995). However, it is important to note that children with SLI do use inflections occasionally, and then often correctly.

A number of different theories have been proposed to account for the difficulty that children with SLI have with inflectional morphology. Early theories proposed a type of "blindness" to grammatical features, leading children with SLI to learn grammatical constructions as unanalyzed wholes (Gopnik, 1990), or to an inability on their behalf to acquire implicit rules to mark tense, aspect, number, person, case, and so on (Gopnik & Crago, 1991). Much of the evidence was tied into a wider debate regarding single- versus dual-route accounts of inflectional morphology. According to dual-route theories (e.g., Pinker, 1999), irregular verbs are learned by rote and stored on an item-by-item basis in an associative memory system, and their retrieval is consequently susceptible to the effects of frequency (more frequently occurring items should be retrieved more quickly and accurately). Regular verbs, on the other hand, should be impervious to the effects of frequency, because they are inflected by the implicit rule "Add -ed." However, claims of an inability to learn grammatical rules in SLI are threatened when behavior associated with rule use is found in individuals with SLI. It follows that the overapplication of the past-tense rule should not be found in SLI; contrary to this, such overgeneralization has been reported by Leonard et al. (1992) and Vargha-Khadem, Watkins, Alcock, Fletcher, and Passingham (1995).

Structural Relationship Accounts

A different type of linguistic approach to SLI emphasizes a higher-level deficit in relating morphological paradigms correctly, rather than in acquiring them. This deficit, referred to as the *representational deficit for dependent relations* (RDDR; van der Lely, 1994), predicts difficulties with agreement and tense marking. It also predicts problems in the use and comprehension of sentences that rely on long-distance syntactic relationships, such as passives (e.g., "The boy is chased by the girl") and those containing pronouns (e.g., "Baloo Bear says Mowgli is tickling him" (van der Lely & Harris, 1990). Children with SLI have striking difficulties with these types of sentence (Norbury, Bishop, & Briscoe, 2002; van der Lely & Stollwerck, 1997). A recent development of the RDDR account broadens its remit to include deficits in other components of language—specifically, those that are structurally complex and hierarchically organized. According to the *computational grammatical complexity* hypothesis (van der Lely, 2005), the heterogeneity seen in SLI is due to deficits in complex computation in at least one of three rule-governed systems. Thus, although syntactic, morphological, and phonological deficits are independent, deficits in these systems may have cumulative effects. For example, Marshall and van der Lely (2006) showed that inflected verb forms containing consonant clusters (e.g., *jumped*—/pt/) are more likely to have the inflection omitted than forms without a cluster (e.g., *sewed*).

The Extended Optional Infinitive Hypothesis

The *extended optional infinitive* (EOI) hypothesis for SLI has its roots in the pattern of typical linguistic development. It follows from Wexler's (1994, 1996) observation that tense marking is a part of the grammar that is particularly slow to emerge in typically-developing children; thus children remain within what is known at the *optional infinitive* stage, during which time the use of these markers is an optional feature in the child's grammar. The EOI hypothesis makes specific predictions about the types of morphemes that will be affected in SLI, primarily the past-tense inflection -ed and the third person singular.

According to Rice and Wexler (1996), children with SLI use immature grammar for a longer period than unaffected children do; they also ultimately use tense-marking morphemes correctly about 50% of the time, compared to over 90% for age-matched controls. Moreover, children with SLI do not catch up to their peers in their use of tense-marking morphemes, so that while most children reach adult levels of usage by 5 years of age, one might still hear a child with SLI at age 8 say, "Granny see me" (Rice, Wexler, & Hershberger, 1998). Problems with tense-marking morphemes are present in comprehension (as tested by grammaticality judgments) as well as production (Rice, Wexler, & Redmond, 1999). Rice and colleagues go on to propose that children with SLI can be identified with high accuracy according to their performance on tests that require the generation of these morphemic markers. A recent independent evaluation of four different types of markers for SLI indeed found the elicitation of past-tense inflection to be particularly sensitive (Conti-Ramsden et al., 2001).

The EOI approach provides quite a convincing account of the patterns of morphosyntactic deficits reported for SLI in English. However, the last decade has seen a burgeoning of cross-linguistic research, and much of the resulting evidence does not sit comfortably either with the original formulation of the EOI hypothesis or with other linguistic accounts of SLI that have focused on English.

Cross-Linguistic Evidence

One of the most striking findings to emerge from studies of SLI in different languages is that although verb morphology is central to the SLI phenotype in English and other Germanic languages, it is relatively unaffected in the Romance languages. For example, Italian-speaking children with SLI are similar to younger MLU-matched children in their comprehension and use of verb inflections, as well as adjective agreement and noun plural inflections, although this level is lower than that of age-matched controls (Leonard et al., 1992). Rather than inflections, the areas of particular difficulty for Italian-speaking children with SLI are function words, such as articles (the, a, an) (Leonard et al., 1992).

In a similar vein, the use of verb inflections is relatively robust for Spanish-speaking children with SLI (Bedore & Leonard 2001, 2005); in contrast, these children have problems with noun-related morphemes, such as inflections indicating adjective agreement. Interestingly, in Spanish, errors are often substitutions that share most of the target's features, rather than the omissions usually reported in other languages. Interesting parallels also emerge from the study of Hebrew, which is an inflectionally rich language that is very different from Romance and Germanic languages in the form of its inflections (e.g., Dromi, Leonard, Adam, & Zadunaisky-Ehrlich, 1999; Dromi, Leonard, & Shteiman, 1993).

In general, evidence from a wide range of languages—including Italian, Spanish, and Hebrew, but also French, German, Greek, Swedish, and most recently Cantonese—suggests that many of these languages pose far fewer problems in inflectional morphology for children with SLI than English does. This creates a challenge for linguistic accounts of SLI if the proximal deficit is to be placed at the level of universal grammatical structures. The concept of the extended unique checking constraint (EUCC; Wexler, 1998) is an elaboration of the EOI hypothesis that attempts to take the differing grammatical profiles of languages other than English into account. While still focusing on the optional marking of tense and agreement, it suggests that children with SLI are able to "check" only one of these two features at any given time. The consequences differ across languages, because the relationship between tense and agreement marking differs. Recent work has tested some of the specific predictions made by the EUCC hypothesis in Swedish and Spanish, and the results have been generally compatible with this account (Bedore & Leonard, 2005; Leonard, Hansson, Nettelbladt, & Deevy, 2004).

The Surface Hypothesis

Based in cross-linguistic research on typical language acquisition (Bates & MacWhinney, 1987), the surface hypothesis suggests that "surface" factors, such as perceptual salience, redundancy, relative frequency, pronounceability, and regularity, are important in determining which aspects of a particular language will be most robust in the face of limited processing resources. In English, many grammatical morphemes are low in surface features, and appear in the speech of normally developing children acquiring English later than in children acquiring other languages. It seems plausible, then, that these morphemes are already vulnerable in English because of their surface properties, and that the problems children with SLI have with them are attributable to these same surface properties rather than to their grammatical identity.

Even within grammatical morphology, some morphemes are more vulnerable than others. As discussed above, it is well documented that English-speaking children with SLI have particular problems with the past-tense -ed and third-person-singular -s inflections (Leonard, 1989). These are all morphemes with short duration relative to the words surrounding them. Contrastingly, the progressive inflection -ing does not seem to pose particular difficulty; it is of much longer duration than the morphemes noted above, especially when it is in phrase-final position (which occurs far more frequently than for the other morphemes).

The typology of the language (and the consequent predictions of which elements are likely to be most vulnerable) is only half of the equation, however. The other half is the presumed mental processing limitation in the child. The surface hypothesis posits a reduced speed of processing, which prevents the morpheme in question from being fully processed before the next element in the speech stream comes along; this is particularly important for morphemes of brief duration.

Support for the surface hypothesis has come from a range of studies, both in English and across languages (Leonard, 1998). A neat illustration in English contrasts morphemes of low phonetic substance (past-tense -ed and third-person-singular -s) and high phonetic substance (present-progressive -ing). In both an online reaction time (RT) task and an offline grammaticality judgment task, children with SLI demonstrated sensitivity to morphemes with high but not low phonetic substance (Montgomery & Leonard, 1998). This pattern was particularly marked in the online task, and it is possible that school-age children with SLI may be able to form a normal morphological paradigm including nonsalient morphemes, but that the pressure of online processing is what causes these fragile morphemes to drop off in production and real-time processing (e.g., Leonard & Deevy, 2003).

Cognitive Accounts

General processing accounts of SLI are concerned with the efficiency with which complex mental operations—such as language—can be carried out. The two interacting elements of efficiency are capacity and speed; the faster an operation can be carried out, the less mental space it occupies. An inefficient system (such as that posited in SLI) can be constrained in terms of either speed or capacity.

Capacity Limitation

Much of the evidence used to argue for a general capacity limitation in SLI comes from tradeoffs between performance and task complexity observed during language-processing tasks. In spoken language production, word omissions and errors increase with sentence complexity, and this effect is more marked in children with SLI than in younger children with similar language levels. In experimental tasks, children with SLI show difficulties with fast mapping and novel word learning, and these difficulties are exacerbated at faster rates of presentation (Ellis Weismer & Hesketh, 1996). They are also slower at word recognition and demonstrate inefficient sentence comprehension (Montgomery, 2000). One of the most thoroughly explored areas of weakness is verbal and phonological working memory (discussed in more detail below), and it is now well established that many children with SLI have difficulty with nonword repetition and listening span tasks (Ellis Weismer, Evans, & Hesketh, 1999).

If a general capacity limitation rather than a language-specific impairment is involved in SLI, then deficits should also be apparent in complex nonlinguistic tasks in this population. This possibility has been underexplored, but there are some recent results pointing to poor visual–spatial recall in SLI, and to poor coordination of resources across modalities in a dual-processing paradigm, suggesting limitations in central executive function (Hoffman & Gillam, 2004).

Reduced Speed of Information Processing

Complementing the evidence suggestive of general capacity limitations, there is also a substantial amount of research showing that children with SLI tend to be slower (generally as gauged with an RT measure) than their peers on a wide range of tasks. Nonverbal examples range from mental rotation to peg moving (Johnston & Ellis Weismer, 1983), whereas verbal tasks include word monitoring (Stark & Montgomery, 1995), picture naming (Lahey & Edwards, 1996), and grammaticality judgments (Bates, Dick, & Wulfeck, 1999).

These findings led to the proposal of a generalized slowing hypothesis (Kail, 1994), which suggests that children with SLI are slower by a constant proportion than their typically developing peers at processing each component of any given task. For example, picture naming may be broken down into a number of different steps: recognizing the picture, retrieving its name, and producing the phonological output. In two meta-analyses of RT data from children with SLI, it was shown that a proportional function could account for 96% of the variance across a range of linguistic and nonlinguistic tasks; the proportion of general slowing was estimated at between 20% and 30% (Kail, 1994). In the largest study to date to examine the issue of generalized slowing, Miller, Kail, Leonard, and Tomblin (2001) directly compared RT data across a range of linguistic and nonlinguistic tasks for the same group of children. These authors compared children with SLI and IQ-matched controls, as well as a group of children with nonspecific language impairment (NLI). Both language-impaired groups were slower than the control group across the board, but the group with NLI showed significantly greater slowing (at 30%) than the group with SLI (20%).

If reduced speed of processing is causally involved in SLI, it should be possible to influence language performance by manipulating the speed of stimulus presentation. There is a limited amount of evidence that slowing the input rate is an effective means of boosting children's performance. For example, expanding the speech signal can improve performance of children with SLI on both an online word recognition task and an offline sentence comprehension task (Montgomery, 2004, 2005), although contrary results have been reported by Bishop, Adams, and Rosen (2006). Perhaps the best-known example of this general approach is the FastForWord intensive intervention program, in which the least salient parts of the speech signal are selectively expanded and amplified (Scientific Learning Corporation, 1997). However, there are mixed reports on the efficacy of this program, and particularly on whether it is more effective than intervention programs that do not manipulate the input rate (e.g., Gillam et al., 2008; Gillam, Loeb, & Friel-Patti, 2001).

A novel experimental approach was recently used to "model" SLI in children with typically developing language (Hayiou-Thomas, Bishop, & Plunkett, 2004). Using compressed speech stimuli in a grammaticality judgment task resulted in the pattern of errors reported in SLI: good performance on noun morphology (plural –s), and very poor performance on verb morphology (past-tense -ed, and third-person-singular -s). Similar results were obtained in a condition increasing memory load. The finding that an SLI-like pattern of performance can be induced in children with intact linguistic systems by increasing processing demands provides strong support for the idea that a processing deficit may underlie language performance in SLI.

In summary, the available evidence suggests that many children with SLI do have reduced processing capacity and speed, and it also seems plausible that such a reduction could in principle have an impact on language acquisition and function.

Auditory Processing Deficits

One of the most influential accounts of SLI proposes low-level auditory processing deficits, which negatively affect language development by compromising speech perception. Much of the work in this area was originally motivated by the research of Tallal and colleagues, who used a procedure now known as the *auditory repetition task* (ART), in which children repeat a sequence of tones by using a button-press response. Children with SLI had difficulty with this task when the tones were brief (75 ms) and the interstimulus interval between the tones was short (150 ms or less; Tallal & Piercy, 1973). This finding was interpreted as evidence for a temporal processing deficit in SLI, which impairs integration of sensory information that impinges on the nervous system in rapid succession. Speech, which by its nature comprises rapidly changing sequences of auditory information, is thus very vulnerable. Consistent with this idea, Tallal (1980) went on to show that children with SLI had difficulty repeating sequences of stop consonants (e.g., /ba/ and /da/), in which the critical contrast occurs in the first few milliseconds of voicing, but performed better on sequences of vowels that were longer in duration.

A different paradigm that has been useful in this area is *auditory backward recognition masking* (ABRM). In this task, a masking sound interrupts the processing of features of the test tones that have preceded it; this effect is particularly strong when the interval between test tone and masker is short. In a comparison of 8-year-old children with SLI and age-matched controls, Wright et al. (1997) found a dramatic group difference in ABRM thresholds. However, when the frequency difference between the tone and the masker was increased, the performance of the group with SLI improved to control levels. This raises the possibility that the auditory deficit in SLI is in the processing of spectral (frequency) information, rather than—or in addition to—temporal information. In support of this proposition, there have been several recent reports that frequency discrimination may be problematic for at least a subgroup of children with SLI (Hill, Hogben, & Bishop, 2005; McArthur & Bishop, 2004; Mengler, Hogben, Michie, & Bishop, 2005).

One of the few studies to look at several indices of central auditory processing in the same individuals was reported by Bishop, Carlyon, Deeks, and Bishop (1999b), who estimated thresholds for detecting backward-masked tones, frequency modulation, and pitch discrimination using temporal cues, and compared these with earlier performance on the ART. A reliable relationship was found, suggesting that the measures were tapping into the same auditory process, which remained stable over time. However, none of the measures (apart from the ART) were able to discriminate between children with SLI and controls.

In short, psychoacoustic studies have been suggestive of a deficit in SLI in processing either temporal or spectral information, but there have also been many negative findings; furthermore, the link between poor auditory processing skills and language outcome is far from clear (Rosen, 2003). A similarly mixed picture emerges from the literature using electrophysiological measures to examine the neural correlates of auditory processing in SLI. Some groups have reported group differences in components of the event-related potential (ERP) that correspond to detection of an auditory stimulus (e.g., Tonnquist-Uhlen, 1996), while others have failed to find reliable differences (e.g., Marler, Champlin, & Gillam, 2002; Neville, Coffey, Holcomb, & Tallal, 1993). A different component of the ERP, the mismatch negativity, indexes the ability to distinguish between two different sounds, rather than just to detect them. Here too, results have been inconsistent, with some groups reporting a diminished mismatch negativity in SLI and others not (see Bishop, 2007, for a review).

There are a number of possible reasons why the literature in this field is so inconsistent. The first is that SLI is a heterogeneous disorder, and it is possible that auditory deficits are implicated in some but not all children with SLI. For example, both behavioral evidence (Heath, Hogben, & Clark, 1999) and ERP evidence (Bishop & McArthur, 2004) suggest that auditory deficits may be most apparent in children who have difficulties in both oral language and literacy. A second possibility is that the profile of auditory deficits may depend on the age at which children are tested, since the auditory system continues to mature into adolescence. Following findings that the brain waveforms of many children with SLI resemble those of younger children, Bishop and McArthur (2005) have suggested that there may be a maturational delay in cortical processing of auditory stimuli. In this context, it is particularly interesting to note that at least two independent longitudinal studies have found auditory processing deficits in infancy to be predictive of later language skills (Benasich, Curtiss, & Tallal, 1993). A third possibility is that the auditory deficits in SLI do not involve low-level perception per se, but rather efficient extraction of speech-critical features from a noisy background; it may be that many studies underestimate such effects because stimuli are typically presented in optimal listening conditions, which lack ecological validity (Ziegler, Pech-George, George, Alario, & Lorenz, 2005). Finally, it is possible that auditory processing deficits may be a "synergistic risk factor" for language impairment (Bishop et al., 1999a). That is, they may be neither necessary nor sufficient to explain language difficulties, but they may exert a moderating influence when children are already at genetic risk of language disorder.

Phonological Memory Deficit

In contrast to accounts proposing general processing deficits, the phonological memory account of SLI focuses on an information-processing system that is specific to language. This account was first proposed by Gathercole and Baddeley (1990), who examined the proficiency of verbal working memory processes in SLI. The performance of a group of children with SLI was unimpaired on tests of speech discrimination and articulation rate, and they showed the normal effect of word length, with memory for long words poorer than that for short words. However, the group with SLI was less sensitive to the phonetic similarity effect at longer list lengths than either age-matched or younger vocabulary-matched controls. They also showed impairments of nonword repetition relative to the age-matched, but not the vocabulary-matched, controls. The authors concluded that the central deficit in SLI was in the ability to represent material in phonological form in working memory. In subsequent work, Gathercole and colleagues have argued that children need the capacity to store phonological material in short-term memory to learn new words (Baddeley, Gathercole, & Papagno, 1998). Thus individual differences in phonological memory are predictors of the ability to learn new vocabulary in the native language, as well as to learn a foreign language (Service, 1992). The corollary of this is that the phonological memory impairments observed in SLI will constrain vocabulary development with consequences for language comprehension.

In the last decade, research from several different groups has confirmed the presence of nonword repetition deficits in many children with SLI (Bishop et al., 1995; Dollaghan & Campbell, 1998). In line with Gathercole's proposal, poor performance on nonword repetition, even when low-level auditory processing skills are controlled for, accounts for significant variance in a range of language measures, including Wechsler Intelligence Scale for Children—Third Edition (WISC-III) Comprehension (a measure of the ability to explain social conventions, which loads on the Verbal Comprehension factor of the WISC-III), receptive grammar, and expressive language tests tapping word finding and sentence repetition (Bishop et al., 1999a). Along with past-tense elicitation, nonword repetition has been found to be an excellent marker of SLI, discriminating children diagnosed with SLI with a high degree of accuracy (Conti-Ramsden et al., 2001); it is also a more effective marker of language impairment than standardized language tests for ethnic minority populations and for those who speak nonstandard dialects (Dollaghan & Campbell, 1998). Nonword repetition tasks not only are good concurrent markers of language problems, but are also sensitive to residual deficits in individuals whose earlier language impairments appear to have resolved, and to subclinical deficits in the family members of children with SLI (Bishop et al., 1995). Finally, nonword repetition ability has been shown to be robustly heritable in twin studies (Bishop et al., 1999a; Kovas et al., 2005), and a chromosomal region likely to be linked to poor nonword repetition has been identified on chromosome 16 (SLI Consortium, 2002, 2004).

Nonetheless, though few would disagree with the conclusion that children with SLI are impaired in the processes involved in phonological representation, the evidence that a phonological memory deficit is central implies a causal relation that is more equivocal.

The link between phonological memory and vocabulary growth could in principle go in either direction. Gathercole's account suggests that in learning new words, children have to hold the item in phonological store without the support of a long-term memory representation (although there would be some support from phonotactic knowledge of permissible phoneme sequences in the language). An alternative view is that with vocabulary growth, phonological representation become more segmental (Metsala, 1999); as a consequence, processes involved in the analysis of words in the incoming speech stream are more finely tuned to allow more effective encoding, and hence better nonword repetition.

Recently, Gathercole, Tiffany, Briscoe, Thorn, and the ALSPAC Team (2005) directly tested the causal hypothesis that nonword repetition taps a primitive learning mechanism critical for word learning by following a cohort of children from age 5 to age 8 years. Contrary to prediction, many children with poor nonword repetition abilities went on to show normal vocabulary at the age of 8. Further evidence refuting the strong version of the hypothesis comes from dissociations between nonword repetition and vocabulary knowledge, and from the finding that nonword repetition deficits are not universal in children with SLI (Catts, Adlof, Hogan, & Ellis Weismer, 2005). In response to these findings, Gathercole (2006) has presented a revised version of the causal hypothesis, emphasizing that nonword repetition performance is subject to constraints in auditory, phonological, and speech–motor processes. She went on to outline a framework comprising the key phonological processes contributing to nonword repetition (and new word learning)—auditory processing, phonological analysis, speech–motor planning, phonological output processes, the quality of phonological representations, and phonological storage—with a range of factors affecting each stage of these processes (hearing loss, phonotactic frequency, stimulus length, and articulatory complexity).

DEVELOPMENTAL COURSE

Language Outcomes

Studies investigating both the relatively short-term and longer-term consequences of SLI suggest that between about 50% and 90% of children continue to exhibit language difficulties through childhood. Nevertheless, in cases where language difficulties are mild or very specific in form (e.g., circumscribed speech difficulties), such outcomes do not appear to be inevitable. Bishop and Edmundson (1987) found that among 87 preschoolers who exhibited speech–language impairments at 4 years, the language impairments of 37% (including those with isolated phonological impairments) had resolved 18 months later, at 5½ years. Among those with SLI (whose nonverbal IQ was in the normal range), there was a good outcome for 44%, whereas 89% of children classified as showing general developmental delays continued to show language difficulties. Three language tests (narrative requiring the expression of semantic relationships, picture naming, and a test of expressive semantics and syntax), together with nonverbal IQ, predicted outcome status correctly for 86% of the children. Given the central role of language skills in educational attainment, it is not surprising that academic difficulties are common in those with a history of speech–language impairment (Aram, Ekelman, & Nation, 1984). This is true even when nonverbal intelligence is within the normal range and oral language difficulties resolve (Snowling, Adams, Bishop, & Stothard, 2001). However, the poorest educational outcomes are observed for children whose language difficulties persist, and for these children, a decline in both verbal and nonverbal IQ scores has been observed (Botting, 2005; Mawhood, Howlin, & Rutter, 2000; Stothard et al., 1998; Tomblin, Freese, & Records, 1992).

Reading Outcomes

Reading disorders are common sequelae of language impairments, and hence there has been a tendency in recent years to group these disorders together under the umbrella term of *language-learning impairments*. This practice fails to take account of the fact that different language impairments are risk factors for different component reading skills (Snowling & Hulme, 2005). First, it is important to separate the effects of speech impairments from those of broader language difficulties; there is good evidence, for example, that peripheral speech difficulties carry a low risk of reading problems. In the case of speech sound disorder affecting the phonological system of language, the literature presents a mixed picture, with some studies finding that the speech disorder affects reading development (Bird et al., 1995; Stackhouse & Snowling, 1992), and others refuting this hypothesis (Bishop & Adams, 1990; Catts, 1993).

In a study aimed at disentangling the effects of speech and of language difficulties on literacy outcome, Nathan et al. (2004) followed the progress of children with primary expressive speech difficulties from the ages of 4 to 6 years, comparing those with pure speech difficulties and those with wider language difficulties. The risk of literacy difficulties was greater in the group with speech and language difficulties, and the literacy problems of these children were mediated by deficits in the development of phoneme awareness (rather than speech perception or speech production processes). Somewhat different results were reported by Raitano et al. (2004), who investigated the preliteracy skills of children with speech sound disorder. In spite of the fact that the speech problems of many of these children had resolved by 5 years, 8 months, many showed deficits in phonological awareness, which arguably presage literacy problems. One possible reason for the discrepancy of findings emerging from different groups may be the types of speech disorders represented in different samples. Importantly, Leitão, Hogben, and Fletcher (1997) found that only those with deviant speech processes showed poor phonological awareness, whereas those who showed normal but delayed speech did not.

In a study of children with more classic forms of SLI, Bishop and Adams (1990) examined reading prognosis at 8½ years in relation to the age at which preschool language impairments resolve. Children whose language impairments had resolved by 5½ years did not show reading difficulties, whereas those with persisting language impairments had reading problems. Interestingly, their problems were not of reading accuracy but of poor reading comprehension scores in relation to Performance IQ (see Catts, Fey, Tomblin, & Zhang, 2002, for similar findings). In a longer-term follow-up of the cohort, Stothard et al. (1998) assessed literacy outcomes at 15 years of age. As a group, adolescents with a preschool history of SLI performed less well on tests of reading, spelling, and reading comprehension than an age-matched control sample, and the proportion of children in the sample who now fulfilled criteria for dyslexia had increased from 6% at 8 years to 24% (Snowling, Bishop, & Stothard, 2000). Thus, even though these children had made a good start with literacy development, their later progress had been less good. The subgroup of children who had persisting SLI at 8½ years had pervasive problems with word-level reading and reading comprehension at 15 years, and their spelling was weak.

In summary, children with SLI are at high risk of reading and spelling problems, but the skills that predict literacy outcomes continue to be debated. Bishop and Snowling (2004) have proposed a two-dimensional model to explain a continuum of risk for literacy impairment. The core dimension of risk for decoding problems is in phonology; however, the impact of phonological difficulties can be modified by broader language skills (e.g., vocabulary and comprehension processes).

Catts et al. (2005) directly tested the hypothesis that there are continuities between SLI and dyslexia in terms of deficiencies in phonological skill. In this study, using research diagnoses of SLI in kindergarten and dyslexia in 4th grade, they contrasted four groups of children: (1) SLI with dyslexia, (2) SLI without dyslexia, (3) dyslexia without SLI, or (4) neither SLI nor dyslexia. In essence, the pattern of performance on tests tapping phoneme awareness and phonological memory skills reflected a dyslexia diagnosis: Children with dyslexia did significantly worse on phonological tasks than children who did not have reading difficulties, regardless of whether or not they had SLI. In contrast, the children with SLI who were free of reading problems did not show phonological difficulties. Catts et al.'s (2005) findings clarify that children with SLI carry the risk of dyslexia if they have problems in phonological processing, whereas children with SLI who do not have phonological impairments are more likely to succumb to reading comprehension impairments (e.g., as seen in PLI).

Psychosocial Outcomes

Evidence from both cross-sectional and prospective longitudinal studies of children with speech–language disorders indicates that there is a heightened risk of psychiatric disorder in children with these disorders (Beitchman, Cohen, Konstantareas, & Tannock, 1996). Moreover, more than half of referrals to psychiatric services are of children with language difficulties, many of whom are previously undiagnosed (Cohen et al., 1993). However, as with reading outcomes, it appears that some forms of language impairment carry greater risk of psychosocial difficulty, and not all psychiatric disorders are prevalent in language-impaired populations. Furthermore, the different trajectories between language impairment and psychiatric outcome may be gender-related, with an increased risk of ADHD in boys and of emotional disorders in girls.

Baker and Cantwell (1982) were the first to report that the risk of psychiatric morbidity is lower in those with speech disorders than in those with language difficulties. There is also some evidence of an association between lack of improvement in speech–language functioning and the development of a psychiatric disorder (Beitchman et al., 1996; Benasich et al., 1993). Similar findings were reported by Snowling, Bishop, Stothard, Chipchase, and Kaplan (2006), who examined the psychosocial outcomes in adolescence of the cohort with SLI recruited by Bishop and Edmundson (1987) at 4 years of age. Overall, the rates of psychopathology were low in this sample, particularly in children whose language difficulties had resolved by the age of 5½ years. The main presenting problems of adolescents with persistent SLI were attention control difficulties and social impairments. These problems were somewhat independent of each other, and the language profiles of affected children differed: Attention problems tended to be associated with specific expressive language difficulties, and social problems with both receptive and expressive impairments. The comorbid pattern of attention and social problems was associated with globally delayed cognitive development. In line with the view that learning difficulties may mediate between SLI and behavioral problems, the children with SLI and the poorest psychosocial outcomes in adolescence also had the poorest literacy skills.

In a similar vein, Mawhood et al. (2000) reported poor prognosis into adulthood for boys with receptive language disorders. None of the young men in this study had passed U.K. national examinations, and although 13 of the 19 had been in prolonged employment, they were mainly engaged in manual or unskilled jobs. A comparison group of children with autistic disorders had a comparatively better prognosis, possibly because they had been educated in specialist settings attuned to their needs. Such placement was rare for the children with SLI (see Clegg, Hollis, Mawhood & Rutter, 2005, for a longer-term study).

In summary, preschool language difficulties are frequently the precursors of language and academic difficulties that persist throughout childhood and adolescence, but there is substantial variation in outcome. Nonverbal IQ appears to be an important protective factor, such that children with higher ability tend to have better outcomes in all domains. More pessimistically, there is accumulating evidence suggesting that nonverbal IQ scores decline with age among children with persistent SLI, and that this lowering of IQ may have wide-ranging consequences for adaptive functioning not only in school but through adult life.

ETIOLOGY

Quantitative Genetics

Behavioural genetic studies of language impairment suggest that it is a heritable disorder, but that the extent of genetic influence differs according to children's language and cognitive profile. Several twin studies have demonstrated that when SLI is considered categorically, more monozygotic twin pairs are concordant for the disorder than dizygotic twins, consistent with genetic influence (Bishop, North, & Donlan, 1995; DeThorne et al., 2006; Lewis & Thompson, 1992; Tomblin & Buckwalter, 1998). However, these studies have drawn primarily on clinically referred samples. A recent report from a large representative study of twins in the U.K. suggests that SLI is strongly heritable *only* in children who have attracted clinical concern and who have speech difficulties in addition to language problems. By contrast, equally severe language difficulties in the absence of speech problems have mainly environmental etiology (Bishop & Hayiou-Thomas, 2008). Nonverbal ability also plays a role: if definitional criteria are broadened to include children with NLI (i.e., children who may have low nonverbal skills in addition to the language deficit) concordance rates are increased for monozygotic pairs and decreased for dizygotic pairs, suggesting even stronger genetic effects (Bishop, 1994; Hayiou-Thomas, Oliver, & Plomin, 2005).

Twin studies have also shown significant genetic influence on quantitatively assessed language skills, both in the normal range and at the low extremes (Bishop, Adams, & Norbury, 2006; Kovas et al., 2005; Spinath, Price, Dale, & Plomin, 2004; Stromswold, 2001). In two recent studies that included a wide range of language measures in large samples of preschool children, there was consistent evidence of at least moderate genetic effects on diverse areas of preschoolers' language skills, from syntax to phonology (Byrne et al., 2002; Kovas et al., 2005). However, there is also some evidence that genetic effects may be weaker, and environmental effects stronger, for vocabulary (Bishop et al., 2005; Byrne et al., 2002) and that some of the strongest genetic effects are apparent for deficits in expressive rather than receptive language skills, and also for deficits in articulation (e.g., Kovas et al. 2005). This is consistent with the findings described above, of higher heritability for SLI in the context of additional speech problems.

Relatively few studies have considered the etiological interrelationships between different components of language. A recent series of multivariate analyses from the Twins Early Development Study in the United Kingdom has found substantial genetic overlap for vocabulary and grammar, both on parental report measures for 2- and 3-year-olds (Dionne, Dale, Bovin, & Plomin, 2003), and in direct psychometric assessments of 4½-year-olds (Hayiou-Thomas et al., 2006). At the same time, it seems that there may be an etiological dissociation between phonology and broader oral language skills, including semantics and syntax; this seems to be the case not only at the individual-differences level, but even more dramatically at the extremes (Bishop et al., 2005). The study by Bishop et al. focused on 6-year-old twins with language impairment, and explicitly compared two of the most sensitive markers for SLI: nonword repetition and the past-tense elicitation task. Although poor performance on both of these was highly heritable, there was no genetic overlap between them, showing striking evidence of etiological heterogeneity in SLI.

Molecular Genetics

Quantitative genetic studies have been informative in confirming that there is genetic influence on SLI, and in pointing to the components of the language system that are most likely to mediate this genetic effect. The next step is to identify the actual genes involved. A dramatic step forward in this quest was the discovery of the FOXP2 mutation in the KE family (Lai, Fisher, Hurst, Vargha-Khadem, & Monaco, 2001). The well-described speech and language deficits in this family have been a transmitted in a way consistent with a single-gene autosomal pattern of inheritance, making the challenge of identifying the mutation a much more tractable one than it otherwise would have been. The FOXP2 mutation on chromosome 7 was present in all 15 family members with the speech and language impairment, and not present in the unaffected family members, thus making it both a necessary and sufficient cause of the language impairment in the KE family. As noted earlier, however, the KE family, although initially described in terms of specific grammatical deficits (Gopnik, 1990), has an unusual type of speech and language impairment that includes deficits in oral–facial motor control and is not typical of SLI.

However, recent work suggests that FOXP2 regulates the expression of a different gene (CNTNAP2) which may be involved in more typical cases of SLI (Vernes et al., 2008). Although FOXP2 will almost certainly provide important clues into the mechanisms underlying speech and language, it is unlikely that any single-gene explanation will account for most common cases of SLI. Instead, it seems increasingly likely that common disorders are complexly determined by multiple genes and multiple environmental factors (Rutter, 2005). This perspective is in line with the quantitative trait locus (QTL) hypothesis, which suggests that a continuum of risk associated with multiple genes underlies a continuum of variation in behavior in the population, and that common disorders (such as SLI) lie at one extreme of this normal variation.

Genome screens in linkage studies of SLI have so far identified four potential QTLs (chromosomal regions linked to a disorder): SLI1 on chromosome 16q, SLI2 on chromosome 19q, SLI3 on chromosome 13q, and SSD on chromosome 3p. These QTLs vary in terms of the phenotype to which they are linked. SLI1 appears to be linked specifically to nonword repetition deficits, a finding that was replicated when the original sample was expanded (SLI Consortium, 2002, 2004). SLI2 was originally linked to more general expressive language deficits, as defined by poor scores on the Clinical Evaluation of Language Fundamentals—Revised (SLI Consortium, 2002), but in a second study it was found to be linked instead to nonword repetition (SLI Consortium, 2004). SSD on chromosome 3p was identified in a sample of children with speech sound disorder rather than SLI; the linkage here was to articulation and phonology (including nonword repetition) factors (Stein et al., 2004). Although it is still early days, this work supports the idea that SLI is a multifactorial disorder, and that some of the heterogeneity seen at the behavioral level may be reflected in the genetic etiology. It also suggests that at least one of the component processes likely to be involved in SLI, phonological memory, may be a promising place to begin tracing the complex pathways from genotype to phenotype (Newbury, Bishop, & Monaco, 2005).

Finally, it is worth noting that genetic evidence may well help to elucidate the causes of comorbidity between SLI and other developmental disorders. For example, at least two of the putative QTLs for SLI have also been linked to autistic symptomatology, an important part of which is communication impairment (Bartlett, Goedken, & Vieland, 2005). Moreover, multivariate analyses of the SLI1 locus on chromosome 16 have shown consistent linkage with nonword repetition, and also linkage to measures of single-word reading and spelling (Newbury et al., 2005). This constitutes some of the earliest molecular genetic evidence for the proposal that SLI and dyslexia share a core phonological deficit, which in SLI is accompanied by additional oral language deficits (Bishop & Snowling, 2004). It also provides a neat illustration of how genetics and cognitive psychology can complement each other in the search for the causes of complex disorders like SLI.

Environmental Factors

Much of the research on environmental factors that influence language development has focused on the normal range of variation, rather than addressing the etiology of SLI directly. Nonetheless, it is likely that at least some of the same variables will contribute to risk status for SLI. One plausible candidate is the quality of the linguistic environment provided in the home: Parents' speaking directly to children, encouraging them to talk, and using decontextualized language and a diverse and complex vocabulary themselves are all linked to larger vocabularies in children (e.g., Hart & Risley, 1995). In addition, maternal responsiveness is predictive of a child's language skills, including the timing of very early milestones in expressive language. Note that the quality of the linguistic environment is often confounded with broader environmental factors like socioeconomic status (SES) (Hart & Risley, 1995), and that SES is not purely environmental, because an individual's SES is partly determined by genetically influenced factors (e.g., intelligence and personality). So the correlation between parent and child language could be partly mediated by genes, as discussed below.

Another frequently cited environmental variable that may affect language development is otitis media with effusion, an infection of the middle ear that is very prevalent among young children. Recurrent bouts of this infection could plausibly affect speech perception and thereby general language acquisition; however, there is no conclusive evidence that it is an important risk factor for SLI, particularly in isolation (Bishop & Edmundson, 1986; Bluestone & Klein, 2005).

Finally, in research assessing the contribution of environmental factors to SLI, it is important to consider that they do not act in isolation, but are likely to interact with genetic influences throughout the course of development (Rutter, 2005). Genetically sensitive research designs are needed to address this confound. A recent example of such an approach demonstrated that parent–child communication is indeed causally related to at least mild language delay (Thorpe, Rutter, & Greenwood, 2003).

TREATMENT

There is a large literature on interventions for children with speech and language impairments. However, many studies are informal, and a recent systematic review identified only 25 studies with adequate methodology to examine the progress of children and adolescents with primary language impairments in response to interventions. The interventions varied in duration and included directive therapies to promote specific linguistic skills, as well as approaches that aimed to foster language skills in natural environments. Interventions that focused on expressive phonology and vocabulary development were found to be effective; there was less evidence of efficacy for interventions tackling expressive syntax or receptive language skills. There was little evidence that therapist-delivered interventions were any more effective than those delivered by parents, or that group therapy was more effective than individual approaches, although one study suggested that the involvement of peers was helpful. In interpreting these findings, we need to bear in mind that the evidence base is limited, and that within each study there was considerable variation in response to the intervention.

One specific form of intervention that has generated considerable research interest as an intervention for SLI because of its theoretical underpinnings is training in rapid auditory processing. According to Tallal and her colleagues (Merzenich et al., 1996; Tallal et al., 1996), the causal connection between auditory processing and language comprehension skills provides a clear rationale for capitalizing on the brain's plasticity for change by training children with SLI in rapid auditory processing skills. In two companion papers, Merzenich et al. (1996) and Tallal et al. (1996) reported very positive results from FastForWord, a training program for children with language-learning impairments that incorporates computerized games and activities to promote rapid auditory processing skills. However, a limitation of these studies was that the experimental group received an intensive period of training to improve a number of related abilities, and it is difficult to know what aspect of the program led to its effectiveness. Initial replications provided converging evidence for the program's efficacy, with the proviso that it increased the length of children's utterances but did not significantly improve their grammaticality (Gillam et al., 2001). Unfortunately, subsequent evaluations using rigorous methodologies have not confirmed the optimistic outcomes originally reported for this treatment approach (e.g., Gillam et al., 2008).

More generally, although it is possible to improve auditory processing skills to within normal limits, transfer to language tasks is often minimal (McArthur, Ellis, Atkinson, & Coltheart, 2008). In particular, poor receptive language skills may be particularly resistant to treatment. Following evaluation of a training approach that combined the use of acoustically modified speech with training in grammatical skills, Bishop et al. (2006) make the important point that children with SLI can comprehend grammatical constructions (often to about 90% accuracy), but persist in making occasional errors. These findings suggest that their difficulty is not one of grammatical competence per se, but of processing limitation. Arguably, the use of language in natural settings may be a more effective approach than the use of computer-based training regimens for children with such difficulties (Fey, Long, & Finestack, 2003). Furthermore, the accepted clinical view that interventions play an important role in improving aspects of socioemotional and behavioral adjustment, and may also reduce parental stress, should not be underestimated.

FUTURE DIRECTIONS: NEW CONCEPTUAL FRAMEWORKS

Connectionism

The connectionist perspective of SLI explains the profile of impairment in terms of a single route. That is, high-level syntactic deficits are thought to be attributable to lower-level deficits in phonological encoding and representation, which in turn are attributable to auditory perceptual deficits. This view is incompatible with theoretical approaches that posit specific syntactic deficits; rather, it is compatible with accounts emphasizing the central role of the phonological system in SLI, including the auditory processing and phonological memory accounts, the surface hypothesis, and indeed the phonological hypothesis of SLI (Chiat, 2001). The unique contribution made by connectionism, however, is the use of implemented models as rigorous tests of whether the hypothesized causal pathway is computationally feasible. In a computational model, one can directly manipulate the quality of the phonological representation and quantify the effect on the learning of particular syntactic structures.

Joanisse and colleagues have applied this approach to examine two structures of particular interest in SLI: pronouns, which have been central to the RDDR hypothesis; and the English past tense, which has been the focus of the influential EOI hypothesis. In the pronoun study, a sentence-processing model learned to associate a pronoun or reflexive to the correct antecedent (in "Baloo Bear says Mowgli is tickling him," the "him" refers to Baloo Bear; in "Baloo Bear says Mowgli is tickling himself," "himself" refers to Mowgli). When a perceptual deficit was simulated by distorting the phonological input to the model, correct performance on pronouns and reflexives decreased significantly. Importantly, the model could still resolve pronouns when additional semantic information (e.g., gender) was available, thus simulating the pattern of performance in SLI (Joanisse & Seidenberg, 2003). In the past-tense study, the model learned to associate the phonological and semantic representations of verbs; a perceptual deficit was simulated by adding random noise to the phonological representations during the training phase. The result again corresponded to the pattern of performance in SLI: Regular, irregular, and nonword past-tense generation were all impaired, but—critically for demonstrating that rule-like behavior can emerge in the absence of explicit rules—the decrement was most marked for nonwords (Joanisse & Seidenberg, 1998).

The Procedural Deficit Hypothesis

Ullman and Pierpont (2005) propose a conceptual framework called the *procedural deficit hypothesis* (PDH), which holds promise for integrating research on the neural, cognitive, and linguistic bases of SLI, and also explains the heterogeneity in the linguistic and non-linguistic deficits found in the disorder. According to the PDH, a substantial number of individuals with SLI have abnormalities of brain structures that constitute the procedural memory system,[1] and these individuals may compensate for these abnormalities to varying degrees by relying on the declarative memory system.

The PDH draws on dual-route views of language processing. It is argued that rule-governed components of language fall under the remit of the procedural memory system, while associative lexical learning is handled by the declarative memory system. In SLI, the PDH proposes that a disordered procedural memory system should impair the development of grammar across domains (syntax, morphology, and phonology) while allowing specific instances of rule-like behavior to be acquired by rote learning, enabled by the intact declarative memory system. Examples would include the ability of some children to rote-learn past-tense forms (e.g., *walked*) without being able to generate novel forms, or the ability to repeat words but not nonwords that require the abstraction of phonological structure. Such compensation would be more likely for high-frequency or particularly salient forms.

Part of the appeal of the PDH as an explanatory framework, however, is that it also addresses the nonlinguistic deficits often observed in SLI. Procedural memory and declarative memory are not language-specific, but rather two domain-general systems that are appropriate for different types of information processing. Therefore, nonlinguistic processes that are mediated by the procedural system, such as the learning and execution of complex sequences and hierarchies across cognitive and motor domains, should also be impaired in SLI. Conversely, functions that rely on declarative memory, such as the acquisition and representation of semantic and declarative knowledge, should be spared. The neural corollary of this approach is that the frequently observed comorbidity between SLI and other developmental disorders, such as ADHD and dyspraxia, may be accounted for by the overlapping brain structures and cognitive processes involved.

In its present form, the PDH is highly productive but speculative. In particular, as pointed out by Thomas (2005), the ability of the language system to compensate for a procedural learning deficit must be constrained in some way, in light of the relatively poor outcome for many children with SLI. Furthermore, more specific predictions are needed with regard to *which* children with SLI have a deficit of the procedural memory system, and what the theory predicts their comorbid conditions should be. The PDH is an intriguing hypothesis, but it remains to be seen how well it can account for the complex etiology of SLI and its manifestations across development.

Finally, the literature we have reviewed in this chapter makes it abundantly clear that SLI is a heterogeneous disorder and that, in common with other developmental disorders, its etiology is multifactorial. It is therefore unlikely that there will be a single account of SLI

---

[1] The subcortical brain structures subserving the procedural system include the basal ganglia and cerebellum; cortical regions include premotor frontal cortex, Broca's area, and portions of parietal and superior temporal cortex. The brain regions subserving the declarative memory system are primarily in the medial temporal lobe (particularly the hippocampus) and have extensive connections with temporal and parietal neocortical regions.

and its developmental course. Rather, there is a move in the field of developmental cognitive neuroscience toward multiple-deficit models that aim to capture the variety of manifestations and developmental outcomes of disorders (e.g., Bishop, 2006; Lyytinen et al., 2006; Pennington, 2005). To take one example, Bishop (2006) has suggested that SLI may arise as the result of separable environmental and genetic risk factors affecting different cognitive mechanisms. Within this view, neither a phonological memory deficit (assumed to be heritable) nor an environmentally mediated auditory perceptual impairment is sufficient to give rise to SLI, but both together might conceivably do so.

CONCLUSIONS

An important aim of research on cognitive-developmental disorders is to trace causal pathways from their biological origins, through brain systems to patterns of social adaptation (Pennington, 2002). This chapter makes it clear that the causal chain from the putative genetic basis of SLI, through neurobiology and cognition, to its educational and psychosocial outcomes is both complex and varied. Indeed, there appear to be several different developmental trajectories, and at present the causal mechanisms are only partly understood. Importantly, genes exert their actions on brain structures through environments (Rutter, 2005), and these aspects of the etiology of SLI are underresearched. However, advances in knowledge of the cognitive and behavioural phenotype of SLI are beginning to bear fruit, in terms of both refining neurobiological research questions and providing a framework for clinical practice.

ACKNOWLEDGMENTS

This chapter was prepared while the first author was supported by a Research Readership from the British Academy. We thank Bruce Pennington for his valuable input and Susannah Witts for assistance.

REFERENCES

American Psychiatric Association. (2000). *Diagnostic and statistical manual of mental disorders* (4th ed., text rev.). Washington, DC: Author.

Aram, D. M., Ekelman, B. L., & Nation, J. E. (1984). Preschoolers with language disorders: 10 years later. *Journal of Speech and Hearing Research, 27,* 232–244.

Baddeley, A., Gathercole, S., & Papagno, C. (1998). The phonological loop as a language learning device. *Psychological Review, 105,* 158–173.

Baker, L., & Cantwell, D. P. (1982). Psychiatric disorder in children with different types of communication disorder. *Journal of Communication Disorders, 15,* 113–126.

Bartlett, C., Goedken, R., & Vieland, V. (2005). Effects of updating linkage evidence across subsets of data: Reanalysis of the Autism Genetic Resource Exchange data set. *American Journal of Human Genetics, 76,* 688–695.

Bates, E., Dick, F., & Wulfeck, B. (1999). Not so fast: Domain-general factors can account for selective deficits in grammatical processing. *Behavioral and Brain Sciences, 22,* 96–97.

Bates, E., & MacWhinney, B. (1987). Competition, variation and language learning. In B. MacWhinney (Ed.), *Mechanisms of language acquisition* (pp. 96–97). Hillsdale, NJ: Erlbaum.

Bedore, L., & Leonard, L. (2001). Grammatical morphology deficits in Spanish-speaking children with specific language impairment. *Journal of Speech, Language, and Hearing Research, 44,* 905–924.

Bedore, L., & Leonard, L. (2005). Spontaneous speech characteristics of Spanish-speaking children with specific language impairment. *Applied Psycholinguistics, 26,* 195–225.

Beitchman, J. H., Cohen, N., Konstantareas, M., & Tannock, R. (Eds.). (1996). *Language, learning and behavior disorders.* Cambridge, UK: Cambridge University Press.

Belton, E., Salmond, C., Watkins, K., Vargha-Khadem, F., & Gadian, D. (2002). Bilateral grey matter abnormalities in a family with mutation in FOXP2. *NeuroImage, 16,* 10144.

Benasich, A. A., Curtiss, S., & Tallal, P. (1993). Language, learning and behavioral disturbances in childhood: A longitudinal perspective. *Journal of the American Academy of Child and Adolescent Psychiatry, 32*(3), 585–594.

Bird, J., Bishop, D. V. M., & Freeman, N. H. (1995). Phonological awareness and literacy development in children with expressive phonological impairments. *Journal of Speech and Hearing Research, 38,* 446–462.

Bishop, D. V. M. (1988). Technical note: Otitis media and developmental language disorder. *Journal of Child Psychology and Psychiatry, 29,* 365–368

Bishop, D. V. M. (1994). Is specific language impairment a valid diagnostic category?: Genetic and psycholinguistic evidence. *Philosophical Transactions of the Royal Society of London, Series B, 34,* 105–111.

Bishop, D. V. M. (1997). *Uncommon understanding.* Hove, Psychology Press.

Bishop, D. V. M. (2003). *The Children's Communication Checklist, Version 2 (CCC-2).* London: Psychological Corporation.

Bishop, D. V. M. (2006). Developmental cognitive genetics: How psychology can inform genetics and vice versa. *Quarterly Journal of Experimental Psychology, 59*(7), 1153–1168.

Bishop, D. V. M. (2007). Using mismatch negativity to study central auditory processing in developmental language and literacy impairments: Where are we, and where should we be going? *Psychological Bulletin, 133,* 651–672.

Bishop, D. V. M., & Adams, C. (1990). A prospective study of the relationship between specific language impairment, phonological disorders and reading retardation. *Journal of Child Psychology and Psychiatry, 31,* 1027–1050.

Bishop, D. V. M., Adams, C., & Norbury, C. F. (2006). Distinct genetic influences on grammar and phonological short-term memory deficits: Evidence from 6-year-old twins. *Genes, Brain and Behavior, 5*(2), 158–169.

Bishop, D. V. M., Adams, C., & Rosen, S. (2006). Resistance of grammatical impairment to computerised comprehension training in children with specific and non-specific language impairments. *International Journal of Language and Communication Disorders, 41,* 19–40.

Bishop, D. V. M., Bishop, S. J., Bright, P., James, C., Delaney, T., & Tallal, P. (1999a). Different origin of auditory and phonological processing problems in children with language impairment: Evidence from a twin study. *Journal of Speech, Language, and Hearing Research, 42*(1), 155–68.

Bishop, D. V. M., Carlyon, R. P., Deeks, J. M., & Bishop, S. J. (1999b). Auditory temporal processing impairment: Neither necessary nor sufficient for causing language impairment in children. *Journal of Speech, Language, and Hearing Research, 42*(6), 1295–310.

Bishop, D. V. M., & Edmundson, A. (1986). Is otitis media a major cause of specific developmental language disorders? *British Journal of Disorders of Communication, 21,* 321–338.

Bishop, D. V. M., & Edmundson, A. (1987). Language-impaired 4-year-olds: Distinguishing transient from persistent impairment. *Journal of Speech and Hearing Disorders, 52,* 156–173.

Bishop, D. V. M., & Hayiou-Thomas, M. E. (2008). Heritability of specific language impairment depends on diagnostic criteria. *Genes, Brain and Behavior, 7,* 365–372.

Bishop, D. V. M., & McArthur, G. M. (2004). Immature cortical responses to auditory stimuli in specific language impairment: Evidence from ERPs to rapid tone sequences. *Developmental Science, 7*(4), F11–F18.

Bishop, D. V. M., & McArthur, G. M. (2005). Individual differences in auditory processing in specific language impairment: A follow-up study using event-related potentials and behavioural thresholds. *Cortex, 41*, 327–341.

Bishop, D. V. M., & Norbury, C. F. (2002). Exploring the borderlands of autistic disorder and specific language impairment: A study using standardised diagnostic instruments. *Journal of Child Psychology and Psychiatry, 43*(7), 917–929.

Bishop, D. V. M., North, T., & Donlan, C. (1995). Genetic basis of specific language impairment: Evidence from a twin study. *Developmental Medicine and Child Neurology, 37*, 56–71.

Bishop, D. V. M., & Snowling, M. J. (2004). Developmental dyslexia and specific language impairment: Same or different? *Psychological Bulletin, 130*, 858–888.

Bluestone, C. D., & Klein, J. O. (2005). *Otitis media in infants and children* (4th ed.). Philadelphia, PA: WB Saunders.

Botting, N. (2005). Non-verbal cognitive development and language impairment. *Journal of Child Psychology and Psychiatry, 46*, 317–326.

Byrne, B., Delaland, C., Fielding-Barnsley, R., Quain, P., Samuelsson, S., Hoien, T., et al. (2002). Longitudinal study of early reading development in three countries: Preliminary results. *Annals of Dyslexia, 52*, 49–73.

Catts, H. W. (1993). The relationship between speech–language and reading disabilities. *Journal of Speech and Hearing Research, 36*, 948–958.

Catts, H. W., Adlof, S. M., Hogan, T. P., & Ellis Weismer, S. (2005). Are specific language impairment and dyslexia distinct disorders? *Journal of Speech, Hearing, and Language Research, 48*, 1378–1396.

Catts, H. W., Fey, M. E., Tomblin, J. B., & Zhang, X. (2002). A longitudinal investigation of reading outcomes in children with language impairments. *Journal of Speech, Hearing, and Language Research, 45*, 1142–1157.

Chiat, S. (2001). Mapping theories of developmental language impairment: Premises, predictions and evidence. *Language and Cognitive Processes, 16*, 113–142.

Clegg, J., Hollis, C., Mawhood, L., & Rutter, M. (2005). Developmental language disorder—a follow up in later adult life: Cognitive, language and psychosocial outcomes. *Journal of Child Psychology and Psychiatry, 46*, 128–149.

Cohen, N. J. (1996). Unsuspected learning impairments in psychiatrically disturbed children: Developmental issues and associated conditions. In J. H. Beichman, M. M. Konstantareas, & R. Tannock (Eds.), *Language, learning, and behaviour disorders: Developmental, biological, and clinical perspectives* (pp. 105–127). New York: Cambridge University Press.

Conti-Ramsden, G., Botting, N., & Faragher, B. (2001). Psycholinguistic markers for specific language impairment (SLI). *Journal of Child Psychology and Psychiatry, 42*, 741–748.

Conti-Ramsden, G., Crutchley, A., & Botting, N. (1997). The extent to which psychometric tests differentiate subgroups of children with specific language impairment. *Journal of Speech, Language, and Hearing Research, 40*, 765–777.

DeThorne, L. S., Hart, S. A., Petrill, S. A., Deater-Deckard, K., Thompson, L. A., Schatschneider, C., & et al. (2006). Children's history of speech-language difficulties: Genetic influences and associations with reading-related measures. *Journal of Speech, Language, and Hearing Research, 49*, 1280–1293.

Dionne, G., Dale, P. S., Bovin, M., & Plomin, R. (2003). Genetic evidence for bi-directional effects of early lexical and grammatical development. *Child Development, 74*, 394–412.

Dollaghan, C., & Campbell, T. F. (1998). Nonword repetition and child language impairment. *Journal of Speech, Language, and Hearing Research, 41*, 1136–1146.

Dromi, E., Leonard, L., Adam, G., & Zadunaisky-Ehrlich, S. (1999). Verb agreement morphology in Hebrew-speaking children with specific language impairment. *Journal of Speech, Language, and Hearing Research, 42*, 1414–31.

Dromi, E., Leonard, L., & Shteiman, M. (1993). The grammatical morphology of Hebrew-speaking children with specific language impairment: Some competing hypotheses. *Journal of Speech and Hearing Research, 36*, 760–771.

Ellis Weismer, S., Evans, J., & Hesketh, L. (1999). An examination of verbal working memory capacity in children with specific language impairment. *Journal of Speech, Language, and Hearing Research, 42*, 1249–1260.

Ellis Weismer, S., & Hesketh, L. (1996). Lexical learning by children with specific language impairment: Effects of linguistic input presented at varying speaking rates. *Journal of Speech and Hearing Research, 39*, 177–190.

Fey, M. E., Long, S. H., & Finestack, L. H. (2003). Ten principles of grammar facilitation for children with specific language impairments. *American Journal of Speech–Language Pathology, 12*, 3–15.

Fodor, J. A. (1983). *The modularity of mind.* Cambridge, MA: MIT Press.

Gathercole, S. E. (2006). Nonword repetition and word learning: The nature of the relationship. *Applied Psycholinguistics, 27*, 513–543.

Gathercole, S. E., & Baddeley, A. D. (1990). Phonological memory deficits in language disordered children: Is there a causal connection? *Journal of Memory and Language 29*, 336–360.

Gathercole, S. E., Tiffany, C., Briscoe, J., Thorn, A. S. C., & ALSPAC Team. (2005). Developmental consequences of poor phonological short-term memory function in childhood: A longitudinal study. *Jounal of Child Psychology and Psychiatry, 46*, 598–611.

Gillam, R. B., Loeb, D. F., & Friel-Patti, S. (2001). Looking back: A summary of five exploratory studies of Fast ForWord. *American Journal of Speech–Language Pathology, 10*, 269–273.

Gillam, R. B., Loeb, D. F., Hoffman, L. M., Bohman, T., Champlin, C. A., Thibodeau, L., et al. (2008). The efficacy of Fast ForWord language intervention in school-age children with language impairment: A randomized controlled trial. *Journal of Speech, Language, and Hearing Research, 51*(1), 97–119.

Gopnik, M. (1990). Feature-blind grammar and dysphasia. *Nature, 344*, 715.

Gopnik, M., & Crago, M. B. (1991). Familial aggregation of a developmental language disorder. *Cognition, 39*, 1–50.

Hart, B., & Risley, T. (1995). *Meaningful differences in the everyday experience of young American children.* Baltimore: Brookes.

Hayiou-Thomas, M. E., Bishop, D. V. M., & Plunkett, M. (2004). Simulating SLI: General cognitive processing stressors can produce a specific linguistic profile. *Journal of Speech, Language, and Hearing Research, 47*, 1347–1362.

Hayiou-Thomas, M. E., Kovas, Y., Harlaar, N., Bishop, D. V. M., Dale, P., & Plomin, R. (2006). Common genetic aetiology for diverse language skills in 4-year-old twins. *Journal of Child Language, 33*, 339–368.

Hayiou-Thomas, M. E., Oliver, B., & Plomin, R. (2005). Genetic influences on specific versus non-specific language impairment in 4-year-old twins. *Journal of Learning Disabilities, 38*, 222–232.

Heath, S. M., Hogben, J. H., & Clark, C. D. (1999). Auditory temporary processing in disabled readers with and without oral language delay. *Journal of Child Psychology and Psychiatry, 40*(4), 637–647.

Hill, E. (2001). Non-specific nature of specific language impairment: A review of the literature with regard to concomitant motor impairments. *International Journal of Language and Communication Disorders, 36*, 149–171.

Hill, P., Hogben, J., & Bishop, D. (2005). Auditory frequency discrimination in children with specific language impairment: A longitudinal study. *Journal of Speech, Language, and Hearing Research, 48*(5), 1136–1146.

Hoffman, Ł. M., & Gillam, R. B. (2004). Verbal and spatial information processing constraints in children with specific language impairment. *Journal of Speech, Language, and Hearing Research, 47*, 114–125.

Joanisse, M., & Seidenberg, M. S. (1998). Specific language impairment: A deficit in grammar or processing? *Trends in Cognitive Sciences, 2*(7), 240–247.

Joanisse, M., & Seidenberg, M. (2003). Phonology and syntax in specific language impairment: Evidence from a connectionist model. *Brain and Language, 86*, 40–56.

Johnston, J. R., & Ellis Weismer, S. (1983). Mental rotation abilities in language-impaired children. *Journal of Speech and Hearing Research, 26*, 397–403

Kail, R. (1994). A method for studying the generalized slowing hypothesis in children with specific language impairment. *Journal of Speech and Hearing Research, 37*, 418–421.

Kail, R., & Salthouse, T. A. (1994). Processing speed as a mental capacity. *Acta Psychologica*, 86, 199–225.

Karmiloff-Smith, A. (1998). Is atypical development necessarily a window on the normal mind/brain?: The case of Williams syndrome. *Developmental Science*, 1(2), 273–277.

Kovas, Y., Hayiou-Thomas, M. E., Oliver, B., Dale, P. S., Bishop, D. V. M., & Plomin, R. (2005). Genetic influences in different aspects of language development: The etiology of language skills in 4.5-year-old twins. *Child Development*, 76, 632–651.

Lahey, M., & Edwards, J. (1996). Why do children with specific language impairment name pictures more slowly than their peers? *Journal of Speech and Hearing Research*, 39, 1081–1098.

Lai, C. S., Fisher, S. E., Hurst, J. A., Vargha-Khadem, F., & Monaco, A. P. (2001). A forkhead-domain gene is mutated in severe speech and language disorder. *Nature*, 413, 519–523.

Leitão, S., Hogben, J., & Fletcher, J. (1997). Phonological processing skills in speech and language impaired children. *European Journal of Disorders of Communication*, 32, 73–93.

Leonard, C. M., Eckert, M., & Bishop, D. (2005). The neurobiology of developmental disorders. *Cortex*, 41, 277–281.

Leonard, C. M., Lombardino, L. J., Walsh, K., Eckert, M. A., Mockler, J. L., & Rowe, L. A., et al. (2002). Anatomical risk factors that distinguish dyslexia from SLI predict reading skill in normal children. *Journal of Communication Disorders*, 35, 501–531.

Leonard, L. B. (1989). Language learnability and specific language impairment in children. *Applied Psycholinguistics*, 10, 179–202.

Leonard, L. B. (1998). *Children with specific language impairment*. Cambridge, MA: MIT Press.

Leonard, L. B., Bortolini, U., Caselli, M. C., McGregor, K., & Sabbadini, L. (1992). Morphological deficits in children with specific language impairment: The status of features in the underlying grammar. *Language Acquisition*, 2, 151–179.

Leonard, L. B., & Deevy, P. (2003). Lexical deficits in specific language impairment. In L. Verhoeven & H. van Balkom (eds.), *Classification of developmental language disorders: Theoretical issues and clinical implications*. Mahwah, NJ: Erlbaum.

Leonard, L. B., Hansson, K., Nettelbladt, U., & Deevy, P. (2004). Specific language impairment in children: A comparison of English and Swedish. *Language Acquisition*, 12, 219–246.

Lewis, B. A., & Thompson, L. A. (1992). A study of developmental speech and language disorders in twins. *Journal of Speech, Language, and Hearing Research*, 35, 1086–1094.

Lyytinen, H., Erskine, J. M., Tolvanen, A., Torppa, M., Poikkeus, A.-M., & Lyytinen, P. (2006). Trajectories of reading development: A follow-up from birth to school age of children with and without risk for dyslexia. *Merril–Palmer Quarterly*, 52(3), 514–546.

Marler, J. A., Champlin, C. A., & Gillam, R. B. (2002). Auditory memory for backward masking signals in children with language impairment. *Psychophysiology*, 29, 767–780.

Marshall, C., &, van der Lely, H. K. J. (2006). A challenge to current models of past tense inflection: The impact of phonotactics. *Cognition*, 100, 302–320.

Mawhood, L., Howlin, P., & Rutter, M. (2000). Autism and developmental receptive language disorder—a comparative follow-up in early adult life. I: Cognitive and language outcomes. *Journal Child Psychology and Psychiatry*, 41, 547–559.

McArthur, G. M., & Bishop, D. (2004). Which people with specific language impairment have auditory deficits? *Cognitive Neuropsychology*, 21, 79–94.

McArthur, G. M., Ellis, D., Atkinson, C., & Coltheart, M. (2008). Auditory processing deficits in children with reading and language impairments: Can they (and should they) be treated? *Cognition*, 107, 946–977.

Mengler, E. D., Hogben J. H., Michie, P., & Bishop, D. V. M. (2005). Poor frequency discrimination is related to oral language disorder in children: A psychoacoustic study. *Dyslexia*, 11, 155–173.

Merzenich, M. M., Jenkins, W. M., Johnston, P., Schreiner, C., Miller, S. L., & Tallal, P. (1996). Temporal processing deficits of language-learning itmpaired children ameliorated by training. *Science*, 271, 77–80.

Metsala, J. L. (1999). Young children's phonological awareness and nonword repetition as a function of vocabulary development. *Journal of Educational Psychology*, 91, 3–19.

Miller, C. A., Kail, R., Leonard, L. B., & Tomblin, J. B. (2001). Speed of processing in children with specific language impairment. *Journal of Speech, Language, and Hearing Research*, *44*(2), 416–433.

Mills, D., & Neville, H. (1997). Electrophysiological studies of language and language impairment. *Seminars in Paediatric Neurology*, *4*, 125–134.

Montgomery, J. W. (2000). Relation of working memory to off-line and real-time sentence processing in children with specific language impairment. *Applied Psycholinguistics*, *21*, 117–148.

Montgomery, J. W. (2004). Sentence comprehension in children with specific language impairment: Effects of input rate and phonological working memory. *International Journal of Language and Communication Disorders*, *39*(1), 115–133.

Montgomery, J. W. (2005). Effects of input rate and age on the real-time language processing of children with specific language impairment. *International Journal of Language and Communication Disorders*, *40*, 171–188.

Montgomery, J. W., & Leonard, L. B. (1998). Real-time inflectional processing by children with specific language impairment: Effects of phonetic substance. *Journal of Speech, Language, and Hearing Research*, *41*(6), 1432–1443.

Morton, J., & Frith, U. (1995). Causal modelling: A structural approach to developmental psychopathology. In D. Cicchetti & D. Cohen (Eds.), *Developmental psychopathology* (Vol. 1, pp. 357–390). New York: Wiley. Nathan, E., Stackhouse, J., Goulandris, N., & Snowling, M. J. (2004). The development of early literacy skills among children with speech difficulties: A test of the "critical age hypothesis." *Journal of Speech, Hearing, and Language Research*, *47*, 377–391.

Neville, H., Coffey, S., Holcomb, P. J., & Tallal, P. (1993). The neurobiology of sensory and language processing in language impaired children. *Journal of Cognitive Neuroscience*, *5*, 235–253.

Newbury, D., Bishop, D., & Monaco, A. P. (2005). Genetic influences of language impairment and phonological short-term memory. *Trends in Cognitive Sciences*, *9*, 528–534.

Norbury, C. F., Bishop, D. V. M., & Briscoe, J. (2002). Does impaired grammatical comprehension provide evidence for an innate grammar module? *Applied Psycholinguistics*, *23*, 247–268.

Pennington, B. F. (2002). *The development of psychopathology: Nature and nurture*. New York: Guilford Press.

Pennington, B. F. (2005). Toward a neuropsychological model of attention-deficit/hyperactivity disorder: Subtypes and multiple deficits. *Biological Psychiatry*, *57*, 1221–1223.

Pennington, B. F. (2009a). *Diagnosing learning disorders: A neuropsychological framework* (2nd ed.). New York: Guilford Press.

Pennington, B. F. (2009b). Relations among speech, language, and reading disorders. *Annual Review of Psychology*, *60*(7), 7.1–7.24.

Pinker, S. (1999). *Words and rules: The ingredients of language*. New York: Basic Books.

Raitano, N. A., Pennington, B. F., Tunick, R. A., Boada, R., & Shriberg, L. D. (2004). Pre-literacy skills of subgroups of children with phonological disorder. *Journal of Child Psychology and Psychiatry*, *45*, 821–835.

Rice, M. L., Oetting, J. B., Marquis, J., Bode, J., & Pae, S. (1994). Frequency of input effects on word comprehension of children with specific language impairment. *Journal of Speech and Hearing Research*, *37*, 106–122.

Rice, M., & Wexler, K. (1996). Toward tense as a clinical marker of specific language impairment in English-speaking children. *Journal of Speech and Hearing Research*, *39*, 850–863.

Rice, M. L., Wexler, K., & Cleave, P. L. (1995). Specific language impairment as a period of extended optional infinitive. *Journal of Speech and Hearing Research*, *38*, 850–863.

Rice, M. L., Wexler, K., & Hershberger, S. (1998). Tense over time: The longitudinal course of tense acquisition in children with specific language impairment. *Journal of Speech, Language, and Hearing Research*, *41*(6), 1412–1431.

Rice, M. L., Wexler, K., & Redmond, S. M. (1999). Grammaticality judgments of an extended optional infinitive grammar: Evidence from English-speaking children with specific language impairment. *Journal of Speech, Language, and Hearing Research*, *42*, 943–961.

Rosen, S. (2003). Auditory processing in dyslexia and specific language impairment: Is there a deficit? What is its nature? Does it explain anything? *Journal of Phonetics, 31,* 509–527.

Rutter, M. (2005). *Genes and behavior.* Oxford: Blackwell.

Scientific Learning Corporation (1997). Fast ForWord. Retrieved from *www.scilearn.com*

Semel, E., Wiig, E. H., & Secord, W. (2006). *Clinical Evaluation of Language Fundamentals—Fourth Edition UK (CELF-4UK).* London: Harcourt Assessment.

Service, E. (1992). Phonology, working memory and foreign-language learning. *Quarterly Journal of Experimental Psychology, 45A*(1), 21–50.

SLI Consortium. (2002). A genome wide scan identifies two novel loci involved in specific language impairment. *American Journal of Human Genetics 70,* 384–398.

SLI Consortium. (2004). Highly significant linkage to SLI1 locus in an expanded sample of individuals affected by specific language impairment (SLI). *American Journal of Human Genetics, 94,* 1225–1238.

Snowling, M., & Hulme, C. (Eds.). (2005). *The science of reading: A handbook.* Oxford: Blackwell.

Snowling, M. J., Adams, J. W., Bishop, D. V. M., & Stothard, S. E. (2001). Educational attainments of school leavers with a preschool history of speech–language impairments. *International Journal of Language and Communication Disorders, 36*(2), 173–183.

Snowling, M. J., Bishop, D. V. M., & Stothard, S. E. (2000). Is pre-school language impairment a risk factor for dyslexia in adolescence? *Journal of Child Psychology and Psychiatry, 41,* 587–600.

Snowling, M. J., Bishop, D. V. M., Stothard, S. E., Chipchase, B., & Kaplan, C. (2006). Psycho-social outcomes at 15 years of children with a pre-history of speech–language impairment. *Journal of Child Psychology and Psychiatry, 47,* 759–765.

Spinath, F. M., Price, T. S., Dale, P. S., & Plomin, R. (2004). The genetic and environmental origins of language disability and ability: A study of language at 2, 3 and 4 years of age in a large community sample of twins. *Child Development, 75,* 445–454.

Stackhouse, J., & Snowling, M. J. (1992). Barriers to literacy development in two cases of developmental verbal dyspraxia. *Cognitive Neuropsychology, 9,* 273–299.

Stark, R. E., & Montgomery, J. W. (1995). Sentence processing in language impaired children under conditions of filtering and time compression. *Applied Psycholinguistics, 16,* 137–154.

Stein, C. M., Schick, J., Taylor, G., Shriberg, L., Millard, C., Kundtz-Kluge, A., et al. (2004). Pleiotropic effects of a chromosome 3 locus on speech-sound disorder and reading. *American Journal of Human Genetics, 74,* 283–297.

Stothard, S. E., Snowling, M. J., Bishop, D. V. M., Chipchase, B., & Kaplan, C. (1998). Language impaired pre-schoolers: A follow-up in adolescence. *Journal of Speech, Language, and Hearing Research, 41,* 407–418.

Stromswold, K. (2001). The heritability of language: A review and metaanalysis of twin, adoption, and linkage studies. *Language Acquisition, 77,* 647–723.

Tallal, P. (1980). Auditory temporal perception, phonics, and reading disabilities in children. *Brain and Language, 9,* 182–198.

Tallal, P., Miller, S. L., Bedi, G., Byma, G., Wang, X., Nagarajan, S. S., et al. (1996). Language comprehension in language-learning impaired children improved with acoustically modified speech. *Science, 271,* 81–84.

Tallal, P., & Piercy, M. (1973). Developmental aphasia: Impaired rate of non-verbal processing as a function of sensory modality. *Neuropsychologia, 11,* 389–398.

Thomas, M. S. C. (2005). Characterising compensation. *Cortex, 41,* 434–442.

Thorpe, K., Rutter, M., & Greenwood, M. (2003). Twins as a natural experiment to study the causes of mild language delay: II. Family interaction risk factors. *Journal of Child Psychology and Psychiatry, 44*(3), 342–355.

Tomblin, J. B., & Buckwalter, P. (1998). The heritability of poor language achievement among twins. *Journal of Speech and Hearing Research, 41,* 188–199.

Tomblin, J. B., Freese, P. R., & Records, N. L. (1992). Diagnosing specific language impairment in adults for the purpose of pedigree analysis. *Journal of Speech and Hearing Research, 35,* 832–843.

Tomblin, J. B., Records, N. L., Buckwalter, P., Zhang, X., Smith, E., & O'Brien, M. (1997). Prevalence of specific language impairment in kindergarten children. *Journal of Speech and Hearing Research, 40*, 1245–1260.

Tonnquist-Uhlen, I. (1996). Topography of auditory evoked cortical potentials in children with severe language impairment. *Scandinavian Audiology Supplement, 44*, 1–40.

Ullman, M. T., & Pierpont, E. I. (2005). Specific language impairment is not specific to language: The procedural deficit hypothesis. *Cortex, 41*, 399–433.

van der Lely, H. K. J. (1994). Canonical linking rules: Forward versus linking in normally developing and specifically language-impaired children. *Cognition, 51*, 29–72.

van der Lely, H. K. J. (2005). Grammatical-SLI and the computational grammatical complexity hypothesis. *Revue Fréquences, 17*, 13–20.

van der Lely, H. K. J., & Harris, M. (1990). Comprehension of reversible sentences in specifically language impaired children. *Journal of Speech and Hearing Disorders, 55*, 101–117.

van der Lely, H. K. J., & Stollwerck, L. (1997). Binding theory and specifically language impaired children. *Cognition, 62*, 245–290.

van Weerdenburg, M., Verhoeven, L., & van Balkom, H. (2006). Towards a typology of specific language impairment. *Journal of Child Psychology and Psychiatry, 47*, 176–189.

Vargha-Khadem, F., Watkins, K., Alcock, K., Fletcher, P., & Passingham, R. (1995). Praxic and nonverbal cognitive deficits in a large family with a genetically transmitted speech and language disorder. *Proceedings of the National Academy of Sciences USA, 92*, 930–933.

Vargha-Khadem, F., Watkins, K. E., Price, C. J., Ashburner, J., Alcock, K., Connelly, A., et al. (1998). Neural basis of an inherited speech and language disorder. *Proceedings of the National Academy of Sciences USA, 95*, 12695–12700.

Vernes, S. C., Newbury, D. F., Abrahams, B. S., Winchester, L., Nicod, J., Groszer, M., et al. (2008). A functional genetic link between distinct developmental language disorders. *The New England Journal of Medicine, 359*(22), 2337–2345.

Watkins, K., Vargha-Khadem, F., Ashburner, J., Passingham, R., Connelly, A., Friston, K. J., et al. (2002). MRI analysis of an inherited speech and language disorder: Structural brain abnormalities. *Brain, 125*, 465–478.

Webster, R. I., & Shevell, M. I. (2004). Neurobiology of specific language impairment. *Journal of Child Neurology, 19*, 471–481.

Wexler, K. (1994). Optional infinitives, head movement and the economy of derivation. In D. Lightfoot & N. Hornstein (Eds.), *Verb movement* (pp. 305–350). Cambridge, UK: Cambridge University Press.

Wexler, K. (1996). The development of inflection in a biologically based theory of language acquisition. In M. L. Rice (Ed.), *Toward a genetics of language* (pp. 113–144). Mahwah, NJ: Erlbaum.

Wexler, K. (1998). Very early parameter setting and the unique checking constraint: A new explanation of the optional infinitive stage. *Lingua, 106*, 23–79.

World Health Organization. (1993). *International statistical classification of diseases and related health problems* (10th rev.). Geneva: Author.

Wright, B. A., Lombardino, L. J., King, W. M., Puranik, C. S., Leonard, C. M., & Merzenich, M. M. (1997). Deficits in auditory temporal and spectral resolution in language-impaired children. *Nature, 387*, 176–178.

Ziegler, J. C., Pech-George, C., George, F., Alario, F.-X., & Lorenz, C. (2005). Deficits in speech perception predict language learning impairment. *Proceedings of the National Academy of Sciences USA, 102*, 14110–14115.

CHAPTER 14

Attention-Deficit/ Hyperactivity Disorder

Erik G. Willcutt

DEFINITION AND PREVALENCE

Approximately 5% of children meet the diagnostic criteria for attention-deficit/hyperactivity disorder (ADHD) as defined in the fourth edition, text revision, of the *Diagnostic and Statistical Manual of Mental Disorders* (DSM-IV-TR; American Psychiatric Association, 2000). ADHD is one of the most common disorders of childhood (e.g., Angold et al., 2002), with a prevalence far higher than that for many of the other syndromes described in this book.

Diagnostic Subtypes

Based on factor-analytic studies (e.g., DuPaul et al., 1997) and results of the DSM-IV clinical field trials for the disruptive behavior disorders (Lahey et al., 1994), the DSM-IV-TR diagnostic criteria for ADHD describe three subtypes based on differential elevations in symptoms of inattention and disorganization versus symptoms of hyperactivity and impulsivity. The nine DSM-IV-TR inattention symptoms include such behaviors as "difficulty sustaining attention," "easily distracted," and "difficulty organizing tasks and activities," whereas the hyperactivity–impulsivity symptom list includes such behaviors as "runs about or climbs . . . [when] it is inappropriate," "talks excessively," and "blurts out answers before questions have been completed" (American Psychiatric Association, 2000, p. 92). The criteria for ADHD specify that a child must exhibit six or more symptoms of inattention or six or more symptoms of hyperactivity–impulsivity. DSM-IV-TR then subdivides

ADHD into subgroups of individuals who exhibit maladaptive levels of both inattention and hyperactivity-impulsivity (combined type), maladaptive levels of inattention only (predominantly inattentive type), and maladaptive levels of hyperactivity–impulsivity alone (predominantly hyperactive–impulsive type).

In virtually all community samples, the proportion of individuals who meet DSM-IV-TR symptom criteria for the inattentive type (approximately 50% across all samples) is higher than the proportion who meet symptom criteria for the hyperactive–impulsive type (20%) or combined type (30%; for a review, see Willcutt & Carlson, 2005). In contrast, samples recruited through clinics typically include a much higher proportion of individuals with the combined type (approximately 60% across samples) than with the inattentive type (30%) or hyperactive–impulsive type (10%). This difference suggests that although more children and adolescents in the population meet symptom criteria for the inattentive type, individuals who meet symptom criteria for the combined type are more likely to receive clinical services.

Sex, Ethnic, and Cross-National Prevalence Differences

Females are significantly less likely than males to meet criteria for DSM-IV-TR ADHD in both clinic-referred and community samples (e.g., Biederman et al., 2002; Gaub & Carlson, 1997). Cross-national studies suggest that the prevalence of ADHD based on symptom criteria may be higher in several other countries (i.e., Colombia, Germany, Ukraine) than in the United States (Baumgaertel, Wolraich, & Dietrich, 1995; Gadow et al., 2000; Pineda et al., 1999), and the few available studies that have compared the prevalence of ADHD in different U.S. ethnic groups suggest that African American children may receive higher ratings of ADHD symptoms from parents and teachers than European American or Hispanic children (e.g., DuPaul, Power, Anastopoulos, & Reid, 1998; Reid et al., 1998). In contrast, a recent study of treatment rates suggests that African American and Hispanic children are less likely than European American children to receive treatment for ADHD (Rowland et al., 2002). The reasons for these sex, ethnic, and cross-national differences in the prevalence and treatment of ADHD are currently unknown. Future studies that test competing explanations of these differences will have critical implications for the validity of ADHD, and are likely to facilitate valid diagnosis and treatment in all populations.

THE VALIDITY OF DSM-IV-TR ADHD

Currently, ADHD and virtually all other DSM-IV-TR mental disorders are necessarily defined on the basis of observable or reportable behaviors. From a clinical perspective, diagnostic validity hinges on a straightforward question: Do the behavioral symptoms of ADHD impair an individual's functioning sufficiently to warrant treatment? Evidence of diagnostic validity is provided if a disorder leads to significant functional impairment, and a disorder has discriminant validity if these associated impairments remain significant when symptoms of comorbid disorders and other confounding variables are controlled for (e.g., Lahey et al., 1994; Widiger & Clark, 2000).

Despite substantial evidence that has accumulated to support the diagnostic validity of ADHD (e.g., Barkley, 2006; Lahey & Willcutt, 2002), some in the popular press continue to suggest that ADHD symptoms may simply describe the exuberant behavior of normal children (e.g., Breeding, 2000). Others argue that ADHD is a valid diagnosis in the sense that it that identifies children and adults who are likely to benefit from treatment, but they question the validity of the specific subtype scheme provided in DSM-IV-TR (e.g., Barkley, 2001; Milich, Balentine, & Lynam, 2001). Because the validity of ADHD remains controversial, we recently completed a comprehensive meta-analysis of over 100 published studies in which we critically examined the internal and external validity of DSM-IV-TR ADHD (Willcutt & Carlson, 2005; Willcutt et al., 2009c). In this section, I briefly summarize these results and their implications before turning to a more detailed overview of the neuropathology and neuropsychology of ADHD.

Symptom Dimensions

Previous studies provide strong support for the internal and external validity of the inattention and hyperactivity–impulsivity symptom dimensions described by DSM-IV-TR. Both exploratory and confirmatory factor analyses consistently support the distinction between inattention and hyperactivity–impulsivity symptoms (e.g., DuPaul et al., 1997), and both symptom dimensions are associated with multiple aspects of global, academic, and social impairment (e.g., Lahey et al., 1994). The discriminant validity of the symptom dimensions was demonstrated by multiple-regression analyses showing that inattention symptoms were more strongly associated with internalizing symptoms, academic difficulties, and neurocognitive weaknesses, whereas hyperactive–impulsive symptoms more strongly predicted comorbid externalizing behaviors, peer rejection, and accidental physical injuries (Lahey & Willcutt, 2002).

Diagnostic Subtypes

Existing data also strongly support the diagnostic validity of the DSM-IV-TR combined and inattentive types (Willcutt & Carlson, 2005). Both groups exhibit significant impairment on measures of global, academic, and social functioning; the average effect size is moderate to large in each of these domains ($d = 0.5$–1.5); and these impairments are not explained by comorbid mental disorders or low intelligence (e.g., Lahey et al., 1998). The discriminant validity of the inattentive and combined subtypes is less clear. Children with the combined type are more likely to be disliked by peers, exhibit higher rates of oppositional defiant disorder and conduct disorder, and experience more frequent accidental injuries sufficiently severe to require care from a physician, whereas individuals with the inattentive type are more likely to be socially passive or isolated (e.g., Lahey et al., 1998; Maedgen & Carlson, 2000). On the other hand, the inattentive and combined types exhibit similar weaknesses on nearly all academic and neurocognitive measures, and etiologically informative studies generally suggest that these subtypes are due at least in part to common familial and genetic influences (e.g., Graetz, Sawyer, Hazell, Arney, & Baghurst, 2001; Hinshaw, Carte, Sami, Treuting, & Zupan, 2002; Lowe et al., 2004; Todd et al., 2001; Willcutt, Pennington, & DeFries, 2000). Overall, these results provide some support for the distinction between the inattentive and combined types, but are most consistent with a gradient-of-severity model, in which the inattentive type falls at a less extreme point on the same continuum of liability as the combined type.

In contrast to the inattentive and combined types, evidence of diagnostic validity is far weaker for the hyperactive–impulsive type. Only 2 of 24 comparisons on measures of academic functioning revealed significant differences between the hyperactive–impulsive type and a comparison group without ADHD or other diagnoses, and fewer than half of the individuals in the hyperactive–impulsive group exhibited significant social impairment (e.g., Gaub & Carlson, 1997; Graetz et al., 2001). Although these results must be interpreted with caution, due to relatively small samples with the hyperactive–impulsive type, they indicate that additional research is sorely needed to test whether the hyperactive–impulsive type is a valid diagnosis that should be retained in its current form.

In summary, the existing literature provides strong support for the overall validity of ADHD as a syndrome that leads to significant impairment for most individuals who meet symptom criteria for the diagnosis. Additional research is needed, however, to understand the causes of the significant sex, ethnic, and national differences in prevalence, and to clarify the validity of the specific subtype taxonomy described in DSM-IV-TR.

NEURAL MECHANISMS OF ADHD

Why Study the Neuropsychology of ADHD?

Although the studies reviewed in the preceding section demonstrate the diagnostic validity of ADHD for clinical purposes, the validity of a behaviorally defined disorder such as ADHD will always be constrained by the difficulties inherent in the measurement of behavior. The long-term objective of research on psychopathology is to understand all disorders at each of the four levels of analysis described by Pennington (2002): (1) behavior, (2) neuropsychology/cognitive processes, (3) brain development, and (4) etiology. The field is not yet at the point at which etiological or neuropsychological markers can be identified and used to improve clinical diagnosis and treatment, but neuropsychological research has the potential to facilitate important advancements in these areas by helping to pinpoint the specific neural systems that are compromised in ADHD.

The voluminous existing literature on the neuropsychology and neurophysiology of ADHD includes over 300 studies with over 10,000 participants. At least one of these studies reported a significant difference between groups with and without ADHD on measures of most cognitive domains, including general intelligence (e.g., Nigg, Hinshaw, Carte, & Treuting, 1998), verbal and nonverbal skills (e.g., Willcutt, Pennington, Chhabildas, Olson, & Hulslander, 2005c), memory (e.g., Seidman, Biederman, Monuteaux, Doyle, & Faraone, 2001), and sensory–motor functioning (e.g., Hinshaw et al., 2002).

Due to space constraints, I focus here on five theoretical constructs emphasized by the most prominent current neuropsychological theories of ADHD. These include executive functions (EFs); aversion to delay; modulation of behavior in response to reward and punishment cues; response variability and related deficits in short-duration temporal processing; and overall cognitive processing speed. In the remainder of this section, I first summarize findings from neuroimaging studies of ADHD, then review neuropsychological studies of the five constructs, and finally integrate these findings and describe the key implications for the field.

Neuroimaging Studies

Frontal–Striatal Networks

Neuropsychological, neuroimaging, and lesion studies suggest that ADHD and other forms of disinhibitory psychopathology are associated with dysfunction in one or more neural circuits involving the prefrontal cortex (PFC; e.g., Barkley, 1997; Pennington & Ozonoff, 1996). One primary PFC circuit includes the thalamus, basal ganglia, and dorsolateral and ventrolateral regions of the PFC. Human and primate studies suggest that this network is especially important for executive control processes, such as response selection and inhibition, maintenance and manipulation of information, and planning and organization of behavior (see Pennington, 2002, for an overview). All structural magnetic resonance imaging (MRI) studies that measured frontal regions reported reduced volume in PFC, and several studies reported volume reductions in the caudate nucleus of the basal ganglia, a structure with close connections to dorsolateral and ventrolateral PFC (Seidman, Valera, & Makris, 2005). These structural results are supported by studies using a variety of functional imaging techniques to demonstrate reduced dorsolateral and ventrolateral PFC activation (e.g., Ernst et al., 2003; Rubia et al., 1999; Vaidya et al., 1998).

Orbitofrontal Cortex

A second PFC network, one central to the delay aversion theory of ADHD, includes feedback loops among ventromedial PFC, limbic structures, and other areas of PFC (e.g., Sonuga-Barke, 2003). Several lines of research suggest that this circuit may coordinate the interface between motivation and cognition during decision-making processes, and may therefore play a role in aversion to delay. Primate studies suggest that ventromedial PFC neurons play a role in prediction of and response to rewards (e.g., Schultz, Tremblay, & Hollerman, 2000). Humans with damage to ventromedial PFC frequently exhibit difficulty in attaching an emotional valence to a behavior based on positive or negative feedback from the environment, leading to difficulty in learning from mistakes, delaying gratification, and monitoring subtle shifts in reward and punishment probabilities to maximize overall outcome (e.g., Bechara, Damasio, & Damasio, 2000; Elliott, Dolan, & Frith, 2000; Rolls, 2004). Few neuroimaging studies of ADHD have examined regions involved in this network, but one study reported significantly reduced left orbital PFC volume in a group with ADHD (Hesslinger et al., 2002).

Other Regions of Interest

Although neural circuits involving PFC have received the most attention in cognitive theories of ADHD, several related neural systems have also been explicitly incorporated in recent theoretical models. These include the role of the anterior cingulate cortex in response selection (e.g., Bush et al., 1999); timing processes mediated by the cerebellum (e.g., Castellanos & Tannock, 2002); and basic neural mechanisms for the regulation of cognitive arousal (e.g., Sergeant, Geurts, Huijbregts, Scheres, & Oosterlaan, 2003). Functional MRI (fMRI) studies have consistently reported underactivation of dorsal anterior cingulate cortex in individuals with ADHD during tasks that require selection of an appropriate response from multiple competing options (e.g., Bush et al., 1999). A subset of studies reported reduced volume and activity in the cerebellum (e.g., Schulz et al., 2004), and one study found that the cerebellum was the only region in which the volume reduction remained significant when total cerebral volume was controlled for (Castellanos et al., 2002).

Conclusions from Neuroimaging Studies

Brain imaging studies generally suggest that ADHD is associated with a small but significant reduction in global brain volume and activation. More specifically, these studies support the hypothesis that ADHD may be attributable to dysfunction in networks involving frontal–striatal structures, the anterior cingulate cortex, and the cerebellum. Additional research is needed to clarify the role of the orbitofrontal cortex in ADHD, but initial results are promising.

Executive Functions

Based on similarities between ADHD symptoms and the behavioral sequelae of frontal lobe injuries (e.g., Fuster, 1997; Stuss & Benson, 1986), one of the most prominent cognitive theories of ADHD suggests that ADHD symptoms arise from a primary deficit in EFs (e.g., Barkley, 1997; Nigg, 2001; Pennington & Ozonoff, 1996). EFs are defined as cognitive functions that serve to maintain an appropriate problem-solving set to attain a future goal (e.g., Welsh & Pennington, 1988). In a simplified model of decision-making processes, EFs represent "top-down" cognitive inputs that facilitate decision making by maintaining information about possible choices in working memory, and integrating this knowledge with information about the current context to identify the optimal action for the current situation. Although executive control processes involve several distributed brain networks, the primary neural circuit includes the thalamus, basal ganglia, and prefrontal cortex (e.g., Casey, Durston, & Fossella, 2001; Pennington, 2002).

Many theoretical models of ADHD have invoked the notion of *executive control* as a single unified construct that encompasses many potentially separable cognitive functions (e.g., Pennington & Ozonoff, 1996). However, exploratory and confirmatory factor analyses and recent fMRI studies suggest that EFs are more accurately characterized as a collection of related but separable abilities (e.g., Collette et al., 2005; Friedman et al., 2006; Miyake, Friedman, Emerson, Witzki, & Howerter, 2000; Willcutt et al., 2005c). Nearly all of these studies obtained factors of response inhibition, working memory/updating, and set shifting, and some studies also found evidence for separable domains of vigilance/sustained attention, planning/organization, interference control, and fluency. Based on evidence of the separability of these different EFs, several neuropsychological theories of ADHD have posited a more focal weakness in a specific aspect of executive control, such as response inhibition (e.g., Barkley, 1997; Nigg, 2001).

EF tasks have been included in far more studies of ADHD than measures of any other neuropsychological construct have been. To synthesize this extensive literature, my colleagues and I completed a meta-analysis of all published studies that administered at least one EF measure (Willcutt et al., 2005a; Willcutt, Doyle, Nigg, Faraone, & Pennington, 2005b), and for this chapter I have added studies published since our initial reviews were completed (Table 14.1). Significant group differences were obtained for 63% of all compari-

TABLE 14.1. Meta-Analysis of Studies That Administered Measures of Key Neuropsychological Domains to Groups with and without ADHD

Neuropsychological domain	Representative task	Number of studies[a] Total *N*	*N* with ADHD main effect	Mean effect size[b] (95% confidence interval)
Executive functions				
Response inhibition	Stop signal task	57	42 (74%)	0.60 (0.06)
Working memory	Span tasks, *N*-back	28	19 (68%)	0.57 (0.09)
Set shifting	Wisconsin Card Sorting Test	31	11 (35%)	0.38 (0.09)
Planning	Tower of Hanoi/London	31	20 (65%)	0.53 (0.12)
Interference control	Stroop	16	5 (31%)	0.29 (0.12)
Vigilance	Continuous-performance test omission errors	35	27 (77%)	0.59 (0.07)
Response speed				
Simple reaction time (RT)	Two-choice RT tasks	26	15 (58%)	0.33 (0.09)
Processing/naming speed	Rapid automatized naming	36	28 (78%)	0.72 (0.08)
Response variability	Intrasubject *SD* of RT	18	15 (83%)	0.69 (0.10)
Motivational processes				
Delay aversion	Delay aversion/discounting	6	4 (67%)	0.53 (0.15)
Response to contingencies	Go/no-go with contingencies	22	Mixed results; see text	

[a]Number of studies as of September 2006.
[b]Mean effect size weighted by the sample size of each study (see Willcutt et al., 2005a, 2005b, for detailed descriptions of this method).

sons on EF tasks in the studies in the meta-analysis, and the weighted mean effect size across all measures was 0.53 (95% confidence interval = 0.50–0.56). The most consistent group differences and largest effect sizes were obtained for measures of inhibition, working memory, vigilance, and planning, and each of these effects fell in the range considered a medium effect (d = 0.53–0.60). Similarly, correlations between ADHD symptoms and dimensional EF measures are typically significant but small to moderate in magnitude (r = .15–.35; e.g., Nigg et al., 1998; Willcutt et al., 2001). Taken together, these results indicate that ADHD is clearly associated with weak executive control, but also suggest that the majority of the variance in ADHD symptoms is independent from variation in EF performance.

Motivational Processes/Response to Contingencies

Motivational explanations of ADHD have several variants, but all of these models suggest that ADHD is attributable to a dysfunctional response to reward and punishment contingencies (e.g., Hartung, Milich, Lynam, & Martin, 2002; Luman, Oosterlaan, & Sergeant, 2006). Because studies of motivational processes have used a wide range of tasks and experimental designs that are difficult to combine for a pooled analysis, these tasks are not included in the meta-analysis summarized in Table 14.1.

Studies that tested motivational hypotheses by manipulating reward and punishment have yielded mixed results (for a comprehensive review, see Luman et al., 2006). Some studies found that response contingencies improved or normalized task performance in individuals with ADHD, particularly on tasks with a strong motivational component (e.g., Carlson & Tamm, 2000; Slusarek, Velling, Bunk, & Eggers, 2001). In contrast, other studies found a main effect of reinforcement or response cost on the task performance of all groups, but no differential effect on individuals with ADHD (e.g., Scheres, Oosterlaan, & Sergeant, 2001; Shanahan, Willcutt, & Pennington, 2008). A third set of studies found that the simultaneous presence of both reward and punishment cues was associated with a significant increase in impulsive responses by individuals with elevations of ADHD symptoms, whereas no group differences were detected in the condition with response cost alone (e.g., Farmer & Rucklidge, 2006; Hartung et al., 2002). Taken together, these results suggest that ADHD may be associated with motivational dysfunction, but additional research is needed to specify the nature of this relation, as well as the relation between response to contingencies and weaknesses in other cognitive domains such as EFs.

Delay Aversion

An intriguing variant of the motivational hypothesis suggests that individuals with ADHD find delay so aversive that they make choices that will minimize delay even when presented with other options that take longer to complete but maximize long-term gains (e.g., Sonuga-Barke, Taylor, Sembi, & Smith, 1992). A series of initial studies demonstrated that children with ADHD were more delay-averse than children without ADHD (Kuntsi, Oosterlaan, & Stevenson, 2001; Solanto et al., 2001; Sonuga-Barke et al., 1992). Furthermore, Solanto et al. (2001) compared the performance of children with ADHD on a delay aversion task and a stop signal task (a widely used measure of response inhibition), and found that aversion to delay predicted ADHD status independently and more strongly than weak response inhibition.

In contrast to these promising initial results, group differences in delay aversion have not been reported in some subsequent studies (Scheres et al., 2006; Willcutt et al., 2009), and the mean effect size across all studies is only moderate (Table 14.1). These inconsistent results suggest that the relation between delay aversion and ADHD may be highly sensitive to developmental changes or to the specific magnitude and timing of reinforcers available in the environment. Scheres et al. (2006) provide a detailed discussion of these issues, and suggest that future studies should systematically manipulate the timing and magnitude of rewards in tasks based on this paradigm, to clarify the relation between delay aversion and ADHD.

Response Variability

One of the most ubiquitous results in cognitive studies of ADHD is the finding that the responses of individuals with ADHD are slower and more variable than those of individuals without ADHD (e.g., Castellanos & Tannock, 2002), but until recently this pattern received little theoretical or empirical attention. Most previous studies have operationalized response variability as the standard deviation of an individual's reaction time (RT) across all task trials. Although Castellanos et al. (2005) recently demonstrated that the standard deviation of RT may be less sensitive than other measures of response variability, group differences on even this relatively coarse measure have a large effect size and are replicated consistently across studies (Table 14.1).

One key theoretical issue is whether increased response variability is a unique weakness that is separable from the other cognitive weaknesses associated with ADHD, or whether inconsistent responses are a secondary consequence of another dysfunctional cognitive process. For example, increased response variability could plausibly result from weak executive control or differential sensitivity to response contingencies, or could be a simple consequence of slow primary reaction time. Several authors have recently attempted to address this concern, and have obtained results suggesting that the greater intraindividual variability exhibited by individuals with ADHD may indeed reflect a dysfunctional physiological mechanism that is distinct from the processes described by existing models.

Elsewhere (Frank, Santamaria, O'Reilly, & Willcutt, 2007), we describe data from neuropsychological tasks, psychopharmacological manipulations, and neurocomputational models suggesting that weaknesses in executive control may reflect reduced striatal dopamine, whereas increased response variability may be an independent weakness that is attributable to noradrenaline dysfunction. A second study conducted a detailed analysis of RT data on a flanker task, and suggested that response variability exhibited by individuals with ADHD primarily reflected systematic low-frequency fluctuations in neuronal activity that could plausibly lead to the forgetfulness and careless errors characteristic of ADHD (Castellanos et al., 2005). In combination with the large effect sizes observed in previous studies, these promising initial results suggest that additional research is sorely needed to assess the relation between ADHD and different measures of response variability. Of particular importance will be studies that also measure constructs such as EFs, delay aversion, and response to motivational contingencies, facilitating a direct test of whether response variability is independent from these other processes.

Cognitive Processing Speed

Finally, recent evidence from our laboratory and others suggests that groups with ADHD exhibit large and consistent deficits on measures of naming speed and more general cognitive processing speed (e.g., Rucklidge & Tannock, 2002; Shanahan, Yerys, Scott, Willcutt, & Pennington, 2006). No theoretical model of ADHD posits processing speed as a single core weakness that is necessary and sufficient to cause ADHD, and neural models of processing speed are less advanced than models of executive control processes, delay aversion, and response to reward or punishment. Nonetheless, the magnitude and consistency of these effects indicates that a comprehensive model of the neuropsychology of ADHD must explain these weaknesses. Future research is also needed to test whether slow processing speed is specific to certain cognitive domains or is a ubiquitous phenomenon that cuts across tasks, and to clarify the relations between slow processing speed and weak executive control, aversion to delay, and response variability.

Integration and Implications: The Need for Multiple-Deficit Models

The results summarized in this section clearly confirm that groups with ADHD differ from groups without ADHD in multiple neuropsychological domains. To examine how these group differences apply to individuals with the disorder, we extended our previous collaborative analyses (Nigg, Willcutt, Doyle, & Sonuga-Barke, 2005b) by calculating the proportion of individuals with ADHD who exhibited significant impairment on measures of each of the five key domains in our ongoing Colorado Learning Disabilities Research Center (CLDRC) twin study (impairment was quantified as a score below the 10th percentile of the comparison group without ADHD or a learning disorder). Individuals with ADHD were more likely than individuals without ADHD to exhibit a significant deficit on all measures except delay aversion (Figure 14.1). However, fewer than half of the individuals with ADHD exhibited a significant deficit on any specific measure, clearly indicating that no neuropsychological weakness is necessary and sufficient to cause all cases of ADHD.

In summary, both dimensional and categorical analyses argue strongly against a primary-deficit model of ADHD. Instead, the models that best fit the data are multifactorial models explicitly hypothesizing that ADHD is a complex, neuropsychologically heterogeneous disorder, with no core neurocognitive weakness that is sufficient to explain all cases. A comprehensive neuropsychological model of ADHD must explain weaknesses in several EF domains, significant aversion to delay, differential sensitivity to some motivational contingencies, and slower and more variable responses on both individual task trials and across entire measures. Below, I describe two plausible types of models that incorporate multiple deficits, to illustrate different ways in which such models can be conceptualized.

1. *Independent-pathway models*. These models suggest that disruption in any one of two or more pathophysiological substrates can independently lead to the same final behavioral manifestation of ADHD (e.g., Sonuga-Barke, 2003). Therefore, independent-pathway models propose *neuropsychological subtypes* of ADHD. For example, Sonuga-Barke (2003) proposes a dual-pathway model in which some individuals exhibit ADHD symptoms due

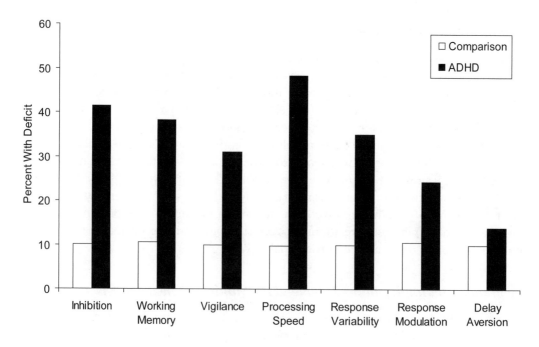

FIGURE 14.1. Percentage of individuals with and without ADHD who scored below the 10th percentile of the comparison sample on each neuropsychological measure.

to significant aversion to delay, whereas others with ADHD have weak inhibitory control. Although much more research is needed to test this model, it has received initial support from studies finding that delay aversion and response inhibition predicted ADHD symptoms independently in both a clinical sample (Solanto et al., 2001) and an unselected community sample of preschool children (Sonuga-Barke, Dalen, & Remington, 2003).

2. *The multiple-deficit model.* The multiple-deficit model suggests that ADHD symptoms arise from an additive and interactive combination of multiple neuropsychological weaknesses in an individual. Specific clusters of weaknesses may then differ across individuals, leading to neuropsychological and clinical heterogeneity. For example, individuals with weaknesses in executive control and processing speed may be most likely to exhibit significant inattention and comorbid learning difficulties (e.g., Willcutt et al., 2005c), whereas EF weaknesses coupled with aversion to delay or disruption in other motivational processes may lead to impulsive behaviors and comorbidity with other disruptive disorders (such as conduct disorder).

The independent-pathway and multiple-deficit models each received some support in our most recent analyses from our ongoing twin study. Figure 14.2 depicts the percentage of individuals in the ADHD and comparison groups who exhibited no significant weakness on any neurocognitive task in our battery; a weakness in only one neuropsychological domain; or significant weaknesses in two, three, or four or more neurocognitive domains. Nearly one in four individuals who met full DSM-IV-TR criteria for ADHD did not exhibit a significant weakness on any of the neuropsychological measures in our battery, and an

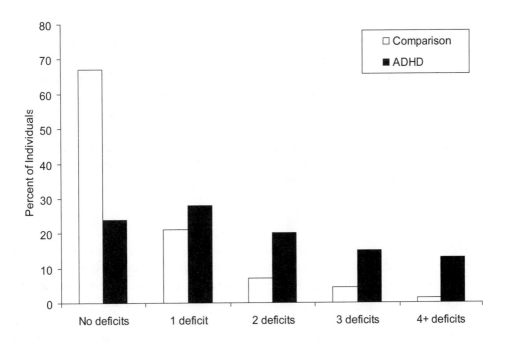

FIGURE 14.2. Percentage of individuals with and without ADHD who exhibited significant weaknesses in no, one, two, three, or four or more neuropsychological domains.

additional 29% exhibited a specific weakness in a single cognitive domain. In contrast, nearly half of all individuals with ADHD exhibited significant weaknesses in at least two distinct neuropsychological domains, and 27% of individuals exhibited weaknesses in three or more domains.

In summary, the correct neurocognitive model of ADHD is likely to involve dysfunction in multiple neural networks distributed across many locations in the brain. Further research is needed to test whether dysfunction in these different networks leads to distinct neuropsychological subtypes within the overall group of individuals with ADHD, or whether dysfunctional processes in multiple processes act in combination to increase susceptibility to ADHD. Perhaps the most likely scenario is that both types of models may be partially correct, such that some cases of ADHD may be attributable to a primary deficit in a relatively specific neurocognitive process, whereas other cases may be caused by the combined effects of dysfunction in multiple neural substrates.

KEY REMAINING ISSUES AND DIRECTIONS FOR FUTURE RESEARCH

The transition from models positing a single primary deficit to multiple-deficit models represents a paradigm shift in the way that the neuropsychology of ADHD is conceptualized (Sonuga-Barke, 2003). In this section, I describe several key remaining issues for the field, and then highlight future directions for studies of the neuropsychology of ADHD within a multiple-deficit framework.

Clinical Heterogeneity

In addition to the neuropsychological heterogeneity described in the preceding section, existing data clearly indicate that ADHD is also heterogeneous at the level of the behavioral phenotype (Lahey & Willcutt, 2002). The most obvious example of behavioral heterogeneity is the DSM-IV-TR distinction among three diagnostic subtypes of ADHD. In addition to subtype differences, the neuropsychological correlates of ADHD could vary as a function of sex, age, race/ethnicity, comorbidity, or the presence of specific etiological risk factors. The potential importance of clinical heterogeneity is illustrated by the results we recently obtained when we subdivided our overall ADHD sample according to the DSM-IV-TR subtypes and various comorbidities.

Diagnostic Subtypes

Although relatively few studies have examined the neuropsychological correlates of the DSM-IV-TR ADHD subtypes, a generally consistent pattern has emerged in both the most recent results from our sample (Figure 14.3; Willcutt et al., 2009) and a meta-analysis of the published literature (Willcutt et al., 2005a, 2005c). The combined and inattentive types differ from comparison groups without ADHD or other related disorders on measures of response inhibition, planning, vigilance, processing and naming speed, and some aspects of motor functioning; these effects are typically not explained by group differences in intelligence, academic achievement, or comorbid mental disorders (e.g., Chhabildas, Pennington, & Willcutt, 2001; Hinshaw et al., 2002; Nigg, Blaskey, Huang-Pollock, & Rappley, 2002).

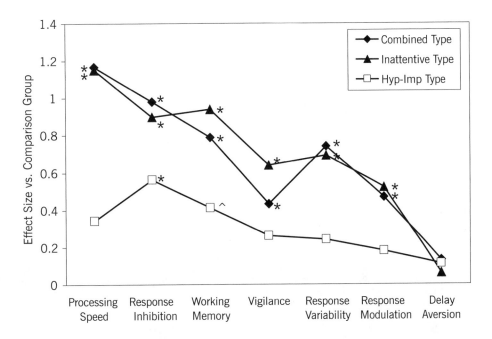

FIGURE 14.3. Neuropsychological performance of the DSM-IV-TR ADHD subtypes. Scores are scaled so that increasing effect sizes indicate greater impairment for all measures. $*p < .05$; $^\wedge p < .10$.

In contrast, the combined and inattentive types do not usually differ significantly from one another.

In contrast to the results for the inattentive and combined types, the hyperactive–impulsive type differed from controls on only 1 of 18 neurocognitive tasks in the meta-analysis, and was only impaired on the response inhibition composite in our current sample (Figure 14.3). Although additional research is needed with larger samples, these results suggest that the inattentive and combined types may share a common neuropsychological etiology, whereas the absence of consistent neuropsychological dysfunction underscores the remaining questions regarding the diagnostic validity of the hyperactive–impulsive type.

Comorbid Mental Disorders

Individuals with ADHD are more likely than expected by chance to meet criteria also for other disruptive behavior disorders (oppositional defiant and conduct disorders), learning disorders, anxiety disorders, and mood disorders (e.g., Faraone, Biederman, Weber, & Russell, 1998; Waschbusch, 2002; Willcutt, Pennington, Chhabildas, Friedman, & Alexander, 1999). However, few previous studies have tested whether the neuropsychological profile of ADHD differs as a function of these comorbidities. Table 14.2 summarizes results in our sample when the group with ADHD is subdivided on the basis of comorbidity with disorders in each of these four domains.

ADHD is associated with significant weaknesses on measures of inhibition, working memory, and processing speed even when all of these comorbidities are statistically controlled for. On the other hand, comorbidity may moderate the association between

TABLE 14.2. Neuropsychological Performance of Groups with DSM-IV-TR ADHD with and without Comorbidity

Measure[c]	Overall ADHD effect size[a]	Effect size of the difference between groups with ADHD with and without the comorbid disorder[a,b]			
		Reading disorder[d]	Conduct disorder[e]	Anxiety disorder[f]	Depression/dysthymia[f]
Response inhibition	0.88***	0.25*	0.10	0.11	0.38*
Vigilance	0.55***	0.30**	0.05	0.07	0.17
Working memory	0.84***	0.74***	−0.02	0.23	0.53**
Processing speed	1.14***	0.58***	−0.05	0.02	0.29*
Response variability	0.68***	0.37***	0.09	−0.12	0.10
Delay aversion	0.11	0.02	0.05	−0.02	0.03
Response modulation	0.39***	0.17	0.36*	0.29*	0.42**

[a]*Effect size* = d (Cohen, 1988).
[b]All effects are scaled so that positive scores indicate that the comorbid group performed worse on the measure.
[c]Measures in composite scores (described in detail by Shanahan et al., 2008, and Willcutt et al., 2005b): Response inhibition = stop signal reaction time and continuous-performance test (CPT) commission errors; vigilance = CPT omission errors; working memory = sentence span, counting span, digits backward, Cambridge Neuropsychological Test Automated Battery (CANTAB) spatial working memory; processing speed = rapid automatized naming, Stroop color and word naming, Wechsler Coding and Symbol Search, Educational Testing Service Identical Pictures, Colorado Perceptual Speed; response variability = stop-signal task go trials reaction time standard deviation; delay aversion = task described by Solanto et al. (2001); response modulation = commission errors on a go/no-go task with rewards and response cost.
[d]Based on a composite of the Peabody Individual Achievement Test Reading Recognition, Reading Comprehension, and Spelling subtests.
[e]Based on parent ratings on the DSM-IV Diagnostic Interview for Children and Adolescents (DICA).
[f]Based on parent and self-report ratings on the DSM-IV DICA.
*$p < .05$; **$p < .01$; ***$p < .001$.

ADHD and some of these weaknesses, such that groups with ADHD and comorbidity exhibit greater impairment than groups with ADHD alone. For example, consistent with previous studies (e.g., Rucklidge & Tannock, 2002; Seidman et al., 2001; Willcutt et al., 2001, 2005c), the magnitude of the ADHD deficit is larger in the group with ADHD and comorbid reading disorder than in the group with ADHD without reading disorder on measures of EFs, processing speed, and response variability (see Willcutt, Sonuga-Barke, Nigg, & Sergeant, 2008, for a more detailed review of the current literature). A similar pattern is evident for comorbidity with depression, although the effect sizes are substantially smaller. In contrast, the profile of the ADHD group does not differ as a function of comorbid anxiety or conduct disorder on the EF, processing speed, or response variability measures, but these comorbidities are associated with higher rates of impulsive errors on a go/no-go task with rewards for correct responses and punishment for commission errors. The latter result is consistent with research on psychopathy and neuroticism in adults (e.g., Patterson & Newman, 1993).

Implications and Recommendations for Future Studies of Clinical Heterogeneity

The current literature indicates that ADHD is associated with significant neuropsychological weaknesses that are not artifacts of the nearly ubiquitous comorbidity that characterizes samples with ADHD. On the other hand, the severity of neuropsychological dysfunction may differ as a function of comorbidity and diagnostic subtype of ADHD. Therefore, future studies of the neuropsychological correlates of ADHD should carefully consider all potential sources of heterogeneity.

One common approach to addressing clinical heterogeneity is to apply stringent exclusionary criteria at the beginning of a study, to maximize the homogeneity of the ADHD sample. However, the a priori exclusion of a subset of individuals with ADHD makes extremely strong assumptions about the meaning of heterogeneity that are not easily justified by existing knowledge, and may even be counterproductive. For example, the exclusion of children with a comorbid reading disability is likely to inadvertently eliminate the subset of individuals with the greatest neuropsychological impairment. For most purposes, the optimal approach is to include all individuals with ADHD, while carefully assessing comorbidities and other potential heterogeneity markers. These markers can then be included in analyses to test directly whether they influence the neuropsychological profile of ADHD.

Direct Tests of Competing Neuropsychological Models

Most previous studies have examined the neuropsychological correlates of ADHD from a single theoretical perspective, making it difficult or impossible to test competing theories in the same study. Although effect sizes from multiple studies can be used to conduct preliminary comparisons between theories, interpretation of such comparisons is inevitably complicated by differences in study design and sampling procedures. Therefore, studies are needed that test multiple competing theoretical models in the same sample, such as the study by Solanto et al. (2001) that suggested significant independent effects of delay aversion and response inhibition. Two recent results from our ongoing studies further illustrate the potential utility of this approach.

The first set of analyses tested whether different EFs are differentially correlated with attention problems in the Colorado Longitudinal Twin Study, an unselected community sample of 586 twins who are now in their early 20s (Friedman et al., 2007). Attention problems measured from ages 7 to 17 correlated significantly with latent trait measures of response inhibition ($r = .55$), updating/working memory ($r = .42$), and shifting ($r = .20$). However, only inhibition predicted ADHD independently of the other EFs. This result is consistent with the predictions of several prominent theoretical models (e.g., Barkley, 1997; Nigg, 2001), and helps to specify the nature of the executive control weaknesses in ADHD.

We conducted the second set of analyses in a sample of twins with and without ADHD from the CLDRC twin study (Willcutt et al., 2009b). Composite measures of response inhibition, working memory, processing speed, response variability, response modulation, and delay aversion were included as predictors of ADHD in a multiple-regression model. Although all constructs except delay aversion were significantly associated with ADHD when analyzed separately, only response inhibition and processing speed made a significant independent prediction in the multiple-regression model ($p < .01$). Response variability and working memory were marginally significant ($p < .10$), whereas response modulation and delay aversion did not make an independent contribution.

Refinement of Neuropsychological Measures

The neuropsychological measures used in previous studies of ADHD are often complex tasks that involve multiple cognitive processes, making it difficult to determine which component of the task is responsible for a group difference. Moreover, the predictive power of many of these tasks is constrained by their relatively modest reliability in children. In addition to procedures that may help to refine each individual task (see Willcutt et al., 2005a), both of these concerns may also be mitigated in future studies by administering multiple measures of key constructs to facilitate the creation of latent trait or factor scores. These scores are based on the common variance across multiple measures of a construct, separate from the variance associated with measurement error or other processes that are idiosyncratic to a particular measure. The potential utility of this measurement approach is also illustrated by recent results in both of our twin samples. The effect size for the relation between attention problems and inhibition was substantially higher for an inhibition latent trait score ($r = .55$; Friedman et al., 2007) or composite score ($d = 0.98$; Willcutt et al., 2009b) than for any individual inhibition measure ($r = .20–.34$; $d = 0.50–0.73$); similar results were obtained for processing speed, shifting, and working memory.

Developmental Stability

The onset of ADHD is in early childhood; levels of ADHD symptoms are relatively stable across development for most individuals (particularly symptoms of inattention); and ADHD is associated with many of the same aspects of functional impairment in childhood, adolescence, and adulthood. As a result, there can be little doubt that ADHD is a valid diagnosis in adulthood for individuals with a history of childhood ADHD (e.g., Barkley, 2002; Lahey & Willcutt, 2002). The few studies of the neuropsychological correlates of ADHD in adults have generally found similar weaknesses in executive control and processing speed (e.g., Nigg et al., 2005a), and a recent longitudinal study suggests that early attention problems predict EF weaknesses in young adulthood (Friedman et al., 2007). Although additional data are needed regarding delay aversion and the influence of reward and punishment contingencies in adults, the current literature suggests that the neuropsychological profile of ADHD is stable across development for most individuals.

Multiple Levels of Analysis

Finally, perhaps the most exciting future direction for studies of the neuropsychology of ADHD is the increasing opportunity to feasibly incorporate multiple levels of analysis in a single study. In the remainder of this section, I briefly describe how neuropsychological studies might interface with four other levels of analysis that show great promise as tools for future research on the pathophysiology of ADHD.

Etiologically Informative Designs

Twin studies of ADHD consistently indicate that genetic influences account for 75–80% of the group deficit in ADHD symptoms (e.g., Levy, Hay, McStephen, Wood, & Waldman,

1997; Willcutt, Pennington, Olson, & DeFries, 2007). The high heritability of ADHD suggests that the neuropsychological weaknesses influencing ADHD are also likely to be due at least in part to genetic influences. One of the goals of our ongoing twin study is to test the etiology of deficits on the five constructs that have been proposed as neuropsychological weaknesses in ADHD. The white bars in Figure 14.4 indicate the extent to which performance on each neuropsychological measure is due to genetic influences (Willcutt et al., 2009b). These results suggest that moderate to strong genetic influences contribute to performance on EF and processing speed tasks, consistent with other twin studies of individual differences in the entire population (e.g., Ando, Ono, & Wright, 2001; Swan & Carmelli, 2002). In contrast, genetic effects are weaker for response variability and response modulation, and individual differences in delay aversion appear to be attributable to environmental influences.

After ADHD symptoms and performance on a specific neuropsychological task have been shown to be heritable, the next step is to test whether their correlation is due to the same genetic influences. Estimates of bivariate heritability (dark bars in Figure 14.4) provide an index of the extent to which ADHD symptoms are due to genetic influences that also lead to neuropsychological impairment. Our current findings suggest that common genetic influences account for nearly all of the covariance between ADHD symptoms and response inhibition, working memory, and processing speed (Willcutt et al., 2009b). These results are promising for future studies that attempt to identify the specific genetic mechanisms influencing ADHD symptoms, neuropsychological performance, and their covariation.

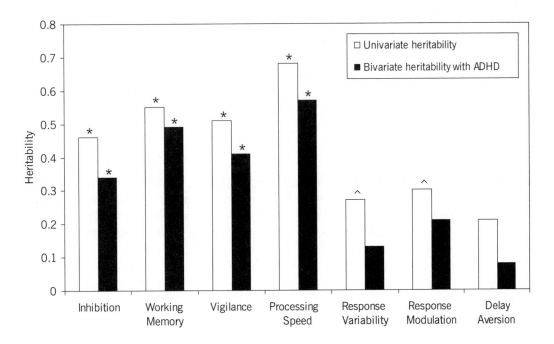

FIGURE 14.4. Univariate heritability of group deficits on neuropsychological composite scores, and bivariate heritability of elevations of ADHD symptoms and each neuropsychological weakness. *$p < .05$; ^$p < .10$.

Neurocomputational Modeling

Computational cognitive neuroscience is a relatively new field that uses powerful computer simulations to understand the neural mechanisms that underlie human cognition (see O'Reilly & Munakata, 2000, for an excellent introduction to this approach). Neurocomputational models simulate specific cognitive processes by using neuron-like units organized in neural networks that are consistent with the brain's known anatomical and physiological properties. Biologically plausible computational models have been developed for several cognitive processes that may be relevant to ADHD, including working memory, inhibition, cognitive control, and response to reward and punishment contingencies (e.g., Cohen & Servan-Schreiber, 1992; Frank, Loughry, & O'Reilly, 2001; O'Reilly & Frank, 2006).

In addition to providing a resource for understanding normative cognitive functioning, computational models can be used to simulate the impact of brain damage or dysfunction through manipulations that would not be possible with human participants. For example, clusters of neuron units in the model can be turned off completely, to enable researchers to examine the effect of a simulated lesion to a component of a neural network. Alternatively, more subtle changes to the sensitivity of individual neuron units or the strength of the associations between units can be used to simulate the impact of abnormally low or high levels of a particular neurotransmitter, or individual differences in patterns of interconnectivity among neurons.

Neurocomputational modeling techniques are likely to provide an important tool for understanding the pathophysiology of complex disorders such as ADHD. Theoretical models of the neurophysiology of ADHD can be instantiated in computational models; then the results of the simulations can be used to derive and constrain new predictions, which can be tested by using neuropsychological tasks or other behavioral measures. Neuropsychological results will then provide new data that the computational models must explain, leading to further refinements to the theoretical model. The potential utility of this iterative approach is demonstrated in a recent study that used a neurocomputational model and psychopharmacological manipulation to begin to tease apart the differential influence of dopamine and noradrenaline on neuropsychological dysfunction in ADHD (Frank et al., 2007).

Brain Imaging

Similar to neurocomputational modeling, the collection of neuroimaging and neuropsychological measures in the same sample will allow these methods to inform and constrain one another. Theoretical models make specific predictions regarding the brain regions and neurotransmitter systems that are likely to be implicated in ADHD. Neuropsychological measures can then be developed that recruit these specific regions of the brain, facilitating direct tests of the theoretical predictions via structural MRI and fMRI, event-related potentials, or other measures of neurophysiology (e.g., Aron & Poldrack, 2005; Bush, Valera, & Seidman, 2005).

Treatment Response

The ongoing National Institute of Mental Health (NIMH) Collaborative Multimodal Treatment Study of Children with ADHD (the MTA; e.g., Arnold et al., 1997; MTA Cooperative

Group, 1999) is the largest treatment study ever conducted for a childhood disorder. Results of the MTA and many other previous studies clearly demonstrate that psychostimulant medication is an effective intervention for children with ADHD (e.g., MTA Cooperative Group, 1999), and subsequent studies suggest that at least a subset of individuals with ADHD may benefit from atomoxetine, a nonstimulant medication (e.g., Michelson et al., 2002). In addition to medication, structured behavioral interventions in the home and classroom may lead to improvement in some domains of functioning (e.g., Pelham & Fabiano, 2008).

The long-term goal of neuropsychological research on ADHD and other clinical disorders is to inform and improve diagnostic assessment and treatment methods, but few studies have examined the relation between neuropsychological functioning and treatment outcome. The inclusion of neuropsychological measures in future treatment studies may help to clarify the neurophysiological mechanisms that underlie an effective treatment. For example, changes in symptoms in response to stimulant medication may be accompanied by concomitant changes in an underlying neuropsychological weakness such as executive control.

A second key issue for future treatment studies is heterogeneous treatment response. For example, although stimulants are an effective treatment for 70–90% of children with ADHD, a subset of children either fail to respond adequately to these medications or exhibit significant side effects (e.g., MTA Cooperative Group, 1999). Similarly, behavioral interventions may be most effective for specific subgroups of children with ADHD. Incorporating measures of neuropsychological functioning in future treatment studies may eventually make it possible to use these tasks to predict the treatment most likely to be helpful for a specific individual with ADHD.

CONCLUSIONS

The neuropsychology of ADHD is clearly complex and multifactorial, with no single deficit that is necessary or sufficient to explain all cases of ADHD. A comprehensive neuropsychological model of ADHD must incorporate weaknesses in response inhibition and other aspects of executive control, increased aversion to delay, and slower and more variable response speed. Additional research is needed to clarify the relations among these complex domains, as well as to understand the impact of diagnostic and neuropsychological heterogeneity. Multidisciplinary studies that incorporate neuropsychological measures as one of several levels of analysis show great promise as an important new approach to continue to refine our understanding of the pathophysiology of ADHD.

ACKNOWLEDGMENTS

I was supported in part during the preparation of this chapter by National Institutes of Health R01 Grant Nos. MH 62120, MH 63941, and HD 47264 (Erik G. Willcutt) and National Institute of Child Health and Human Development Center Grant No. P50 HD 27802 (Center Director: Richard K. Olson). I thank Bruce F. Pennington, John C. DeFries, and Richard K. Olson for sharing a portion of the data presented in this chapter, and I am grateful to Nomita Chhabildas for helpful comments on an earlier version of the chapter.

REFERENCES

American Psychiatric Association. (2000). *Diagnostic and statistical manual of mental disorders* (4th ed., text rev.). Washington, DC: Author.

Ando, J., Ono, Y., & Wright, M. J. (2001). Genetic structure of spatial and working memory. *Behavioral Genetics, 31,* 615–624.

Angold, A., Erkanli, A., Farmer, E. M. Z., Fairbank, J. A., Burns, B. J., Keeler, G., et al. (2002). Psychiatric disorder, impairment, and service use in rural African American and White youth. *Archives of General Psychiatry, 59,* 893–901.

Arnold, L. E., Abikoff, H. B., Cantwell, D. P., Conners, C. K., Elliott, G., Greenhill, L. L., et al. (1997). National Institute of Mental Health Collaborative Multimodal Treatment study of Children with ADHD (the MTA). *Archives of General Psychiatry, 54,* 865–870.

Aron A. R., & Poldrack R. A. (2005). The cognitive neuroscience of response inhibition: Relevance for genetic research in attention-deficit/hyperactivity disorder. *Biological Psychiatry, 57,* 1285–1292.

Barkley, R. A. (1997). Behavioral inhibition, sustained attention, and executive function: Constructing a unified theory of ADHD. *Psychological Bulletin, 121,* 65–94.

Barkley, R. A. (2001). The inattentive type of ADHD as a distinct disorder: What remains to be done. *Clinical Psychology: Science and Practice, 8,* 489–493.

Barkley, R. A. (2002). Major life activity and health outcomes associated with attention-deficit/hyperactivity disorder. *Journal of Clinical Psychiatry, 63*(Suppl. 12), 10–15.

Barkley, R. A. (2006). *Attention-deficit hyperactivity disorder: A handbook for diagnosis and treatment* (3rd ed.). New York: Guilford Press.

Baumgaertel, A., Wolraich, M. L., & Dietrich, M. (1995). Comparison of diagnostic criteria for attention deficit disorders in a German elementary school sample. *Journal of the American Academy of Child and Adolescent Psychiatry, 34,* 629–638.

Bechara, A., Damasio, H., & Damasio, A. R. (2000). Emotion, decision making and the orbitofrontal cortex. *Cerebral Cortex, 10,* 295–307.

Biederman, J., Mick, E., Faraone, S. V., Braaten, E., Doyle, A., Spencer, T., et al. (2002). Influence of gender on attention-deficit hyperactivity disorder in children referred to a psychiatric clinic. *American Journal of Psychiatry, 159,* 36–42.

Breeding, J. (2000, July–August). Does ADHD even exist?: The Ritalin sham. *Mothering,* pp. 43–47.

Bush, G., Frazier, J. A., Rauch, S. L., Seidman, L. J., Whalen, P. J., Jenike, M. A., et al. (1999). Anterior cingulate cortex dysfunction in attention-deficit hyperactivity disorder revealed by fMRI and the counting Stroop. *Biological Psychiatry, 45,* 1542–1552.

Bush, G., Valera, E. M., & Seidman, L. J. (2005). Functional neuroimaging of attention-deficit/hyperactivity disorder: A review and suggested future directions. *Biological Psychiatry, 57,* 1273–1284.

Carlson, C. L., & Tamm, L. (2000). Responsiveness of children with attention deficit-hyperactivity disorder to reward and response cost: Differential impact on performance and motivation. *Journal of Consulting and Clinical Psychology, 68,* 73–83.

Casey, B. J., Durston, S., & Fossella, J. A. (2001). Towards a mechanistic model of cognitive control. *Clinical Neuroscience Research, 1,* 267–282.

Castellanos, F. X., Lee, P. P., Sharp, W., Jeffries, N. O., Greenstein, D. K., Clasen L. S., et al. (2002). Developmental trajectories of brain volume abnormalities in children and adolescents with attention-deficit/hyperactivity disorder. *Journal of the American Medical Association, 288,* 1740–1748.

Castellanos, F. X., Sonuga-Barke, E. J. S., Scheres, A., Di Martino, A., Hyde, C., & Walters, J. R. (2005). Varieties of attention-deficit/hyperactivity disorder-related intra-individual variability. *Biological Psychiatry, 57,* 1416–1423.

Castellanos, F. X., & Tannock, R. (2002). Neuroscience of attention-deficit/hyperactivity disorder: The search for endophenotypes. *Nature Reviews Neuroscience, 3,* 617–628.

Chhabildas, N. A., Pennington, B. F., & Willcutt, E. G. (2001). A comparison of the cognitive deficits in the DSM-IV subtypes of ADHD. *Journal of Abnormal Child Psychology, 29,* 529–540.

Cohen, J. (1988). *Statistical power analysis for the behavioral sciences*. Hillsdale, NJ: Erlbaum.

Cohen, J. D., & Servan-Schreiber, D. (1992). Context, cortex and dopamine: A connectionist approach to behavior and biology in schizophrenia. *Psychological Review, 99*, 45–77.

Collette, F., Van der Linden, M., Laureys, S., Delfiore, G., Degueldre, C., Luxen, A., et al. (2005). Exploring the unity and diversity of the neural substrates of executive functioning. *Human Brain Mapping, 25*, 409–423.

DuPaul, G. J., Anastopoulos, A. D., McGoey, K. E., Power, T. J., Reid, R., & Ikeda, M. J. (1997). Teacher ratings of attention deficit hyperactivity disorder symptoms: Factor structure and normative data. *Psychological Assessment, 9*, 436–444.

DuPaul, G. J., Power, T. P., Anastopoulos, A. D., & Reid, R. (1998). *ADHD Rating Scale–IV*. New York: Guilford Press.

Elliott, R., Dolan, R. J., & Frith, C. D. (2000). Dissociable functions in the medial and lateral orbitofrontal cortex: Evidence from human neuroimaging studies. *Cerebral Cortex, 10*, 308–317.

Ernst, M., Kimes A. S., London, E. D., Matochik, J. A., Eldreth, D., Tata, S., Contoreggi, C., et al. (2003). Neural substrates of decision making in adults with attention deficit hyperactivity disorder. *American Journal of Psychiatry, 160*, 1061–1070.

Faraone, S. V., Biederman, J., Weber, W., & Russell, R. L. (1998). Psychiatric, neuropsychological, and psychosocial features of DSM-IV subtypes of attention-deficit/hyperactivity disorder: Results from a clinically-referred sample. *Journal of the American Academy of Child and Adolescent Psychiatry, 37*, 185–193.

Farmer, R. F., & Rucklidge, J. J. (2006). An evaluation of the response modulation hypothesis in relation to attention-deficit/hyperactivity disorder. *Journal of Abnormal Child Psychology, 34*, 545–557.

Frank, M. J., Loughry, B., & O'Reilly, R. C. (2001). Interactions between frontal cortex and basal ganglia in working memory: A computational model. *Cognitive, Affective, and Behavioral Neuroscience, 1*, 137–160.

Frank, M., Santamaria, A., O'Reilly, R., & Willcutt, E. G. (2007). Testing computational models of dopamine and noradrenaline dysfunction in attention deficit/hyperactivity disorder. *Neuropsychopharmacology, 32*, 1583–1599.

Friedman, N. P., Haberstick, B. C., Willcutt, E. G., Miyake, A., Young, S. E., Corley, R. P., et al. (2007). Greater attention problems during childhood predict poorer executive functioning in late adolescence. *Psychological Science, 18*, 893–900.

Friedman, N. P., Miyake, A., Corley, R. P., Young, S. E., DeFries, J. C., & Hewitt, J. K. (2006). Not all executive functions are related to intelligence. *Psychological Science, 17*, 172–179.

Fuster, J. M. (1997). *The prefrontal cortex: Anatomy, physiology, and neuropsychology of the frontal lobe* (2nd ed.). Philadelphia: Lippincott-Raven.

Gadow, K. D., Nolan, E. E., Litcher, L., Carlson, G. A., Panina, N., Golovakha, E., et al. (2000). Comparison of attention-deficit/hyperactivity disorder symptom subtype in Ukrainian schoolchildren. *Journal of the American Academy of Child and Adolescent Psychiatry, 39*, 1520–1527.

Gaub, M., & Carlson, C. L. (1997). Behavioral characteristics of DSM-IV ADHD subtypes in a school-based population. *Journal of Abnormal Child Psychology, 25*, 103–111.

Graetz, B. W., Sawyer, M. G., Hazell, P. L., Arney, F., & Baghurst, P. (2001). Validity of DSM-IV ADHD subtypes in a nationally representative sample of Australian children and adolescents. *Journal of the American Academy of Child and Adolescent Psychiatry, 40*, 1410–1417.

Hartung, C. M., Milich, R., Lynam, D. R., & Martin, C. A. (2002). Understanding the relations among gender, disinhibition, and disruptive behavior in adolescents. *Journal of Abnormal Psychology, 111*, 659–664.

Hesslinger, B., Tebartz van Elst, L., Thiel, T., Haegele, K., Hennig, J., & Ebert, D. (2002). Frontoorbital volume reductions in adult patients with attention deficit hyperactivity disorder. *Neuroscience Letters, 328*, 319–321.

Hinshaw, S. P., Carte, E. T., Sami, N., Treuting, J. J., & Zupan, B. A. (2002). Preadolescent girls with attention-deficit/hyperactivity disorder: II. Neuropsychological performance in relation to subtypes and individual classification. *Journal of Consulting and Clinical Psychology, 70,* 1099–1111.

Kuntsi, J., Oosterlaan, J., & Stevenson, J. (2001). Psychological mechanisms in hyperactivity: I. Response inhibition deficit, working memory impairment, delay aversion, or something else? *Journal of Child Psychology and Psychiatry, 42,* 199–210.

Lahey, B. B., Applegate, B., McBurnett, K., Biederman, J., Greenhill, L., Hynd, G. W., et al. (1994). DSM-IV field trials for attention deficit hyperactivity disorder in children and adolescents. *American Journal of Psychiatry, 151,* 1673–1685.

Lahey, B. B., Pelham, W. E., Stein, M., Loney, J., Trapani, C., Nugent, K., et al. (1998). Validity of DSM-IV attention-deficit/hyperactivity disorder for young children. *Journal of the American Academy of Child and Adolescent Psychiatry, 37,* 695–702.

Lahey, B. B., & Willcutt, E. (2002). Validity of the diagnosis and dimensions of attention deficit hyperactivity disorder. In P. S. Jensen & J. R. Cooper (Eds.), *Attention deficit hyperactivity disorder: State of the science* (pp. 1-1–1-23). New York: Civic Research Institute.

Levy, F., Hay, D., McStephen, M., Wood, C., & Waldman, I. (1997). Attention-deficit hyperactivity disorder: A category or a continuum? A genetic analysis of a large-scale twin study. *Journal of the American Academy of Child and Adolescent Psychiatry, 36,* 737–744.

Lowe, N., Kirley, A., Hawi, Z., Sham, P., Wickham, H., Kratochvil, C. J., et al. (2004). Joint analysis of the DRD5 marker concludes association with attention-deficit/hyperactivity disorder confined to the predominantly inattentive and combined subtypes. *American Journal of Human Genetics, 74,* 348–356.

Luman, M., Oosterlaan, J., & Sergeant, J. A. (2006). The impact of reinforcement contingencies on AD/HD: A review and theoretical appraisal. *Clinical Psychology Review, 25,* 183–213.

Maedgen, J. W., & Carlson, C. L. (2000). Social functioning and emotional regulation in the attention deficit hyperactivity disorder subtypes. *Journal of Clinical Child Psychology, 29,* 30–42.

Michelson, D., Allen, A. J., Busner, J., Casat, C., Dunn, D., Kratochvil, C., et al. (2002). Once-daily atomoxetine treatment for children and adolescents with attention deficit hyperactivity disorder: A randomized, placebo-controlled study. *American Journal of Psychiatry, 159,* 1896–1901.

Milich, R., Balentine, A. C., & Lynam, D. R. (2001). ADHD combined type and ADHD predominately inattentive type are distinct and unrelated disorders. *Clinical Psychology: Science and Practice, 8,* 463–488.

Miyake, A., Friedman, N. P., Emerson, M. J., Witzki, A. H., & Howerter, A. (2000). The unity and diversity of executive functions and their contributions to complex frontal lobe tasks: A latent variable analysis. *Cognitive Psychology, 41,* 49–100.

MTA Cooperative Group. (1999). A 14-month randomized clinical trial of treatment strategies for attention-deficit/hyperactivity disorder. *Archives of General Psychiatry, 56,* 1073–86, 1097–1009.

Nigg, J. T. (2001). Is ADHD a disinhibitory disorder? *Psychological Bulletin, 127,* 571–598.

Nigg, J. T., Blaskey, L. G., Huang-Pollock, C. L., & Rappley, M. D. (2002). Neuropsychological executive functions and DSM-IV ADHD subtypes. *Journal of the American Academy of Child and Adolescent Psychiatry, 41,* 59–66.

Nigg, J. T., Hinshaw, S. P., Carte, E., & Treuting, J. (1998). Neuropsychological correlates of childhood attention-deficit/hyperactivity disorder: Explainable by comorbid disruptive behavior or reading problems? *Journal of Abnormal Psychology, 107,* 468–480.

Nigg, J. T., Stavro, G., Ettenhofer, M., Hambrick, D. Z., Miller, T., & Henderson, J. M. (2005a). Executive functions and ADHD in adults: Evidence for selective effects on ADHD symptom domains. *Journal of Abnormal Psychology, 114,* 706–717.

Nigg, J. T., Willcutt, E. G., Doyle, A. E., & Sonuga-Barke, E. J. S. (2005b). Heterogeneous causality in ADHD: The need for a neuropsychologically impaired subtype. *Biological Psychiatry, 57,* 1231–1238.

O'Reilly, R. C., & Frank, M. J. (2006). Making working memory work: A computational model of learning in the prefrontal cortex and basal ganglia. *Neural Computation, 18,* 283–328.

O'Reilly, R. C., & Munakata, Y. (2000). *Computational explorations in cognitive neuroscience: Understanding the mind by simulating the brain*. Cambridge, MA: MIT Press.

Patterson, C. M., & Newman, J. P. (1993). Reflectivity and learning from aversive events: Toward a psychological mechanism for the syndromes of disinhibition. *Psychological Review, 100*, 716–736.

Pelham, W. E., & Fabiano, G. A. (2008). Evidence-based psychosocial treatments for attention-deficit/hyperactivity disorder. *Journal of Clinical Child and Adolescent Psychology, 37*, 184–214.

Pennington, B. F. (2002). *The development of psychopathology*. New York: Guilford Press.

Pennington, B. F., & Ozonoff, S. (1996). Executive functions and developmental psychopathology. *Journal of Child Psychology and Psychiatry, 37*, 51–87.

Pineda, D. A., Ardila, A., Roselli, M., Arias, B. E., Henao, G. C., Gomez, L. F., et al. (1999). Prevalence of attention-deficit/hyperactivity disorder symptoms in 4- to 17-year-old children in the general population. *Journal of Abnormal Child Psychology, 27*, 455–462.

Reid, R., DuPaul, G., Power, T. J., Anastopoulos, A. D., Rogers-Adkinson, D., Noll, M., et al. (1998). Assessing culturally different students for attention deficit hyperactivity disorder using behavior rating scales. *Journal of Abnormal Child Psychology, 26*, 187–198.

Rolls, E. T. (2004). The functions of the orbitofrontal cortex. *Brain and Cognition, 55*, 11–29.

Rowland, A. S., Umbach, D. M., Stallone, L., Naftel, A. J., Bohlig, E. M., & Sandler, D. P. (2002). Prevalence of medication treatment for attention deficit-hyperactivity disorder among elementary school children in Johnstone County, North Carolina. *American Journal of Public Health, 92*, 231–234.

Rubia, K., Overmeyer, S., Taylor, E., Brammer, M., Williams, S.C., Simmons, A., et al. (1999). Hypofrontality in attention deficit hyperactivity disorder during higher-order motor control: A study with functional MRI. *American Journal of Psychiatry, 156*, 891–896.

Rucklidge, J. J., & Tannock, R. (2002). Neuropsychological profiles of adolescents with ADHD: Effects of reading difficulties and gender. *Journal of Child Psychology and Psychiatry, 43*, 988–1003.

Scheres, A., Dijkstra, M., Ainslie, E., Balkan, J., Reynolds, B., Sonuga-Barke, E., et al. (2006). Temporal and probabilistic discounting of rewards in children and adolescents: Effects of age and ADHD symptoms. *Neuropsychologia, 44*, 2092–2103.

Scheres, A., Oosterlaan, J., & Sergeant, J. A. (2001). Response execution and inhibition in children with AD/HD and other disruptive disorders: The role of behavioural activation. *Journal of Child Psychology and Psychiatry, 42*, 347–357.

Schultz, W., Tremblay, L., & Hollerman, J. R. (2000). Reward processing in primate orbitofrontal cortex and basal ganglia. *Cerebral Cortex, 10*, 272–283.

Schulz, K. P., Fan, J., Tang, C. K., Newcorn, J. H., Buchsbaum, M. S., Cheung, A. M., et al. (2004). Response inhibition in adolescents diagnosed with attention deficit hyperactivity disorder: An event-related fMRI study. *American Journal of Psychiatry, 156*, 891–896.

Seidman, L. J., Biederman, J., Monuteaux, M. C., Doyle, A. E., & Faraone, S. V. (2001). Learning disabilities and executive dysfunction in boys with attention-deficit/hyperactivity disorder. *Neuropsychology, 15*, 544–556.

Seidman, L. J., Valera, E. M., & Makris, N. (2005). Structural brain imaging of attention-deficit/hyperactivity disorder. *Biological Psychiatry, 57*, 1263–1272.

Sergeant, J. A., Geurts, H., Huijbregts, S., Scheres, A., & Oosterlaan, J. (2003). The top and bottom of ADHD: a neuropsychological perspective. *Neuroscience and Biobehavioral Reviews, 27*, 583–592.

Shanahan, M., Willcutt, E. G., & Pennington, B. F. (2008). Do motivational incentives reduce the inhibition deficit in ADHD? *Developmental Neuropsychology, 33*, 137–159.

Shanahan, M., Yerys, B., Scott, A., Willcutt, E. G., & Pennington, B. F. (2006). Processing speed deficits in attention-deficit/hyperactivity disorder and reading disability. *Journal of Abnormal Child Psychology, 34*, 585–602.

Slusarek, M., Velling, S., Bunk, D., & Eggers, C. (2001). Motivational effects on inhibitory control in children with ADHD. *Journal of the American Academy of Child and Adolescent Psychiatry, 40,* 355–363.

Solanto, M. V., Abikoff, H., Sonuga-Barke, E. J. S., Schachar, R., Logan, G. D., Wigal, T., et al. (2001). The ecological validity of delay aversion and response inhibition as measures of impulsivity in AD/HD: A supplement to the NIMH multimodal treatment study of AD/HD. *Journal of Abnormal Child Psychology, 29,* 215–228.

Sonuga-Barke, E. J. S. (2003). The dual pathway model of ADHD: An elaboration of neurodevelopmental characteristics. *Neuroscience and Biobehavioral Reviews, 27,* 593–604.

Sonuga-Barke, E. J. S., Dalen, L., & Remington, B. (2003). Do executive deficits and delay aversion make independent contributions to preschool attention-deficit/hyperactivity disorder symptoms? *Journal of the American Academy of Child and Adolescent Psychiatry, 42,* 1335–1342.

Sonuga-Barke, E. J. S., Taylor, E., Sembi, S., & Smith, J. (1992). Hyperactivity and delay aversion: I. The effect of delay on choice. *Journal of Child Psychology and Psychiatry, 33,* 387–398.

Stuss, D. T., & Benson, D. F. (1986). *The frontal lobes.* New York: Raven Press.

Swan, G. E., & Carmelli, D (2002). Evidence for genetic mediation of executive control: A study of aging male twins. *Journal of Gerontology: B. Psychological Science and Social Science, 57,* 133–143.

Todd, R. D., Rasmussen, E. R., Neuman, R. J., Reich, W., Hudziak, J. J., Bucholz, K. K., et al. (2001). Familiality and heritability of subtypes of attention deficit hyperactivity disorder in a population sample of adolescent female twins. *American Journal of Psychiatry, 158,* 1891–1898.

Vaidya, C. Y., Austin, G., Kirkorian, G., Ridlehuber, H. W., Desmond, J. E., Glover, G. H., et al. (1998). Selective effects of methylphenidate in attention deficit hyperactivity disorder: A functional magnetic resonance study. *Proceedings of the National Academy of Sciences USA, 95,* 14494–14499.

Waschbusch, D. A. (2002). A meta-analytic examination of comorbid hyperactive–impulsive–attention problems and conduct problems. *Psychological Bulletin, 128,* 118–150.

Welsh, M. C., & Pennington, B. F. (1988). Assessing frontal lobe functioning in children: Views from developmental psychology. *Developmental Neuropsychology, 4,* 199–230.

Widiger, T. A., & Clark, L. A. (2000). Toward DSM-V and the classification of psychopathology. *Psychological Bulletin, 126,* 946–963.

Willcutt, E. G., Bidwell, L. C., Hartung, C. M., Santerre-Lemmon, L., Shanahan, M., Barnard, H., et al. (2009a). *The neuropsychology of ADHD.* Manuscript submitted for publication.

Willcutt, E. G., Brodsky, K., Chhabildas, N., Shanahan, M., Yerys, B., Scott, A., et al. (2005a). The neuropsychology of ADHD: Validity of the executive function hypothesis. In D. Gozal & D. L. Molfese (Eds.), *Attention deficit hyperactivity disorder: From genes to patients* (pp. 185–213). Totowa, NJ: Humana Press.

Willcutt, E. G., & Carlson, C. L. (2005). Diagnostic validity of attention-deficit/hyperactivity disorder. *Clinical Neuroscience Review, 5,* 219–232.

Willcutt, E. G., Chhabildas, N., Betjemann, R., Bidwell, L. C., DeFries, J. C., & Pennington, B. F. (2009b). *A twin study of the validity of the executive function theory of ADHD.* Manuscript submitted for publication.

Willcutt, E. G., Doyle, A. E., Nigg, J. T., Faraone, S. V., & Pennington, B. F. (2005b). A meta-analytic review of the executive function theory of ADHD. *Biological Psychiatry, 57,* 1336–1346.

Willcutt, E. G., Lahey, B. B., Pennington, B. F., Carlson, C. L., Nigg, J. T., & McBurnett, K. (2009c). *Validity of attention-deficit/hyperactivity disorder.* Manuscript submitted for publication.

Willcutt, E. G., Pennington, B. F., Boada, R., Tunick, R. A., Ogline, J., Chhabildas, N. A., et al. (2001). A comparison of the cognitive deficits in reading disability and attention-deficit/hyperactivity disorder. *Journal of Abnormal Psychology, 110,* 157–172.

Willcutt, E. G., Pennington, B. F., Chhabildas, N. A., Friedman, M. C., & Alexander, J. (1999). Psychiatric comorbidity associated with DSM-IV ADHD in a nonreferred sample of twins. *Journal of the American Academy of Child and Adolescent Psychiatry, 38,* 1355–1362.

Willcutt, E. G., Pennington, B. F., Chhabildas, N. A., Olson, R. K., & Hulslander, J. L. (2005c). Neuropsychological analyses of comorbidity between RD and ADHD: In search of the common deficit. *Developmental Neuropsychology, 27,* 35–78.

Willcutt, E. G., Pennington, B. F., & DeFries, J. C. (2000). Etiology of inattention and hyperactivity/impulsivity in a community sample of twins with learning difficulties. *Journal of Abnormal Child Psychology, 28,* 149–159.

Willcutt, E. G., Pennington, B. F., Olson, R. K., & DeFries, J. C. (2007). Understanding comorbidity: A twin study of reading disability and attention-deficit/hyperactivity disorder. *American Journal of Medical Genetics: Part B. Neuropsychiatric Genetics, 8,* 709–714.

Willcutt, E. G., Sonuga-Barke, E. J. S., Nigg, J. T., & Sergeant, J. A. (2008). Recent developments in neuropsychological models of childhood psychiatric disorders. *Advances in Biological Psychiatry, 24,* 195–226.

CHAPTER 15

Autism Spectrum Disorders

SALLY OZONOFF

Autism, first described only 60+ years ago, was once thought to be a rare disorder. Knowledge about it—the condition itself; its diagnosis and management; and its causes, course, and outcome—was not considered necessary for most psychologists and other mental health professionals. In many communities, autism was evaluated by a small group of specialists, and treatments were not readily available. Now, however, with the number of affected children increasing, the responsibility of practitioners to recognize, evaluate, and refer these children is high. It is clear that autism involves brain changes at both the structural and functional levels, making knowledge about it even more imperative for neuropsychologists. In this chapter, I first give background about autism and related disorders, diagnosis, epidemiology, course, and outcome. Then the neural substrates of autism spectrum disorders (ASD), as they have come to be called, and their neuropsychological consequences are summarized. I end with a review and critique of existing cognitive theories of ASD and suggestions for future directions.

SYMPTOMS AND DIAGNOSTIC DEFINITIONS

As specified in the *Diagnostic and Statistical Manual of Mental Disorders*, fourth edition, text revision (DSM-IV-TR; American Psychiatric Association, 2000), there are five pervasive developmental disorders (PDD): autistic disorder, Asperger's disorder, Rett's disorder, childhood disintegrative disorder, and PDD not otherwise specified (PDD-NOS). Symptoms of autistic disorder fall into the three areas of social relatedness, communication, and behaviors and interests. In the social domain, symptoms include impaired use of nonverbal behaviors (e.g., eye contact, facial expression, gestures) to regulate social interaction; failure to develop age-appropriate peer relationships; little seeking to share enjoyment or interests with other people; and limited social-emotional reciprocity. Communication deficits include delay in or absence of spoken language; difficulty initiating or sustaining conversation; idiosyncratic or repetitive language; and deficits in imitation and pretend play. In the domain of behaviors and interests, there are often all-encompassing, unusual interests; inflexible adherence to nonfunctional routines; stereotyped body movements; and preoccupation with parts or sensory qualities of objects (American Psychiatric Association, 2000). To meet criteria for autistic disorder, an individual must demonstrate at least 6 of the 12 symptoms, with at least 2 coming from the social domain and 1 each from the communication and restricted behaviors/interests categories. At least 1 symptom must have been present before 36 months of age.

Asperger's disorder (or Asperger syndrome, as I refer to it hereafter) shares the social disabilities and restricted, repetitive behaviors of autism, but language is well developed and intellectual functioning is not impaired. Its symptoms are identical to those just listed for autistic disorder, except that there is no requirement of any difficulties in the second category, communication. Although described well over 60 years ago by Austrian pediatrician Hans Asperger (1944), the Asperger syndrome diagnosis was not included in the DSM until the fourth edition. The main point of differentiation from autistic disorder, especially the higher-functioning subtype, is that those with Asperger syndrome do not exhibit significant delays in the onset or early course of language. As specified in DSM-IV-TR, nonechoed, communicative use of single words must be demonstrated by age 2 and meaningful phrase speech by age 3. Most parents of children with Asperger syndrome are not concerned about early language development and may even report precocious language abilities, such as a large vocabulary and adult-like phrasing. Autistic disorder must be ruled out before a diagnosis of Asperger syndrome is justified. DSM-IV-TR mandates that the diagnosis of autistic disorder always takes precedence over that of Asperger syndrome. Thus, if a child meets criteria for autistic disorder, the diagnosis must be autism even if he or she displays excellent structural language, average or better cognitive skills, and other "typical" features of Asperger syndrome.

Individuals who meet criteria for autistic disorder and are intellectually normal are considered "high-functioning." Research comparing Asperger syndrome and high-functioning autism (HFA) provides mixed evidence of their external validity. Early history differences are evident between the disorders, with children with Asperger syndrome showing fewer and less severe symptoms and better language in the preschool years than children with HFA, but these group differences are likely to be artifacts of the diagnostic definitions (Ozonoff, South, & Miller, 2000). Follow-up studies demonstrate similar adaptive and functional outcomes (Ozonoff & Griffith, 2000; Szatmari et al., 2000). Recent neuropsychological research suggests that the two conditions are more similar than different (Macintosh & Dissanayake, 2004).

Two other conditions also appear in DSM-IV-TR within the PDD category: Rett's disorder and childhood disintegrative disorder. Both involve a period of typical development, followed by a regression in development. The classic symptoms of Rett's disorder, seen primarily in females, include unsteady gait; lack of language and functional hand use; almost constant stereotyped hand movements, including repetitive wringing, "washing," twisting, clapping, or rubbing of the hands in the midline; very severe cognitive deficits; and lack of typical social interaction. A gene that appears responsible for most cases of Rett's disorder, MECP2, has been isolated on the X chromosome (Amir et al., 1999). In childhood disintegrative disorder, an abrupt and severe regression occurs after at least 2 (and up to 10) years of normal development. After the loss of skills, the child has all the characteristics of severe autism and severe mental retardation; unlike in typical autism, however, there is little developmental growth after treatment, and the condition continues as a chronic, severe developmental disability.

The fifth and final condition that falls within the PDD category is PDD-NOS. This label is used for children who experience difficulties in at least two of the three autism-related symptom clusters, but who do not meet criteria for any other PDD. The same list of 12 symptoms outlined above is used to diagnose PDD-NOS, but only one difficulty within the "reciprocal social interaction" domain and one symptom from either the "communication deficits" or "repetitive, restricted behaviors" domains is required. Children with PDD-NOS display autistic-like behaviors and difficulties, but either have too few symptoms or a different pattern of symptoms than the other conditions in the PDD category. For example, a child may be diagnosed with PDD-NOS if he or she displays only 4 of the DSM-IV-TR symptoms (ruling out autistic disorder), displays a delay in language onset (ruling out Asperger syndrome), and shows no regression in development (ruling out both Rett's and childhood disintegrative disorders).

Before I conclude this section on clinical characteristics, it is important to note that ASDs can co-occur with a variety of additional psychiatric and behavioral disturbances. The most common comorbid conditions in the population with ASD are anxiety disorders and depressed mood (Kim, Szatmari, Bryson, Streiner, & Wilson, 2000; Lainhart & Folstein, 1994). There is general agreement that rates are higher than expected (e.g., greater than the 10% lifetime rate in the general population), but few epidemiological studies of comorbidity prevalence have been done. Other common comorbidities are disturbances in attention and activity level (Goldstein & Schwebach, 2004). DSM-IV-TR does not permit the diagnosis of attention-deficit/hyperactivity disorder (ADHD) in individuals with ASD, but it has been suggested that this exclusion should be changed in future versions of the DSM, and many clinicians do diagnose both conditions in the same individual (Frazier et al., 2001). Other common comorbidities include tics, aggression, and problems with sleep and appetite (Deprey & Ozonoff, 2009).

DEVELOPMENTAL COURSE

The onset of autistic disorder always occurs before age 3, at two peak periods. The majority of children (approximately two-thirds) display developmental abnormalities within the first 2 years of life. A smaller group of children with autism display a period of normal or mostly normal development, followed by a loss of communication and social skills and onset of autism (Lord, Shulman, & DiLavore, 2004). Onset, parental recognition, and clinical diagnosis do not always (or even usually) coincide. For example, in a large epidemiological study in the United Kingdom, the average age of first symptom recognition by parents was 18.6 months, age at referral was 32.4 months, and age at diagnosis was 37.8 months (Chakrabarti & Fombonne, 2005). Parents often begin to be concerned when language fails to develop as expected (De Giacomo & Fombonne, 1998). However, several other behavioral differences, particularly social ones, appear to predate the language abnormalities that parents report at the time of recognition. These include less looking at faces, responding to name, pointing, and sharing enjoyment and interests with others (Lord, 1995; Nadig et al., 2007; Osterling & Dawson, 1994; Wetherby et al., 2004; Zwaigenbaum et al., 2005).

In the regressive pattern of onset, there is a period of mostly typical development, followed by a loss of previously acquired behavior and onset of autistic symptoms. The average age of regression is consistently described across studies as between 14 and 24 months (Fombonne & Chakrabarti, 2001). Regression typically progresses gradually, although onset can be sudden in a minority of cases. It is important to distinguish *regression* from *developmental plateau*, in which children fail to progress as expected and do not gain new skills. This form of onset is not considered a regression, as there is no loss of previously acquired skills. Loss of language is the most commonly described and perhaps most salient manifestation of regression (Goldberg & Osann, 2003; Siperstein & Volkmar, 2004). Virtually all children who lose language lose social behaviors as well, such as eye contact, social interest, and engagement with others (Hansen et al., 2008; Lord et al., 2004; Ozonoff, Williams, & Landa, 2005).

ASDs are considered lifelong, chronic conditions. There may be periods of waxing or waning of particular symptoms and improvement with age and development, however. Some studies suggest that improvement is most marked in preschool and early childhood, with functioning levels remaining stable and sometimes even worsening in adolescence and adulthood (Sigman & McGovern, 2005). Once diagnosed with an ASD, the vast majority of children will retain this diagnosis into adulthood (Gonzalez, Murray, Shay, Campbell, & Small, 1993; Piven, Harper, Palmer, & Arndt, 1996b) and present with functional impairment throughout life (Billstedt, Gillberg, & Gillberg, 2005; Howlin, 2003; Seltzer et al., 2003). In a very small proportion of cases, there are children who appear to "grow out of" an ASD diagnosis (Lovaas, 1987; Perry, Cohen, & DeCarlo, 1995), although some do retain difficulties in other areas (Fein, Dixon, Paul, & Levin, 2005). Diagnosis at age 2 is remarkably reliable and stable, with 85–90% of children diagnosed at this age retaining the diagnosis over time (Lord, 1995; Moore & Goodson, 2003). Later functional and adaptive outcome is highly related to overall cognitive ability. Across all studies conducted to date, the most powerful predictors of outcome continue to be two factors identified several decades years ago: IQ scores and verbal ability at age 5 (Lotter, 1974; Rutter, 1984).

EPIDEMIOLOGY

Early research suggested that autism (strictly defined as meeting full criteria for autistic disorder) occurred at the rate of 4–6 affected individuals per 10,000 (Lotter, 1966). A study conducted in the mid-1980s broadened diagnostic criteria and found a rate of 10 per 10,000 in a total population screening of a circumscribed geographical region in Canada (Bryson, Clark, & Smith, 1988). Newer studies using standardized diagnostic measures and active ascertainment techniques have yielded prevalence estimates of 60–70 per 10,000 or approximately 1 per 150 across the spectrum of autism, and 1 per 500 for children with the full syndrome of autistic disorder (Rice et al., 2007). One obvious reason for the rise in rates is that more recent research has examined all ASD, whereas early surveys looked at rates of only strictly defined autism. However, in studies that have broken down the rates by specific DSM-IV-TR subtypes, it is clear that the prevalence of classic autism itself is higher. Chakrabarti and Fombonne (2001) reported a rate of 16.8 per 10,000 for autistic disorder, which is three to four times higher than suggested in the 1960s and 1970s, and over 1.5 times higher than thought in the 1980s and 1990s.

Several reasons for the rising prevalence rates have been proposed, from methodological artifacts to potentially emerging risk factors. In the first category are increased awareness among clinicians and the public, better identification/referral practices, more sensitive diagnostic tools, broader classification systems, and more active case ascertainment in epidemiological studies. Whether these changes alone can account for the large increase is uncertain, and hypotheses abound about environmental factors that may have emerged in the last few decades to put infants and young children at greater risk for developing ASD. These are covered, along with other etiological factors, in the next section.

Very few studies have examined the prevalence of ASD as a function of race and ethnic group. It has occasionally been suggested that the rate of ASD is higher in immigrant than in native populations (Gillberg, Steffenburg, & Schaumann, 1991). For example, one study observed an elevated rate of ASD in immigrants from Pakistan to the United Kingdom (Morton, Sharma, Nicholson, Broderick, & Poyser, 2002), suggesting that the increase was due to high rates of consanguinity. However, a large California study using a similar database analysis of prevalence described the rates as very similar across race and ethnic groups during an 8-year period (Croen, Grether, Hoogstrate, & Selvin, 2002). The current consensus is that there is no relationship between ethnicity or race and ASD in large studies with adequate sampling and statistical controls (Fombonne, 2005).

Kanner (1943), who provided the first description of autism, was the first to identify the much greater preponderance of affected boys. A recent meta-analysis suggests that the widely reported 4:1 ratio of boys to girls is quite consistent across studies, geographical regions, ethnicities, and time (Fombonne, 2003). Sex differences in ASD have received little attention except for the purpose of examining differences in prevalence (Koenig & Tsatsanis, 2005; Thompson, Caruso, & Ellerbeck, 2003). Of the few studies that have been done, most describe greater severity in females. For example, studies consistently report lower IQ and mental age in females with autism (Pilowsky, Yirmiya, Shulman, & Dover, 1998; Volkmar, Szatmari, & Sparrow, 1993). Some investigators have suggested that females with autism have a different phenotype and present with different referral issues than boys do (Kopp & Gillberg, 1992), but this position is controversial and has not been studied enough.

ETIOLOGIES

Genetic Mechanisms

Kanner (1943) suggested that autistic children were born with "an innate inability to form the usual, biologically provided affective contacts with people" (p. 42). Later, however, his thinking came into line with that of his psychoanalytic contemporaries in suggesting that autism was the result of inadequate nurturance by emotionally cold, rejecting parents (Bettelheim, 1967)—a theory that prevailed until the late 1960s. It is now well accepted, however, that ASD has clear genetic and neurological origins.

The recurrence risk for ASD after the birth of one child with the disorder is usually reported as between 3% and 6%, a rate that far exceeds the general population risk

(Bailey, Palferman, Heavey, & Le Couteur, 1998b); recent studies of younger siblings have found rates exceeding 10% (Zwaigenbaum et al., 2005). The concordance rate of 60% for strictly defined autism in monozygotic (MZ) twins is greatly elevated, relative to that of 5% for dizygotic (DZ) pairs. MZ concordance rates of up to 90% are reported when social and communication abnormalities broader than autistic disorder are included. Twin studies yield a heritability estimate greater than .90 (Bailey et al., 1995; Le Couteur et al., 1996). And there is evidence for familial transmission of an extended set of cognitive and social anomalies that are milder than but qualitatively similar to autism (the so-called "broader autism phenotype" or BAP; Bailey et al., 1998b). Family members also suffer from higher-than-average rates of anxiety and mood disorders and of learning disabilities. Collectively, these features of the BAP have been found in 15–45% of family members of people with ASD in different samples (Bailey et al., 1998b).

Twin studies also make it clear that ASD is not a purely genetic disorder, since concordance rates among identical twins fall short of 100%. There can be tremendous phenotypic variability even among MZ twins, with one twin displaying severe autism and the other the BAP, for example. Fifty-point IQ differences within MZ pairs have been reported (Rutter, 1999). The search for other factors that influence the development and severity of ASD is intense. Several pre- and perinatal risk factors have been shown to increase risk for ASD, presumably in genetically vulnerable children. They include advanced maternal and paternal age, low birthweight, premature birth, and intrapartum hypoxia (Kolevzon, Gross, & Reichenberg, 2007). These factors are not specific to ASD, but also increase risk for several other adverse developmental outcomes.

Environmental Factors

It has also been suggested that environmental factors—including vaccination, heavy-metal or pesticide exposure, viral agents, and food products—may interact with genetic susceptibility to trigger ASD, to cause it alone, or to mediate the expression and severity of the disorder (Hornig & Lipkin, 2001). The potential environmental etiological agent that has received the most attention is immunization. Wakefield et al. (1998) described a case series of 12 children with gastrointestinal disturbances that were reported to begin at about the time when autistic behaviors became evident. He postulated that these children had a new subtype of "regressive autism" that was induced by the measles–mumps–rubella (MMR) vaccination. Subsequent studies have not supported this hypothesis, however. Taylor et al. (1999, 2002) identified 498 children with autism born since 1979 and linked clinical records to independently recorded immunization data. No evidence of a change in trend in incidence or age at diagnosis was associated with the introduction of the MMR vaccine in 1988. Other recent studies that examined large cohorts of children born in Japan and Denmark failed to find any increase in vaccinated relative to unvaccinated children, and any temporal clustering of cases of autism after immunization (Honda, Shimizu, & Rutter, 2005; Madsen et al., 2002). A related environmental hypothesis is that mercury exposure can cause ASD, through either environmental exposures or thimerosal, an ethyl-mercury-based preservative included in some vaccines to prevent bacterial contamination. This is a controversial theory that has provoked strong reactions on both sides, but current scientific evidence does not support a link between ASD and thimerosal exposure (Madsen et al., 2003).

Brain Mechanisms

Kanner's (1943) original description noted unusually large head size in a proportion of children, and macrocephaly (head circumference > 97th percentile) has been confirmed in approximately 20% of individuals with ASD (Lainhart et al., 1997). The increase in head volume reflects an increase in brain volume, which is not apparent at birth but is present by the first birthday (Courchesne, Carper, & Akshoomoff, 2003), and is hypothesized to be due to both overgrowth and the failure of normal pruning mechanisms (Piven, Arndt, Bailey, & Andreasen, 1996a). Thus there is evidence that the brains of children with ASD are different from very early in life. The neuropathological changes that have been found, summarized in this section, are developmental in origin. Acquired lesions or brain insults are not known etiologies of ASD.

Aside from macrocephaly, structural neuroimaging studies have yielded inconsistent results, possibly stemming from methodological issues such as small samples, inappropriate or no control groups, and inconsistent use of covariates (such as age, gender, IQ, and total brain volume) in analyses. Studies have demonstrated decreased volume of the cerebellar vermis, particularly lobules VI and VII (Courchesne, Yeung-Courchesne, Press, Hesselink, & Jernigan, 1988), but this finding has not always been replicated by other research teams (Hardan, Minshew, Harenski, & Keshavan, 2001; Piven, Bailey, Ranson, & Arndt, 1997). The body and posterior portions of the corpus callosum have been reported to be significantly smaller than normal (Piven et al., 1997). Saitoh, Karns, and Courchesne (2001) found that the area dentata (dentate gyrus and CA4) of the hippocampus was significantly smaller in magnetic resonance imaging (MRI) scans of children with autism than in those of normal children, while Sparks et al. (2002) reported increased hippocampal and amygdala volumes in children with ASD.

Although structural MRI results are variable across studies and do not point to any signature abnormality characteristic of ASD, regional volumetric changes do not measure brain function and thus are not the most sensitive indices of the brain-level mechanisms operative in ASD. Functional brain imaging studies have more consistently demonstrated differences in samples of children with ASD (Cody, Pelphrey, & Piven, 2002). Two studies found reduced cerebral blood flow bilaterally in the superior temporal gyrus and left frontal cortex (Ohnishi et al., 2000; Zilbovicius et al., 2000) in children with autism at rest (e.g., not engaged in task performance). In activation studies that examine brain regions used to perform specific tasks, several research groups have found that individuals with ASD show reduced or different patterns of brain activity from those of controls. In one study in which participants had to identify facial expressions of emotion, those with ASD activated the fusiform gyrus (part of the temporal lobes), the left amygdala, and the left cerebellum significantly less than controls did (Critchley et al., 2000). Two other studies, discussed in more detail in the next section, found reduced or absent activation of similar brain regions during social reasoning tasks (Baron-Cohen et al., 1999; Schultz et al., 2000). Different patterns of activation were also found in a study that examined brain function during a visual search task that is often a strength for individuals with ASD. Participants demonstrated reduced activation of prefrontal cortex, but increased activation of ventral occipitotemporal networks, relative to controls (Ring et al., 1999). Thus, even when performance is not deficient, the brains of people with ASD show functional differences from typical patterns.

The changes present in detailed autopsy studies of a limited number of individuals with autism (most of whom also had significant mental retardation and seizures) consist of increased neuronal density, particularly in the hippocampus; olivary dysplasia; scattered areas of cortical and white matter dysplasia, including neuronal ectopias; and other nonspecific developmental abnormalities in the brainstem and cerebellum (Bailey et al., 1998a). Bauman and Kemper (1988) reported increased cell packing, reduced cell size, and reduced dendritic connections in the limbic system. One research group developed a computer program to quantify the size and density of the parallel vertical columns that organize the human neocortex (Casanova, Buxhoeveden, Switala, & Roy, 2002). The basic unit is the minicolumn, a chain of neurons oriented perpendicular to the cortical surface, surrounded by axons and dendrites that make lateral connections. Casanova et al. (2002) found smaller, less compact, and more numerous minicolumns in the superior and middle temporal gyrus and superior and middle frontal gyrus, relative to those of controls with either typical development or dyslexia. As I discuss in the next section, these findings have potential implications for neuropsychological theories of ASD.

NEUROPSYCHOLOGY

Research at the neuropsychological level of analysis has been very active, perhaps because the profile of strengths and weaknesses in individuals with ASD is an interesting and unusual one. In Kanner's (1943) original paper, he highlighted both deficits and talents. He mentioned precocious reading, prodigious memory, and well-developed visual–spatial skills, alongside a fundamental inability to relate to others, a failure to use language to convey meaning, and an obsessive desire for sameness. As detailed below, several subsequent studies have confirmed the uneven profile of neuropsychological function in ASD.

General Intellectual Function

Autism is often associated with mental retardation. In an initial study, DeMyer et al. (1974) reported that close to half their sample functioned in the severe to profound range of mental retardation (IQ < 35); one-quarter demonstrated abilities in the moderately range (IQ = 35–50); a fifth functioned in the mild range (IQ = 50–70); and only 6% obtained IQ scores in the range above mental retardation (IQ > 70). More recent estimates suggested that approximately a quarter of children with autism function intellectually in the borderline range or above (Freeman, Ritvo, Needleman, & Yokota, 1985; Lord & Schopler, 1988). A recent epidemiological study of a preschool-age sample found that 31% with autism and 94% with other ASDs (such as Asperger syndrome and PDD-NOS) demonstrated IQ scores above the mental retardation range (Chakrabarti & Fombonne, 2001), suggesting that the higher-functioning forms of ASD, with IQ > 70, may in fact now be the more common form.

Children with ASD demonstrate a wide scatter of skills on intellectual testing (Green, Fein, Joy, & Waterhouse, 1995; Lincoln, Allen, & Kilman, 1995). They perform least well on intellectual tasks that require language, abstract reasoning, integration, and sequencing, and best on tasks that require visual–spatial processing, attention to detail, and rote memory abilities. This general pattern of strengths and weaknesses contributes to a characteristic profile on intellectual testing. On standard intelligence tests such as the Wechsler scales, most studies report higher Performance than Verbal IQ, with substantial variability among subtests. Block Design, Object Assembly, and Digit Span subtests are often the highest in a profile, while Comprehension is often the lowest (Dennis et al., 1999; Goldstein, Beers, Siegel, & Minshew, 2001; Lincoln et al., 1995). These patterns appear to be independent of IQ level and severity of autistic symptomatology (Fein, Waterhouse, Lucci, & Snyder, 1985; Freeman et al., 1985) and differentiate individuals with ASD from those with learning disabilities (Goldstein et al., 2001). Similar patterns are obtained on other intelligence tests as well. For example, on the Kaufman Assessment Battery for Children, high scores are obtained on both the Triangles subtest, a measure analogous to the Wechsler Block Design task, and Number Recall, similar to Digit Span (Allen, Lincoln, & Kaufman, 1991). Similarly, profile patterns on the Stanford–Binet Intelligence Scales demonstrate highest performance on the Pattern Analysis subtest, a measure of visual–spatial function, and lowest performance on the Absurdities subtest, a measure of verbal conceptual reasoning and social judgment (Carpentieri & Morgan, 1994; Harris, Handleman, & Burton, 1990).

These intellectual profiles have been suggested to be so consistent and universal in children with autism that they can be used for diagnostic purposes. Lincoln, Courchesne, Kilman, Elmasian, and Allen (1988) wrote that

> the pattern of subtest scaled scores should not provide the exclusive criteria to make the diagnosis of autism. It does appear, however, that the pattern of subtest scaled scores is robust enough to support history and other test results in developing a diagnosis in nonretarded children, adolescents, and adults suspected of having a disorder of autism. (pp. 521-522)

However, in a large (N = 81) sample of high-functioning adults (Full Scale IQ > 70) meeting research criteria for autism, only 20% had a significantly higher Performance IQ than Verbal IQ, and almost as many (16%) showed the opposite pattern (Siegel, Minshew, & Goldstein, 1996). Block Design was the highest subtest for only 22%, and Comprehension was the lowest for 33% of this sample. Similarly, in a group of 47 children with ASD (all but 5 of whom met research criteria for autism), 62% demonstrated verbal–nonverbal intelligence discrepancies, which occurred equally in both directions (Tager-Flusberg & Joseph, 2003). So, although there appear to be profiles that are common within ASD, they should never be used for diagnostic purposes.

There has been some suggestion that the cognitive profile in Asperger syndrome may differ from that in autistic disorder. In his initial description of the syndrome, Asperger (1944) stated that the children he was studying were extremely clumsy and demonstrated delays in both gross and fine motor development. Motor deficits have been shown to correlate with poor visual–spatial skills (Henderson, Barnett, & Henderson, 1994), stimulating recent exploration of visual–spatial functions in individuals with Asperger syndrome. One study found that Verbal IQ was significantly higher than Performance IQ in a sample with Asperger syndrome (Klin, Volkmar, Sparrow, Cicchetti, & Rourke, 1995)—the opposite of typical findings in autism. In addition, subjects with Asperger syndrome in this study showed deficits on tests of fine and gross motor ability, visual–motor integration, visual–spatial perception, visual memory, and nonverbal concept formation. Conversely, subjects with HFA and similar overall IQ performed well on these tests, but demonstrated deficits on measures of auditory perception, verbal memory, articulation, vocabulary, and verbal output (Klin et al., 1995). However, several research teams have failed to replicate these findings (Ghaziuddin, Butler, Tsai, & Ghaziuddin, 1994; Manjiviona & Prior, 1995; Mayes & Calhoun, 2003a; Miller & Ozonoff, 2000; Szatmari, Archer, Fisman, Streiner, & Wilson, 1995), so I reiterate the warning that IQ or cognitive profiles should not be used for differential diagnosis purposes.

The IQ scores of individuals with ASD are relatively stable across time and development. Correlations of IQ scores obtained in preschool and school age are generally statistically significant and similar to values seen in children without disability (Lord & Schopler, 1988). The older a child is at initial assessment, the more stable and predictive scores are (Lord & Schopler, 1989). Scores can and do change, however, with a proportion of children changing IQ grouping levels as they age (Freeman et al., 1991; Lord & Schopler, 1989; Mayes & Calhoun, 2003a) and in response to early intervention (Rogers, 1998). Thus categorization of intellectual level based on early IQ scores is not appropriate. However, IQ scores remain among the best predictors of later outcome, with both early studies (Lotter, 1974; Rutter, 1984) and more recent investigations conducted during the era of widespread early intervention (Freeman, Del'Homme, Guthrie, & Zhang, 1999; Harris & Handleman, 2000; Stevens et al., 2000) upholding the finding that intelligence during preschool predicts later functional outcome.

Language

In most children with autism, impairment in language is apparent early in life. Use of gesture to communicate is also notably restricted. Language does not always develop, and even when it does, its onset is often delayed. For those who do speak, phonology and syntax are often consistent with mental age, but abnormalities in pragmatics (Tager-Flusberg & Anderson, 1991) are characteristic. Even mildly affected children show difficulty in adapting their discourse to a listener's response or perspective and taking turns in conversation. Although children with HFA are willing to engage in conversation, they often give no response, repeat questions and comments, and do not spontaneously elaborate; their conversational exchanges with others are marked by disjointedness, lack of reciprocity, and noncontextual utterances (Adams, Green, Gilchrist, & Cox, 2002; Capps, Kehres, & Sigman, 1998). Although autism was at one time considered a disorder of language (Rutter, 1978), more recent theories emphasize impairments in social cognition and attribute the universal difficulties with pragmatic language to higher-order social information-processing deficits.

Nonverbal Skills

Individuals with ASD often perform well on tasks that require visual–spatial processing and attention to visual detail (Green et al., 1995). Recent research suggests, in fact, that they may perform better on some tasks in this domain than typically developing individuals do. Mottron and colleagues, in a programmatic series of studies, have demonstrated that individuals with ASD are superior at detecting, matching, and reproducing visual elements, yielding superior performance on visual–spatial tasks (Caron, Mottron, Rainville, & Chouinard, 2004). Prowess at processing visual material may not come without costs, however. Individuals with ASD have been described as displaying *weak central coherence* (Frith & Happé, 1994), or difficulty processing information in context. The information processing of typically developing individuals is motivated by a "drive" to achieve higher-level meaning and a preference for global processing. By contrast, the processing of people with ASD appears to be very detail-focused. Central coherence theory predicts that people with ASD will perform poorly on tasks that require integration of constituent parts into coherent wholes, but perform normally (or even in a superior fashion) on tasks that require a focus on detail-oriented or local processing. They should also show preserved or enhanced performance on tasks in which the typical tendency to use contextual information actually interferes with performance, since central coherence theory predicts that people with ASD should be relatively impervious to context effects.

Several studies have supported central coherence theory. Shah and Frith (1983) found that children with autism were significantly more accurate in discovering figures embedded within complex pictures than controls matched on mental and chronological age. This research team also found evidence that weak central coherence played a role in the strong performance of people with ASD on the Wechsler Block Design subtest (Shah & Frith, 1993). They found that presegmenting the designs significantly improved performance for participants without ASD (both those with typical development and those with mental retardation), presumably because of the strong tendency to process the unsegmented designs as a gestalt. The performance of people with ASD was not, however, enhanced in this way by presegmentation, suggesting that this group had a natural tendency to see the stimuli in terms of parts rather than as a whole and did not need the parts to be explicitly highlighted. Later studies have not fully confirmed these results, however. Subsequent investigations have used the Embedded Figures Test, with one study finding no superiority in accuracy (Ozonoff, Pennington, & Rogers, 1991); another failing to replicate the accuracy results, but demonstrating significantly faster reaction time on the part of people with ASD (Jolliffe & Baron-Cohen, 1997); and a third failing to find superiority in either accuracy or reaction time (Rodgers, 2000). So although it is not yet certain whether this neuropsychological domain truly represents a superiority for individuals with ASD, newer research questions if this is an area of impairment.

Attention

Many investigations have documented attentional abnormalities in individuals with ASD (for a review, see Allen & Courchesne, 2001), but the deficits are variable across different components of attention and present a different profile from those seen in other disorders. It has been noted in case studies and in the clinical literature for many years that individuals with ASD appear to have "overfocused" attention, responding to only a subset of environmental cues during learning situations (e.g., Lovaas, Koegel, & Schreibman, 1979). Deficits relative to controls have been found in the shifting of attention between sensory modalities. In one study, adults with autism and average IQ performed as well as typical controls on a task that required no shifting of attention, but performance was over six standard deviations below that of controls when rapid alternation of attention between auditory and visual channels was required (Courchesne et al., 1994). Several studies using the visual–spatial orienting task of Posner (1980) have documented that people with ASD take longer to disengage and move attention than controls matched on ability (e.g., Wainwright-Sharp & Bryson, 1993). In contrast, a number of studies have suggested that the ability to *sustain* attention is a relatively spared ability in ASD, with normal function on continuous-performance tests found in several investigations (Garretson, Fein, & Waterhouse, 1990; Goldstein, Johnson, & Minshew, 2001; Noterdaeme, Amorosa, Mildenberger, Sitter, & Minow, 2001). This profile of attentional strengths and weaknesses distinguishes children with ASD from those with ADHD. Whereas children with ADHD have less difficulty with disengaging and shifting attention (Swanson et al., 1991), they demonstrate severe impairment in sustaining attention and controlling impulses.

Memory

The memory of people with ASD has been extensively studied, stimulated by early research that likened autism to amnesia (Boucher & Warrington, 1976). This analogy has received some support from neuroanatomical research (Aylward et al., 1999; Bauman & Kemper, 1988; Saitoh et al., 2001; Salmond, de Haan, Friston, Gadian, & Vargha-Khadem, 2003) and renewed interest, due to the recent popularity of an "amygdala" theory of autism (Baron-Cohen et al., 2000). Proposed similarity at the neuropsychological level has been more controversial. Subjects with amnesia typically demonstrate three patterns: (1) intact immediate and short-term memory, but deficient long-term memory; (2) reduced primacy but normal recency effects; and (3) a flatter learning curve. Similar patterns have been hypothesized to exist in ASD (Bachevalier, 1994; Boucher & Warrington, 1976; DeLong, 1992).

In the opening paragraphs of his seminal paper describing the syndrome of autism, Kanner (1943) commented upon the extraordinary memories of the children he was studying, particularly their ability to recite long lists of items or facts. Experimental investigations have confirmed this observation. Hermelin and Frith (1971) demonstrated that children with autism were as able as mental-age controls to repeat back strings of words, and Prior and Chen (1976) demonstrated typical recall of both single items and lists in a visual memory task.

Another piece of the autism–amnesia analogy concerns primacy and recency effects. O'Connor and Hermelin (1967) were the first to note that primacy effects in list learning tended to be weaker than recency effects in autism; these results were replicated by Boucher (1981). This pattern is also characteristic of adults with amnesia (Baddeley & Warrington, 1970). Hermelin and Frith (1971) attempted, unsuccessfully, to attenuate strong recency effects by composing sentences in which the beginning part of the word string was made up of meaningful sentence fragments, while the latter part was composed of random verbal material. The children with autism continued to demonstrate strong recency and weak primacy effects even under these conditions. Deficient primacy but intact recency memory has been replicated more recently by Renner, Klinger, and Klinger (2000). As recency effects rely more purely on rote auditory mechanisms, whereas recall of the first part of a list requires further processing and encoding of the material, less developed primacy effects in ASD may be secondary to organizational and encoding impairments rather than to memory deficits per se—an issue to which I return below.

In a pioneering series of experiments, Hermelin, O'Connor, and colleagues found that the advantage in remembering meaningful over random material typically seen in normally developing individuals is not apparent in ASD; that is, individuals with ASD do not appear to use the syntactic and semantic cues that aid others in recalling material. For example, two studies demonstrated that children with autism were just as capable of recalling random verbal material (e.g., unconnected words) as they were of remembering meaningful sentences (Hermelin & Frith, 1971; Hermelin & O'Connor, 1967). Later experiments clarified that children with ASD are not incapable of using semantic cues in recall, but do appear to be less efficient in doing so and less likely to use this strategy spontaneously. Fyffe and Prior (1978) failed to replicate earlier results, finding that children with autism recalled sentences significantly better than random word lists. Relative to that of controls, however, recall of sentences was deficient, whereas recall of random material was adequate. Thus, although the group with autism did appear to make use of meaning in recall, their advantage was not as great as in controls with mental retardation or typical development. Tager-Flusberg (1991) replicated this pattern, finding that recall of related and unrelated word lists was equivalent within the group with autism; however, their memory for meaningful material was less efficient than that of controls.

Deficits in working memory have sometimes been found in autism. *Working memory* is defined as the ability to maintain information in an activated, online state to guide cognitive processing (Baddeley, 1986), and is thought to be subserved by prefrontal cortex. An initial study found that subjects with autism were significantly impaired relative to controls on working memory tasks, but not on measures of short- and long-term recognition memory, cued recall, or new learning ability (Bennetto, Pennington, & Rogers, 1996). Later studies have been less consistent. In an investigation by Russell, Jarrold, and Henry (1996), a group with both autism and mental retardation did not differ from matched controls on three measures of verbal working memory. In another study, no group differences were found in a higher-functioning sample, relative to matched comparison groups with Tourette syndrome and typical development, on three tasks of working memory (Ozonoff & Strayer, 2001).

The evidence reviewed here suggests that ASD is not a primary disorder of long-term memory. Rather, difficulty appears to occur at the stage of encoding and organizing material. It is the overlay or additional requirement of higher-order processing that makes certain memory tasks difficult for people with autism.

Executive Function

Investigating aspects of executive function (EF) has been another active area of research in ASD. Beginning with Rumsey (1985), many studies have documented deficient performance on tests of EF. The dysfunction most often found is perseveration of behavior—that is, continuing to perform actions that are no longer appropriate or relevant, given the context. An example of this is sorting by previously correct rules, despite feedback that these strategies are incorrect in the present situation (Prior & Hoffmann, 1990; Rumsey & Hamburger, 1988). Several research groups have found that EF deficits are apparent in persons with ASD, even relative to controls with other neurodevelopmental disorders (Ozonoff et al., 1991; Szatmari, Tuff, Finlayson, & Bartolucci, 1990). Shu, Lung, Tien, and Chen (2001) reported significant deficits on Wisconsin Card Sorting Test (WCST) performance in a sample of 26 Taiwanese children with ASD, relative to matched controls. Since these children were raised in a completely different culture and environment from those of the Western children who participate in most EF studies, the authors suggested that executive dysfunction may be a core impairment in ASD. In a review of the EF literature, Pennington & Ozonoff (1996) reported that 13 out of the 14 studies existing at the time of publication demonstrated impaired performance on at least 1 EF task in autism, including 25 of the 32 EF tasks used across those empirical studies. The magnitude of group differences tended to be quite large, with an average effect size (Cohen's *d*) across all studies of 0.98, marked by especially large effect sizes for the Tower of Hanoi (*d* = 2.07) and the WCST (*d* = 1.04). More recently, significant group differences on the Intradimensional–Extradimensional Shift task of the Cambridge Neuropsychological Test Automated Battery were found in a very large sample of individuals with autism and matched controls, recruited from the Collaborative Programs of Excellence in Autism network funded by the National Institutes of Health (Ozonoff et al., 2004). This work was important in replicating the flexibility impairment of autism across samples collected at seven independent sites, in individuals ranging in age from 6 to 47 years.

Two research groups have tested age-related EF development in very young children with autism. McEvoy, Rogers, and Pennington (1993) studied preschool-age children with autism (mean age = 5 years) and matched developmentally delayed and typically developing control groups. Significant group differences were found on the spatial reversal task, a measure of flexibility developed for infants and nonhuman primates, but no group differences were evident on three other EF measures. It was suggested that these tasks may have been less developmentally appropriate for the sample. However, in another investigation by the same research team (Griffith, Pennington, Wehner, & Rogers, 1999), studying even younger preschool children with autism (mean age = 4 years), there were no differences in performance on any of eight EF tasks (including the spatial reversal task), compared to a developmentally delayed group matched on chronological age and both verbal and nonverbal mental age. Likewise, in a larger study of even younger children with autism (mean age = 3 years), Dawson et al. (2002) reported no significant differences on six EF tasks (again including spatial reversal), relative to developmentally delayed and typically developing control groups matched on mental age. This work raises the possibility that EF deficits in children with autism emerge with age and are not present (at least relative to other samples with delayed development) early in the preschool range. Since aspects of EF are just beginning to develop during the early preschool period in all children, a relative lack of variance across groups may explain this apparent developmental discontinuity. Differences in the way EF is measured at different ages may also contribute to this finding.

It has become clear that various non-EF skills, such as language and intelligence, may contribute to EF deficits. Liss et al. (2001) gave a battery of EF tests to children with HFA and a control group of children with language disorders. The only group difference, more perserverative errors on the WCST by the group with HFA, disappeared when Verbal IQ was statistically controlled for. My colleagues and I have also identified significant relations between IQ and EF performance in people with ASD (Miller & Ozonoff, 2000; Ozonoff & McEvoy, 1994; Ozonoff & Strayer, 2001).

Finally, it is apparent that EF deficits are not specific to ASD, but are found in many other disorders, including ADHD (Shallice et al., 2002), obsessive–compulsive disorder (Spitznagel & Suhr, 2002), and schizophrenia (Bustini et al., 1999). Thus the EF account of ASD has failed as a grand cognitive theory of autism. EF deficits are not specific to ASD, universal within individuals with the condition, or precedent in development.

Motor Skills

Evidence that children with ASD show motor abnormalities has gathered steadily over the years. Early descriptions of these children suggested that they were graceful and had few signs of motor impairment. Later systematic studies of motor performance uncovered clear signs of delayed or abnormal motor development, however. Motor milestones are reported to be slow in a substantial proportion of cases (DeMyer, Hingtgen, & Jackson 1981). Noterdaeme, Mildenberger, Minow, and Amorosa (2002) compared children with ASD to those with language disorder and to controls on a neurological examination. They found motor problems across balance and coordination, as well as fine, gross, and oral–motor functions. In studies using standardized tests of motor impairment and including children with Asperger syndrome and HFA as subjects (Ghaziuddin et al., 1994; Goldstein et al., 2001; Manjiviona & Prior, 1995), it has been shown that both groups show signs of neuromotor clumsiness across a range of motor systems. These findings have been of particular interest, given the belief that clumsiness is a marked feature of Asperger syndrome rather than autism, and that it might be a diagnostically differentiating sign. It appears that this belief is questionable (Prior, 2003).

Social Cognition

Problems in perceiving faces and emotions have been documented in several studies of children with ASD. Using a cross-modal paradigm in which subjects had to match affective and nonaffective auditory and visual stimuli, Hobson (1986) found that a group with autism committed significantly more errors than controls with similar nonverbal IQ when matching affective material, but performed as well as the controls on nonaffective cross-modal matching. Other researchers using different paradigms have replicated the finding that individuals with ASD are selectively impaired on affect-matching tasks, relative both to performance of comparison subjects matched on nonverbal IQ and to their own performance on nonaffective control tasks (Bormann-Kischkel, Vilsmeier, & Baude, 1995; MacDonald et al., 1989). Language ability and verbal IQ account for large amounts of variance in emotion perception scores, with intercorrelations in the .60–.70 range (Fein, Lucci, Braverman, & Waterhouse, 1992). It should be noted that the emotion tasks used have all been poor approximations of naturalistic, real-world opportunities for emotion perception. Structured laboratory tests of this type are susceptible to compensation. Better tasks that measure basic, "online" affective processes, particularly those that develop early in life, are needed to fully test emotion-related hypotheses in ASD.

Several studies have also explored potential differences in more basic processes involved in understanding faces. New techniques that have only recently become available suggest that the mechanisms underlying face processing, regardless of accuracy, may be different in people with and without ASD. Recent eye-tracking and behavioral studies have demonstrated that individuals with autism use an atypical and disorganized approach to viewing faces, including an unusual focus on areas of the face such as the mouth (Joseph & Tanaka, 2003; Klin, Jones, Schultz, Volkmar, & Cohen, 2002; Pelphry et al., 2002), instead of the normal focus on the eyes. Dawson et al. (2002) studied the event-related potential (ERP) response to familiar faces (i.e., their mothers') and unfamiliar faces in young children with ASD and matched controls. Only those with ASD failed to show a difference in ERP response to the familiar versus unfamiliar face, although they did show the expected response to familiar versus unfamiliar objects. Another important study, by Schultz et al. (2000), found that people with autism or Asperger syndrome use the inferior temporal gyrus, the part of the brain that normally makes sense of objects, when they look at faces;

they do not activate typical face-processing structures, such as the fusiform gyrus. These studies suggest that even when people with ASD can figure out what someone's eyes or face conveys, they do so in a different and possibly less efficient manner.

Another aspect of social cognition in autism that has received a great deal of research attention is the theory-of-mind hypothesis, which became prominent in autism research in the 1980s and 1990s and has been posited as able to explain many characteristics of the disorder. Early studies demonstrated that children with autism have specific difficulties in understanding such states of mind as false belief, ignorance, and second-order belief (beliefs about beliefs) in other people (Baron-Cohen, Leslie, & Frith, 1985). More recent functional imaging research has examined the neural foundations of theory-of-mind skills. Baron-Cohen et al. (1999) used functional MRI while participants looked at pictures of eyes and made judgments about what mental states the eyes conveyed. They found that typical adults relied heavily on both the amygdala and the frontal lobes to perform this task. In contrast, adults with either HFA or Asperger syndrome used the frontal lobes much less than the normal adults, and did not activate the amygdala at all, when looking at the pictures of eyes. Instead, they used the superior temporal gyrus, which is not typically active during this task in people without ASD (Baron-Cohen et al., 1999). Happé et al. (1996) found that adults with Asperger syndrome used different regions of prefrontal cortex than typical controls did when engaged in reasoning about mental states. A recent report found significantly less activation in medial prefrontal cortex and the superior temporal sulcus, relative to controls, in adults with ASD. Activation in extrastriate cortex was high (and equivalent) in both groups, but the group with ASD alone showed reduced connectivity between this region and the superior temporal sulcus, suggesting an information transfer bottleneck within this mentalizing network (Castelli, Frith, Happé, & Frith, 2002).

A limitation of the theory-of-mind hypothesis of autism is that theory-of-mind skills do not begin to emerge in typical development until after symptoms of ASD are already present. Thus they lack the developmental precedence necessary for causal explanatory power. Some work has focused on potential precursors of later theory-of-mind development. One purported precursor is joint attention behavior, which typically emerges by about the first birthday and involves sharing attention to an object with another person. It is usually evident through pointing, referential looking, and shared affect. Many studies have demonstrated a paucity or absence of joint attention behaviors in young children with autism (Baron-Cohen, 1989; Mundy & Sigman, 1989), and some have hypothesized that this is the earliest sign of the failure to appreciate the minds of others exhibited by children with autism (Baron-Cohen, 1991; Mundy, Sigman, & Kasari, 1993).

Rogers and Pennington (1991) proposed that the symptoms of ASD might stem from impairment in another very early social process, that of imitation. Based on a theoretical model of early interpersonal processes developed by Stern (1985) and evidence that newborns are capable of imitating some facial movements (Meltzoff & Moore, 1977), it has been proposed that infants and young children come to understand the behavior, subjective experiences, and mental states of other people through imitation, social mirroring, and affect sharing (Meltzoff & Gopnik, 1993; Rogers & Pennington, 1991). An early impairment in motor imitation could have cascading consequences that profoundly alter later social development. Many studies have documented imitation deficits in young children with autism (e.g., Jones & Prior, 1985; Rogers, Hepburn, Stackhouse, & Wehner, 2003) and even in older, higher-functioning individuals with ASD (Rogers, Bennetto, McEvoy, &

Pennington, 1996). More work examining the developmental emergence and relationships among joint attention, imitation, other early social processes, and later theory of mind is needed.

Another limitation of the theory-of-mind hypothesis is that not all children with ASD lack a theory of mind. Studies have shown that higher-functioning individuals are often able to pass theory-of-mind tests (Bowler, 1992; Ozonoff et al., 1991). Nor are theory-of-mind deficits specific to autism. A meta-analysis found significant theory-of-mind deficits in individuals with mental retardation, as well as those with ASD (Yirmiya, Erel, Shaked, & Solomonica-Levi, 1998). Other children with linguistic disabilities, including those who are deaf (Peterson & Siegal, 1995), may show theory-of-mind deficits, but not the other social and pragmatic impairments. Some studies have failed to find deficits in the understanding of simple mental states, such as intentions, in young children with autism (Carpenter, Pennington, & Rogers, 2001). These findings collectively have tempered early claims to have discovered the "core" psychological defect of autism—as has the inability of this theory to account for the repetitive and stereotyped behaviors of autism, as well as the cognitive strengths in visual–spatial processing that are often evident (Hughes, 2002). Researchers are increasingly debating and reevaluating the theory, especially in terms of claims regarding its modularity or componential quality in brain development and dysfunction (Garfield, Peterson, & Perry, 2001; Tager-Flusberg, 2001).

Academic Skills

There is a characteristic pattern of strengths and weaknesses in academic functioning that parallels the intellectual profile in ASD (Mayes & Calhoun, 2003b). Academic areas that require good memory or concrete skills are often better preserved than areas that require integration, abstraction, or generalization. Some children with high-functioning ASD have precocious reading skills and can decode words at a higher level than others of the same age and functional ability. The good memory of children with ASD may mean that spelling lists and multiplication tables will be learned more easily. Conversely, specific areas of weakness also exist, with the most consistently demonstrated ones being in reading comprehension and written language (Mayes & Calhoun, 2003b). This academic profile is quite different from the problem patterns most teachers and school psychologists are trained to detect (e.g., the poor decoding but good comprehension often seen in dyslexia).

Adaptive Function

Adaptive abilities largely determine whether an individual requires constant supervision or is capable of some independence. As such, adaptive function is an important measure of outcome that has been used in many longitudinal and treatment studies (e.g., Freeman et al. 1999; Szatmari, Bryson, Boyle, Streiner, & Duku, 2003). Children with ASD consistently demonstrate adaptive behavior levels that are lower than their intelligence, and this pattern is most pronounced for individuals with normal IQ (Bolte & Poustka, 2002). As summarized by Howlin (2005), outcomes for adults with ASD have improved over the last 25 years: Approximately 20% of adults with ASD have good social and functional outcomes. Although highly variable across studies, the average percentage of individuals with ASD attending college in these studies was 12%. Across studies, approximately one in four were employed; however, most of their jobs were relatively menial and included food service, unskilled factory work, and warehouse work. Employment stability also was low. On all dimensions, individuals with higher cognitive abilities fared better. This is highlighted by the results of a prospective population-based follow-up study of 120 adults diagnosed with autism and mental retardation in childhood (Billstedt et al., 2005). In this lower-functioning sample, 80% of the sample had poor or very poor outcomes, defined as displaying obvious, severe handicaps, without the possibility of independent living or satis-fying social relationships.

CONCLUSIONS

Individuals with ASD present with a broad array of neuropsychological strengths and weak-nesses. Despite active research for the past four decades, none of the theories put forth so far are capable of organizing the behavioral and cognitive strengths and weaknesses of autism within one unifying model. So we do not have a convincing single-deficit theory of autism. Part of the puzzle of autism is that it involves multiple neuropsychological deficits, but at the same time there is specificity in the profile of strengths and weaknesses. There are several broad solutions to this puzzle, but we do not yet know enough to distinguish among them. One possibility is a *developmental cascade* model (e.g., Fein, Pennington, Markowitz, Braver-man, & Waterhouse, 1986; Rogers & Pennington, 1991), in which one early deficit disrupts the enculturation through which many distinctive human cognitive capacities develop. Another is that there are neuropsychological subtypes of autism, each with its own primary deficit. A third possibility is that the notion of a single primary neuropsychological deficit is too simple, and that two or more interacting primary deficits are required. A final possibil-ity is that the seemingly disparate multiple deficits that have been observed all share some general underlying cognitive characteristic (e.g., complex information processing), and that the deficit in that cognitive process is primary.

Let us evaluate these possibilities in light of the empirical findings just reviewed. It remains possible that some early-developing aspect of basic affective or interpersonal pro-cessing is the primary deficit in infants with autism, and that this deficit "unhooks" these infants from normal socialization, thus producing a cascade of deficits in the domains reviewed here: attention, memory, language, social cognition, EF, and central coherence. Unfortunately, our knowledge of affective processes in typical infants, and especially infants with autism, is very sparse, so it is difficult to critically examine this hypothesis at the pres-ent time. None of the three other possible solutions to the puzzle of the neuropsychology of autism—subtypes with their own primary deficits, multiple interacting deficits, or a deeper core cognitive deficit—can be clearly rejected at this point. The evidence reviewed in this chapter suggests it is unlikely that deficits in memory will be on the list for subtype or multiple-interacting-deficit causal theories of autism. It is possible, although not probable, that difficulties in attention shifting, theory of mind, imitation, affective processes, EF, and central coherence may define different subtypes of autism. It is more plausible, but equally undetermined, that some or all of these impairments are components of a set of interacting deficits that, as a configuration, are primary to autism. Complicating matters is the typical failure of studies to correlate individual differences in symptom severity with deficits in various domains (e.g., theory of mind, language, etc.). The typical case–control study compares two groups on a set of measures, but does not examine whether severity of symptoms is correlated with the magnitude of the deficit in the group with ASD. The absence of such correlations could argue against any one impairment being central to autism.

Finally, let us turn to the fourth possible solution to the puzzle—that of a deeper core cognitive deficit. Minshew, Goldstein, and Siegel (1997) have proposed that the central cognitive deficit in autism is one of complex information processing. Any neuropsychological task (be it perceptual, spatial, verbal, or motor) that requires less information processing will be spared, according to this account, while those that require higher-order information processing will be impaired. The review of the ASD literature across many neuropsychological domains appears to support this theory. We have summarized the relative sparing of simple language processes (e.g., phonology, syntax), simple executive functions (e.g., inhibition), simple attentional processes (e.g., selective and focused attention), and simple memory functions (e.g., rote and recognition), with complementary dysfunction in each of these domains at the level of more complex processes (e.g., language pragmatics, attention shifting, working memory, cognitive flexibility, abstraction). The complex-information-processing theory is also compatible with recent neurological findings of enlarged brains (Courchesne et al., 2003) with increased numbers of cortical columns, of reduced size and density (Casanova et al., 2002); these could significantly disrupt neural networks, increase "noise" in the computational system, and lower efficiency of information processing (Casanova et al., 2002).

There is an important conceptual challenge for this theory, however, which is the need for a more detailed and principled account of what makes a cognitive task complex or not. Does complexity just equal difficulty? Chapman and Chapman (1973) argued that many demonstrations of apparently specific cognitive deficits in schizophrenia did not equate the experimental and comparison tasks for difficulty. It is not too surprising that subjects with an extreme neurodevelopmental disorder like schizophrenia would perform differentially worse on difficult cognitive tasks. A similar pattern would be expected in mental retardation syndromes and in autism. So for the complex-information-processing theory to work, we need an explicit definition of cognitive complexity that is derived independently of the empirical results in autism, yet explains the specific pattern of cognitive strengths and weaknesses found in autism, which differ from those found in schizophrenia or mental retardation.

A second challenge to the complex-information-processing theory of autism is that it does not adequately explain the very early symptoms of autism that are often apparent before the first birthday (Osterling & Dawson, 1994). Autism is particularly interesting because impairments in very basic interpersonal processes coexist with spared abilities in certain cognitive domains, such as memory and visual–spatial processes. The complex-information-processing theory cannot explain why a 2-year-old with autism can put together puzzles at a 3-year mental age level, but is not able to point—a developmentally simpler skill normally apparent by 1 year of age.

Recent genetic advances make it clear that a number of interacting genes may be needed for the development of ASD. It is implausible that all genes (and other potential environmental factors) confer susceptibility for a single specific neuropsychological deficit. Moreover, such modular hypotheses are unable to account for the variations across ASD in severity and pattern of symptoms and deficits. These variations make subtypes and multiple-deficit theories more likely, but more work is needed to identify the relevant deficits. Although research on the neuropsychology of autism has been very active, it is far from definitive at this point. As in the legend of the blind men describing the elephant, the theories proposed depend largely on the characteristics of the participants and the neuropsychological domains being studied. Researchers who study young children focus on early interpersonal deficits, while those who study older and higher-functioning individuals focus on cognitive impairments. No model accounts for everything. A major test of any viable future model will be its ability to explain early-appearing infant symptoms. Research on the very early development of infants at family risk for autism will help identify such deficits, as will a more careful dissection of the typical development of early social cognition. Until we have a better model of typical very early social-emotional development (before joint attention develops), answers to the autism puzzle may remain elusive.

REFERENCES

Adams, C., Green, J., Gilchrist, A., & Cox, A. (2002). Conversational behaviour of children with Asperger syndrome and conduct disorder. *Journal of Child Psychology and Psychiatry, 43,* 679–690.

Allen, G., & Courchesne, E. (2001). Attention function and dysfunction in autism. *Frontiers in Bioscience, 6,* 105–119.

Allen, M. H., Lincoln, A. J., & Kaufman, A. S. (1991). Sequential and simultaneous processing abilities of high-functioning autistic and language-impaired children. *Journal of Autism and Developmental Disorders, 21,* 483–502.

American Psychiatric Association. (2000). *Diagnostic and statistical manual of mental disorders* (4th ed., text rev.). Washington, DC: American Psychiatric Press.

Amir, R. E., Van Den Veyver, I. B., Wan, M., Tran, C. Q., Franke, U., & Zoghbi, H. (1999). Rett syndrome is caused by mutations in X-linked MECP2, encoding methyl CpG binding protein 2. *Nature Genetics, 23,* 185–188.

Asperger, H. (1944). "Autistic psychopathy" in childhood. *Archiv für Psychiatrie und Nervenkrankheiten, 117,* 76–136.

Aylward, E. H., Minshew, M. J., Goldstein, G., Honeycutt, N. A., Augustine, A. M., Yates, K. O., et al. (1999). MRI volumes of amygdala and hippocampus in non-mentally retarded autistic adolescents and adults. *Neurology, 52,* 2145–2150.

Bachevalier, J. (1994). Medial temporal lobe structures and autism: A review of clinical and experimental findings. *Neuropsychologia, 32,* 627–648.

Baddeley, A. D. (1986). *Working memory.* Oxford: Clarendon Press.

Baddeley, A. D., & Warrington, E. K. (1970). The distinction between long and short-term memory. *Journal of Verbal Learning and Verbal Behavior, 9,* 176–189.

Bailey, A., Le Couteur, A., Gottesman, I., Bolton, P., Simonoff, E., Yuzda, E., et al. (1995). Autism as a strongly genetic disorder: Evidence from a British twin study. *Psychological Medicine, 25,* 63–77.

Bailey, A., Luthert, P., Dean, A., Harding, B., Janota, I., Montgomery, M., et al. (1998a). A clinicopathological study of autism. *Brain, 121,* 889–905.

Bailey, A., Palferman, S., Heavey, L., & Le Couteur, A. (1998b). Autism: The phenotype in relatives. *Journal of Autism and Developmental Disorders, 28,* 369–392.

Baron-Cohen, S. (1989). Perceptual role taking and protodeclarative pointing in autism. *British Journal of Developmental Psychology, 7,* 113–127.

Baron-Cohen, S. (1991). Precursors to a theory of mind: Understanding attention in others. In A. Whiten (Ed.), *Natural theories of mind: The evolution, development and simulation of everyday mind-reading* (pp. 233–251). Oxford: Blackwell.

Baron-Cohen, S., Leslie, A. M., & Frith, U. (1985). Does the autistic child have a "theory of mind"? *Cognition, 21,* 37–46.

Baron-Cohen, S., Ring, H., Wheelwright, S., Bullmore, E., Brammer, M., Simmons, A., et al. (1999).

Social intelligence in the normal and autistic brain: An fMRI study. *European Journal of Neuroscience, 11,* 1891–1898.

Baron-Cohen, S., Ring, H. A., Bullmore, E. T., Wheelwright, S., Ashwin, C., & Williams, S. C. (2000). The amygdala theory of autism. *Neuroscience and Biobehavioral Reviews, 24,* 355–364.

Bauman, M., & Kemper, T. L. (1988). Limbic and cerebellar abnormalities: Consistent findings in infantile autism. *Journal of Neuropathology and Experimental Neurology, 47,* 369.

Bennetto, L., Pennington, B. F., & Rogers, S. J. (1996). Impaired and intact memory functions in autism: A working memory model. *Child Development, 67,* 1816–1835.

Bettelheim, B. (1967). *The empty fortress.* New York: Free Press.

Billstedt, E., Gillberg, C., & Gillberg, C. (2005). Autism after adolescence: Population-based 13- to 22-year follow-up study of 120 individuals with autism diagnosed in childhood. *Journal of Autism and Developmental Disorders, 35,* 351–360.

Bolte, S., & Poustka, F. (2002). The relation between general cognitive level and adaptive behavior domains in individuals with autism with and without co-morbid mental retardation. *Child Psychiatry and Human Development, 33,* 165–172.

Bormann-Kischkel, C., Vilsmeier, M., & Baude, B. (1995). The development of emotional concepts in autism. *Journal of Child Psychology and Psychiatry, 36,* 1243–1259.

Boucher, J. (1981). Immediate free recall in early childhood autism: Another point of behavioral similarity with the amnesic syndrome. *British Journal of Psychology, 72,* 211–215.

Boucher, J., & Warrington, E. K. (1976). Memory deficits in early infantile autism: Some similarities to the amnesic syndrome. *British Journal of Psychology, 67,* 73–87.

Bowler, D. M. (1992). "Theory of mind" in Asperger's syndrome. *Journal of Child Psychology and Psychiatry, 33,* 877–893.

Bryson, S. E., Clark, B. S., & Smith, I. M. (1988). First report of a Canadian epidemiological study of autistic syndromes. *Journal of Child Psychology and Psychiatry, 29,* 433–445.

Bustini, M., Stratta, P., Daneluzzo, E., Pollice, R., Prosperini, P., & Rossi, A. (1999). Tower of Hanoi and WCST performance in schizophrenia: Problem-solving capacity. *Journal of Psychiatric Research, 33,* 285–290.

Capps, L., Kehres, J., & Sigman, M. (1998). Conversational abilities among children with autism and children with developmental delays. *Autism, 2,* 325–344.

Caron, M. J., Mottron, L., Rainville, C., & Chouinard, S. (2004). Do high functioning persons with autism present superior spatial abilities? *Neuropsychologia, 42,* 467–481.

Carpenter, M., Pennington, B. F., & Rogers, S. J. (2001). Understanding of others' intentions in children with autism. *Journal of Autism and Developmental Disorders, 31,* 589–599.

Carpentieri, S. C., & Morgan, S. B. (1994). Brief report: A comparison of patterns of cognitive functioning of autistic and nonautistic retarded children on the Stanford–Binet Fourth Edition. *Journal of Autism and Developmental Disorders, 24,* 215–223.

Casanova, M. F., Buxhoeveden, D. P., Switala, A. E., & Roy, E. (2002). Minicolumnar pathology in autism. *Neurology, 58,* 428–432.

Castelli, F., Frith, C., Happé, F., & Frith, U. (2002). Autism, Asperger syndrome and brain mechanisms for the attribution of mental states to animated shapes. *Brain, 125,* 1839–1849.

Chakrabarti, S., & Fombonne, E. (2001). Pervasive developmental disorders in preschool children. *Journal of the American Medical Association, 285,* 3093–3099.

Chakrabarti, S., & Fombonne, E. (2005). Pervasive developmental disorders in preschool children: Confirmation of high prevalence. *American Journal of Psychiatry, 162,* 1133–1141.

Chapman, L. J., & Chapman, J. P. (1973). Problems in the measurement of cognitive deficit. *Psychological Bulletin, 79,* 380–385.

Cody, H., Pelphrey, K., & Piven, J. (2002). Structural and functional magnetic resonance imaging of autism. *International Journal of Developmental Neuroscience, 20,* 421–438.

Courchesne, E., Carper, R., & Akshoomoff, N. (2003). Evidence of brain overgrowth in the first year of life in autism. *Journal of the American Medical Association, 290,* 337–344.

Courchesne, E., Townsend, J., Akshoomoff, N. A., Saitoh, O., Yeung-Courchesne, R., Lincoln, A. J., et al. (1994). Impairment in shifting attention in autistic and cerebellar patients. *Behavioral Neuroscience, 108,* 848–865.

Courchesne, E., Yeung-Courchesne, R., Press, G. A., Hesselink, J. R., & Jernigan, T. L. (1988). Hypoplasia of cerebellar vermal lobules VI and VII in autism. *New England Journal of Medicine, 318,* 1349–1354.

Critchley, H. D., Daly, E. M., Bullmore, E. T., Williams, S. C. R., Van Amelsvoort, T., Robertson, D. M., et al. (2000). The functional neuroanatomy of social behaviour: Changes in cerebral blood flow when people with autistic disorder process facial expressions. *Brain, 123,* 2203–2212.

Croen, L. A., Grether, J. K., Hoogstrate, J., & Selvin, S. (2002). The changing prevalence of autism in California. *Journal of Autism and Developmental Disorders, 32,* 207–215.

Dawson, G., Munson, J., Estes, A., Osterling, J., McPartland, J., Toth, K., et al. (2002). Neurocognitive function and joint attention ability in young children with autism spectrum disorder versus developmental delay. *Child Development, 73,* 345–358.

De Giacomo, A., & Fombonne, E. (1998). Parental recognition of developmental abnormalities in autism. *European Child and Adolescent Psychiatry, 7,* 131–136.

DeLong, G. R. (1992). Autism, amnesia, hippocampus, and learning. *Neuroscience and Biobehavioral Reviews, 16,* 63–70.

DeMyer, M. K., Barton, S., Alpern, G. D., Kimberlin, C., Allen, J., Yang, E., et al. (1974). The measured intelligence of autistic children. *Journal of Autism and Childhood Schizophrenia, 4,* 42–60.

DeMyer, M. K., Hingtgen, J. N., & Jackson, R. K. (1981). Infantile autism reviewed: A decade of research. *Schizophrenia Bulletin, 7,* 388–451.

Dennis, M., Lockyer, L., Lazenby, A. L., Donnelly, R. E., Wilkinson, M., & Schoonheyt, W. (1999). Intelligence patterns among children with high-functioning autism, phenylketonuria, and childhood head injury. *Journal of Autism and Developmental Disorders, 29,* 5–17.

Deprey, L., & Ozonoff, S. (2009). Assessment of comorbid psychiatric conditions in autism spectrum disorders. In S. Goldstein, J. Naglieri, & S. Ozonoff (Eds.), *Assessment of autism spectrum disorders* (pp. 290–317). New York: Guilford Press.

Fein, D., Dixon, P., Paul, J., & Levin, H. (2005). Pervasive developmental disorder can evolve into ADHD: Case illustrations. *Journal of Autism and Developmental Disorders, 35,* 525–534.

Fein, D., Lucci, D., Braverman, M., & Waterhouse, L. (1992). Comprehension of affect in context in children with pervasive developmental disorders. *Journal of Child Psychology, 33,* 1157–1167.

Fein, D., Pennington, B. F., Markowitz, P., Braverman, M., & Waterhouse, L. (1986). Toward a neuropsychological model of infantile autism: Are the social deficits primary? *Journal of the American Academy of Child Psychiatry, 25,* 198–212.

Fein, D., Waterhouse, L., Lucci, D., & Snyder, D. (1985). Cognitive subtypes in developmentally disabled children: A pilot study. *Journal of Autism and Developmental Disorders, 15,* 77–95.

Fombonne, E. (2003). Epidemiological surveys of autism and other pervasive developmental disorders: An update. *Journal of Autism and Developmental Disorders, 33,* 365– 382.

Fombonne, E. (2005). Epidemiological studies of pervasive developmental disorders. In F. R. Volkmar, R. Paul, A. Klin, & D. Cohen (Eds.), *Handbook of autism and pervasive developmental Disorders* (3rd ed., Vol. 1, pp. 42–69). Hoboken, NJ: Wiley.

Fombonne, E., & Chakrabarti, S. (2001). No evidence for a new variant of measles–mumps–rubella-induced autism. *Pediatrics, 108,* 1–8.

Frazier, J. A., Biederman, J., Bellordre, C. A., Garfield, S. B., Geller, D. A., Coffey, B. J., et al. (2001). Should the diagnosis of attention-deficit/hyperactivity disorder be considered in children with pervasive developmental disorder? *Journal of Attention Disorders, 4,* 203–211.

Freeman, B. J., Del'Homme, M., Guthrie, D., & Zhang, F. (1999). Vineland Adaptive Behavior Scale scores as a function of age and initial IQ in 210 autistic children. *Journal of Autism and Developmental Disorders, 29,* 379–384.

Freeman, B. J., Rahbar, B., Ritvo, E. R., Bice, T. L., Yokota, A., & Ritvo, R. (1991). The stability of cognitive and behavioral parameters in autism: A 12-year prospective study. *Journal of the American Academy of Child and Adolescent Psychiatry, 30,* 479–482.

Freeman, B. J., Ritvo, E. R., Needleman, R., & Yokota, A. (1985). The stability of cognitive and linguistic parameters in autism: A five-year prospective study. *Journal of the American Academy of Child Psychiatry, 24,* 459–464.

Frith, U., & Happé, F. (1994). Autism: Beyond theory of mind. *Cognition, 50,* 115–132.

Fyffe, C., & Prior, M. (1978). Evidence for language recoding in autistic, retarded and normal children: A re-examination. *British Journal of Psychology, 69,* 393–402.

Garfield, J. L., Peterson, C. C., & Perry, T. (2001). Social cognition, language acquisition, and the development of the theory of mind. *Mind and Language, 16,* 494–541.

Garretson, H. B., Fein, D., & Waterhouse, L. (1990). Sustained attention in children with autism. *Journal of Autism and Developmental Disorders, 20,* 101–114.

Ghaziuddin M., Butler, E., Tsai, L., & Ghaziuddin, M. (1994). Is clumsiness a marker for Asperger syndrome? *Journal of Intellectual Disability Research, 38,* 519–527.

Gillberg, C., Steffenburg, S., & Schaumann, H. (1991). Is autism more common now than ten years ago? *British Journal of Psychiatry, 158,* 403–409.

Goldberg, W. A., & Osann, K. (2003). Language and other regression: Assessment and timing. *Journal of Autism and Developmental Disorders, 33,* 607–615.

Goldstein, G., Beers, S. R., Siegel, D. J., & Minshew, N. J. (2001). A comparison of WAIS-R profiles in adults with high-functioning autism or differing subtypes of learning disability. *Applied Neuropsychology, 8,* 148–154.

Goldstein, G., Johnson, C. R., & Minshew, N. J. (2001). Attentional process in autism. *Journal of Autism and Developmental Disorders, 31,* 433–440.

Goldstein, S., & Schwebach, A. J. (2004). The comorbidity of pervasive developmental disorder and attention deficit hyperactivity disorder: Results of a retrospective chart review. *Journal of Autism and Developmental Disorders, 34,* 329–339.

Gonzalez, N. M., Murray, A., Shay, J., Campbell, M., & Small, A. M. (1993). Autistic children on follow-up: Change of diagnosis. *Psychopharmacology Bulletin, 29,* 353–358.

Green, L., Fein, D., Joy, S., & Waterhouse, L. (1995). Cognitive functioning in autism: An overview. In E. Schopler & G. B. Mesibov (Eds.), *Learning and cognition in autism* (pp. 13–31). New York: Plenum Press.

Griffith, E. M., Pennington, B. F., Wehner, E. A., & Rogers, S. J. (1999). Executive functions in young children with autism. *Child Development, 70,* 817–832.

Hansen, R. L., Ozonoff, S., Krakowiak, P., Angkustsiri, K., Jones, C., Deprey, L. J., et al. (2008). Regression in autism: Definitions, prevalence, and associated factors in the CHARGE study. *Ambulatory Pediatrics, 8,* 25–31.

Happé, F. G. E., Ehlers, S., Fletcher, P., Frith, U., Johansson, M., Gillberg, C., et al. (1996). 'Theory of mind' in the brain. Evidence from a PET scan study of Asperger syndrome. *NeuroReport, 8,* 197–201.

Hardan, A. Y., Minshew, N. J., Harenski, K., & Keshavan, M. S. (2001). Posterior fossa magnetic resonance imaging in autism. *Journal of the American Academy of Child and Adolescent Psychiatry, 40,* 666–672.

Harris, S. L., & Handleman, J. S. (2000). Age and IQ at intake as predictors of placement for young children with autism: A four- to six-year follow-up. *Journal of Autism and Developmental Disorders, 30,* 137–142.

Harris, S. L., Handleman, J. S., & Burton, J. B. (1990). The Stanford Binet profiles of young children with autism. *Special Services in the School, 6,* 135–143.

Henderson, S. E., Barnett, A., & Henderson, L. (1994). Visuospatial difficulties and clumsiness: On the interpretation of conjoined deficits. *Journal of Child Psychology and Psychiatry, 35,* 961–969.

Hermelin, B., & Frith, U. (1971). Psychological studies of childhood autism: Can autistic children make sense of what they see and hear? *Journal of Special Education, 5,* 107–117.

Hermelin, B., & O'Connor, N. (1967). Remembering of words by psychotic and subnormal children. *British Journal of Psychology, 58,* 213–218.

Hobson, R. P. (1986). The autistic child's appraisal of expressions of emotion. *Journal of Child Psychology and Psychiatry, 27,* 321–342.

Honda, H., Shimizu, Y., & Rutter, M. (2005). No effect of MMR withdrawal on the incidence of autism: A total population study. *Journal of Child Psychology and Psychiatry, 46,* 572–570.

Hornig, M., & Lipkin, W. I. (2001). Infectious and immune factors in the pathogenesis of neurodevelopmental disorders: Epidemiology, hypotheses, and animal models. *Mental Retardation and Developmental Disabilities Research Reviews, 7,* 200–210.

Howlin, P. (2003). Outcome in high-functioning adults with autism with and without early language delays: Implications for the differentiation between autism and Asperger syndrome. *Journal of Autism and Developmental Disorders, 33,* 3–14.

Howlin, P. (2005). Outcomes in autism spectrum disorders. In F. R. Volkmar, R. Paul, A. Klin, & D. Cohen (Eds.), *Handbook of autism and pervasive developmental disorders* (3rd ed., Vol. 1, pp. 201–220). Hoboken, NJ: Wiley.

Hughes, C. (2002). Executive functions and development: Emerging themes. *Infant and Child Development, 11,* 201–209.

Jolliffe, T., & Baron-Cohen, S. (1997). Are people with autism and Asperger syndrome faster than normal on the Embedded Figures Test? *Journal of Child Psychology and Psychiatry, 38,* 527–534.

Jones, V., & Prior, M. R. (1985). Motor imitation abilities and neurological signs in autistic children. *Journal of Autism and Developmental Disorders, 15,* 37–46.

Joseph, R. M., & Tanaka, J. (2003). Holistic and part-based faced recognition in children with autism. *Journal of Child Psychology and Psychiatry, 44,* 529–542.

Kanner, L. (1943). Autistic disturbances of affective content. *Nervous Child, 2,* 217–250.

Kim, J. A., Szatmari, P., Bryson, S. E., Streiner, D. L., & Wilson, F. J. (2000). The prevalence of anxiety and mood problems among children with autism and Asperger syndrome. *Autism, 4,* 117–132.

Klin, A., Jones, W., Schultz, R., Volkmar, F., & Cohen, D. (2002). Visual fixation patterns during viewing of naturalistic social situations as predictors of social competence in individuals with autism. *Archives of General Psychiatry, 59,* 809–816.

Klin, A., Volkmar, F. R., Sparrow, S. S., Cicchetti, D. V., & Rourke, B. P. (1995). Validity and neuropsychological characterization of Asperger syndrome: Convergence with nonverbal learning disabilities syndrome. *Journal of Child Psychology and Psychiatry, 36,* 1127–1140.

Koenig, K., & Tsatsanis, K. D. (2005). Pervasive developmental disorder in girls. In D. J. Bell, S. L. Foster, & E. J. Mash (Eds.), *Handbook of emotional and behavioral disorders in girls* (pp. 211–237). New York: Kluwer Academic.

Kolevzon, A., Gross, R., & Reichenberg, A. (2007). Prenatal and perinatal risk factors for autism: A review and integration of findings. *Archives of Pediatrics and Adolescent Medicine, 161,* 326–333.

Kopp, S., & Gillberg, C. (1992). Girls with social deficits and learning problems: Autism, atypical Asperger syndrome or a variant of these conditions. *European Child and Adolescent Psychiatry, 1,* 89–99.

Lainhart, J. E., & Folstein, S. E. (1994). Affective disorders in people with autism: A review of published cases. *Journal of Autism and Developmental Disorders, 24,* 587–601.

Lainhart, J. E., Piven, J., Wzorek, M., Landa, R., Santangelo, S. L., Coon, H., et al. (1997). Macrocephaly in children and adults with autism. *Journal of the American Academy of Child and Adolescent Psychiatry, 36,* 282–290.

Le Couteur, A., Bailey, A. J., Goode, S., Pickles, A., Robertson, S., & Gottesman, I. (1996). A broader phenotype of autism: The clinical spectrum in twins. *Journal of Child Psychology and Psychiatry, 37,* 785–801.

Lincoln, A. J., Allen, M. H., & Kilman, A. (1995). The assessment and interpretation of intellectual abilities in people with autism. In E. Schopler & G. B. Mesibov (Eds.), *Learning and cognition in autism* (pp. 89–117). New York: Plenum Press.

Lincoln, A. J., Courchesne, E., Kilman, B. A., Elmasian, R., & Allen, M. (1988). A study of intellectual abilities in high-functioning people with autism. *Journal of Autism and Developmental Disorders, 18,* 505–524.

Liss, M., Fein, D., Allen, D., Dunn, M., Feinstein, C., Morris, R., et al. (2001). Executive functioning in high-functioning children with autism. *Journal of Child Psychology and Psychiatry, 42,* 261–270.

Lord, C. (1995). Follow-up of two-year-olds referred for possible autism. *Journal of Child Psychology and Psychiatry, 36,* 1365–1382.

Lord, C., & Schopler, E. (1988). Intellectual and developmental assessment of autistic children from pre-school to schoolage: Clinical implications of two follow-up studies. In E. Schopler & G. B. Mesibov (Eds.), *Diagnosis and assessment in autism* (pp. 167–181). New York: Plenum Press.

Lord, C., & Schopler, E. (1989). The role of age at assessment, developmental level, and test in the stability of intelligence scores in young autistic children. *Journal of Autism and Developmental Disorders, 19,* 483–499.

Lord, C., Shulman, C., & DiLavore, P. (2004). Regression and word loss in autistic spectrum disorders. *Journal of Child Psychology and Psychiatry, 45,* 936–955.

Lotter, V. (1966). Epidemiology of autistic conditions in young children. I. Prevalence. *Social Psychiatry, 1,* 124–137.

Lotter, V. (1974). Factors related to outcome in autistic children. *Journal of Autism and Childhood Schizophrenia, 4,* 263–277.

Lovaas, O. I. (1987). Behavioral treatment and normal educational and intellectual functioning in young autistic children. *Journal of Consulting and Clinical Psychology, 55,* 3–9.

Lovaas, O. I., Koegel, R. L., & Schreibman, L. (1979). Stimulus overselectivity in autism: A review of research. *Psychological Bulletin, 86,* 1236–1254.

MacDonald, H., Rutter, M., Howlin, P., Rios, P., Le Couteur, A., Evered, C., et al. (1989). Recognition and expression of emotional cues by autistic and normal adults. *Journal of Child Psychology and Psychiatry, 30,* 865–877.

Macintosh, K. E., & Dissanayake, C. (2004). The similarities and differences between autistic disorder and Asperger disorder: A review of the empirical evidence. *Journal of Child Psychology and Psychiatry, 45,* 410–434.

Madsen, K. M., Hviid, A., Vestergaard, M., Schendel, D., Wohlfahrt, J., Thorsen, P., et al. (2002). A population-based study of measles, mumps, and rubella vaccination and autism. *New England Journal of Medicine, 347,* 1477–1482.

Madsen, K. M., Lauritsen, M. B., Pedersen, C. B., Thorsen, P., Plesner, A. M., Andersen, P. H., et al. (2003). Thimerosal and the occurrence of autism: Negative ecological evidence from Danish population-based data. *Pediatrics, 112,* 604–606.

Manjiviona, J., & Prior, M. (1995). Comparison of Asperger syndrome and high-functioning autistic children on a test of motor impairment. *Journal of Autism and Developmental Disorders, 25,* 23–39.

Mayes, S. D., & Calhoun, S. L. (2003a). Ability profiles in children with autism: Influence of age and IQ. *Autism, 6,* 83–98.

Mayes, S. D., & Calhoun, S. L. (2003b). Analysis of WISC-III, Stanford-Binet:IV, and academic achievement test scores in children with autism. *Journal of Autism and Developmental Disorders, 33,* 329–341.

McEvoy, R. E., Rogers, S. J., & Pennington, B. F. (1993). Executive function and social communication deficits in young autistic children. *Journal of Child Psychology and Psychiatry, 34,* 563–578.

Meltzoff, A., & Gopnik, A. (1993). The role of imitation in understanding persons and developing a theory of mind. In S. Baron-Cohen, H. Tager-Flusberg, & D. J. Cohen (Eds.), *Understanding other minds: Perspectives from autism* (pp. 335–366). New York: Oxford University Press.

Meltzoff, A., & Moore, M. K. (1977). Imitation of facial and manual gestures by human neonates. *Science, 198,* 75–78.

Miller, J. N., & Ozonoff, S. (2000). The external validity of Asperger disorder: Lack of evidence from the domain of neuropsychology. *Journal of Abnormal Psychology, 109,* 227–238.

Minshew, N. J., Goldstein, G., & Siegel, D. J. (1997). Neuropsychologic functioning in autism: Profile of a complex information processing disorder. *Journal of the International Neuropsychological Society, 3,* 303–316.

Moore, V., & Goodson, S. (2003). How well does early diagnosis of autism stand the test of time?: Follow-up study of children assessed for autism at age 2 and development of an early diagnostic service. *Autism, 7,* 47–63.

Morton, R., Sharma, V., Nicholson, J., Broderick, M., & Poyser, J. (2002). Disability in children from different ethnic populations. *Child: Care, Health and Development, 28,* 87–93.

Mundy, P., & Sigman, M. (1989). The theoretical implications of joint attention deficits in autism. *Development and Psychopathology, 1,* 173–183.

Mundy, P., Sigman, M., & Kasari, C. (1993). The theory of mind and joint-attention deficits in autism. In S. Baron-Cohen, H. Tager-Flusberg, & D. Cohen (Eds.), *Understanding other minds: perspectives from autism* (pp. 181–203). New York: Oxford University Press.

Nadig, A. S., Ozonoff, S., Young, G. S., Rozga, A., Sigman, M., & Rogers, S. J. (2007). A prospective study of response to name in infants at risk for autism. *Archives of Pediatrics and Adolescent Medicine, 161,* 378–383.

Noterdaeme, M., Amorosa, H., Mildenberger, K., Sitter, S., & Minow, F. (2001). Evaluation of attention problems in children with autism and children with a specific language disorder. *European Child and Adolescent Psychiatry, 10,* 58–66.

Noterdaeme, M., Mildenberger, K., Minow, F., & Amorosa, H. (2002). Evaluation of neuromotor deficits in autism and children with a specific speech and language disorder. *European Child and Adolescent Psychiatry, 11,* 219–225.

O'Connor, N., & Hermelin, B. (1967). Auditory and visual memory in autistic and normal children. *Journal of Mental Deficiency Research, 11,* 126–131.

Ohnishi, T., Matsuda, H., Hashimoto, T., Kunihiro, T., Nishikawa, M., Uema, T., et al. (2000). Abnormal regional blood flow in childhood autism. *Brain, 123,* 1838–1844.

Osterling, J., & Dawson, G. (1994). Early recognition of children with autism: A study of first birthday home video tapes. *Journal of Autism and Developmental Disorders, 24,* 247–259.

Ozonoff, S., Coon, H., Dawson, G., Joseph, R., Klin, A., McMahon, W. M., et al. (2004). Performance on CANTAB subtests sensitive to frontal lobe function in people with autistic disorder: Evidence from the CPEA network. *Journal of Autism and Developmental Disorders, 34,* 139–150.

Ozonoff, S., & Griffith, E. M. (2000). Neuropsychological function and the external validity of Asperger syndrome. In A. Klin, F. Volkmar, & S. S. Sparrow (Eds.), *Asperger syndrome* (pp. 72–96). New York: Guilford Press.

Ozonoff, S., & McEvoy, R. E. (1994). A longitudinal study of executive function and theory of mind development in autism. *Development and Psychopathology, 6,* 415–431.

Ozonoff, S., Pennington, B. F., & Rogers, S. J. (1991). Executive function deficits in high-functioning autistic individuals: Relationship to theory of mind. *Journal of Child Psychology and Psychiatry, 32,* 1081–1105.

Ozonoff, S., South, M., & Miller, J. N. (2000). DSM-IV-defined Asperger syndrome: Cognitive, behavioral, and early history differentiation from high-functioning autism. *Autism, 4,* 29–46.

Ozonoff, S., & Strayer, D. L. (2001). Further evidence of intact working memory in autism. *Journal of Autism and Developmental Disorders, 31,* 257–263.

Ozonoff, S., Williams, B. J., & Landa, R. (2005). Parental report of the early development of children with regressive autism. *Autism, 9,* 461–486.

Pelphrey, K. A., Sasson, N. J., Reznick, J. S., Paul, G., Goldman, B. D., & Piven, J. (2002). Visual scanning of faces in autism. *Journal of Autism and Developmental Disorders, 32,* 249–261.

Pennington, B. F., & Ozonoff, S. (1996). Executive functions and developmental psychopathologies. *Journal of Child Psychology and Psychiatry, 37,* 51–87.

Perry, R., Cohen, I., & DeCarlo, R. (1995). Case study: Deterioration, autism, and recovery in two siblings. *Journal of the American Academy of Child and Adolescent Psychiatry, 34,* 232–237.

Peterson, C. C., & Siegal, M. (1995). Deafness, conversation and theory of mind. *Journal of Child Psychology and Psychiatry, 36,* 459–474.

Pilowsky, T., Yirmiya, N., Shulman, C., & Dover, R. (1998). The Autism Diagnostic Interview—Revised and the Childhood Autism Rating Scale: Differences between diagnostic systems and comparison between genders. *Journal of Autism and Developmental Disorders, 28,* 148–151.

Piven, J., Arndt, S., Bailey, J., & Andreasen, N. (1996a). Regional brain enlargement in autism: A magnetic resonance imaging study. *Journal of the American Academy of Child and Adolescent Psychiatry,* *35,* 530–536.

Piven, J., Bailey, J., Ranson, B. J., & Arndt, S. (1997). An MRI study of the corpus callosum in autism. *American Journal of Psychiatry, 154,* 1051–1056.

Piven, J., Harper, J., Palmer, P., & Arndt, S. (1996b). Course of behavioral change in autism: A retrospective study of high-IQ adolescents and adults. *Journal of the American Academy of Child and Adolescent Psychiatry, 35,* 523–529.

Posner, M. I. (1980). Orienting of attention. *Quarterly Journal of Experimental Psychology, 32,* 3–25.

Prior, M. (2003). What do we know and where should we go? In M. Prior (Ed.), *Learning and behavior problems in Asperger syndrome* (pp. 295–319). New York: Guilford Press.

Prior, M. R., & Chen, C. S. (1976). Short-term and serial memory in autistic, retarded, and normal children. *Journal of Autism and Childhood Schizophrenia, 6,* 121–131.

Prior, M. R., & Hoffmann, W. (1990). Neuropsychological testing of autistic children through an exploration with frontal lobe tests. *Journal of Autism and Developmental Disorders, 20,* 581–590.

Renner, P., Klinger, L. G., & Klinger, M. R. (2000). Implicit and explicit memory in autism: Is autism an amnesic disorder? *Journal of Autism and Developmental Disorders, 30,* 3–14.

Rice, C. E., Baio, J., Van Naarden Braun, K., Doernberg, N., Meaney, F. J., Kirby, R. S., et al. (2007). A public health collaboration for the surveillance of autism spectrum disorders. *Pediatric and Perinatal Epidemiology, 21,* 179–190.

Ring, H. A., Baron-Cohen, S., Wheelwright, S., Williams, S. C., Brammer, M., Andrew, C., et al. (1999). Cerebral correlates of preserved cognitive skills in autism: A functional MRI study of embedded figures task performance. *Brain, 122,* 1305–1315.

Rodgers, J. (2000). Visual perception and Asperger syndrome: Central coherence deficit or hierarchization deficit? *Autism, 4,* 321–329.

Rogers, S. J. (1998). Empirically supported comprehensive treatments for young children with autism. *Journal of Clinical Child Psychology, 27,* 167–178.

Rogers, S. J., Bennetto, L., McEvoy, R., & Pennington, B. F. (1996). Imitation and pantomime in high functioning adolescents with autism spectrum disorders. *Child Development, 67,* 2060–2073.

Rogers, S. J., Hepburn, S. L., Stackhouse, T., & Wehner, E. (2003). Imitation performance in toddlers with autism and those with other developmental disorders. *Journal of Child Psychology and Psychiatry, 44,* 763–781.

Rogers, S. J., & Pennington, B. F. (1991). A theoretical approach to the deficits in infantile autism. *Development and Psychopathology, 3,* 137–162.

Rumsey, J. M. (1985). Conceptual problem-solving in highly verbal, nonretarded autistic men. *Journal of Autism and Developmental Disorders, 15,* 23–36.

Rumsey, J. M., & Hamburger, S. D. (1988). Neuropsychological findings in high-functioning men with infantile autism, residual state. *Journal of Clinical and Experimental Neuropsychology, 10,* 201–221.

Russell, J., Jarrold, C., & Henry, L. (1996). Working memory in children with autism and with moderate learning difficulties. *Journal of Child Psychology and Psychiatry, 37,* 673–686.

Rutter, M. (1978). Language disorder and infantile autism. In M. Rutter & E. Schopler (Eds.), *Autism: A reappraisal of concepts and treatment* (pp. 85–104). New York: Plenum Press.

Rutter, M. (1984). Autistic children growing up. *Developmental Medicine and Child Neurology, 26,* 122–129.

Rutter, M. (1999). Two-way interplay between research and clinical work. *Journal of Child Psychology and Psychiatry, 40,* 169–188.

Saitoh, O., Karns, C. M., & Courchesne, E. (2001). Development of the hippocampal formation from 2 to 42 years: MRI evidence of smaller area dentata in autism. *Brain, 124,* 1317–1324.

Salmond, C. H., de Haan, M., Friston, K. J., Gadian, D. G., & Vargha-Khadem, F. (2003). Investigating individual differences in brain abnormalities in autism. *Philosophical Transactions of the Royal Society of London, 358,* 405–413.

Schultz, R. T., Gauthier, I., Klin, A., Fulbright, R. K., Anderson, A. W., Volkmar, F., et al. (2000). Abnormal ventral temporal cortical activity during face discrimination among individuals with autism and Asperger syndrome. *Archives of General Psychiatry, 57,* 331–340.

Seltzer, M. M., Krauss, M. W., Shattuck, P. T., Orsmond, G., Swe, A., & Lord, C. (2003). The symptoms of autism spectrum disorders in adolescence and adulthood. *Journal of Autism and Developmental Disorders, 33,* 565–581.

Shah, A., & Frith, U. (1983). An islet of ability in autistic children. *Journal of Child Psychology and Psychiatry, 24,* 613–620.

Shah, A., & Frith, U. (1993). Why do autistic individuals show superior performance on the block design task? *Journal of Child Psychology and Psychiatry, 34,* 1351–1364.

Shallice, T., Marzocchi, G. M., Coser, S., Del Savio, M., Meuter, R. F., & Rumiati, R. I. (2002). Executive function profile of children with attention deficit hyperactivity disorder. *Developmental Neuropsychology, 21,* 43–71.

Shu, B. C., Lung, F.-W., Tien, A. Y., & Chen, B.-C. (2001). Executive function deficits in non-retarded autistic children. *Autism, 5,* 165–174.

Siegel, D. J., Minshew, N. J., & Goldstein, G. (1996). Wechsler IQ profiles in diagnosis of high-functioning autism. *Journal of Autism and Developmental Disorders, 26,* 389–406.

Sigman, M., & McGovern, C. W. (2005). Improvement in cognitive and language skills from preschool to adolescence in autism. *Journal of Autism and Developmental Disorders, 35,* 15–23.

Siperstein, R., & Volkmar, F. (2004). Parental reporting of regression in children with pervasive developmental disorders. *Journal of Autism and Developmental Disorders, 34,* 731–734.

Sparks, B. F., Friedman, S. D., Shaw, D. W., Aylward, E. H., Echelard, D., Artru, A. A., et al. (2002). Brain structural abnormalities in young children with autism spectrum disorder. *Neurology, 59,* 184–192.

Spitznagel, M. G., & Suhr, J. A. (2002). Executive function deficits associated with symptoms of schizotypy and obsessive–compulsive disorder. *Psychiatry Research, 110,* 151–163.

Stern, D. N. (1985). *The interpersonal world of the infant.* New York: Basic Books.

Stevens, M. C., Fein, D. A., Dunn, M., Allen, D., Waterhouse, L. H., Feinstein, C., et al. (2000). Subgroups of children with autism by cluster analysis: A longitudinal examination. *Journal of the American Academy of Child and Adolescent Psychiatry, 39,* 346–352.

Swanson, J. M., Posner, M., Potkin, S. G., Bonforte, S., Youpa, D., Fiore, C., et al. (1991). Activating tasks for the study of visual–spatial attention in ADHD children: A cognitive anatomic approach. *Journal of Child Neurology, 6,* S119–S127.

Szatmari, P., Archer, L., Fisman, S., Streiner, D. L., & Wilson, F. (1995). Asperger's syndrome and autism: Differences in behavior, cognition, and adaptive functioning. *Journal of the American Academy of Child and Adolescent Psychiatry, 34,* 1662–1671.

Szatmari, P., Bryson, S. E., Boyle, M. H., Streiner, D. L., & Duku, E. (2003). Predictors of outcome among high functioning children with autism and Asperger syndrome. *Journal of Child Psychology and Psychiatry, 44,* 520–528.

Szatmari, P., Bryson, S. E., Streiner, D. L., Wilson, F., Archer, L., & Ryerse, C. (2000). Two-year outcome of preschool children with autism or Asperger's syndrome. *American Journal of Psychiatry, 157,* 1980–1987.

Szatmari, P., Tuff, L., Finlayson, M. J. A., & Bartolucci, G. (1990). Asperger's syndrome and autism: Neurocognitive aspects. *Journal of the American Academy of Child and Adolescent Psychiatry, 29,* 130–136.

Tager-Flusberg, H. (1991). Semantic processing in the free recall of autistic children: Further evidence for a cognitive deficit. *British Journal of Developmental Psychology, 9,* 417–430.

Tager-Flusberg, H. (2001). A re-examination of the theory of mind hypothesis of autism. In J. Burack, T. Charman, N. Yirmiya, & P. Zelazo (Eds.), *The development of autism: Perspectives from theory and research* (pp. 173–193). Mahwah, NJ: Erlbaum.

Tager-Flusberg, H., & Anderson, M. (1991). The development of contingent discourse ability in autistic children. *Journal of Child Psychology and Psychiatry, 32,* 1123–1134.

Tager-Flusberg, H., & Joseph, R. M. (2003). Identifying neurocognitive phenotypes in autism. *Philosophical Transactions of the Royal Society of London, 358,* 303–314.

Taylor, B., Miller, E., Farrington, C. P., Petropoulos, M. C., Favot-Mayaud, I., Li, J., et al. (1999). Autism and measles, mumps, and rubella vaccine: No epidemiological evidence for a causal association. *Lancet, 353,* 2026–2029.

Taylor, B., Miller, E., Lingam, R., Andrews, N., Simmons, A., & Stowe, J. (2002). Measles, mumps, and rubella vaccination and bowel problems or developmental regression in children with autism: Population study. *British Medical Journal, 324,* 393–396.

Thompson, T., Caruso, M., & Ellerbeck, K. (2003). Sex matters in autism and other developmental disabilities. *Journal of Learning Disabilities, 7,* 345–362.

Volkmar, F. R., Szatmari, P., & Sparrow, S. S. (1993). Sex differences in pervasive developmental disorders. *Journal of Autism and Developmental Disorders, 23,* 579–591.

Wainwright-Sharp, J. A., & Bryson, S. E. (1993). Visual orienting deficits in high-functioning people with autism. *Journal of Autism and Developmental Disorders, 23,* 1–13.

Wakefield, A. J., Murch, S. H., Anthony, A., Linnell, J., Casson, D. M., Malik, M., et al. (1998). Ileal-lymphoid-nodular hyperplasia, non-specific colitis, and pervasive developmental disorder in children. *Lancet, 351,* 637–641.

Wetherby, A. M., Woods, J., Allen, L., Cleary, J., Dickinson, H., & Lord, C. (2004). Early indicators of autism spectrum disorders in the second year of life. *Journal of Autism and Developmental Disorders, 34,* 473–493.

Yirmiya, N., Erel, O., Shaked, M., & Solomonica-Levi, D. (1998). Meta-analyses comparing theory of mind abilities of individuals with autism, individuals with mental retardation, and normally developing individuals. *Psychological Bulletin, 124,* 283–307.

Zilbovicius, M., Boddaert, N., Belin, P., Poline, J. B., Remy, P., Mangin, J. F., et al. (2000). Temporal lobe dysfunction in childhood autism: A PET study. *American Journal of Psychiatry, 157,* 1988–1993.

Zwaigenbaum, L., Bryson, S., Rogers, T., Roberts, W., Brian, J., & Szatmari, P. (2005). Behavioral manifestations of autism in the first year of life. *International Journal of Developmental Neuroscience, 23,* 143–152.

CHAPTER 16

Intellectual Disability Syndromes

CAROLYN B. MERVIS
ANGELA E. JOHN

People differ substantially in their ability to understand abstract ideas, adapt to their environments, learn from experience, and engage in different forms of reasoning (Neisser et al., 1996). These characteristics of intelligence reflect the accumulation of an individual's learning (Wesman, 1968). There are significant differences both among and within cultures in beliefs about what intelligence is and how it should be measured (see the chapters in Sternberg, 2004).

INTELLECTUAL DISABILITY: AN OVERVIEW

The first intelligence test was designed and constructed by Binet and Simon (1911) in response to a charge from the French Ministry of Public Instruction to develop a fast and reliable way to identify any child who "because of the state of his intelligence, was unable to profit, in a normal manner, from the instruction given in ordinary schools" (Binet & Simon, 1905, p. 163; translation from Mackintosh, 1998). Children who were identified were to be assigned to special classes.

Modern intelligence tests yield IQ scores based on a bell curve model, with a mean of 100 and standard deviation of 15. Approximately 95% of the population scores within two standard deviations of the mean (70–130), with ~2.5% scoring <70 and ~2.5% scoring >130. Current IQ tests are standardized on samples that are carefully stratified to reflect recent census data with regard to gender, racial/ethnic group, socioeconomic status (SES) and/or educational attainment of the parent(s), and the population density of the community. Typically ~100 children (50 girls, 50 boys) are tested in each age group. As indicated in the definitions provided below, an IQ score at the bottom of the normal distribution is one criterion that must be met for a person to be classified as having intellectual disability (mental retardation).

Definitions of Intellectual Disability (Mental Retardation)

The most commonly used definition of mental retardation is provided by the fourth edition, text revision, of the *Diagnostic and Statistical Manual of Mental Disorders* (DSM-IV-TR; American Psychiatric Association, 2000). According to this definition, individuals are considered to have mental retardation if:

1. Their current IQ, based on an individually administered test, is at least two standard deviations below the mean (≤~70).
2. They have significant limitations, relative to those expected for their chronological age (CA) and sociocultural background, in at least two of the following adaptive behavior domains: communication, social/interpersonal skills, self-care, home living, self-direction, leisure, functional academic skills, use of community resources, work, health, and safety.
3. These difficulties were first evidenced prior to age 18 years.

Each of the other major organizations involved in the treatment of individuals with intellectual disability—the American Association on Intellectual and Developmental Disabilities (AAIDD), the American Psychological Association, and the World Health Organization (WHO)—accepts the same criteria but implements them in slightly different ways (see American Psychological Association, 1996; Luckasson et al., 2002; WHO, 1996). Note that because the confidence interval around an IQ score is ~5 points, individuals who have IQs between 70 and 75 but who also have significant adaptive behavior limitations may be classified as having mental retardation (e.g., Luckasson et al., 2002).

For many years, the term *intellectual disability* has been preferred to the term *mental retardation* in Europe. Recently, the AAIDD has strongly endorsed the use of *intellectual disability*, and this term is thus starting to be used in the United States as well. In the present chapter, we have used *intellectual disability* (hereafter abbreviated as ID), except when providing definitions that were explicitly stated as definitions of *mental retardation*.

Prevalence

Estimates of the prevalence of ID vary as a function of the specific definition, as well as of age, sex, and SES. According to the bell curve model, ~2.5% of the population would be expected to have an IQ ≤70 (and 5% an IQ ≤75). However, some of these individuals would have adaptive behavior within the normal range and therefore would not be classified as having ID. Zigler (1967) has argued that there is an excess of individuals with IQ ≤70 (and especially IQ ≤55) relative to the predictions of the bell curve model, due to individuals whose low IQ is due to organic rather than familial causes. In a summary of several epidemiological studies, Batshaw, Shapiro, and Farber (2007) note that the lowest reported prevalence of ID is for children under 5 years old (<1%), and that the highest is for children ages 10–14 years (9.7%). Much of the discrepancy is probably attributable to increases in the diagnosis of mild ID during the early school years, as these mild impairments may not be as noticeable in younger children. In addition, the reported school-age prevalence is based solely on IQ; some of the children thus identified would have normal adaptive skills, and so would not meet standard criteria for ID (Leonard & Wen, 2002).

Winnepenninckx, Rooms, and Kooy (2003) state that ~50% of cases of ID are due primarily to genetic causes and ~50% primarily to environmental causes. They note that on average, epidemiological studies have identified specific causes for ID for about half of the presumed environmental cases and half of the presumed genetic cases. The 25% of cases of ID for which a specific genetic cause is known can be accounted for as follows: 12% are due to chromosomal abnormalities, 6% to subtelomeric abnormalities, 4% to known genetic syndromes, and 3% to metabolic disorders. More than 1,000 genetic causes of ID have been identified (King, Hodapp, & Dykens, 2005). Environmental causes include prenatal exposure to alcohol, maternal infection during pregnancy, extremely low birthweight and/ or extreme prematurity, malnutrition, environmental toxins, and head injury (see McDermott, Durkin, Schupf, & Stein, 2007, for further discussion).

Classification Systems

Historically, individuals with ID have been classified into four groups based on level of severity. More recently, many researchers have classified individuals with ID on the basis of their syndrome rather than on the severity of their ID.

Classification by Level of ID

All of the definitions of mental retardation discussed above also include subdivisions based on level of severity. The American Psychological Association and WHO subdivisions are based on IQ, as follows: *mild* (IQ between 50–55 and ~70), *moderate* (IQ between 35–40 and 50–55), *severe* (IQ between 20–25 and 35–40), and *profound* (IQ below 20–25). The AAIDD subdivisions are based on the intensity of support required to enhance independence, productivity, and community integration (Luckasson et al., 2002). Information about level of severity may be used to obtain a clearer picture regarding likely outcome and level of functioning (see Table 16.1). Historically, psychologists and educators have focused on level of ID rather than etiology, both for educational interventions and for research. A traditional research design for studies of cognitive aspects of ID included two groups of participants: individuals with ID and individuals with normal intelligence. In determining the individuals to be assigned to the group with ID, etiology was characteristically ignored; individuals with cultural–familial mental retardation, individuals with ID due to environmental causes, and individuals with various genetic syndromes were all likely to be included within the same group. This decision was based on the common assumption that individuals with ID differed from individuals with normal intelligence in specific and fundamental ways, beyond simply intellectual slowness. Proposed bases for these differences included behavioral rigidity, deficits in verbal mediation ability, deficits in short-term memory, and deficits in attention (see, e.g., Burack, Hodapp, & Zigler, 1998; Zigler & Balla, 1982). This type of position is now referred to as the *difference approach*.

Classification by Syndrome

The first major break from the difference approach was provided by Zigler (1967), who offered the initial formal proposal of the *developmental approach* (see Burack et al., 1998).

TABLE 16.1. Characteristics Associated with Individuals of Differing Levels of ID

Level of ID	% of population with ID	Language development	Academic skills	Living skills and employment
Mild	~85%	Some delay; fluent by adolescence (minimal impairment)	May acquire academic skills up to sixth-grade level	May need supervision or guidance
Moderate	~10%	Functional language by adolescence	May acquire academic skills up to second-grade level	Moderate supervision required
Severe	~3–4%	Limited	May become familiar with alphabet and simple counting	Close supervision required
Profound	~1–2%	May learn single words	None	Pervasive supervision required

Note. Based on American Psychiatric Association (2000) and World Health Organization (1996).

Zigler argued that individuals whose ID was due to cultural–familial causes should follow the same developmental path as individuals with normal intelligence, although each step might take longer, and later steps might not be attained. Furthermore, when matched to individuals with normal intelligence of the same mental age (MA), individuals with cultural–familial ID (as a group) should show no particular areas of cognitive strength or weakness (*similar-structure hypothesis*).

Beginning in the early 1980s, the developmental approach began to be extended to individuals with ID due to organic causes (e.g., Cicchetti & Pogge-Hesse, 1982). More recent studies have often confirmed the similar sequence hypothesis for a wide range of syndromes (e.g., Hodapp & Burack, 1990). However, the similar-structure hypothesis has consistently been disconfirmed. Syndrome-specific intellectual profiles (patterns of relative intellectual strengths and weaknesses) and behavioral profiles have been identified for a variety of syndromes associated with ID, including Down syndrome (DS) (e.g., Fidler, Hodapp, & Dykens, 2002; Fidler & Nadel, 2007; Silverman, 2007), fragile X syndrome (e.g., Cornish, Levitas, & Sudhalter, 2007; Hagerman, 2002), Smith–Magenis syndrome (see Shelley & Robertson, 2005, for a review), and Williams syndrome (WS) (Klein-Tasman & Mervis, 2003; Mervis et al., 2000; Mervis & Morris, 2007). For this reason, treating ID as a monolith is inappropriate. Instead, we focus in the remainder of this chapter on a single illustrative genetic disorder associated with ID: WS. Where contrasts with other syndromes (especially DS) are available, these are briefly presented.

WILLIAMS SYNDROME: AN ILLUSTRATIVE ID SYNDROME

WS is a neurodevelopmental disorder caused by a hemizygous 1.6-megabase microdeletion of ~25 genes on chromosome 7q11.23 (Hillier et al., 2003) and is associated with a recognizable pattern of physical characteristics, including a specific set of facial features, heart disease (most commonly supravalvar aortic stenosis), connective tissue abnormalities, failure to thrive, and growth deficiency (Mervis & Morris, 2007; Morris, 2006). About 95%

of individuals with WS have the same set of genes deleted ("classic deletion"). Individuals with WS have developmental delay; this typically leads to mild to moderate ID or learning difficulties, although some individuals have low-average to average intelligence, and a small proportion has severe ID. The syndrome is characterized by a specific cognitive profile (Mervis et al., 2000), with relative strengths in verbal short-term memory and language, and extreme weakness in visual–spatial construction; it is also characterized by a specific personality profile (Klein-Tasman & Mervis, 2003), including high levels of sociability and empathy, eagerness to interact with others, and high levels of tension and sensitivity.

Epidemiology

WS has a prevalence of 1 per 7,500 (Strømme, Bjørnstad, & Ramstad, 2003). The deleted region is flanked by low-copy repeats, which predispose it to unequal crossing over during meiosis, increasing the likelihood of deletion, duplication, or inversion. Approximately 7% of the general population has an inversion of the WS region; individuals with this inversion have a fivefold increased chance of having a child with WS (Morris, 2006). However, most children with WS are born to parents who do not have inversions.

Neuropathology/Neural Substrates

The study of the associations among genes, brain, and behavior in genetic syndromes offers an opportunity to examine these relations in cases in which the underlying genetics are well characterized. Most neuroimaging studies have focused on individuals with WS who have ID and compared them to individuals with typical development (TD). This design makes it difficult to interpret significant between-group differences, as effects due to the core disabilities in WS are difficult to separate from more general effects of ID. A few studies have restricted the group with WS to individuals with low-average or average intelligence and included a control group of individuals from the general population with similar CA and IQ. In this section, we focus on these studies.

Structural Abnormalities

Structural magnetic resonance imaging (MRI) studies of individuals with WS and ID have identified reductions in the parietal lobule (Eckert et al., 2005) and occipital gray matter (Reiss et al., 2000). Cerebellar size is preserved (Wang, Hesselink, Jernigan, Doherty, & Bellugi, 1992). Reiss et al. (2004) found pronounced gray matter reduction in the intraparietal sulcus, but increases in gray matter in the orbital and medial prefrontal cortices, anterior cingulate, insular cortex, and superior temporal gyrus. Structural MRI studies of individuals with WS and normal IQ have identified symmetrical gray matter reductions in three regions: the intraparietal sulcus, the area around the third ventricle, and the orbitofrontal cortex (OFC) (Meyer-Lindenberg et al., 2004). No volume increases were found. A diffusion tensor imaging study of individuals with WS and normal IQ indicated abnormal white matter integrity, including alteration in directionality of white matter fibers, deviation in posterior fiber tract course (including that underlying the intraparietal sulcus), and reduced lateralization of fiber coherence (Marenco et al., 2007). Marenco et al. note that these findings indicate a likely role for two of the deleted genes (LIMK1 and CYLN2) in axon guidance and neuronal migration.

Functional Abnormalities

Severe impairment in visual–spatial construction is a neuropsychological hallmark of WS (Farran & Jarrold, 2003; Mervis et al., 2000). This finding, coupled with relatively good face- and object-processing skills (e.g., Landau, Hoffman, & Kurz, 2006), suggests a neural processing abnormality in the dorsal stream (e.g., Atkinson et al., 2003; Paul, Stiles, Passarotti, Bavar, & Bellugi, 2002) with relatively intact ventral stream function. This hypothesis has been confirmed by Meyer-Lindenberg et al. (2004) in a study of individuals with WS and normal intelligence. A hierarchical assessment of visual processing using functional MRI (fMRI) indicated isolated hypoactivation in the parietal portion of the dorsal stream, immediately adjacent to the gray matter reduction in the intraparietal sulcus identified by structural neuroimaging. Path analysis demonstrated that the functional abnormalities could be attributed to impaired input from this structurally altered region.

WS has also been associated with deficits in spatial navigation (O'Hearn, Landau, & Hoffman, 2005) and long-term memory (Nichols et al., 2004; Vicari, Bellucci, & Carlesimo, 2005)—cognitive domains that have been linked to hippocampal function. Positron emission tomography, fMRI, and spectropic studies of this region in individuals with WS and normal IQ found profound reduction in resting blood flow and absent differential response to visual stimuli and reduced measures of N-acetylaspartate, a marker of synaptic activity (Meyer-Lindenberg et al., 2005b). Hippocampal size was preserved, but there were subtle alterations in shape. These findings suggest that hippocampal dysfunction may contribute to neurocognitive abnormalities in WS.

WS is associated with a unique personality profile, characterized in part by high levels of gregariousness (social disinhibition) accompanied by high rates of nonsocial anxiety. In an fMRI study of individuals with WS and normal IQ, Meyer-Lindenberg et al. (2005a) found that amygdala activation was significantly reduced to angry or fearful faces but significantly increased to threatening or fearful scenes, suggesting abnormal regulation. This pattern is consistent with findings of indiscriminate approach to people combined with specific phobias of a nonsocial nature. Using path analysis, a statistical method allowing the assessment of functional interregional interactions, Meyer-Lindenberg et al. showed that for individuals with WS and normal IQ, the region in the OFC previously found to have reduced gray matter was not regulating the amygdala. In the general population, OFC–amygdala interactions have been shown to link sensory representations of stimuli with social judgments about them based on their motivational value (Adolphs, 2003). Meyer-Lindenberg et al. (2005a; Meyer-Lindenberg, Mervis, & Berman, 2006) argued that this lack of regulation of the amygdala by the OFC even for individuals with WS who have normal IQ contributes to the social disinhibition, reduced reactivity to social cues, and increased tendency to approach strangers that characterize this syndrome.

Neuropsychological Consequences

General Intellectual Functioning

For school-age children with WS, mean IQ on a full-scale intelligence test is toward the bottom of the mild ID range. Mervis and Morris (2007) have reported a mean General Conceptual Ability (GCA; similar to IQ) score on the Differential Ability Scales (DAS; Elliott, 1990) of 58.29 (SD = 12.77, range = 24–94) for a sample of 119 children ages 8–17 who had the classic deletion. This overall GCA is misleading, however. As mentioned earlier, WS is associated with a distinct cognitive profile including relative strengths in verbal short-term memory and language, and extreme weakness in visual–spatial construction. Given this profile, one would expect that performance on full-scale IQ tests that include a separate scale measuring visual–spatial construction would typically indicate large between-scale differences in ability. As shown in Figure 16.1, this is exactly the pattern found on the DAS. Mean Cluster standard scores were as follows: Verbal, 70.18; Nonverbal Reasoning, 67.43, and Spatial, 55.54 (very close to floor). This pattern is seen even more dramatically on the second edition of the DAS (DAS-II; Elliott, 2007), on which the floor for the subtests has been substantially lowered. On the DAS-II, 72% of a sample of 53 children and youth ages 4–17 scored significantly higher on the Verbal Cluster than the Spatial Cluster, and 75% scored significantly higher on the Nonverbal Reasoning Cluster than the Spatial Cluster (Mervis & Morris, 2007). Thus, for the majority of children with WS, overall IQ is not an appropriate measure of intellectual ability. Instead, verbal, nonverbal reasoning abilities, and spatial abilities need to be considered separately.

This same pattern of intellectual strengths and weaknesses is apparent even in toddlers and preschoolers with WS. On the Mullen Scales of Early Learning (Mullen, 1995), the mean Early Learning Composite (similar to developmental quotient) for 79 children ages 2–4 with the classic deletion was 63.44 (SD = 11.97; range = 49 [lowest possible]–109). Mean T scores for the scales were as follows: Visual Reception (nonverbal reasoning), 30.46; Fine Motor (measuring primarily visual–spatial construction), 21.48 (floor = 20); Receptive Language, 31.81; and Expressive Language, 34.59 (Mervis & Morris, 2007).

Language

WS initially came to the attention of psychological researchers because of the claim that it offered a paradigmatic case of the independence of language from cognition. In particular, Bellugi, Marks, Bihrle, and Sabo (1988) argued that individuals with WS had excellent language skills in the face of severe mental retardation. Although Bellugi and her colleagues (e.g., Bellugi, Lichtenberger, Jones, Lai, & St. George, 2000) and Clahsen and his colleagues (e.g., Clahsen & Almazan, 1998) continue to argue that language is selectively spared in WS, recent findings suggest that overall language abilities are approximately at the level expected for IQ (see reviews by Brock, 2007; Mervis, 2006; Mervis & Becerra, 2007).

Within the language domain, children with WS evidence a consistent pattern of relative strengths and weaknesses. The greatest strength is in concrete vocabulary; mean standard score on the Peabody Picture Vocabulary Test–III (PPVT-III; Dunn & Dunn, 1997) for 238 children and youth ages 4–17 was 79.85 (low-average for the general population), and 78% scored in the normal range for the general population (Mervis & Becerra, 2007). The greatest weakness is in relational vocabulary (spatial, temporal, quantitative, and dimensional concepts), with a mean standard score on the Test of Relational Concepts (Edmonston & Litchfield Thane, 1988) ~30 points below the mean standard score on the PPVT-III and approximately at the same level as performance on DAS Pattern Construction (Mervis & John, 2008). By age 6 years, most children with WS speak in complete sentences. Syntactic abilities are typically at about the same level as those of MA-matched children with TD or MA-matched children with ID of mixed or unknown etiology (e.g., Gosch, Städing, & Pankau, 1994; Udwin & Yule, 1990; Volterra, Capirci, Pezzini, Sabbadini, & Vicari,

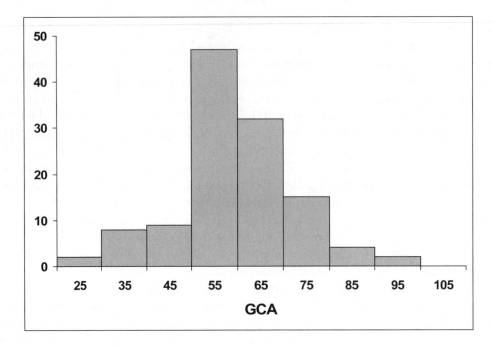

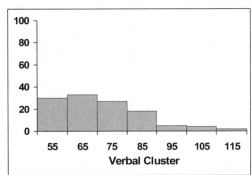

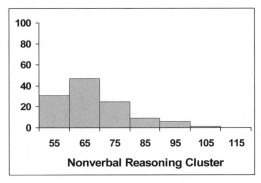

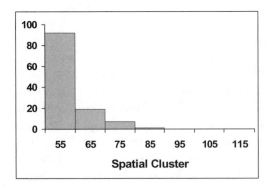

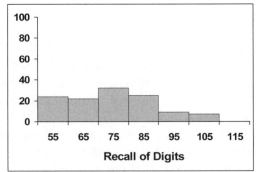

FIGURE 16.1. Differential Ability Scales (DAS) General Conceptual Ability (GCA) and Verbal Cluster, Nonverbal Reasoning Cluster, Spatial Cluster, and Recall of Digits standard scores for 119 children with WS ages 8–17 years who completed the School-Age Level of the DAS. Recall of Digits *T* scores have been converted to the same scale as GCA and Cluster standard scores. All children have the classic deletion, and none has been diagnosed with an autism spectrum disorder. From Mervis and Morris (2007). Copyright 2007 by the Massachusetts Institute of Technology. Reprinted by permission.

1996; Zukowski, 2004). The syntactic abilities of children with WS are typically (e.g., Bellugi et al., 1988, 2000; Klein & Mervis, 1999) significantly stronger than those of CA- and IQ- or MA-matched children with DS; this probably reflects the relative weakness children with DS have in expressive language (e.g., Mervis, 2006). In languages with relatively complex morphology, children with WS perform below the level of MA-matched children with TD (e.g., for French, Karmiloff-Smith et al., 1997; for Hebrew, Levy & Hermon, 2003; for Hungarian, Lukács, 2005; Lukács, Racsmány, & Pléh, 2001).

Despite their social nature, individuals with WS have considerable difficulty with pragmatics, as evidenced by the results of studies of standardized questionnaires completed by parents (Laws & Bishop, 2004; Philofsky, Fidler, & Hepburn, 2007) and studies of conversational abilities (e.g., Stojanovik, 2006). This difficulty is presaged in early childhood by the extremely delayed onset of comprehension and production of referential pointing gestures. In contrast to the pattern shown by children with TD, children with DS, and children with ID of mixed etiology, referential pointing almost always begins after the onset of referential language in children with WS (Mervis, 2006; Mervis & Bertrand, 1997). Even after the onset of pointing, young children with WS have more difficulty following pointing gestures and are less likely to produce pointing gestures than MA-matched children with TD (Laing et al., 2002). Using a semistructured play-based assessment designed to evaluate communication and reciprocal social interaction skills in young children with limited or no expressive language (Autism Diagnostic Observation Schedule—Module 1; Lord et al., 2000), Klein-Tasman, Mervis, Lord, and Phillips (2007) found that the majority of preschoolers with WS who had limited expressive language had significant difficulties with pointing, giving objects, showing objects, and appropriate use of eye contact. Many also had difficulties with initiation of joint attention, response to the examiners' bids for joint attention, and integration of gaze with other behaviors.

Visual–Spatial Skills

Consistent with Meyer-Lindenberg et al.'s (2006) hypothesis that ventral stream processing in WS is appropriate for IQ, the results of studies of object recognition (e.g., Landau et al., 2006) have shown that visual-perceptual ability is at MA level (see review in Farran & Jarrold, 2003). Jordan, Reiss, Hoffman, and Landau (2002) found that children with WS were as good as MA-matched children with TD at perceiving biological motion in moving point–light displays.

In contrast, visual–spatial construction is the signature weakness for individuals with WS. On tests of drawing ability (e.g., the Developmental Test of Visual–Motor Integration; Beery, 1989), individuals with WS score significantly lower than either MA-matched individuals with DS (Wang & Bellugi, 1994) or MA-matched children with TD (Bertrand, Mervis, & Eisenberg, 1997). As discussed above, performance on tests of pattern construction is similar (e.g., Bellugi et al., 1988, 2000; Mervis et al., 2000). Bellugi et al. have argued that the pattern of difficulties is consistent with a focus on local (rather than global) processing. However, Pani, Mervis, and Robinson (1999) demonstrated that individuals with WS showed a global (rather than local) precedence effect, and Bertrand and Mervis (1996; Bertrand et al., 1997) argued that the pattern of errors produced by children with WS was consistent with the normal process of learning to draw. They also presented longitudinal data showing clear improvement in drawing ability for children with WS when tested 4 years later. Hoffman, Landau, and Pagani (2003) used eye-tracking data to argue that the basic executive functions involved in pattern construction were at MA level for patterns that were not too difficult for the children with WS. However, their spatial representational skills as measured by matching of block orientation and block placement were well below MA level. Overall, the pattern of findings for WS is consistent with a severe delay in the development of visual–spatial construction, rather than with deviance.

Attention

The early studies addressing the possibility of attention problems in WS were based on parental responses to the Child Behavior Checklist (CBCL; Achenbach, 1991). Significantly elevated scores on the Attention Problems subscale were reported for 67% of the children studied by Dilts, Morris, and Leonard (1990) and 73% of the children studied by Greer, Brown, Pai, Choudry, and Klein (1997). Einfeld and Tonge (Einfeld, Tonge, & Florio, 1997; Tonge & Einfeld, 2003) reported that parents of children with WS were significantly more likely to endorse the items "overactive" and "short attention span" than were the parents of the epidemiological control group for the Developmental Behavior Checklist (Einfeld & Tonge, 1995). Leyfer, Woodruff-Borden, Klein-Tasman, Fricke, and Mervis (2006) administered the Anxiety Disorders Interview Schedule—Parent (ADIS-P; Silverman & Albano, 1996)—a structured interview that provides DSM-IV-TR diagnoses for all anxiety and related disorders, including attention-deficit/hyperactivity disorder (ADHD)—to parents of 119 children and youth ages 4–16 with WS. The results indicated that 65% met criteria for ADHD, most for the predominantly inattentive type. The proportion diagnosed with the combined type of ADHD decreased significantly with age, and the predominantly hyperactive–impulsive type was very rare. This pattern is similar to that for the general population. Prevalence of ADHD was much higher than for children in the general population (3–7%; American Psychiatric Association, 2000), children with ID of mixed etiology (6.8% in Dekker & Koot, 2003), or children with DS (6.1%; Myers & Pueschel, 1991), but similar to that for boys with fragile X syndrome (72%; Backes et al., 2000).

Memory

Given the pattern of relative intellectual strengths and weaknesses associated with WS, individuals with this syndrome would be predicted to have significantly better verbal memory than spatial memory. This prediction has been confirmed (e.g., Jarrold, Baddeley, & Hewes, 1999; Wang & Bellugi, 1994). Individuals with WS might also be expected to have significantly better verbal memory and significantly weaker spatial memory than CA- and IQ-matched individuals who have other forms of ID. Results are consistent with this expectation for memory tasks that do not require mental manipulation. Thus individuals with WS perform significantly better on measures of forward digit recall than do CA- and IQ-/MA-matched groups with DS (Edgin, 2003; Jarrold et al., 1999; Klein & Mervis, 1999; Wang & Bellugi, 1994) or with ID of mixed or unknown etiology (Devenny et al., 2004; Udwin & Yule, 1991). The same pattern holds for the first trial of word list recall (Nichols et al., 2004). In contrast, children and adults with WS perform significantly worse than CA- and IQ-/MA-matched individuals with other forms of ID on forward Corsi (spatial) recall (Jarrold et al., 1999; Wang & Bellugi, 1994).

Several studies comparing the memory abilities of individuals with WS to much younger groups of MA-matched children (whether with TD or with other forms of disability) have been conducted. Interpreting the results of these studies is difficult for methodological reasons. In particular, use of this matching procedure assumes similar rates of development for both the control and target variables, which is often not the case. If development of the control and target variables proceeds at different rates, then differences in CA will confound the matching design, because the differences in raw scores (and therefore age equivalent [AE] scores) will not be stable across CA. In such cases, one cannot predict that two groups with identical AEs on control variables but different CAs should be expected to have similar scores on the target variable. As demonstrated by Mervis and colleagues, younger children with the same MA (or verbal ability) as older children with ID should be predicted to have better verbal memory abilities (see Figure 1 in Mervis & Robinson, 2005, and further discussion in Rowe & Mervis, 2006). The results of studies using this type of design indicate that the performance of the group with WS is at or above the level of the contrast group. Furthermore, the performance of the group with WS is affected by the same semantic and phonological factors as for the general population (see review in Rowe & Mervis, 2006).

When mental manipulation is required, however, differences between individuals with WS and the contrast group(s) are considerably reduced. On backward digit recall tasks, groups of individuals with WS consistently demonstrate longer spans than CA- and IQ-/MA-matched groups with other forms of ID (e.g., Devenny et al., 2004; Edgin, 2003; Wang & Bellugi, 1994), but the between-group differences are not significant. In the only study that compared backward Corsi span, mean span for the groups with WS and with DS was almost identical (Edgin, 2003). In contrast to expectations based on the initial characterization of WS as demonstrating the independence of language from cognition (e.g., Bellugi et al., 1988), the verbal memory abilities of children with WS have consistently been found to be strongly related to both grammatical and vocabulary abilities (Grant et al., 1997; Mervis, 2006; Mervis & Becerra, 2007; Pléh, Lukács, & Racsmány, 2002; Robinson, Mervis, & Robinson, 2003).

Executive Functions

Despite the clear importance of executive functioning, such functions (apart from attention and working memory) have been directly addressed in only one study of children with WS. Atkinson et al. (2003) reported findings for one verbal executive function task (Day and Night, modeled on the Stroop task) and two spatial executive function tasks (Detour Box and Pointing/Counterpointing). All three tasks require the inhibition of a prepotent response. Comparisons were made both to CA-based expectations and to expectations based on vocabulary age from the British form of the PPVT. Performance on the verbal task was at or above the level expected for vocabulary age; a subset of children performed at the level expected for CA. For most of the children with WS, performance on the spatial executive function tasks was well below the level expected for vocabulary age, although a small subset of children (some of whom used a verbal mediation strategy) performed at the level expected for CA. There was a significant correlation between performance on the Detour Box and performance on the Day and Night task.

Sensory–Motor Skills

Another area that has received little attention in WS is sensory–motor development. Although retrospective reports of ages at attainment of sensory–motor milestones for individuals with WS have been collected (e.g., Dilts et al., 1990), there has only been one prospective study. Masataka (2001) followed the development of eight young children with WS every 2 weeks from 6 to 20 months of age. Results indicated significant delays in the attainment of all early sensory–motor milestones. Mean CAs were as follows: reaching for objects, 40.25 weeks; rolling from stomach to back, 47.50 weeks; sitting unsupported, 59.25 weeks; pulling to a stand, 88.25 weeks; first steps, 100.00 weeks. This delay in motor skill attainment is ongoing, as indicated by the adaptive behavior findings reported next.

Adaptive Functioning

Most studies of the adaptive behavior skills of children with WS have used a version of the Vineland Scales of Adaptive Behavior (Sparrow, Balla, & Cicchetti, 1984), a semi-structured interview conducted with a caregiver (in these studies, a parent). The Vineland includes four scales: Communication, Socialization, Daily Living Skills, and Motor Skills. Gosch and Pankau (1994) included a CA- and IQ-matched contrast group with nonspecific ID; the children in the contrast group performed significantly better overall. The authors suggested that the difference was due primarily to the large number of items that required fine motor skills—an area of considerable weakness for individuals with WS.

The remaining studies did not include a contrast group. Greer et al. (1997) reported that performance on the Vineland Socialization and Communication scales was significantly stronger than on Daily Living Skills or Motor Skills. Mervis, Klein-Tasman, and Mastin (2001), reporting on a larger sample, found significant differences in performance between all pairs of Vineland scales, with performance ordered as follows: (1) Socialization, (2) Communication, (3) Daily Living Skills, (4) Motor Skills. Mervis and Morris (2007) examined the adaptive behavior of 122 children and adolescents with WS, using the Scales of Independent Behavior—Revised (Bruininks, Woodcock, Weatherman, & Hill, 1996). Performance on the Social Interaction and Communication Skills scale was significantly better than on the remaining scales, all of which depend heavily on fine motor, time management, or money skills. In all three studies, mean adaptive behavior standard score was similar to mean IQ.

Emotional and Behavioral Adjustment

The paradoxical nature of social behavior and emotional adjustment of individuals with WS was aptly described by von Arnim and Engel (1964, p. 376) in one of the first reports of children with WS (at the time called *idiopathic infantile hypercalcemia*): "They show outstanding loquacity and a great ability to establish interpersonal contacts. This stands against a background of insecurity and anxiety." Almost 40 years later, Klein-Tasman and Mervis (2003) quantified the WS personality profile, demonstrating very high sensitivity and high specificity relative to a CA- and IQ-matched group of children with developmental disability of mixed etiology. This profile is composed of high levels of approach, sociability, and empathy as measured by the Children's Behavior Questionnaire (Rothbart &

Ahadi, 1994), and high levels of gregariousness, people orientation, tenseness, sensitivity, and visibility as measured by the parent report version of the Multidimensional Personality Questionnaire (MPQ; Tellegen, 1985). The MPQ profile has high sensitivity (>.90) for individuals with WS ages 5–20 years, after which the sensitivity decreases considerably (Mervis & Morris, 2007).

One of the most striking aspects of the WS personality profile is the extreme willingness of children with WS to approach other people, even strangers. Most parents of children with WS report that they "never met a stranger." Stranger anxiety is extremely rare; infants and toddlers are typically willing to be left with anyone (Doyle, Bellugi, Korenberg, & Graham, 2004). An unusual type of staring behavior that is not found in infants and toddlers with other genetic disorders, and that leaves a recipient feeling as if a child's eyes were boring into him or her, also characterizes the early reaction of these children to strangers (Mervis et al., 2003). A recent parent report study of the approach behaviors of American and Japanese children with WS in comparison to children with TD from the same cultures confirmed that within each culture, the children with WS were more likely to approach strangers than the children with TD were. A possible effect of culture was also found: The ratings of likelihood of approaching strangers provided by the Japanese parents were significantly lower than the ratings provided by the American parents (Zitzer-Comfort, Doyle, Masataka, Korenberg, & Bellugi, 2007). The authors note that an alternative explanation, given that the qualitative descriptions of approach to strangers provided by Japanese and American parents of children with WS were very similar, is that Japanese parents are more conservative in their ratings than American parents.

The question of why individuals with WS are more willing to approach strangers has been addressed in two studies involving approachability ratings based on photos of strangers' faces. In the original study, Bellugi, Adolphs, Cassady, and Chiles (1999) found that individuals with WS consistently rated photos of strangers (all of whom showed positive emotion) as more approachable than did a CA-matched group with TD. In a second study that included both photos showing positive emotion and photos showing negative emotion, Frigerio et al. (2006) found that the ratings of approachability made by persons with WS were significantly higher than those made by the CA-matched and the MA-matched control groups (both composed of individuals with TD) for the faces showing positive emotion, and significantly lower (less approachable) for the faces showing negative emotion. Nevertheless, stranger approach is consistently reported by parents to be indiscriminate; this is likely to reflect disinhibition (Davies, Udwin, & Howlin, 1998; Frigerio et al., 2006), suggesting possible frontal lobe impairment. This proposal is consistent with Meyer-Lindenberg et al.'s (2005a, 2006) finding of reduced gray matter in the OFC of adults with WS and normal IQ, resulting in dysregulation of the amygdala.

Results of studies using a simulated distress procedure, in which the researcher pretends to injure him- or herself and then displays appropriate facial and vocal expressions for ~30 seconds, have confirmed that children with WS show significantly more empathy, comforting behavior, and overall level of concern than CA- and IQ-matched children with Prader–Willi syndrome (Plesa-Skwerer & Tager-Flusberg, 2006) or developmental disability of mixed etiology (Thomas, Becerra, & Mervis, 2002), or CA-matched children with TD (Thomas et al., 2002).

Despite the many positive characteristics reflected in the WS personality profile, individuals with WS frequently demonstrate difficulty with peer relationships (e.g., Sullivan,

Winner, & Tager-Flusberg, 2003), and their families are often highly stressed (Fidler, Hodapp, & Dykens, 2000). Mothers of children with WS have a rate of generalized anxiety disorder (GAD) about three times that of women their age in the general population, despite (based on retrospective report) having a rate of GAD similar to that of women in the general population prior to the birth of their children with WS (Leyfer, Woodruff-Borden, & Mervis, 2009). These problems are likely to be due at least in part to the difficult temperamental characteristics associated with WS. Tomc, Williamson, and Pauli (1990) reported, based on parental responses to questionnaires based on Thomas and Chess's (1977) model of temperament, that relative to both CA- and MA-based expectations, children with WS were rated significantly higher on approach, intensity, negative mood, and distractibility, and significantly lower on persistence and threshold of excitability. These characteristics suggest that children with WS tend to overreact—a finding consistently confirmed by parents' indications during the Vineland interview that their children overdramatize in reaction to a wide variety of situations, both positive and negative (Mervis, 2008). Unusually high levels of problem behavior were also documented by Fidler et al. (2000), who found that 75% of the group with WS (compared to 10% of the group with DS) scored in the clinically significant range on the CBCL for Total Problems. Children and adolescents with WS have significant difficulties with theory of mind, performing at or below the level of CA-, IQ-, and language-age-matched groups with Prader–Willi syndrome or developmental disability of mixed etiology (see review in Plesa-Skwerer & Tager-Flusberg, 2006); such difficulties would be expected to have a negative impact on peer relationships. The previously described difficulties with pragmatics, attention, and adaptive behavior also negatively impact the social success of children with WS and increase the stress/anxiety experienced by their families.

A further significant difficulty is caused by the very high levels of anxiety experienced by children with WS. Leyfer et al. (2006) used the ADIS-P to identify DSM-IV-TR diagnoses for anxiety in 119 children and youth ages 4–16 with WS. The prevalence for any anxiety disorder was 57%, which is considerably higher than reported in the two population-based studies of psychopathology in children with ID (10.5% in Dekker & Koot, 2003, and 8.7% in Emerson, 2003). The most common anxiety disorder was specific phobia (54%); the most common type of phobia was for loud noises (28%). GAD diagnoses significantly increased with age, occurring in 0% of 4- to 6-year-olds, 14% of 7- to 10-year-olds, and 23% of 11- to 16-year-olds. Leyfer et al. argue that in their clinical experience, the DSM-IV-TR criteria for GAD often do not capture the nature of worrying in children with WS; if the criteria reflected this type of worrying, the prevalence of GAD would be much higher. Most children with WS worry in anticipation of both events they expect to dislike and events they expect to enjoy. The worry is perseverative, is typically manifested by repeated questions about upcoming activities, and causes significant interference in daily life.

Developmental Considerations

WS is present from conception and results in initial developmental delays in all intellectual and behavioral domains. A few researchers have suggested that the pattern of cognitive strengths and weaknesses varies significantly over time. For example, Paterson and her colleagues (Paterson, 2001; Paterson, Brown, Gsödl, Johnson, & Karmiloff-Smith, 1999) argued that although CA- and IQ-matched young children with WS or DS have equivalent vocabulary abilities, individuals with WS have significantly better vocabularies than matched individuals with DS by early adulthood. Jarrold and his colleagues (Jarrold, Baddeley, & Hewes, 1998; Jarrold, Baddeley, Hewes, & Phillips, 2001) have argued that the pattern of relative strength in vocabulary and weakness in pattern construction becomes more pronounced over time. Both sets of arguments are based on AE scores rather than standard scores and involve treating AE scores as though they are interval data. Problems with the interpretation of AE scores are highlighted in the manuals for most standardized assessments, and methodological issues involved in the use of these scores in psychological research are discussed in Mervis and Robinson (1999, 2005). Comparisons involving standard scores do not suggest changes in developmental trajectories over time for children with WS (see Mervis, 2006, for a more extensive discussion). Karmiloff-Smith (e.g., 2007) has raised a further developmental consideration that deserves serious study: She has argued that even when children with WS (or any other genetic disorder) appear to show the same sequences of development as children with TD, or appear to be performing in the normal range in some domain, the developmental processes that led to the apparently normal sequence or performance may be very different from those for children with TD, due to the impact of the genetic deletion on developmental processes during embryogenesis and postnatal brain development.

Predictors and Moderators of Outcome

Because WS is caused by a microdeletion, a major predictor of outcome is the specific set of genes that is deleted. Most individuals with WS (~95%) have the same ("classic") deletion. However, a few individuals with WS with shorter deletions have been reported. In addition, several kindred groups with members who have very short deletions in the WS region (too short to be classified as WS) have been described. Individuals whose deletion does not include GFT2I, the most telomeric gene in the classic deletion, have higher general intelligence, although most of them still fit the WS cognitive profile (Morris et al., 2003). Several individuals who have longer deletions have also been reported; for individuals whose deletions extended to HIP1 (also referred to as HSP27), overall level of intelligence was significantly lower than for individuals with the classic deletion (Stock et al., 2003). Studies of a kindred group with some members who had a deletion encompassing only part of ELN and all of LIMK1 found that almost all members who had this deletion, but none of the other members, fit the WS cognitive profile, suggesting that deletion of LIMK1 plays a role in the visual–spatial construction weakness characteristic of individuals with WS (Frangiskakis et al., 1996; Morris et al., 2003; but see Tassabehji et al., 1999). For a more complete discussion of WS as a genomic disorder, see Mervis and Morris (2007).

Long-term outcomes for individuals with WS who have the classic deletion vary dramatically. For example, some individuals with WS never learn to read, whereas others read at the high school level. A few individuals have passed state exit exams in both English and mathematics and graduated with regular diplomas, having fulfilled the same requirements as students in the general population. These individuals have had overall IQs ranging from the top of the mild ID range to the lower part of the average range. Some adults (including both those who passed the high school exit exams and others who were considerably less successful academically) are employed full-time in competitive employment, and others are in supported employment, but the majority are not employed (although some are involved in volunteer work).

Unfortunately, there are no published studies on factors that influence adult outcomes. From our research, however, it is clear that strong family support—accompanied by a focus (beginning in early childhood) on taking responsibility for oneself to the extent possible, and leading to the development of strong adaptive skills and the discipline to try one's best—has a major impact on the likelihood of positive adult outcomes (Mervis & Morris, 2007). Although the most successful adults tend to have average to above-average IQs for WS, they are not necessarily the individuals with the highest IQs. The most striking characteristic of these individuals is their adaptive behavior, which is reliably near the top of the range for WS.

There is only one published study on educational strategies that affect outcomes for children with WS (Mervis, 2009). As indicated in this study children with WS who are taught to read using an intensive phonics approach typically decode words at or above the level expected for IQ, whereas children with WS who are taught to read using a whole-word (sight word) approach almost always decode words at a level below that expected for IQ. Reading comprehension is generally more limited, but is significantly higher relative to IQ for the phonics group than the whole-word group (Mervis, 2009). Studies on factors affecting adult outcomes, academic skill development, and positive psychosocial outcomes at all ages are needed.

Summary and Future Directions

WS is a genetic disorder, and the impact of the deleted genes on cognition, personality, and behavior is clear, demonstrating the inappropriateness of treating ID as a monolith. Although the overall IQ of individuals with WS is typically in the range of mild to moderate ID, the uneven cognitive profile associated with the syndrome—including relative strengths in verbal short-term memory and language (primarily concrete vocabulary), and extreme weakness in visual–spatial construction—typically invalidates the overall IQ. The extreme weakness in visual–spatial construction has been related to deletion of LIMK1. It has also been linked to reduced gray matter in the intraparietal sulcus and alteration in directionality of white matter fibers, including deviation in the posterior fiber tract course underlying the intraparietal sulcus even of individuals with WS who have normal IQ, leading to impaired input to upstream components of the dorsal pathway. This same impairment probably also contributes to the extreme difficulty individuals with WS have with relational language, and to the great difficulty children with WS have in acquiring adaptive behavior skills that depend on visual–motor integration. Deletion of GTF2I probably relates to the reduced general intellectual ability of individuals with WS relative to their family members, reflected in performance across all cognitive domains. Deletion of HIP1 in individuals who have longer-than-usual deletions probably leads to further cognitive limitation.

The personality profile associated with WS includes sociability, high approach, and high levels of empathy combined with oversensitivity and anxiety. Although no specific gene has yet been related to this profile or its components, neuroimaging findings demonstrate brain alterations that are likely to underlie the findings of both indiscriminate approach and specific phobia: Structural MRI findings for individuals with WS and normal IQ indicate an area of reduced gray matter in the OFC that, based on fMRI findings, leads to dysregulation of the amygdala.

Continued neuroimaging and behavioral studies of both individuals with the classic deletion and individuals with well-characterized smaller deletions in the WS region are critical for further characterization of genotype–phenotype relations, which are informative not only about WS but about the role played by the genes deleted in WS in normal development. Recently, the first cases of duplication of the WS region were identified (see review in Osborne & Mervis, 2007). The major phenotypic characteristic associated with the duplication is severe expressive speech delay. Neuroimaging, genetic, and behavioral studies contrasting individuals with deletions and duplications will also allow for further understanding of the roles played by the genes in the WS region, in transaction with genes outside the deleted region and with the environment, in human development.

Continued behavioral studies of children with classic deletions are also important, especially longitudinal studies incorporating both experimental and observational paradigms designed to clarify the subtleties of the cognitive and personality profiles associated with WS. Developmental computational models (e.g., connectionist models) of cognition, behavior, personality, and brain development would also be helpful (see Thomas & Karmiloff-Smith, 2003, for an example). Finally, carefully designed treatment studies addressing both behavioral and psychopharmacological therapies for ADHD, anxiety, mastery motivation, and improvement of social skills are critical. These studies have the potential not only to increase scientific understanding of development, but also to make a critical difference in the lives of children with WS and their families.

ACKNOWLEDGMENTS

Preparation of this chapter was supported by Grant No. R37 HD29957 from the National Institute of Child Health and Human Development and Grant No. R01 NS35102 from the National Institute of Neurological Disorders and Stroke. We thank the individuals and their families whose participation in research has made progress in understanding ID possible.

REFERENCES

Achenbach, T. M. (1991). *Child Behavior Checklist/4–18*. Burlington: University of Vermont, Department of Psychiatry.

Adolphs, R. (2003). Cognitive neuroscience of human social behavior. *Nature Reviews Neuroscience, 4,* 165–178.

American Psychiatric Association. (2000). *Diagnostic and statistical manual of mental disorders* (4th ed., text rev.). Washington, DC: Author.

American Psychological Association. (1996). Definition of mental retardation. In J. W. Jacobson & J. D. Mulick (Eds.), *Manual of diagnosis and professional practice in mental retardation* (pp. 13–54). Washington, DC: American Psychological Association.

Atkinson, J., Braddick, O., Anker, S., Curran, W., Andrew, R., Wattam-Bell, J., et al. (2003). Neurobiological models of visuospatial cognition in children with Williams syndrome: Measures for dorsal-stream and frontal function. *Developmental Neuropsychology, 23,* 139–172.

Backes, M., Genc, B., Schreck, J., Doerfler, W., Lehmkuhl, G., & von Gontard, A. (2000). Cognitive and behavioral profile of fragile X boys: Correlations to molecular data. *American Journal of Medical Genetics, 95,* 150–156.

Batshaw, M. L., Shapiro, B., & Farber, M. L. Z. (2007). Developmental delay and intellectual disability. In M. L. Batshaw, L. Pellegrino, & N. J. Roizen (Eds.), *Children with disabilities* (6th ed., pp. 245–261). Baltimore: Brookes.

Beery, K. M. (1989). *The Beery–Buktenica Developmental Test of Visual–Motor Integration* (3rd ed.). Parsippany, NJ: Modern Curriculum Press.

Bellugi, U., Adolphs, R., Cassady, C., & Chiles, M. (1999). Towards the neural basis for hypersociability in a genetic syndrome. *NeuroReport, 10,* 1653–1657.

Bellugi, U., Lichtenberger, L., Jones, W., Lai, Z., & St. George, M. (2000). The neurocognitive profile of Williams syndrome: A complex pattern of strengths and weaknesses. *Journal of Cognitive Neuroscience, 12*(Suppl. 1), 7–29.

Bellugi, U., Marks, S., Bihrle, A., & Sabo, H. (1988). Dissociation between language and cognitive functions in Williams syndrome. In D. Bishop & K. Mogford (Eds.), *Language development in exceptional circumstances* (pp. 177–189). London: Churchill Livingstone.

Bertrand, J., & Mervis, C. B. (1996). Longitudinal analysis of drawings by children with Williams syndrome: Preliminary results. *Visual Arts Research, 22,* 19–34.

Bertrand, J., Mervis, C. B., & Eisenberg, J. D. (1997). Drawing by children with Williams syndrome: A developmental perspective. *Developmental Neuropsychology, 13,* 41–67.

Binet, A., & Simon, T. (1911). *A method of measuring the development of the intelligence of young children.* Lincoln, IL: Courier.

Brock, J. (2007). Language abilities in Williams syndrome: A critical review. *Developmental Psychopathology, 19,* 97–127.

Bruininks, R. H., Woodcock, R. W., Weatherman, R. F., & Hill, B. K. (1996). *Scales of Independent Behavior—Revised.* Itasca, IL: Riverside.

Burack, J. A., Hodapp, R. M., & Zigler, E. (Eds.). (1998). *Handbook of mental retardation and development.* Cambridge, UK: Cambridge University Press.

Cicchetti D., & Pogge-Hesse, P. (1982). Possible contributions of the study of organically retarded persons to developmental theory. In E. Zigler & D. Balla (Eds.), *Mental retardation: The developmental-difference controversy* (pp. 277–318). Hillsdale, NJ: Erlbaum.

Clahsen, H., & Almazan, M. (1998). Syntax and morphology in Williams syndrome. *Cognition, 68,* 167–198.

Cornish, K. M., Levitas, A., & Sudhalter, V. (2007). Fragile X syndrome: Journey from genes to behavior. In M. M. Mazzocco & J. L. Ross (Eds.), *Neurogenetic developmental disorders: Variation of manifestation in childhood* (pp. 73–103). Cambridge, MA: MIT Press.

Davies, M., Udwin, O., & Howlin, P. (1998). Adults with Williams syndrome: Preliminary study of social, emotional, and behavioral difficulties. *British Journal of Psychiatry, 172,* 273–276.

Dekker, M. C., & Koot, H. M. (2003). DSM-IV disorders in children with borderline to moderate intellectual disability: I. Prevalence and impact. *Journal of the American Academy of Child and Adolescent Psychiatry, 42,* 915–922.

Devenny, D. A., Krinsky-McHale, S. J., Kittler, P. M., Flory, M., Jenkins, E., & Brown, W. T. (2004). Age-associated memory changes in adults with Williams syndrome. *Developmental Neuropsychology, 26,* 691–706.

Dilts, C., Morris, C. A., & Leonard, C. O. L. (1990). A hypothesis for the development of a behavioral phenotype in Williams syndrome. *American Journal of Medical Genetics Supplement, 6,* 126–131.

Doyle, T. F., Bellugi, U., Korenberg, J. R., & Graham, J. (2004). "Everybody in the world is my friend": Hypersociability in young children with Williams syndrome. *American Journal of Medical Genetics, 124A,* 263–273.

Dunn, L. E., & Dunn, L. E. (1997). *Peabody Picture Vocabulary Test* (3rd ed.). Circle Pines, MN: American Guidance Service.

Eckert, M. A., Hu, D., Eliez, S., Bellugi, U., Galaburda, A., Korenberg, J., et al. (2005). Evidence for superior parietal impairment in Williams syndrome. *Neurology, 64,* 152–153.

Edgin, J. O. (2003). A neuropsychological model for the development of the cognitive profiles in mental retardation syndromes: Evidence from Down syndrome and Williams syndrome. *Dissertation Abstracts International, 64*(3), 1522B.

Edmonston, N. K., & Litchfield Thane, N. (1988). *TRC: Test of Relational Concepts*. Austin, TX: PRO-ED.

Einfeld, S. L., & Tonge, B. J. (1995). The Developmental Behavior Checklist: The development and validation of an instrument to assess behavioral and emotional disturbance in children and adolescents with mental retardation. *Journal of Autism and Developmental Disorders, 25*, 81–104.

Einfeld, S. L., Tonge, B. J., & Florio, T. (1997). Behavioral and emotional disturbance in individuals with Williams syndrome. *American Journal on Mental Retardation, 102*, 45–53.

Elliott, C. D. (1990). *Differential Ability Scales*. San Antonio, TX: Psychological Corporation.

Elliott, C. D. (2007). *Differential Ability Scales–II*. San Antonio, TX: Harcourt Assessment.

Emerson, E. (2003). Prevalence of psychiatric disorders in children and adolescents with and without intellectual disability. *Journal of Intellectual Disability Research, 47*, 51–58.

Farran, E. K., & Jarrold, C. (2003). Visuospatial cognition in Williams syndrome: Reviewing and accounting for the strengths and weaknesses in performance. *Developmental Neuropsychology, 23*, 173–200.

Fidler, D. J., Hodapp, R. M., & Dykens, E. M. (2000). Stress in families of young children with Down syndrome, Williams syndrome, and Smith–Magenis syndrome. *Early Education and Development, 11*, 395–406.

Fidler, D. J., Hodapp, R. M., & Dykens, E. M. (2002). Behavioral phenotypes and special education: Parent report of educational issues for children with Down syndrome, Prader–Willi syndrome, and Williams syndrome. *Journal of Special Education, 36*, 80–88.

Fidler, D. J., & Nadel, L. (2007). Education and children with Down syndrome: Neuroscience, development, and intervention. *Mental Retardation and Developmental Disabilities Research Reviews, 13*, 262–271.

Frangiskakis, J. M., Ewart, A. K., Morris, C. A., Mervis, C. B., Bertrand, J., Robinson, B. F., et al. (1996). LIM-kinase 1 hemizygosity implicated in impaired visuospatial constructive cognition. *Cell, 86*, 59–69.

Frigerio, E., Burt, D., Gagliardi, C., Cioffi, G., Martelli, S., Perrett, D., et al. (2006). Is everybody always my friend?: Perception of approachability in Williams syndrome. *Neuropsychologia, 44*, 254–259.

Gosch, A., & Pankau, R. (1994). Social-emotional and behavioral adjustment in children with Williams–Beuren syndrome. *American Journal of Medical Genetics, 53*, 335–339.

Gosch, A., Städing, G., & Pankau, R. (1994). Linguistic abilities in children with Williams–Beuren syndrome. *American Journal of Medical Genetics, 52*, 291–296.

Grant, J., Karmiloff-Smith, A., Gathercole, S. A., Paterson, S., Howlin, P., Davies, M., et al. (1997). Phonological short-term memory and its relationship to language in Williams syndrome. *Cognitive Neuropsychiatry, 2*, 81–99.

Greer, M. K., Brown, R. R., Pai, G. S., Choudry, S. H., & Klein, A. J. (1997). Cognitive, adaptive, and behavioral characteristics of Williams syndrome. *American Journal of Medical Genetics: Part B. Neuropsychiatric Genetics, 74*, 521–525.

Hagerman, R. J. (2002). The physical and behavioral phenotype. In R. J. Hagerman & P. J. Hagerman (Eds.), *Fragile X syndrome: Diagnosis, treatment, and research* (pp. 3–109). Baltimore: Johns Hopkins University Press.

Hillier, L. W., Fulton, R. S., Fulton, L. A., Graves, T. A., Pepin, K. H., Wagner-McPherson, C., et al. (2003). The DNA sequence of chromosome 7. *Nature, 424*, 157–164.

Hodapp, R. M., & Burack, J. A. (1990). What mental retardation tells us about typical development: The examples of sequences, rates, and cross-domain relations. *Development and Psychopathology, 2*, 213–225.

Hoffman, J. E., Landau, B., & Pagani, B. (2003). Spatial breakdown in spatial construction: Evidence from eye fixations in children with Williams syndrome. *Cognitive Psychology, 46*, 260–301.

Jarrold, C., Baddeley, A. D., & Hewes, A. K. (1998). Verbal and nonverbal abilities in the Williams syndrome phenotype: Evidence for diverging developmental trajectories. *Journal of Child Psychology and Psychiatry, 39,* 511–523.

Jarrold, C., Baddeley, A. D., & Hewes, A. K. (1999). Genetically dissociated components of working memory: Evidence from Down's and Williams syndrome. *Neuropsychologia, 37,* 637–651.

Jarrold, C., Baddeley, A. D., Hewes, A. K., & Phillips, C. (2001). A longitudinal assessment of diverging verbal and non-verbal abilities in the Williams syndrome phenotype. *Cortex, 37,* 423–431.

Jordan, H., Reiss, J. E., Hoffman, J. E., & Landau, B. (2002). Intact perception of biological motion in the face of profound spatial deficits: Williams syndrome. *Psychological Science, 13,* 162–167.

Karmiloff-Smith, A. (2007). Atypical epigenesis. *Developmental Science, 10,* 84–88.

Karmiloff-Smith, A., Grant, J., Berthoud, I., Davies, M., Howlin, P., & Udwin, O. (1997). Language and Williams syndrome: How intact is "intact"? *Child Development, 68,* 246–262.

King, B. H., Hodapp, R. M., & Dykens, E. M. (2005). Mental retardation. In H. I. Kaplan & B. J. Sadock (Eds.), *Comprehensive textbook of psychiatry* (8th ed., Vol. 2, pp. 3076–3106). Baltimore: Williams & Wilkins.

Klein, B. P., & Mervis, C. B. (1999). Cognitive strengths and weaknesses of 9- and 10-year-olds with Williams syndrome or Down syndrome. *Developmental Neuropsychology, 16,* 177–196.

Klein-Tasman, B. P., & Mervis, C. B. (2003). Distinctive personality characteristics of 8-, 9-, and 10-year-old children with Williams syndrome. *Developmental Neuropsychology, 23,* 271–292.

Klein-Tasman, B. P., Mervis, C. B., Lord, C., & Phillips, K. D. (2007). Socio-communicative deficits in young children with Williams syndrome: Performance on the Autism Diagnostic Observation Schedule. *Child Neuropsychology, 13,* 444–467.

Laing, E., Butterworth, G., Ansari, D., Gsödl, M., Longhi, E., Panagiotaki, G., et al. (2002). Atypical development of language and social communication in toddlers with Williams syndrome. *Developmental Science, 5,* 233–246.

Landau, B., Hoffman, J. E., & Kurz, N. (2006). Object recognition with severe spatial deficits in Williams syndrome: Sparing and breakdown. *Cognition, 100,* 483–510.

Laws, G., & Bishop, D. V. M. (2004). Pragmatic language impairment and social deficits in Williams syndrome: A comparison with Down's syndrome and specific language impairment. *International Journal of Language and Communication Disorders, 39,* 45–64.

Leonard, H., & Wen, X. (2002). The epidemiology of mental retardation: Challenges and opportunities in the new millennium. *Mental Retardation and Developmental Disabilities Research Reviews, 8,* 117–134.

Levy, Y., & Hermon, S. (2003). Morphological abilities in Hebrew-speaking adolescents with Williams syndrome. *Developmental Neuropsychology, 23,* 59–83.

Leyfer, O. T., Woodruff-Borden, J., Klein-Tasman, B. P., Fricke, J. S., & Mervis, C. B. (2006). Prevalence of psychiatric disorders in 4 to 16-year-olds with Williams syndrome. *American Journal of Medical Genetics: Part B. Neuropsychiatric Genetics, 141B,* 615–622.

Leyfer, O., Woodruff-Borden, J., & Mervis, C. B. (2009). Anxiety disorders in children with Williams syndrome, their mothers, and their siblings: Implications for the etiology of anxiety disorders. *Journal of Neurodevelopmental Disorders, 1,* 4–14.

Lord, C., Risi, S., Lambrecht, L., Cook, E., Leventhal, B., DiValore, P., et al. (2000). The Autism Diagnostic Observation Schedule—Generic: A standard measure of social and communication deficits associated with the spectrum of autism. *Journal of Autism and Developmental Disorders, 30,* 205–223.

Luckasson, R., Borthwick-Duffy, S., Buntinx, W. H. E., Coulter, D. L., Craig, E. M., Reeve, A., et al. (2002). *Mental retardation: Definition, classification, and system of supports* (10th ed.). Washington, DC: American Association on Mental Retardation.

Lukács, Á. (2005). *Language abilities in Williams syndrome.* Budapest, Hungary: Akadémiai Kiadó.

Lukács, Á., Racsmány, M., & Pléh, C. (2001). Vocabulary and morphological patterns in Hungarian children with Williams syndrome: A preliminary report. *Acta Linguistica Hungarica, 48,* 243–269.

Mackintosh, N. J. (1998). *IQ and human intelligence.* Oxford: Oxford University Press.

Marenco, S., Siuta, M. A., Kippenhan, J. S., Grodofsky, S., Chang, W.-L., Kohn, P., et al. Genetic contributions to white matter architecture revealed by diffusion tensor imaging in Williams syndrome. *Proceedings of the National Academy of Sciences USA, 104,* 15117–15122.

Masataka, N. (2001). Why early linguistic milestones are delayed in children with Williams syndrome: Late onset of hand banging as a possible rate-limiting constraint on the emergence of canonical babbling. *Developmental Science, 4,* 158–164.

McDermott, S., Durkin, M. S., Schupf, N., & Stein, Z. A. (2007). Epidemiology and etiology of mental retardation. In J. W. Jacobson, J. A. Mulick, & J. Rojann (Eds.), *Handbook of intellectual and developmental disabilities* (pp. 3–40). New York: Springer.

Mervis, C. B. (2006). Language abilities in Williams–Beuren syndrome. In C. A. Morris, H. M. Lenhoff, & P. P. Wang (Eds.), *Williams–Beuren syndrome: Research, evaluation, and treatment* (pp. 159–206). Baltimore, MD: Johns Hopkins University Press.

Mervis, C. B. (2008). Unpublished data.

Mervis, C. B. (2009). Language and literacy development of children with Williams syndrome. *Topics in Language Disorders, 29,* 149–169.

Mervis, C. B., & Becerra, A. M. (2007). Language and communicative development in Williams syndrome. *Mental Retardation and Developmental Disabilities Research Reviews, 13,* 3–15.

Mervis, C. B., & Bertrand, J. (1997). Developmental relations between cognition and language: Evidence from Williams syndrome. In L. B. Adamson & M. A. Romski (Eds.), *Communication and language acquisition: Discoveries from atypical development* (pp. 75–106). Baltimore: Brookes.

Mervis, C. B., & John, A. E. (2008). Vocabulary abilities of children with Williams syndrome: Strengths, weaknesses, and relation to visuospatial construction. *Journal of Speech, Language, and Hearing Research, 51,* 967–982.

Mervis, C. B., Klein-Tasman, B. P., & Mastin, M. E. (2001). Adaptive behavior of 4- through 8- year old children with Williams syndrome. *American Journal on Mental Retardation, 106,* 82–93.

Mervis, C. B., & Morris, C. A. (2007). Williams syndrome. In M. M. Mazzocco & J. L. Ross (Eds.), *Neurogenetic developmental disorders: Variation of manifestation in childhood* (pp. 199–262). Cambridge, MA: MIT Press.

Mervis, C. B., Morris, C. A., Klein-Tasman, B. P., Bertrand, J., Kwitny, S., Appelbaum, L. G., et al. (2003). Attentional characteristics of infants and toddlers with Williams syndrome during triadic interactions. *Developmental Neuropsychology, 23,* 245–270.

Mervis, C. B., & Robinson, B. F. (1999). Methodological issues in cross-syndrome comparisons: Matching procedures, sensitivity (*Se*), and specificity (*Sp*). [Commentary on M. Sigman & E. Ruskin, Continuity and change in the social competence of children with autism, Down syndrome, and developmental delays.] *Monographs of the Society for Research in Child Development, 64*(1, Serial No. 256), 115–130.

Mervis, C. B., & Robinson, B. F. (2005). Designing measures for profiling and genotype/phenotype studies of individuals with genetic syndromes or developmental language disorders. *Applied Psycholinguistics, 26,* 41–64.

Mervis, C. B., Robinson, B. F., Bertrand, J., Morris, C. A., Klein-Tasman, B. P., & Armstrong, S. C. (2000). The Williams syndrome cognitive profile. *Brain and Cognition, 44,* 604–628.

Meyer-Lindenberg, A., Hariri, A. R., Munoz, K E., Mervis, C. B., Mattay, V. S., Morris, C. A., et al. (2005a). Neural correlates of genetically abnormal social cognition in Williams syndrome. *Nature Neuroscience, 8,* 991–993.

Meyer-Lindenberg, A., Kohn, P., Mervis, C. B., Kippenhan, J. S., Olsen, R., Morris, C. A., et al. (2004). Neural basis of genetically determined visuospatial construction deficit in Williams syndrome. *Neuron, 43,* 623–631.

Meyer-Lindenberg, A., Mervis, C. B., & Berman, K. F. (2006). Neural mechanisms in Williams syndrome: A unique window to genetic influences on cognition and behavior. *Nature Reviews Neuroscience, 7,* 380–393.

Meyer-Lindenberg, A., Mervis, C. B., Sarpal, D., Koch, P., Steele, S., Kohn, P., et al. (2005b). Functional, structural, and metabolic abnormalities of the hippocampal formation in Williams syndrome. *Journal of Clinical Investigations, 115,* 1888–1895.

Morris, C. A. (2006). The dysmorphology, genetics, and natural history of Williams–Beuren syndrome. In C. A. Morris, H. M., Lenhoff, & P. P. Wang (Eds.), *Williams–Beuren syndrome: Research, evaluation, and treatment* (pp. 3–17). Baltimore: Johns Hopkins University Press.

Morris, C. A., Mervis, C. B., Hobart, H. H., Gregg, R. G., Bertrand, J., Ensing, G. J., et al. (2003). *GTF2I* hemizygosity implicated in mental retardation in Williams syndrome: Genotype–phenotype analysis of 5 families with deletions in the Williams syndrome region. *American Journal of Medical Genetics: Part A, 123,* 45–59.

Mullen, E. M. (1995). *Mullen Scales of Early Learning.* Circle Pines, MN: American Guidance Service.

Myers, B. A., & Pueschel, S. M. (1991). Psychiatric disorders in persons with Down syndrome. *Journal of Nervous and Mental Disease, 179,* 609–613.

Neisser, U., Boodoo, G., Bouchard, T. J., Boykin, A. W., Brody, N., Ceci, S. J., et al. (1996). Intelligence: Knowns and unknowns. *American Psychologist, 51,* 77–101.

Nichols, S., Jones, W., Roman, M. J., Wulfeck, B., Delis, D. C., Reilly, J., et al. (2004). Mechanisms of verbal memory impairment in four neurodevelopmental disorders. *Brain and Language, 88,* 180–189.

O'Hearn, K., Landau, B., & Hoffman, J. E. (2005). Multiple object tracking in people with Williams syndrome and in normally developing children. *Psychological Science, 16,* 905–912.

Osborne, L. R., & Mervis, C. B. (2007). Rearrangements of the Williams–Beuren syndrome locus: molecular basis and implications for speech and language development. *Expert Reviews in Molecular Medicine, 9*(15), 1–16.

Pani, J. R., Mervis, C. B., & Robinson, B. F. (1999). Global spatial organization by individuals with Williams syndrome. *Psychological Science, 10,* 453–458.

Paterson, S. (2001). Language and number in Down syndrome: The complex trajectory from infancy to adulthood. *Down Syndrome Research and Practice, 7,* 79–86.

Paterson, S., Brown, J. H., Gsödl, M. K., Johnson, M. H., & Karmiloff-Smith, A. (1999). Cognitive modularity and genetic disorders. *Science, 286*(5448), 2355–2358.

Paul, B. M., Stiles, J., Passarotti, A., Bavar, N., & Bellugi, U. (2002). Face and place processing in Williams syndrome: Evidence for a dorsal–ventral dissociation. *NeuroReport, 13,* 1115–1119.

Philofsky, A., Fidler, D. J., & Hepburn, S. (2007). Pragmatic language profiles of school-age children with autism spectrum disorders and Williams syndrome. *American Journal of Speech and Language Pathology, 16,* 368–380.

Pléh, C., Lukács, A., & Racsmány, M. (2002). Morphological patterns in Hungarian children with Williams syndrome and the rule debates. *Brain and Language, 86,* 377–383.

Plesa-Skwerer, D., & Tager-Flusberg, H. (2006). Social cognition in Williams–Beuren syndrome. In C. A. Morris , H. M. Lenhoff, & P. P. Wang (Eds.), *Williams–Beuren syndrome: Research, evaluation, and treatment* (pp. 237–253). Baltimore: Johns Hopkins University Press.

Reiss, A. L., Eckert, M., Rose, F. E., Karchemskiy, A., Kesler, S., Chang, M., et al. (2004). An experiment of nature: Brain anatomy parallels cognition and behaviour in Williams syndrome. *Journal of Neuroscience, 24,* 5009–5015.

Reiss, A. L., Eliez, S., Schmitt, E., Straus, E., Lai, Z., Jones, W., et al. (2000). Neuroanatomy of Williams syndrome: A high-resolution MRI study. *Journal of Cognitive Neuroscience, 12*(Suppl. 1), 65–73.

Robinson, B. F., Mervis, C. B., & Robinson, B. W. (2003). Roles of verbal short-term memory and working memory in the acquisition of grammar by children with Williams syndrome. *Developmental Neuropsychology, 23,* 13–31.

Rothbart, M. K., & Ahadi, S. A. (1994). Temperament and the development of personality. *Journal of Abnormal Psychology, 103,* 55–66.

Rowe, M. L., & Mervis, C. B. (2006). Working memory in Williams syndrome. In T. P. Alloway & S. E. Gathercole (Eds.), *Working memory and neurodevelopmental disorders* (pp. 267–293). Hove, UK: Psychology Press.

Shelley, B. P., & Robertson, M. M. (2005). The neuropsychiatry and multisystem features of the Smith–Magenis syndrome: A review. *Journal of Neuropsychiatry and Clinical Neurosciences, 17,* 91–97.

Silverman, W. (2007). Down syndrome: Cognitive phenotype. *Mental Retardation and Developmental Disabilities Research Reviews, 13,* 228–236.

Silverman, W. K., & Albano, A. M. (1996). *The Anxiety Disorders Interview Schedule for DSM-IV: Parent interview schedule.* San Antonio, TX: Graywind.

Sparrow, S. S., Balla, D. A., & Cicchetti, D. V. (1984). *Vineland Adaptive Behavior Scales—Interview Edition.* Circle Pines, MN: American Guidance Service.

Sternberg, R. J. (Ed.). (2004). *International handbook of intelligence.* New York: Cambridge University Press.

Stock, A. D., Spallone, P. A., Dennis, T. R., Netski, D., Morris, C. A., Mervis, C. B., et al. (2003). Heat shock protein 27 gene: Chromosomal and molecular location and relationship to Williams syndrome. *American Journal of Medical Genetics: Part A, 120,* 320–325.

Stojanovik, V. (2006). Social interaction deficits and conversational inadequacy in Williams syndrome. *Journal of Neurolinguistics, 19,* 157–173.

Strømme, P., Bjørnstad, P. G., & Ramstad, K. (2002). Prevalence estimation of Williams syndrome. *Journal of Childhood Neuropsychology, 17,* 269–271.

Sullivan, K., Winner, E., & Tager-Flusberg, T. (2003). Can adolescents with Williams syndrome tell the difference between lies and jokes? *Developmental Neuropsychology, 23,* 85–104.

Tassabehji, M., Metcalfe, K., Karmiloff-Smith, A., Carette, M. J., Grant, J., Dennis, N. et al. (1999). Williams syndrome: Use of chromosomal microdeletions as a tool to dissect cognitive and physical phenotypes. *American Journal of Human Genetics, 64,* 118–125.

Tellegen, A. (1985). Structures of mood and personality and their relevance to assessing anxiety, with an emphasis on self-report. In A. H. Tuma & J. Maser (Eds.), *Anxiety and the anxiety disorders* (pp. 681–706). Hillsdale, NJ: Erlbaum.

Thomas, A., & Chess, S. (1977). *Temperament and development.* New York: Brunner/Mazel.

Thomas, M. L., Becerra, A. M., & Mervis, C. B. (2002, July). *Empathic behavior of 4-year-olds with Williams syndrome, other forms of developmental delay, or typical development.* Paper presented at the International Professional Meeting of the Williams Syndrome Association, Long Beach, CA.

Thomas, M. S. C., & Karmiloff-Smith, A. (2003). Modeling language acquisition in atypical phenotypes. *Psychological Review, 110,* 647–682.

Tomc, S. A., Williamson, N. K., & Pauli, R. M. (1990). Temperament in Williams syndrome. *American Journal of Medical Genetics, 36,* 345–352.

Tonge, B. J., & Einfeld, S. L. (2003). Psychopathology and intellectual disability: The Australian Child to Adult Longitudinal Study. *International Review of Research in Mental Retardation, 26,* 61–91.

Udwin, O., & Yule, W. (1990). Expressive language of children with Williams syndrome. *American Journal of Medical Genetics Supplement, 6,* 108–114.

Udwin, O., & Yule, W. (1991). A cognitive and behavioral phenotype in Williams syndrome. *Journal of Clinical and Experimental Neuropsychology, 13,* 232–244.

Vicari, S., Bellucci, S., & Carlesimo, G. A. (2005). Visual and spatial long-term memory: Differential pattern of impairments in Williams and Down syndromes. *Developmental Medicine and Child Neurology, 47,* 305–311.

Volterra, V., Capirci, O., Pezzini, G., Sabbadini, L., & Vicari, S. (1996). Linguistic abilities in Italian children with Williams syndrome. *Cortex, 32,* 663–677.

von Arnim, G., & Engel, P. (1964). Mental retardation related to hypercalcaemia. *Developmental Medicine and Child Neurology, 6,* 366–377.

Wang, P. P., & Bellugi, U. (1994). Evidence from two genetic syndromes for a dissociation between verbal and visual–spatial short term memory. *Journal of Clinical and Experimental Neuropsychology, 16,* 317–322.

Wang, P. P., Hesselink, J. R., Jernigan, T. L., Doherty, S., & Bellugi, U. (1992). Specific neurobehavioral profile of Williams syndrome is associated with neocerebellar hemispheric preservation. *Neurology, 42,* 1999–2002.

Wesman, A. G. (1968). Intelligent testing. *American Psychologist, 23,* 267–274.

Winnepenninckx, B., Rooms, L., & Kooy, R. F. (2003). Mental retardation: A review of the genetic causes. *British Journal of Developmental Disabilities, 96,* 29–44.

World Health Organization (WHO). (1996). *Multiaxial classification of child and adolescent psychiatric disorders: The ICD-10 classification of mental and behavioral disorders in children and adolescents.* Cambridge, UK: Cambridge University Press.

Zigler, E. (1967). Familial mental retardation: A continuing dilemma. *Science, 155,* 292–298.

Zigler, E., & Balla, D. (Eds.). (1982). *Mental retardation: The developmental-difference controversy.* Hillsdale, NJ: Erlbaum.

Zitzer-Comfort, C., Doyle, T., Masataka, N., Korenberg, J., & Bellugi, U. (2007). Nature and nurture: Williams syndrome across cultures. *Developmental Science, 10,* 755–762.

Zukowski, A. (2004). Investigating knowledge of complex syntax: Insights from experimental studies of Williams syndrome. In M. Rice & S. Warren (Eds.), *Developmental language disorders: From phenotypes to etiologies* (pp. 99–119). Cambridge: MIT Press.

PART III

CLINICAL ASSESSMENT AND INTERVENTION

CHAPTER 17

Maxims and a Model for the Practice of Pediatric Neuropsychology

IDA SUE BARON

The goal of conducting a thorough and informative pediatric neuropsychological evaluation may seem like a straightforward objective, but the means to that end are quite involved. A hierarchy of steps must be taken; these include *testing*, the administration of specially designed and standardized tools to measure specific functions or behaviors; *assessment*, a broader process that includes data acquisition from a wide range of sources (history taking) to supplement direct testing and support case formulation; and *evaluation*, the principal summary process that incorporates all preliminary steps, leading to well-formulated conclusions and recommendations for management or treatment. Practitioners who fail to recognize the complexity of pediatric neuropsychological evaluation are likely to encounter significant obstacles that reduce the efficacy of their well-meaning efforts, and may even do harm to patients and their families. This chapter briefly reviews the decades of progress made in neuropsychological practice, presents a summary of applicable maxims that highlight what is unique about pediatric neuropsychological practice, and concludes with thoughts about future directions and continuing challenges.

PROGRESS IN PEDIATRIC NEUROPSYCHOLOGY: A BRIEF REVIEW

The term *neuropsychology* refers to the science concerned with explicating brain–behavior relationships. The profession of clinical neuropsychology was established as a distinctive discipline in the 1950s (Benton, 2000) and was recognized by the American Psychological Association as a specialty area in 1996 (see Barr, 2008, for a review of the historical development of the neuropsychological test battery). Pediatric neuropsychologists have long represented a small subset of all neuropsychologists, but their numbers and influence are rapidly increasing, in parallel with the substantial progress made by the profession over several decades of rapid growth. Despite early concerns that the value of a pediatric clinical neuropsychological evaluation would be underappreciated with the advent of medical and neuroradiological advances, there has been ever-increasing recognition that pediatric neuropsychologists are proficient in a broad range of evaluation, treatment, and research roles that have direct applicability to current patient needs. Pediatric neuropsychologists participate actively in diverse clinical, scientific, educational, academic, and corporate arenas (Baron, 2007b), and make appreciable contributions toward the care, evaluation, and treatment of infants, children, and adolescents with diverse medical and psychological conditions (Anderson, Northam, Hendy, & Wrennall, 2001; Baron, Fennell, & Voeller, 1995; Yeates, Ris, & Taylor, 2000).

Along with the expansion of pediatric neuropsychological services has come more sophisticated methodology for evaluating brain structure–function relationships. These advances support and reinforce the many unique contributions pediatric neuropsychologists make to the evaluation of cerebral function or dysfunction in the dynamically developing organism, and pediatric neuropsychological practice reflects these gains in numerous ways. For example, there has been greater application of experimental techniques and technical advances from allied disciplines in clinical practice, such as those that enable identification of the genetic/molecular bases of developmental disorders and neuroradiological studies of both normal and abnormal populations. These have aided parsing of broad behavioral domains into more discrete subcomponent capacities, and have led to more refined subtype analyses with direct treatment implications. The combined progress achieved across disciplines has also led to more effective means of evaluating and treating not only especially common referral problems—such as learning disabilities (Fletcher, Lyon, Fuchs, & Barnes, 2007) and attention-deficit/hyperactivity disorder (ADHD) (Barkley, 2006; Pennington, 2005) (see Stefanatos & Baron, 2007, for a critical review of obstacles and dilemmas related to ADHD diagnosis)—but many less prevalent central nervous system disorders that now routinely come to the pediatric neuropsychologist's attention. Neuropsychological methods are also employed to elucidate a child's adaptive or preserved functions, and they are increasingly relied on in the design, implementation, and evaluation of interventional strategies that not only aim to ameliorate dysfunction but place an emphasis on using these residual strengths to best advantage. Furthermore, pediatric neuropsychologists more often participate in outcome research, examining the long-term effects of diverse conditions, their clinical course, and their treatments. Thus the pediatric neuropsychologist's initial role as a provider of standardized psychological test results for children primarily experiencing neurological or psychiatric dysfunction has evolved substantially to encompass an ever-expanding range of activities and influence in clinical practice and research investigation (Yeates et al., 2000).

Reflecting this growth, the related literature has expanded exponentially. Journals and textbooks dedicated to the interests of pediatric neuropsychologists have proliferated. Among recent volumes are several focused on specific interests of pediatric practitioners, such as normal brain development (Stiles, 2008), neurobehavioral consequences of early brain disorders (Broman & Fletcher, 1999), early development of psychiatric disorders (Pennington, 2002), learning disabilities (Fletcher et al., 2007), developmental motor disorders (Dewey & Tupper, 2004), pediatric neuropsychological intervention (Hunter & Donders, 2007), and treatment of neurodevelopmental disorders (Farmer, Donders, & Warschausky, 2006). More frequent articulation of pediatric-specific neuropsychological models and emphasis on theory-driven investigation have been additional indicators of the substantial progress occurring in pediatric neuropsychology (Baron, 2007; Cooley & Morris, 1990; Denckla, 1973; Fletcher & Taylor, 1984; Dennis, Landry, Barnes, & Fletcher, 2006a; Rourke, 1989; Taylor & Schatschneider, 1992; Wilson, 1992; Wilson & Finucci, 1986). All these developments encourage diminished reliance on adult models (Bernstein & Waber, 1990; Fennell & Bauer, 1997) and greater appreciation for the unique aspects of pediatric practice.

FIVE MAXIMS OF PEDIATRIC NEUROPSYCHOLOGICAL PRACTICE

Central to responsible pediatric neuropsychological practice is the recognition that the field depends on foundational skills from broader disciplines that preceded the emergence of this specialty area (e.g., clinical psychology, abnormal psychology, and developmental psychology), and that an ability to appreciate complex developmental and maturational factors is a core capacity. Important commonalities exist between adult and pediatric neuropsychological practice, but unique features arise in child evaluation that rarely occur in adult practice. Most of these are directly related to the complexities encountered in attempting to evaluate the integrity of an actively maturing young brain progressing toward its eventual adult arrangement of distributed neural networks or functional neural circuitry. Several of these distinctive differences from adult neuropsychological practice may be regarded as maxims of pediatric neuropsychological practice.

Maxim 1. *Maturation is a paramount force in pediatric neuropsychology.*

The dynamic developmental course of brain maturation is *the* major influence in pediatric neuropsychological practice and research. A practitioner's fundamental tasks are to identify the range and magnitude of behavioral effects related to integrity or disruption of brain maturation, and to clarify those capacities that are preserved or unaffected. Although brain maturation is expected to progress through a consistent series of stages in the absence of any direct brain interference due to illness, injury, or neurodevelopmental disorder, the intricacy of the developmental course toward full maturation has become clearer in recent years. This is due in large part to advances in structural and functional imaging that have visualized the trajectory of normal brain development in novel ways. For example, a longitudinal study using magnetic resonance imaging (MRI) has revealed a nonlinear progression of brain development, with white matter volume increases throughout the brain from childhood through adolescence, along with regionally specific inverted-U-shaped trajectories for gray matter volumes (Giedd et al., 2004). In addition, time lapse sequencing from childhood until early adulthood has found that higher-order association cortices mature after lower-order primary somatosensory and visual cortices, and that phylogenetically older brain areas mature earlier than phylogenetically younger brain areas (Gogtay et al., 2004).

Such advances have also begun to clarify neural system variability across chronological ages and at differing maturational stages. For example, whereas adult models have traditionally emphasized the importance of cortical mantle thickness and integrity for preserved intellectual function, pediatric longitudinal research has found that the *trajectory* of developmental change in cerebral cortex mantle thickness is more closely related to intelligence level than actual cortical thickness is (Shaw et al., 2006a). The Shaw et al. (2006a) study found a developmental shift away from a predominantly negative correlation between intelligence and cortical thickness (primarily in frontal regions normally implicated in the maturation of intellectual activity) in early childhood toward a positive correlation in later childhood and at older ages, providing support for a hypothesis of dynamic neuroanatomical expression of intelligence in children. Gender and diagnostic group differences, as well as age differences, have been studied; brain morphometric measures are highly variable across individuals, but with considerable overlap between boys and girls, between typically developing and neuropsychiatric populations, and between young and old individuals (Lenroot & Giedd, 2006). In a study of puberty-related influences on the underlying neuroanatomy of behavioral change for both typically developing children and adolescents, and those with anomalous hormone or sex chromosome profiles, gender differences were found in the trajectories of brain morphometry; girls reached peak gray matter thickness approximately 1–2 years earlier than boys (Giedd et al., 2006). In addition, neuroimaging data are increasingly informative about regional development and behavioral effects. For example, dorsal lateral prefrontal cortex, a brain region with central importance for inhibition and impulse control, is among the last brain regions to mature, reaching adult dimensions in the early 20s (Giedd, 2004). These data have practical implications, as they suggest that a measurable and direct neurobiological link exists between the often turbulent and confusing adolescent years and incomplete brain development.

Imaging advances have also been increasingly applied to the study of children's capacity for recovery. For example, Shaw et al. (2006b) found that children diagnosed with ADHD had global thinning of the cortex, especially in medial and superior prefrontal and precentral regions. Interestingly, those with poorer outcomes also had a thinner left medial prefrontal cortex (a cerebral region implicated in an anterior attentional network) at baseline compared to those who had more optimal outcomes or were controls. Cortical thickness developmental trajectories enabled by the technology revealed a normalization of cortical thickness in the right parietal cortex, but only for the group with better outcomes, whereas thinning of the left medial prefrontal cortex persisted in those who had poorer outcomes (Shaw et al., 2006b).

Overall, such studies have extended our knowledge well beyond what was envisioned in those formative early years of neuropsychological practice and investigation, when only traditional assessment tools were available for examining brain–behavior function, and archaic methods were the only means of viewing brain structure. Together, the simultaneous advances in neuropsychological methodology and neuroradiological technology serve as an important heuristic regarding temporal (early vs. late) cause–effect relationships of central nervous system insult. They have also aided the unraveling of the intricate dynamic developmental course of brain maturation, and reemphasized that maturation is *the* major influence in pediatric neuropsychological practice and research.

Maxim 2. *Adult brain–behavior relationship rules do not invariably apply to children.*

In the not-so-remote history of the profession, the rules promulgated regarding brain–behavior relationships and methods of assessment were endorsed for children if they were useful in adult evaluation. Yet children react to illness or its treatment quite differently than do adults, and applying the teachings of adult neuropsychology to pediatric neuropsychology frequently resulted in a range of bewildering results across the spectrum of childhood injury, disease, and neurodevelopmental disorder. It became increasingly evident that rules developed and based on adult characteristics could not satisfactorily be extended downward to children, and that typical adult behavioral responses to disease or disorder were not appropriate guidelines. This realization was seminal in the extension of pediatric neuropsychological practice methods and interpretive considerations.

The complications inherent in translation of adult practice to child practice become apparent in consideration of etiologies, response to intervention, and interpretive prognostication. Children often experience a different range of causal factors, and may respond in unpredicted ways to diseases or conditions also found in adults. For example, focal neurological injury in childhood may not lead to circumscribed impairment on tests of function subserved by the damaged brain region, as it would for an adult, whose capacity for recovery is more restricted. Enlistment of brain regions for particular functioning appears more variable between adults and children than was previously recognized. For example, contrary to results from studies of decision making in adults with focal lesions of vascular etiology, children who had focal amygdala lesions after traumatic brain injury (TBI), but not those with ventromedial lesions, were found to have impaired performance on a modified gambling task (Hanten et al., 2006). Outcomes after focal or diffuse cerebral disruption, or for acute or chronic disorder, may be expected to differ between adults and children with similar neurological involvement. The potential for impressive functional ability after substantial brain disruption has been dramatically demonstrated by the remarkable preservation of function after major brain region excision (hemispherectomy) in childhood (Holloway et al., 2000; Vargha-Khadem, Carr, Isaacs, & Brett, 1997). That impairment in children may be only transient, or evident later as merely mild neurobehavioral dysfunction or even nearly or fully complete recovery, continues to be a phenomenon of significant heuristic interest across etiological groups; it has been hypothesized to be due to children's capacity for normal developmental processes to remain functional despite serious neural perturbation (Stiles, Reilly, Paul, & Moses, 2005).

Differential treatment effects are also observed, and these highlight the risks inherent in basing prediction for a child on the typical adult course and outcome. For example, contrary to the usual course for adults with Cushing syndrome, whose cognitive impairments often resolve rapidly once treatment corrects hypercortisolism and reverses cerebral atrophy, the intelligence level of children with this syndrome declined significantly and was accompanied by poor school performance 1 year after surgery for glucocorticoid excess (Merke et al., 2005). Differential susceptibility to the immediate effects of fluctuating intracerebral dynamics provides another example of contrasting course. Whereas hydrocephalus in an adult may become evident only after a prolonged course of slow decompensation, followed by postintervention stability or limited recovery, a very young child may demonstrate a rapid and precipitous deterioration of cognitive function, and then more complete and rapid recovery following successful surgical intervention to correct pressure flow dynamics. Results such as these underscore the importance of formulating and offering discrete prognoses for fully mature adults and for children whose brains are actively maturing.

Consequently, it becomes ever clearer that interpretive rules applicable to adults may often be inaccurate if applied to children. For example, finding a significantly poorer nonverbal IQ than verbal IQ has traditionally been interpreted as a likely indication of lateralized right cerebral dysfunction in an adult. Yet children with neurological impairment have a ubiquitous tendency to demonstrate a similar pattern of results. The implication of the discrepancy score may be quite different, although it is sometimes still misinterpreted as indicative of similar lateralized dysfunction. Instead, this common clinical finding in children may be best interpreted as further evidence of the developing brain's compensatory efforts to preserve verbal over nonverbal capacities, as was concluded in a study of preterm infants who had unilateral cerebral lesions (Vollmer et al., 2006).

Nonetheless, in consideration of a full range of neuropsychological knowledge, adult studies, models, and practice remain pertinent to an understanding of brain–behavior relationships in childhood, just as child studies, models, and practice are relevant for understanding adult brain–behavior relationships. As adult investigations of neural networks and of integrated cortical–subcortical pathways are refined, these have also come under scrutiny with respect to their applicability to children. One example of this progression from adult to child studies relates to the emergence of greater understanding about the cerebellar contribution to cognitive and affective function, beyond its well-substantiated importance for motor function. The cerebellum's importance for nonmotor functions in children is now well documented (Akshoomoff, Courchesne, Press, & Iragui, 1992; Diamond, 2000; Lechtenberg & Gilman, 1978; Leiner, Leiner, & Dow, 1986; Riva & Giorgi, 2000; Schmahmann, 1991). Cerebellar maldevelopment may be especially influential with regard to late cognitive and neurodevelopmental disabilities in preterm children (Limperopoulos et al., 2005), for whom long-term cognitive disabilities have been consistently reported (Anderson & Doyle, 2004; Taylor, 2006). Specification of a *cerebellar cognitive affective syndrome* (CCAS) in adults (Schmahmann & Sherman, 1998), and of the functional contributions made by the hemispheric regions of cerebellar posterior lobes (Allen & Courchesne, 2003; Ravizza et al., 2006), preceded questions about how precisely the constellation of executive function, spatial cognition, language processing, and emotional regulation of behavior associated with the CCAS may also relate to functioning at different stages of childhood and consequent to neurological compromise (Levisohn, Cronin-Golomb, & Schmahmann, 2000; Sadeh & Cohen, 2001). Therefore, as demonstrated in this interesting sequence of studies, pediatric neuropsychologists are well advised to remain cognizant of adult studies, and to consider maturational issues related to the clinical populations seen in their practices. The examples above related to etiology, treatment response, and interpretive conclusions underscore the crucial point that children are not appropriately considered solely within the context of existent adult models.

Maxim 3. *A model of normal development provides critical clinical context.*

A solid foundation in normal child development is essential knowledge for pediatric neuropsychologists, who must offer opinions as to whether behavior falls within or outside a normal range relative to a child's chronological age and specific neurobiological, medical, familial, and socioenvironmental circumstances. Without an informed context for "normal," judgments about whether there is evidence of developmentally delayed brain maturation or of deficit due to adverse events will necessarily be constrained. A model of normal development facilitates appropriate consideration of the extremely wide range of influential factors affecting maturational progression. A model also provides a relevant context of practice parameters that may help a practitioner choose measurement instruments, consider diagnostic criteria, and recommend or implement intervention techniques for a maturing child. A helpful model compresses professional experience into a formulation explanatory for behavior at diverse points along the developmental spectrum. It should be instructive regarding the varied influences potentially affecting the neurodevelopmental course. In an effort to construct a dynamic model whose graphic presentation also conveys the potential for rapidity of change and susceptibility to different critical influences at any point over the course of development, I have proposed a maturational model of child neuropsychological development (Baron, 2008). This model, illustrated in Figure 17.1, provides a clinically useful template (see Figure 17.2) for considering the broad range of influences affecting an infant, child, or adolescent over these respective periods of brain growth and development.

This model emphasizes the dynamic evolution of the developing organism. It highlights the primary influence of neurobiological factors, including genetic predisposition, socioenvironmental factors, family factors, and medical variables that simultaneously influence the maturational course. The model includes a series of modules representing the child's capacities at any point in time, and continues along a trajectory from infancy through a series of active stages of growth and development into childhood and adolescence. Each point in time, or module, represents the integration and persistence of those influences that came before. At any time point, the maturational course may be affected by a child's inherent strengths, relative weaknesses, and any impairment (whether an acquired insult or other stressor). Intervention to lessen impairment may result in residual deficit, improvement but with residual weakness, or improvement sufficient to return the individual to acceptable functional status. Strengths, or preserved abilities, may be recruited to support interventional strategies. Development is further influenced by acquired skills and knowledge (e.g., education) up to and at any time point—a further influence on maturation that helps the child to move forward to the next maturational point in time. As brain maturation proceeds in this dynamic model, the module repeats infinitely, as depicted in Figure 17.2.

Importantly, deviation from normal development (e.g., developmental delay) does not necessarily imply intractable abnormality. Variability occurs in the course of normal development, only to resolve spontaneously with greater elapsed maturational time. It would not be surprising to see separation anxiety in a preschooler whose parent is left behind in the waiting room; to contend with a 2-year-old child who says "no" to most requests or otherwise exhibits defiance; or to observe test results indicative of an adolescent patient's poor social judgment, or to be told of the adolescent's susceptibility to negative peer influences. These behaviors are typical for their developmental course and, by themselves, are not conducive to reaching conclusions of abnormality. Furthermore, notable behaviors that suggest abnormality, such as poor social interaction, inability to sustain attention, or delay in expressive language, may occur in response to factors other than true neuropsychological dysfunction. Knowledge about the acceptable range for consideration of normal variability is crucial to avoid a judgment that a normal response is a worrisome predictor of future abnormality. For example, error interpretation relies on the practical application of this knowledge, as a child may make errors that are entirely acceptable in the course of normal development. For example, certain rotational errors on design copying, writing backward, producing mirror image reversals for letters or numbers, and phonemic substitutions are examples of developmentally appropriate errors often made by a young child, and are natural parts of the process of refining competence. Thus a wide range of normal variability

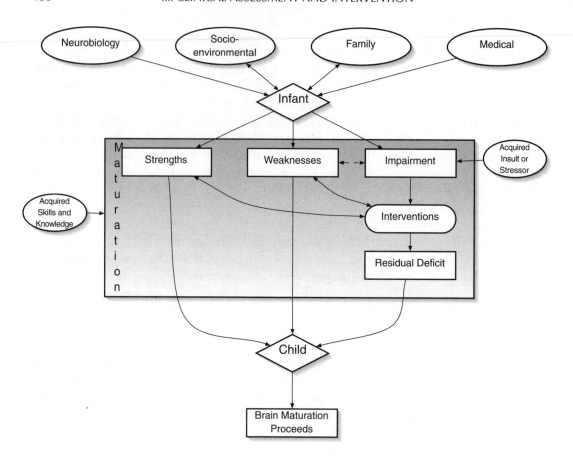

FIGURE 17.1. A maturational model of child neuropsychological development. From Baron (2008a). Copyright 2004 by Oxford University Press. Reprinted by permission.

may be allowable before the clinician concludes that a response is indicative of true deficit. Consideration of the range of potential explanations in synchrony with an internalized model of development is both useful and necessary.

Maxim 4. *Pediatric neuropsychological methods are distinctive.*

To determine precisely where a child falls on the dynamic spectrum of maturational growth, pediatric neuropsychologists enlist a fundamentally different set of examiner skills from those relied on for adult evaluation. Concerns about developmental level pervade every aspect of pediatric neuropsychological evaluation, including how one engages in the mechanics of testing, selection of developmentally appropriate measurement instruments; choosing criteria for evaluation of performance; clinical interpretation of observed behavior; integration of history; formulation of conclusions relative to presumptive brain maturational factors; and specification of recommendations and interventions that will best assist the child to use his or her inherent strengths to optimal advantage at home, in school, and in diverse socioenvironmental circumstances.

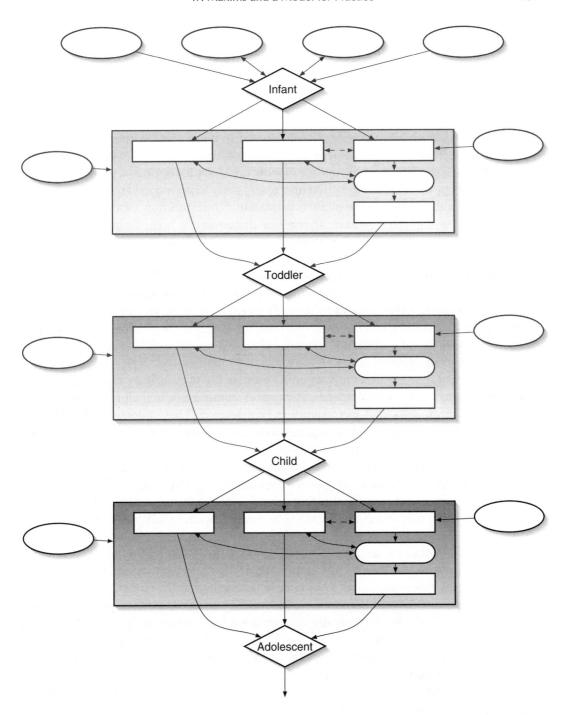

FIGURE 17.2. A template, based on the maturational model of child neuropsychological development, for considering influences affecting development from infancy to adulthood. From Baron (2008a). Copyright 2004 by Oxford University Press. Reprinted by permission.

There are both general (age-specific) and child-specific influences on the evaluative process. Among general influences are those that relate to typically defined periods of child development—infancy; early, middle, or late childhood; and adolescence. Each of these behaviorally distinct maturational stages has associated relatively invariable behaviors, which may either facilitate or interfere with direct evaluation. What constitutes an acceptable range of behavior in the testing environment is determined in part by these broad ranges. For example, a preschool child unused to being alone with someone who is not a family member is liable to experience significant stranger anxiety, which may defeat attempts to build the examiner–examinee rapport necessary for optimal testing, especially of deficient functions. A school-age child may react poorly when required to be absent from school and a familiar daily routine to attend an unfamiliar test session, especially when the administered tests tap those weaknesses causing discomfort at home or at school. Or an adolescent may be especially sensitive to privacy concerns and overtly reluctant to respond to questions about personal life events or peer relationships.

Child-specific influences include consideration of the individual's personality and state. That is, temperament, pain or discomfort, emotional fluctuations, hunger, or fatigue may each directly influence the moment-to-moment interactions with an examiner; they may directly affect cooperation, and therefore outcome. It is necessary in pediatric neuropsychology to allow sometimes for clinical judgment and consideration of child-specific individual circumstances to supersede strict normative test data analysis and interpretation. Therefore, developmental milestones are best considered as broad guidelines that will require adjustment related to the child's specific personal circumstances, including acculturation, state/personality variables, and socioenvironmental context. These interact and modulate behavior (see Figure 17.1), and they require careful consideration before an examiner can conclude that cognitive dysfunction is present.

Building rapport in order to elicit and maintain optimal cooperation for reliable evaluation is often a greater practical complexity in pediatric than in adult evaluation (Baron, 2004). The clinician must consider the most agreeable way to introduce the child to the test setting, debunk any misperceptions regarding testing to facilitate full cooperation, select a test order that does not unduly stress the child by emphasizing weakness too heavily at the start, and apply behavioral techniques effectively to support desired test-taking behavior. Play, a primary means by which a child communicates, is essential to overall healthy physical, cognitive, and socioemotional development (Ginsburg, 2007). Consequently, a more relaxed atmosphere that does not violate standardized test administration procedures can be helpful, along with developmentally appropriate reinforcement techniques (e.g., exuberant hand clapping, positive facial displays, or enthusiastic verbal encouragement). The examiner must also remain alert to intervene quickly at the first sign of tears, resistance, or withdrawal due to anxiety or emotional discomfort, or due to effects of the disorder or disease that initiated the referral. For further detail about eliciting optimal cooperation during behavioral assessment, see Baron (2004).

History taking, an especially critical component of the pediatric neuropsychological evaluation, includes coverage of prenatal and gestational factors; circumstances surrounding birth and delivery; rates of acquisition of developmental milestones, and any deviations from the expected course; review of any preexisting medical factors; impressions of interpersonal adequacy in familial and socioenvironmental settings; levels of educational achievement and teacher impressions; and relevant familial, developmental, neurological, and psychiatric histories (Baron et al., 1995). This knowledge is preparatory for appropriate test selection and administration, case formulation, and report preparation with suitable recommendations (Donders, 2001a, 2001b).

Although skill mastery directly relates to developmental level, it is also heavily dependent on socioenvironmental context—that is, the exposure and opportunities the child has had that have encouraged developmental progress or inhibited development. For example, a child's interpersonal behavior is expected to be contingent in part on the nature and degree of social interaction modeled by other family members. Notably, though birth and developmental histories are especially critical for contemporaneous pediatric neuropsychological evaluation, acquisition of such knowledge is equally important in adult neuropsychological practice. After all, the adult's specific neural network circuitry reflects a culmination of that individual's particular maturational forces and the influences of his or her unique developmental context (i.e., the many interrelated influences on brain function from gestation, birth, and infancy, through the formative childhood years, and into adolescence and adulthood). Clearly, developmental factors are not any less important in consideration of an adult's personal history than in consideration of a child's, but they may well be more elusive, given their occurrence many years earlier and the frequent lack of a knowledgeable third party to confirm the adult's self-report.

Domains assessed by pediatric neuropsychologists are comparable to those assessed by adult neuropsychologists: general intelligence, executive functions, attention/concentration, language, nonverbal skills, learning and recall, sensory and motor functions, mood and personality, and (when needed) symptom validity testing. Fractionating domains into subdomains is leading to enhanced understanding about the normally developing brain. It is no longer advisable to conclude that a child has a problem with attention or some other executive function, without elaborating further regarding the specific type of attentional or executive capacity that is impaired—for example, whether it is a weakness in focused or selective attention (Posner, 1988); sustained attention and vigilance (Barkley, 1997); divided attention (Craik, Govoni, Naveh-Benjamin, & Anderson, 1996; Troyer, Winocur, Craik, & Moscovitch, 1999; Vakil & Hoffman, 2004); attention-shifting capacity (Anderson, Jacobs, & Harvey, 2005b); inhibitory capacity (Barkley, 1997); or self-monitoring, planning, and verbal or nonverbal working memory (Baddeley, 1986; Baddeley & Hitch, 1974; Hitch & Halliday, 1983; Jonides et al., 1993; Pennington, Bennetto, McAleer, & Roberts, 1996).

There is also growing interest in further fractionating subdomains into *microdomains* (Repovs & Baddeley, 2006; Vallar & Baddeley, 1984). For example, working memory may be deconstructed into a collection of distinct component processes, each of which may have a unique neural substrate (e.g., the left inferior frontal gyrus has been implicated in a general, nonmnemonic function of selecting relevant information in the presence of interference; Thompson-Schill et al., 2002). Such finer delineation of capacities is meaningful not only with respect to which brain regions may be implicated as crucial for successful functioning, but also for potential identification of more precise, targeted interventional strategies.

Maxim 5. *Genetic, socioenvironmental, and family factors have primacy.*

How neuropsychological functions in childhood are influenced by perturbation at different developmental stages and different chronological ages is not sufficiently well understood without consideration of genetic, socioenvironmental, and family factors. These affect outcomes in significant ways but are only recently achieving deserved recognition, such as with respect to prematurity (Gross, Mettelman, Dye, & Slagle, 2001; Taylor, Klein, Minich, & Hack, 2001a; Vohr et al., 2003), TBI (Kinsella, Ong, Murtaugh, Prior, & Sawyer, 1999; Taylor et al., 2001b; Yeates et al., 1997, 2004), learning disorders (Wolff & Melngailis, 1994; Wolff, Melngailis, & Kotwica, 1996; Wolff, Melngailis, Obregon, & Bedrosian, 1995), and ADHD (Edwards, Schulz, & Long, 1995; Miller et al., 2006). For example, it has been well documented through adoption, family, and twin studies (Cook, 1999; Doyle & Anderson, 2005; Faraone & Doyle, 2001; Hechtman, 1996) that there is a high family concordance of ADHD, and that there is a high rate of ADHD in children of parents diagnosed with ADHD (Alberts-Corush, Firestone, & Goodman, 1986; Biederman et al., 1995; Epstein et al., 2000). The many hormonal and sex chromosome effects on a developing human brain are only beginning to be understood. For example, brain MRI scans found that boys with congenital adrenal hyperplasia had smaller amygdala volumes than matched controls, as did those with Klinefelter syndrome (47,XXY syndrome), who also had smaller hippocampus volumes than the controls (Rose et al., 2004).

There is also growing recognition of the centrality of socioenvironmental contextual influences on the developing child, and these variables are now more routinely included in research designs (Yeates et al., 2002) and explored in clinical practice. Investigation of the situational context is a necessary component of the evaluative process, since many competing family and socioenvironmental influences that potentially affect a child's behavior must be thoroughly considered before a diagnosis is made or a treatment is recommended. Among these, lower socioeconomic status, fewer family resources, and poorer family functioning have been circumstances associated with more negative social outcomes after TBI (Yeates et al., 2004). Family outcome monitoring and development of interventions for both the child and the stressed family is increasingly recommended (Taylor et al., 2001a).

A significant methodological limitation of early pediatric neuropsychological studies was that comprehensive attention was often not given to these factors along with the emphasis on neurocognitive measurement. Yet the influence of such factors as parental literacy, cultural group, family adversity, family medical history, and socioeconomic status may be particularly important for an individual (Manly, Jacobs, Touradji, Small, & Stern, 2002; Waber, Carlson, Mann, Merola, & Moylan, 1984), and their impact on developmental trajectories is only beginning to receive deserved attention (Lenroot & Giedd, 2006).

Teachers and others knowledgeable about a child may contribute important insights regarding the child's behavior across settings and are increasingly relied on as supplemental informants. Reports about peer interpersonal relationships may be especially crucial sources of information. However, there are other relevant considerations in interpreting these reports. For example, mood symptoms/disorders or reactive stress may decrease informant reliability and negatively affect determination of diagnosis (van der Oord, Prins, Oosterlaan, & Emmelkamp, 2006). Such circumstances as the child's illness, death of a family member or pet, exposure to parental discord or knowledge about parental job stressors, sibling conflicts, and bullying or peer pressure outside the home may result in poor behavior that is inconclusive for a diagnosable mental disorder, although intervention may be a high priority.

The increased volume of neuropsychological investigations related to circumstances once considered outside the purview of pediatric neuropsychology underscores the ever-greater opportunities to investigate neurodevelopment with respect to socioenvironmental variables in innovative ways. Studies of adopted children, children in foster care, and those from impoverished areas are helping us to better understand some of these influences (Faraone & Doyle, 2001). For example, children in foster care may be exposed to neglect, maltreatment, or placement decisions that result in developmental delays; Pears and Fisher (2005) found that foster children showed developmental lags on measures of height, head circumference, visual–spatial functioning, language functioning, and general cognitive functioning, compared to nonmaltreated, same-age children from comparable socioeconomic backgrounds. Also, individual neuropsychological measures may have wider applicability than was previously appreciated in assessment of the influence of socioenvironmental factors on behavioral development. For example, verbal fluency was a useful executive function measure in a study of children challenged by poor nutrition and enteric illness in early life. The negative influence of early childhood diarrhea on language development reinforced the usefulness of early assessment of enteric illnesses to enhance childhood development (Patrick et al., 2005).

FUTURE DIRECTIONS

As pediatric neuropsychology continues to make significant progress, pediatric neuropsychologists continue to assume increasingly diverse and substantial roles in advancing both science and practice, and in clarifying the impact of diverse medical, neurobiological, socioenvironmental, and psychological factors on both healthy children and those with disorder or disease. Recent years have seen the increased application of developmentally appropriate models and theories to guide pediatric practice; attention to developmentally sensitive testing, with methods that have reliability and validity in childhood (including for the youngest ages); refinement of measurement parameters; responsibility taken for reevaluating diagnostic nosology; and an increased forensic presence; expanded neuroscience collaborations in research; and greater consideration of lifespan issues, particularly the concepts of plasticity and reserve.

Developmentally Appropriate Models for Practice

Pediatric neuropsychologists extrapolate from their clinical work to reevaluate existent developmental models that influence their practice, and recognize that developmental models need to be discarded or amended when proven ineffective or incomplete. One example is the reconsideration of a flawed model for identification of learning disabilities, which persisted for many years as a result of wide acceptance of aptitude–achievement discrepancy as definitional. Pediatric neuropsychologists have recognized through their clinical practice and methods that numerous permutations of learning disorders may be apparent, but the definition of these disorders in the *Diagnostic and Statistical Manual of Mental Disorders*, fourth edition, text revision (DSM-IV-TR; American Psychiatric Association, 2000) has been restricted to four types: reading disorder, mathematics disorder, disorder of written expression, and learning disorder not otherwise specified. Consequently, this nosology failed to support identification and treatment of various learning difficulties commonly encountered in practice, and therefore failed to allow for provision of appropriate school-based intervention for children whose impairments fell outside these standard classifications. Children deserving of assistance for their learning problems were found ineligible even when their difficulties were well documented through neuropsychological evaluation. This unsatisfactory course of events has been changed in large part through the influence of neuropsychologists and allied colleagues who were instrumental in supporting the introduction of evidence-based assessment, as well as the response-to-intervention model, which emphasizes outcomes for children requiring interventional services over process and eligibility (Fletcher, Coulter, Reschly, & Vaughn, 2004; Fletcher, Francis, Morris, & Lyon, 2005). This useful reconceptualization and pragmatic redefinition should serve as a model for future corrections related to other diagnoses, when necessary.

Developmentally Sensitive Testing

Pediatric neuropsychologists have increasingly recognized that their expanded roles in serving the needs of very young children have been impeded by a lack of measurement instruments enabling finer discrimination of function at these vulnerable early ages. For more precise examination of structure–function correlations in early childhood, an emphasis needs to be placed on empirical development and application of test instruments that are sensitive to a child's developmental level and that have demonstrated prognostic value. Concepts derived from cognitive-developmental neuroscience and the extensive literature regarding normal child development have been formative in this regard. Consequently, with the acknowledgment that expectations based on adult practice models will not suffice, important steps forward have begun to be taken. Adult methods and paradigms are not the most efficacious for children, and it is increasingly well recognized that these need to be amended or discarded in favor of ones more compatible with the dynamic nature of the developing organism. Formal neuropsychological evaluation has value even for very young children, and a delineation of functioning by domains, subdomains, and microdomains is now increasingly possible (Baron, 2007b).

A number of very promising test instruments have been developed for the youngest age ranges (Baron & Gioia, 1998; Diamond, Carlson, & Beck, 2005; Espy, 2004; Espy, Bull, Martin, & Stroup, 2006; Espy & Cwik, 2004; Kerns, McInerney, & Wilde, 2001; McInerney, Hrabok, & Kerns, 2005), and well-conceptualized test batteries now extend downward to early preschool ages, with increased sensitivity for measurement of early neurocognitive function (e.g., Elliott, 2007; Korkman, Kirk, & Kemp, 1997). Although test development has lagged in part because many pediatric neuropsychologists had less exposure in their education and training to such young populations, and since these children were less often referred for neuropsychological evaluation, the full range of capacities that can be measured in the very young is recently being more fully appreciated and is expected to become a more prominent focus. It is tempting to think that *infant neuropsychological evaluation* may become a valid replacement for the current broad neurodevelopmental evaluation that does not sufficiently address individual variability. (Surely, if a pediatric neuropsychologist examines an infant or very young child and frames the results within a neuropsychological context, then *infant neuropsychological evaluation* would seem to be a valid descriptor). Importantly, neuropsychologists are especially well suited to anticipate later function or dysfunction resulting from early brain insult or systemic medical problems. This should prove to be enormously helpful in working with a medical team, or when counseling parents about which behaviors they need to observe and what they can probably expect as neuromaturation proceeds. Overall, greater attention to infants from a neuropsychological perspective is an exciting area of inquiry, and one that has not yet received sufficient clinical application.

Refinement of Measurement Parameters

Pediatric measures and methods have had several inherent limitations. Quantification of useful qualitative test features remains limited in pediatric practice, so it is often not possible for observed clinical behaviors to be usefully integrated into case formulation and measured repeatedly. Yet such quantification has begun to filter from adult studies to child investigations and practice. For example, tests of inhibition, working memory, and discrete aspects of attentional capacity are being used to greater advantage at younger ages. Adult studies have clarified that it is possible to make finer discriminations that have greater utility for clinical case formulation. For example, the subdomain of verbal fluency has been fractionated further into microdomains of clustering and switching. Adult studies have correlated letter fluency performance with more anterior cerebral function (Martin, Wiggs, Lalonde, & Mack, 1994), noun fluency with more posterior cerebral function (Tranel, Adolphs, Damasio, & Damasio, 2001; Warburton et al., 1996), and verb fluency with frontal–basal ganglia function (Piatt, Fields, Paolo, & Troster, 2004; Woods et al., 2005). The clustering and switching scores computed from verbal fluency test performance in adults (Troyer, Moscovitch, & Winocur, 1997) also have had relevance for appreciating childhood structure–function relationships (Koren, Kofman, & Berger, 2005; Roncadin & Rich, 2002; Sauzeon, Lestage, Raboutet, N'Kaoua, & Claverie, 2004). Whether they will have utility in distinguishing among those discrete neural systems that underlie successful performance in childhood (compared to their efficacy in making such discriminations in adulthood), and whether it will be possible to distinguish similar correlations between structure and function secondary to early insult and at different developmental stages, remain to be determined.

Test selection and interpretation in child evaluation are often made problematic by limited normative data for individual child measures, and for some clinically favored multiple-subtest batteries; such data may be weak or nonexistent when prospective follow-up is needed. Furthermore, although it is expected that children may capably respond to tests constructed for their chronological age, some may experience one or more developmental delays that make them less able to master basal-level performance on the intended measure. There continues to be a clear need for construction and standardization of developmentally appropriate test instruments, especially for the very youngest ages. Many existent child tests do not sufficiently sample those discrete behaviors that are likely to underlie more complex neuropsychological functions, and remain psychometrically weak for functional subdomain partitioning. Others are broad-based instruments and therefore multiply determined; that is, poor performance could be attributed equally well to a number of competing functions required for successful performance, each potentially subserved by a different neural system. Consequently, substantial methodological obstacles remain to be overcome with regard to determining the adequacy of cerebral function after disorder and the impact of disorder on a child's dynamic developmental course of brain maturation.

Reevaluation of Diagnostic Nosology

The ADHD literature provides an example of the contribution of pediatric neuropsychologists and members of allied disciplines to progress in model development, diagnosis, assessment, and treatment. Moving beyond causal models of ADHD based on core (executive function) deficits, investigators have turned toward other contributing factors, such as noncognitive dysregulation. For instance, motivational constructs of delay aversion and altered reward processes are proposed in an alternative model of ADHD that posits neuropathological heterogeneity (Sonuga-Barke, 2003, 2005). Neural networks have begun to be explored in novel ways that often have special relevance for pediatric populations. It is now possible to identify landmarks in the development of brain networks underlying executive attention from infancy and childhood; to use individual differences in network efficiency to examine genetic alleles that are related to performance; and to incorporate training methods to enhance attentional networks (Posner, Sheese, Odludas, & Tang, 2006).

Altogether, the large ADHD literature and clinical experience have led to a conclusion that the DSM-IV-TR diagnostic nosology on which we rely for ADHD diagnosis is outdated and in need of revision. Neuropsychologists need to continue taking direct responsibility for establishing empirically based definitions for neuropsychological disorders, or at least to contribute substantially and directly to those entities responsible for updating current diagnostic and treatment criteria. Their efforts increasingly directed toward reevaluation of diagnostic nosology and practice guidelines as they pertain to their clinical populations are expected to lead to better diagnostic classification systems for neuropsychological conditions. The establishment of definitional criteria by non-neuropsychologists for pediatric neuropsychological disorders has been one obstacle complicating pragmatic attempts to ensure that children are diagnosed correctly and receive needed services. It is a notable feature of pediatric practice that there are definitional problems associated with the current diagnostic nosology for some conditions; in addition to learning disorders and ADHD, these include pervasive developmental disorders and other neurodevelopmental disorders. Consequently, the existing criteria perpetuate older assumptions and models that no longer serve these children well. A notable example pertains to the inadequacy of the DSM-IV-TR criteria on which we rely for the exclusionary ADHD behavioral diagnosis (Baron, 2007a; Stefanatos & Baron, 2007). Yet neuropsychologists' "theoretical conceptualizations regarding ADHD have been enormously influential for decades, their clinical skills [are] highly pertinent to meticulous delineation of ADHD symptomatology and co-morbidity, their participation in clinical trials to reach evidence-based decisions [is] immensely valuable, and they are often front-line consultants to physician-colleagues when an ADHD diagnosis is under consideration" (Baron, 2007a, p. 2). This record of accomplishment needs to be extended to other diagnostic formulations.

Increased Forensic Presence

Pediatric neuropsychological evaluations are increasingly recognized as highly informative, objective, and pertinent in forensic neuropsychological practice, albeit they are currently less of a presence in such practice than adult evaluations are. The importance of neuropsychological evaluations within adult forensic practice is well established, with a rapidly growing literature (Boone, 2007; Bush, 2005; Denney & Sullivan, 2008; Heilbronner, 2005;

Larrabee, 2005). Before they enter the legal arena, pediatric neuropsychologists are well advised to formally consider the type of forensic practice that they wish to pursue. Various ethical and professional issues arise with respect to neuropsychological evaluations conducted for the benefit of (and at the behest of) counsel, compared to those that are conducted as nonforensic clinical referrals; increasingly, pediatric neuropsychologists recruited to serve in these roles will need to educate themselves about these issues. The forces of maturation as they pertain to children's neurodevelopment may not be fully understood by a legal establishment eager to obtain case conclusion. Pediatric neuropsychologists in an advisory capacity are well suited to detailing the likely eventual course of disease, disorder, or injury, and the relevance of monitoring neurocognitive development over time. Pediatric neuropsychological data are especially useful with respect to detailing the advantages and disadvantages of waiting to settle a case until such time as a child has matured sufficiently to make the deficits consequent to the insult most apparent (Baron, 2008). This valuable capacity based on training and experience may encourage some pediatric neuropsychologists to choose to accept an educative role for counsel, and, by extension, counsel's pediatric clients.

Expanded Neuroscience Collaborations in Research

Just as we must wait to see what functions will develop (or fail to develop) with maturational time, we must await future technological advances that will further enable structure–function correlations for both healthy and clinical populations. There is continued interest in determining those neural networks or functional neural systems that are enlisted in the presence of damage, as well as those utilized in a normal developmental progression. Technological advances that are not invasive but that offer opportunities for correlations with neuropsychological data are increasingly becoming available, enabling further insights such as those made possible by longitudinal scanning of healthy children with MRI to understand brain maturation (Giedd et al., 1999). The immense value of the team approach to combining knowledge from allied specialists cannot be overemphasized.

Plasticity, Reserve, and Other Lifespan Issues

Plasticity and reserve are vital factors influencing children's recovery from, or accommodation to, neurological insult. The pediatric neuropsychologist's skills are especially suited for the evaluation of the limits of brain plasticity (the neural response or adaptation to brain insult) and the course of function recovery, and for documenting late neurocognitive and behavioral effects related to specific prophylactic or interventional procedures provided in response to neurological injury or to systemic or central nervous system disease and treatment. As noted above, children often confound the teachings of adult neuropsychology by failing to demonstrate predictable or typical adult behavioral patterns after neurological insult. The adult literature describes the potential protective effects of intelligence and education related to recovery from injury (Satz, 1993; Stern, 2002, 2003; Stern et al., 2003). There is a need to determine which factors may be most protective against dysfunction consequent to a congenital or acquired childhood lesion, and how these factors relate to developmental maturation and the emergence of developmental delay or impairment.

Conceptualizations of children's brain reserve and cognitive reserve have begun to be elaborated (Dennis, Yeates, Taylor, & Fletcher, 2006b) and considered in context with the mechanisms of plasticity for the developing child. The term *brain reserve* is often used as an index of threshold features that are hypothesized but not always amenable to direct quantification, such as total brain mass or number of dendrites. Intelligence has been postulated as an indirect measure of brain reserve capacity (Satz, 1993). In contrast, the term *cognitive reserve* refers to a dynamic involvement of neural networks to effect maximal use of cognitive strategies, in order to bring about the highest level of function possible after brain insult.

Questions regarding cerebral reorganization for different functional capacities remain to be answered. These include whether and to what degree intact homologous or contiguous brain regions are enlisted; whether some combination of recruited regions not yet fully understood is active; and how lesion location affects intra- versus interhemispheric cerebral reorganization. More needs to be understood about alternative profiles of neural organization that can, and often will, result after early brain injury (Stiles et al., 2003). These brain changes may result from either maladaptive or adaptive plasticity. For example, plasticity may confer risk for maladaptation or psychopathology, since children's learning is based on prominent features of their environment even when they are anomalous (Pollak, 2003), and an immature neural circuitry of emotion systems at the time of insult may result in development of psychopathology (Pollak, 2005). Specialized neural substrates may underlie a function, have limited plasticity, and be more strongly lateralized to one or the other cerebral hemisphere. For example, an examination of reading and spelling performance of children with unilateral brain damage found impairment in boys only with a left cerebral lesion, while girls showed no significant impairments regardless of which hemisphere was impaired (Frith & Vargha-Khadem, 2001). In another study, adaptive neural plasticity was invoked as the basis for why children with arteriovenous malformations tolerated surgery and recovered better than adults with similar anatomy, rupture rates, lesion, clinical presentation, and treatment (Sanchez-Mejia et al., 2006). And, as noted above, children's capacity for adaptation may reflect normal developmental processes operating against a backdrop of serious neural perturbation (Stiles et al., 2005). There is a substantial basis for expecting compensatory adaptation in childhood, although this may be tempered by residual problems when a child is expected to engage in higher levels of functioning (e.g., in language or constructional ability). Future outcome studies are expected to provide additional examples of compensatory neural processes, and the limits of such processes. However, and regrettably, compensatory adaptation does not necessarily mean that a child will return to intact functioning if given sufficient time. How to achieve maximum compensatory adaptation remains a stimulus for further study.

In contrast to early teachings, the negative impact of early brain insult may be significant, and very early brain injury may be more incapacitating than injury sustained at a later age (Anderson & Moore, 1995; Aram, 1988; Ewing-Cobbs, 1998; Ewing-Cobbs et al., 1997; Lehnung et al., 2001; Levin et al., 1993; Stiles, Bates, Thal, Trauner, & Reilly, 1998; Taylor & Alden, 1997;). For example, a "double-hazard" model for severe and early brain insults posits that young children who sustain severe TBI in early childhood, or moderate or severe TBI in infancy, may be particularly vulnerable to significant residual cognitive impairment (Anderson, Catroppa, Morse, Haritou, & Rosenfeld, 2005a). It is now better appreciated that the lasting and intrusive effects of early brain damage may only be masked until such time as there is a demand for the function affected—that is, when it is recruited for a task at a more mature stage of development. This is repeatedly evident in clinical practice, and the literature contains numerous examples, such as in a study of reading skill acquisition after injury at the preschool age (Anderson, Catroppa, Morse, Haritou, & Rosenfeld, 2000). Expectation for late-appearing deficit is a prominent consideration in evaluative conclusions and recommendations. Nuances related to timing of insult, age at which the insult was incurred, and nature and extent of the insult make prediction for an individual child a very intricate endeavor—but one that becomes essential in the clinical setting.

SUMMARY AND CONCLUSIONS

In summary, the future of pediatric neuropsychological practice is contingent on the ability of pediatric neuropsychologists to apply their full range of capabilities to effect meaningful change for those children who require their services. Evaluating each child's neurodevelopmental level appropriately; recommending and providing interventions that are timely, targeted appropriately, and applied accurately; and employing valid outcome measurements are all fundamental. Within the profession, practitioners are well aware that clinical neuropsychology is not simply test administration. There is an obligation to extend this message and disseminate the broad range of roles played by pediatric neuropsychologists, especially to those who may inadvertently misuse neuropsychological methods to their patients' disadvantage. Ideally, through work with colleagues concerned with neuropsychological principles and practice, a satisfactory means will emerge to integrate responsible neuropsychological evaluation with the professional responsibilities of allied colleagues for the betterment of children.

REFERENCES

Akshoomoff, N. A., Courchesne, E., Press, G. A., & Iragui, V. (1992). Contribution of the cerebellum to neuropsychological functioning: Evidence from a case of cerebellar degenerative disorder. *Neuropsychologia, 30,* 315–328.

Alberts-Corush, J., Firestone, P., & Goodman, J. T. (1986). Attention and impulsivity characteristics of the biological and adoptive parents of hyperactive and normal control children. *American Journal of Orthopsychiatry, 56*(3), 413–423.

Allen, G., & Courchesne, E. (2003). Differential effects of developmental cerebellar abnormality on cognitive and motor functions in the cerebellum: An fMRI study of autism. *American Journal of Psychiatry, 160*(2), 262–273.

American Psychiatric Association. (2000). *Diagnostic and statistical manual of mental disorders* (4th ed., text rev.). Washington, DC: Author.

Anderson, P. J., & Doyle, L. W. (2004). Executive functioning in school-aged children who were born very preterm or with extremely low birth weight in the 1990s. *Pediatrics, 114*(1), 50–57.

Anderson, V., Catroppa, C., Morse, S., Haritou, F., & Rosenfeld, J. (2000). Recovery of intellectual ability following traumatic brain injury in childhood: Impact of injury severity and age at injury. *Pediatric Neurosurgery, 32,* 282–290.

Anderson, V., Catroppa, C., Morse, S., Haritou, F., & Rosenfeld, J. (2005a). Functional plasticity or vulnerability after early brain injury? *Pediatrics, 116*(6), 1374–1382.

Anderson, V., Jacobs, R., & Harvey, A. S. (2005b). Prefrontal lesions and attentional skills in childhood. *Journal of the International Neuropsychological Society, 11*(7), 817–831.

Anderson, V., & Moore, C. (1995). Age at injury as a predictor of outcome following pediatric head injury: A longitudinal perspective. *Child Neuropsychology, 1,* 187–202.

Anderson, V., Northam, E., Hendy, J., & Wrennall, J. (2001). *Developmental neuropsychology.* Philadelphia: Psychology Press.

Aram, D. (1988). Language sequelae of unilateral brain lesions in children. In F. Plum (Ed.), *Language, communication, and the brain* (pp. 171–197). New York: Raven Press.

Baddeley, A. D. (1986). *Working memory.* New York: Oxford University Press.

Baddeley, A. D., & Hitch, G. J. (1974). Working memory. In G. H. Bower (Ed.), *The psychology of learning and motivation Volume* (Vol. 8, pp. 47–88). New York: Academic Press.

Barkley, R. A. (1997). Behavioral inhibition, sustained attention, and executive functions: Constructing a unifying theory of ADHD. *Psychological Bulletin, 121,* 65–94.

Barkley, R. A. (2006). *Attention-deficit hyperactivity disorder: A handbook for diagnosis and treatment* (3rd ed.). New York: Guilford Press.

Baron, I. S. (2004). *Neuropsychological evaluation of the child.* New York: Oxford University Press.

Baron, I. S. (2007). Attention-deficit/hyperactivity disorder: New challenges for definition, diagnosis, and treatment [Editorial]. *Neuropsychology Review, 17,* 1–3.

Baron, I. S. (2008a). Growth and development of pediatric neuropsychology. In J. E. Morgan & J. H. Ricker (Eds.), *Textbook of clinical neuropsychology* (pp. 91–104). New York: Taylor & Francis.

Baron, I. S. (2008b). Maturation into impairment: The merit of delayed settlement in pediatric forensic neuropsychology cases. In R. L. Heilbronner (Ed.), *Neuropsychology in the courtroom: Expert analysis of reports and testimony* (pp. 66–78). New York: Guilford Press.

Baron, I. S., Fennell, E. B., & Voeller, K. K. S. (1995). *Pediatric neuropsychology in the medical setting.* New York: Oxford University Press.

Baron, I. S., & Gioia, G. A. (1998). Neuropsychology of infants and young children. In G. Goldstein, P. D. Nussbaum, & S. R. Beers (Eds.), *Handbook of human brain function: Assessment and rehabilitation* (Vol. III: Neuropsychology, pp. 9–34). New York: Plenum Press.

Barr, W. B. (2008). Historical development of the neuropsychological test battery. In J. E. Morgan & J. H. Ricker (Eds.), *Textbook of clinical neuropsychology* (pp. 3–17). New York: Taylor & Francis.

Benton, A. (2000). Foreword. In K. O. Yeates, M. D. Ris, & H. G. Taylor (Eds.), *Pediatric neuropsychology: Research, theory, and practice* (p. xv). New York: Guilford Press.

Bernstein, J. H., & Waber, D. (1990). Developmental neuropsychological assessment: The systemic approach. In A. A. Boulton, G. B. Baker, & M. Hiscock (Eds.), *Neuromethods: Vol. 17. Neuropsychology* (pp. 311–371). Clifton, NJ: Humana Press.

Biederman, J., Faraone, S. V., Mick, E., Spencer, T., Wilens, T., Kiely, K., et al. (1995). High risk for attention deficit hyperactivity disorder among children of parents with childhood onset of the disorder: A pilot study. *American Journal of Psychiatry, 152*(3), 431–435.

Boone, K. B. (Ed.). (2007). *Assessment of feigned cognitive impairment: A neuropsychological perspective.* New York: Guilford Press.

Broman, S. H., & Fletcher, J. M. (1999). *The changing nervous system.* New York: Oxford University Press.

Bush, S. S. (Ed.). (2005). *A casebook of ethical challenges in neuropsychology.* New York: Psychology Press.

Cook, E. H., Jr. (1999). The early development of child psychopharmacogenetics. *Journal of the American Academy of Child and Adolescent Psychiatry, 38*(12), 1478–1481.

Cooley, E. L., & Morris, R. D. (1990). Attention in children: A neuropsychologically based model for assessment. *Developmental Neuropsychology, 6,* 239–274.

Craik, F. I. M., Govoni, R., Naveh-Benjamin, M., & Anderson, N. D. (1996). The effects of divided attention on encoding and retrieval processes in human memory. *Journal of Experimental Psychology: General, 125,* 159–180.

Denckla, M. B. (1973). Development of speed in repetitive and successive finger-movements in normal children. *Developmental Medicine and Child Neurology, 15,* 635–645.

Denney, R. L., & Sullivan, J. P. (Eds.). (2008). *Clinical neuropsychology in the criminal forensic setting.* New York: Guilford Press.

Dennis, M., Landry, S. H., Barnes, M., & Fletcher, J. M. (2006a). A model of neurocognitive function in spina bifida over the life span. *Journal of the International Neuropsychological Society, 12*(2), 285–296.

Dennis, M., Yeates, K., Taylor, H. G., & Fletcher, J. M. (2006b). Brain reserve capacity, cognitive reserve capacity, and age-based functional plasticity after congenital and acquired brain injury in children. In Y. Stern (Ed.), *Cognitive reserve.* New York: Psychology Press.

Dewey, D., & Tupper, D. E. (Eds.). (2004). *Developmental motor disorders: A neuropsychological perspective.* New York: Guilford Press.

Diamond, A. (2000). Close interrelation of motor development and cognitive development and of the cerebellum and prefrontal cortex. *Child Development, 71*(1), 44–56.

Diamond, A., Carlson, S. M., & Beck, D. M. (2005). Preschool children's performance in task switching on the dimensional change card sort task: Separating the dimensions aids the ability to switch. *Developmental Neuropsychology, 28*(2), 689–729.

Donders, J. (2001a). A survey of report writing by neuropsychologists: I. General characteristics and content. *The Clinical Neuropsychologist, 15,* 137–149.

Donders, J. (2001b). A survey of report writing by neuropsychologists: II. Test data, report format, and document length. *The Clinical Neuropsychologist, 15,* 150–161.

Doyle, L. W., & Anderson, P. J. (2005). Improved neurosensory outcome at 8 years of age of extremely low birthweight children born in Victoria over three distinct eras. *Archives of Disease in Childhood: Fetal and Neonatal Edition, 90*(6), F484–F488.

Edwards, M. C., Schulz, E. G., & Long, N. (1995). The role of the family in the assessment of attention-deficit hyperactivity disorder. *Clinical Psychology Review, 15,* 375–394.

Elliott, C. D. (2007). *Differential Ability Scales–II.* San Antonio, TX: Harcourt Assessment

Epstein, J. N., Conners, C. K., Erhardt, D., Arnold, L. E., Hechtman, L., Hinshaw, S. P., et al. (2000). Familial aggregation of ADHD characteristics. *Journal of Abnormal Child Psychology, 28*(6), 585–594.

Espy, K. A. (2004). Using developmental, cognitive, and neuroscience approaches to understand executive control in young children. *Developmental Neuropsychology, 26*(1), 379–384.

Espy, K. A., Bull, R., Martin, J., & Stroup, W. (2006). Measuring the development of executive control with the Shape School. *Psychological Assessment 18*(4), 373–381.

Espy, K. A., & Cwik, M. F. (2004). The development of a trail making test in young children: The TRAILS-P. *The Clinical Neuropsychologist, 18*(3), 411–422.

Ewing-Cobbs, L. (1998). Attention after pediatric traumatic brain injury: A multidimensional assessment. *Child Neuropsychology, 4,* 35–48.

Ewing-Cobbs, L., Fletcher, J., Levin, H. S., Francis, D. J., Davidson, K., & Miner, M. E. (1997). Longitudinal neuropsychological outcome in infants and preschoolers with traumatic brain injury. *Journal of the International Neuropsychological Society, 3,* 581–591.

Faraone, S. V., & Doyle, A. E. (2001). The nature and heritability of attention-deficit/hyperactivity disorder. *Child and Adolescent Psychiatric Clinics of North America, 10*(2), 299–316, viii–ix.

Farmer, J. E., Donders, J., & Warschausky, S. (Eds.). (2006). *Treating neurodevelopmental disabilities: Clinical research and practice.* New York: Guilford Press.

Fennell, E. B., & Bauer, R. M. (1997). Models of inference and evaluating brain–behavioral relationships in children. In C. R. Reynolds & E. Fletcher-Janzen (Eds.), *Handbook of clinical child neuropsychology* (2nd ed., pp. 204–215). New York: Plenum Press.

Fletcher, J. M., Coulter, W. A., Reschly, D. J., & Vaughn, S. (2004). Alternative approaches to the definition and identification of learning disabilities: Some questions and answers. *Annals of Dyslexia, 54*(2), 304–331.

Fletcher, J. M., Francis, D. J., Morris, R. D., & Lyon, G. R. (2005). Evidence-based assessment of learning disabilities in children and adolescents. *Journal of Clinical Child and Adolescent Psychology, 34*(3), 506–522.

Fletcher, J. M., Lyon, G. R., Fuchs, L. S., & Barnes, M. A. (2007). *Learning disabilities: From identification to intervention.* New York: Guilford Press.

Fletcher, J. M., & Taylor, H. G. (1984). Neuropsychological approaches to children: Towards a developmental neuropsychology. *Journal of Clinical Neuropsychology, 6*, 39–56.

Frith, U., & Vargha-Khadem, F. (2001). Are there sex differences in the brain basis of literacy related skills?: Evidence from reading and spelling impairments after early unilateral brain damage. *Neuropsychologia, 39*(13), 1485–1488.

Giedd, J. N. (2004). Structural magnetic resonance imaging of the adolescent brain. *Annals of the New York Academy of Sciences, 1021*, 77–85.

Giedd, J. N., Blumenthal, J., Jeffries, N. O., Castellanos, F. X., Liu, H., Zijdenbos, A., et al. (1999). Brain development during childhood and adolescence: A longitudinal MRI study. *Nature Neuroscience, 2*(10), 861–863.

Giedd, J. N., Clasen, L. S., Lenroot, R., Greenstein, D., Wallace, G. L., Ordaz, S., et al. (2006). Puberty-related influences on brain development. *Molecular and Cellular Endocrinology, 254–255*, 154–162.

Giedd, J. N., Rosenthal, M. A., Rose, A. B., Blumenthal, J. D., Molloy, E., Dopp, R. R., et al. (2004). Brain development in healthy children and adolescents: Magnetic resonance imaging studies. In J. K. M. Keshavan & R. Murray (Eds.), *Neurodevelopment and schizophrenia* (pp. 35–44). Cambridge, UK: Cambridge University Press.

Ginsburg, K. R. (2007). The importance of play in promoting healthy child development and maintaining strong parent–child bonds. *Pediatrics, 119*(1), 182–191.

Gogtay, N., Giedd, J. N., Lusk, L., Hayashi, K. M., Greenstein, D., Vaituzis, A. C., et al. (2004). Dynamic mapping of human cortical development during childhood through early adulthood. *Proceedings of the National Academy of Sciences USA, 101*(21), 8174–8179.

Gross, S. J., Mettelman, B. B., Dye, T. D., & Slagle, T. A. (2001). Impact of family structure and stability on academic outcome in preterm children at 10 years of age. *Journal of Pediatrics, 138*(2), 169–175.

Hanten, G., Scheibel, R. S., Li, X., Oomer, I., Stallings-Roberson, G., Hunter, J. V., et al. (2006). Decision-making after traumatic brain injury in children: A preliminary study. *Neurocase, 12*(4), 247–251.

Hechtman, L. (1996). Families of children with attention deficit hyperactivity disorder: A review. *Canadian Journal of Psychiatry, 41*(6), 350–360.

Heilbronner, R. L. (Ed.). (2005). *Forensic neuropsychology casebook.* New York: Guilford Press.

Hitch, G. J., & Halliday, M. S. (1983). Working memory in children. *Philosophical Transactions of the Royal Society of London, 302*, 325–340.

Holloway, V., Gadian, D. G., Vargha-Khadem, F., Porter, D. A., Boyd, S. G., & Connelly, A. (2000). The reorganization of sensorimotor function in children after hemispherectomy: A functional MRI and somatosensory evoked potential study. *Brain, 123*(Pt. 12), 2432–2444.

Hunter, S. J., & Donders, J. (Eds.). (2007). *Pediatric neuropsychological intervention.* Cambridge, UK: Cambridge University Press.

Jonides, J. J., Smith, E. E., Koeppe, R. A., Awh, E., Minoshima, S., & Mintun, M. A. (1993). Spatial working memory in humans as revealed by PET. *Nature, 363*, 623–625.

Kerns, K. A., McInerney, R. J., & Wilde, N. J. (2001). Time reproduction, working memory, and behavioral inhibition in children with ADHD. *Child Neuropsychology, 7*, 21–31.

Kinsella, G., Ong, B., Murtaugh, D., Prior, M., & Sawyer, M. (1999). The role of the family for behavioral outcome in children and adolescents following traumatic brain injury. *Journal of Consulting and Clinical Psychology, 67*, 116–123.

Koren, R., Kofman, O., & Berger, A. (2005). Analysis of word clustering in verbal fluency of school-aged children. *Archives of Clinical Neuropsychology, 20*, 1087–1104.

Korkman, M., Kirk, U., & Kemp, S. (1997). *NEPSY: A developmental neuropsychological assessment.* San Antonio, TX: Psychological Corporation.

Larrabee, G. J. (Ed.). (2005). *Forensic neuropsychology: A scientific approach.* New York: Oxford University Press.

Lechtenberg, R., & Gilman, S. (1978). Speech disorders in cerebellar disease. *Annals of Neurology, 3*, 285–290.

Lehnung, M., Leplow, B., Herzog, A., Benz, B., Ritz, A., Stolze, H., et al. (2001). Children's spatial behavior is differentially affected after traumatic brain injury. *Child Neuropsychology, 7*, 59–71.

Leiner, H. C., Leiner, A. L., & Dow, R. S. (1986). Does the cerebellum contribute to mental skills? *Behavioral Neuroscience, 100*(4), 443–454.

Lenroot, R. K., & Giedd, J. N. (2006). Brain development in children and adolescents: Insights from anatomical magnetic resonance imaging. *Neuroscience and Biobehavioral Reviews, 30*(6), 718–729.

Levin, H. S., Culhane, K. A., Mendelsohn, D., Lilly, M. A., Bruce, D., Fletcher, J. M., et al. (1993). Cognition in relation to magnetic resonance imaging in head-injured children and adolescents. *Archives of Neurology, 50,* 897–905.

Levisohn, L., Cronin-Golomb, A., & Schmahmann, J. D. (2000). Neuropsychological consequences of cerebellar tumour resection in children: Cerebellar cognitive affective syndrome in a paediatric population. *Brain, 123*(5), 1041–1050.

Limperopoulos, C., Soul, J. S., Gauvreau, K., Huppi, P. S., Warfield, S. K., Bassan, H., et al. (2005). Late gestation cerebellar growth is rapid and impeded by premature birth. *Pediatrics, 115,* 688–695.

Manly, J. J., Jacobs, D., Touradji, P., Small, S. A., & Stern, Y. (2002). Reading level attenuates differences in neuropsychological test performance between African American and white elders. *Journal of the International Neuropsychological Society, 8,* 341–348.

Martin, A., Wiggs, C. L., Lalonde, F., & Mack, C. (1994). Word retrieval to letter and semantic cues: A double dissociation in normal subjects using interference tasks. *Neuropsychologia, 32*(12), 1487–1494.

McInerney, R. J., Hrabok, M., & Kerns, K. A. (2005). The children's size-ordering task: A new measure of nonverbal working memory. *Journal of Clinical and Experimental Neuropsychology, 27,* 735–745.

Merke, D. P., Giedd, J. N., Keil, M. F., Mehlinger, S. L., Wiggs, E. A., Holzer, S., et al. (2005). Children experience cognitive decline despite reversal of brain atrophy one year after resolution of Cushing syndrome. *Journal of Clinical Endocrinology and Metabolism, 90*(5), 2531–2536.

Miller, C. J., Miller, S. R., Trampush, J., McKay, K. E., Newcorn, J. H., & Halperin, J. M. (2006). Family and cognitive factors: Modeling risk for aggression in children with ADHD. *Journal of the American Academy of Child and Adolescent Psychiatry, 45*(3), 355–363.

Patrick, P. D., Oria, R. B., Madhavan, V., Pinkerton, R. C., Lorntz, B., Lima, A. A., et al. (2005). Limitations in verbal fluency following heavy burdens of early childhood diarrhea in Brazilian shantytown children. *Child Neuropsychology, 11*(3), 233–244.

Pears, K., & Fisher, P. A. (2005). Developmental, cognitive, and neuropsychological functioning in preschool-aged foster children: Associations with prior maltreatment and placement history. *Journal of Developmental and Behavioral Pediatrics, 26,* 112–122.

Pennington, B. F. (2002). *The development of psychopathology.* New York: Guilford Press.

Pennington, B. F. (2005). Toward a new neuropsychological model of attention-deficit/hyperactivity disorder: Subtypes and multiple deficits. *Biological Psychiatry, 57*(11), 1221–1223.

Pennington, B. F., Bennetto, L., McAleer, O., & Roberts, R. J. (1996). Executive functions and working memory: Theoretical and measurement issues. In G. R. Lyon & N. A. Krasnegor (Eds.), *Attention, memory, and executive function* (pp. 327–348). Baltimore: Brookes.

Piatt, A. L., Fields, J. A., Paolo, A. M., & Troster, A. I. (2004). Action verbal fluency normative data for the elderly. *Brain and Language, 89,* 580–583.

Pollak, S. D. (2003). Experience-dependent affective learning and risk for psychopathology in children. *Annals of the New York Academy of Sciences, 1008,* 102–111.

Pollak, S. D. (2005). Early adversity and mechanisms of plasticity: Integrating affective neuroscience with developmental approaches to psychopathology. *Development and Psychopathology, 17*(3), 735–752.

Posner, M. I. (1988). Structures and functions of selective attention. In T. Boll & B. K. Bryant (Eds.), *Clinical neuropsychology and brain function: Research, measurement, and practice.* Washington, DC: American Psychological Association.

Posner, M. I., Sheese, B. E., Odludas, Y., & Tang, Y. (2006). Analyzing and shaping human attentional networks. *Neural Networks, 19*(9), 1422–1429.

Ravizza, S. M., McCormick, C. A., Schlerf, J. E., Justus, T., Ivry, R. B., & Fiez, J. A. (2006). Cerebellar damage produces selective deficits in verbal working memory. *Brain, 129*(Pt. 2), 306–320.

Repovs, G., & Baddeley, A. (2006). The multi-component model of working memory: Explorations in experimental cognitive psychology. *Neuroscience, 139*(1), 5–21.

Riva, D., & Giorgi, D. (2000). The cerebellum contributes to higher functions during development: Evidence from a series of children surgically treated for posterior fossa tumours. *Brain, 123,* 1051–1061.

Roncadin, C., & Rich, J. B. (2002). Clustering and switching on verbal fluency tasks in childhood and adolescence. *Journal of the International Neuropsychological Society, 8,* 206.

Rose, A. B., Merke, D. P., Clasen, L. S., Rosenthal, M. A., Wallace, G. L., Vaituzis, A. C., et al. (2004). Effects of hormones and sex chromosomes on stress-influenced regions of the developing pediatric brain. *Annals of the New York Academy of Sciences, 1032,* 231–233.

Rourke, B. P. (1989). *Nonverbal learning disabilities: The syndrome and the model.* New York: Guilford Press.

Sadeh, M., & Cohen, I. (2001). Transient loss of speech after removal of posterior fossa tumors: One aspect of a larger neuropsychological entity: The cerebellar cognitive affective syndrome. *Pediatric Hematology and Oncology, 18,* 423–426.

Sanchez-Mejia, R. O., Chennupati, S. K., Gupta, N., Fullerton, H., Young, W. L., & Lawton, M. T. (2006). Superior outcomes in children compared with adults after microsurgical resection of brain arteriovenous malformations. *Journal of Neurosurgery, 105*(2, Suppl.), 82–87.

Satz, P. (1993). Brain reserve capacity on symptom onset after brain injury: A formulation and review of evidence for threshold theory. *Neuropsychology, 7,* 273–295.

Sauzeon, H., Lestage, P., Raboutet, C., N'Kaoua, B., & Claverie, B. (2004). Verbal fluency output in children aged 7–16 as a function of the production criterion: Qualitative analysis of clustering, switching processes, and semantic network exploitation. *Brain and Language, 89*(1), 192–202.

Schmahmann, J. D. (1991). An emerging concept: The cerebellar contribution to higher function. *Archives of Neurology, 48,* 1178–1185.

Schmahmann, J. D., & Sherman, J. C. (1998). The cerebellar cognitive affective syndrome. *Brain, 121* 561–579.

Shaw, P., Greenstein, D., Lerch, J., Clasen, L., Lenroot, R., Gogtay, N., et al. (2006a). Intellectual ability and cortical development in children and adolescents. *Nature, 440*(7084), 676–679.

Shaw, P., Lerch, J., Greenstein, D., Sharp, W., Clasen, L., Evans, A., et al. (2006b). Longitudinal mapping of cortical thickness and clinical outcome in children and adolescents with attention-deficit/hyperactivity disorder. *Archives of General Psychiatry, 63*(5), 540–549.

Sonuga-Barke, E. J. (2003). The dual pathway model of AD/HD: An elaboration of neurodevelopmental characteristics. *Neuroscience and Biobehavioral Reviews, 27*(7), 593–604.

Sonuga-Barke, E. J. (2005). Causal models of attention-deficit/hyperactivity disorder: From common simple deficits to multiple developmental pathways. *Biological Psychiatry, 57*(11), 1231–1238.

Stefanatos, G. A., & Baron, I. S. (2007). Attention deficit hyperactivity disorder (ADHD): A neuropsychological perspective towards DSM-V. *Neuropsychology Review, 17,* 5–38.

Stern, Y. (2002). What is cognitive reserve?: Theory and research application of the reserve concept. *Journal of the International Neuropsychological Society, 8,* 448–460.

Stern, Y. (2003). The concept of cognitive reserve: A catalyst for research. *Journal of Clinical and Experimental Neuropsychology, 25,* 589–593.

Stern, Y., Zarahn, E., Hilton, H. J., Flynn, J., DeLaPaz, R., & Rakitin, B. (2003). Exploring the neural basis of cognitive reserve. *Journal of Clinical and Experimental Neuropsychology, 25,* 691–701.

Stiles, J. (2008). *The fundamentals of brain development: Integrating nature and nurture.* Cambridge, MA: Harvard University Press.

Stiles, J., Bates, E., Thal, D. J., Trauner, D., & Reilly, J. (1998). Linguistic, cognitive, and affective development in children with pre- and perinatal focal brain injury: A ten-year overview from the San Diego Longitudinal Project. In C. Rovee-Collier, L. P. Lipsitt & H. Hayne (Eds.), *Advances in infancy research* (Vol. 12, pp. 131–163). Norwood, NJ: Ablex.

Stiles, J., Moses, P., Roe, K., Trauner, D., Hesselink, J., Wong, E., et al. (2003). Alternative brain organization after prenatal cerebral injury: Convergent fMRI and cognitive data. *Journal of the International Neuropsychological Society, 9,* 604–622.

Stiles, J., Reilly, J., Paul, B., & Moses, P. (2005). Cognitive development following early brain injury: Evidence for neural adaptation. *Trends in Cognitive Sciences*, 9(3), 136–143.

Taylor, H. G. (2006). Children born preterm or with very low birth weight can have both global and selective cognitive deficits. *Journal of Developmental and Behavioral Pediatrics*, 27(6), 485–486.

Taylor, H. G., & Alden, J. (1997). Age-related differences in outcomes following childhood brain insults: An introduction and overview. *Journal of the International Neuropsychological Society*, 3, 555–567.

Taylor, H. G., Klein, N., Minich, N. M., & Hack, M. (2001a). Long-term family outcomes for children with very low birth weights. *Archives of Pediatrics and Adolescent Medicine*, 155, 155–161.

Taylor, H. G., & Schatschneider, C. (1992). Child neuropsychological assessment: A test of basic assumptions. *The Clinical Neuropsychologist*, 6, 259–275.

Taylor, H. G., Yeates, K. O., Wade, S. L., Drotar, D., Stancin, T., & Burant, C. (2001b). Bidirectional child–family influences on outcomes of traumatic brain injury in children. *Journal of the International Neuropsychological Society*, 7, 755–767.

Thompson-Schill, S. L., Jonides, J., Marshuetz, C., Smith, E. E., D'Esposito, M., Kan, I. P., et al. (2002). Effects of frontal lobe damage on interference effects in working memory. *Cognitive, Affective, and Behavioral Neuroscience*, 2(2), 109–120.

Tranel, D., Adolphs, R., Damasio, H., & Damasio, A. R. (2001). A neural basis for the retrieval of words for actions. *Cognitive Neuropsychology*, 18, 655–670.

Troyer, A. K., Moscovitch, M., & Winocur, G. (1997). Clustering and switching as two components of verbal fluency: Evidence from younger and older healthy adults. *Neuropsychology*, 11, 138–146.

Troyer, A. K., Winocur, G., Craik, F. I. M., & Moscovitch, M. (1999). Source memory and divided attention: Reciprocal costs to primary and secondary tasks. *Neuropsychology*, 13, 467–474.

Vakil, E., & Hoffman, Y. (2004). Dissociation between two types of skill learning tasks: The differential effect of divided attention. *Journal of Clinical and Experimental Neuropsychology*, 26, 653–666.

Vallar, G., & Baddeley, A. (1984). Fractionation of working memory: Neuropsychological evidence for a phonological short-term store. *Journal of Verbal Learning and Verbal Behavior*, 23, 151–161.

van der Oord, S., Prins, P. J., Oosterlaan, J., & Emmelkamp, P. M. (2006). The association between parenting stress, depressed mood and informant agreement in ADHD and ODD. *Behaviour Research and Therapy*, 44(11), 1585–1595.

Vargha-Khadem, F., Carr, L. J., Isaacs, E., & Brett, E. (1997). Onset of speech after left hemispherectomy in a nine-year-old boy. *Brain*, 120(Pt. 1), 159–182.

Vohr, B. R., Allan, W., Westerveld, M., Schneider, K., Katz, K., Makuch, R. W., et al. (2003). School-age outcomes of very low birth weight infants in the indomethacin intraventricular hemorrhage prevention trial. *Pediatrics*, 111, e340–e346.

Vollmer, B., Roth, S., Riley, K., O'Brien, F., Baudin, J., De Haan, M., et al. (2006). Long-term neurodevelopmental outcome of preterm children with unilateral cerebral lesions diagnosed by neonatal ultrasound. *Early Human Development*, 82(10), 655–661.

Waber, D. P., Carlson, D., Mann, M., Merola, J., & Moylan, P. (1984). SES-related aspects of neuropsychological performance. *Child Development*, 55, 1878–1886.

Warburton, E., Wise, R. J., Price, C. J., Weiller, C., Hadar, U., Ramsay, S., et al. (1996). Noun and verb retrieval by normal subjects. Studies with PET. *Brain*, 119, 159–179.

Wilson, B. C. (1992). The neuropsychological assessment of the preschool child: A branching model. In I. Rapin & S. Segalowitz (Eds.), *Handbook of neuropsychology: Vol. 6. Child neuropsychology* (pp. 377–394). Amsterdam: Elsevier.

Wilson, B. C., & Finucci, D. H. (1986). A model for clinical-quantitative classification: Application to language-disordered preschool children. *Brain and Language*, 27, 282–309.

Wolff, P. H., & Melngailis, I. (1994). Family patterns of developmental dyslexia: Clinical findings. *American Journal of Medical Genetics*, 54(2), 122–131.

Wolff, P. H., Melngailis, I., & Kotwica, K. (1996). Family patterns of developmental dyslexia: Part III. Spelling errors as behavioral phenotype. *American Journal of Medical Genetics*, 67(4), 378–386.

Wolff, P. H., Melngailis, I., Obregon, M., & Bedrosian, M. (1995). Family patterns of developmental dyslexia: Part II. behavioral phenotypes. *American Journal of Medical Genetics*, 60(6), 494–505.

Woods, S. P., Scott, J. C., Sires, D. A., Grant, I., Heaton, R. K., Troster, A. I., et al. (2005). Action (verb) fluency: Test–retest reliability, normative standards, and construct validity. *Journal of the International Neuropsychological Society, 11*, 408–415.

Yeates, K. O., Ris, M. D., & Taylor, H. G. (Eds.). (2000). *Pediatric neuropsychology: Research, theory, and practice.* New York: Guilford Press.

Yeates, K. O., Swift, E., Taylor, H. G., Wade, S. L., Drotar, D., Stancin, T., et al. (2004). Short- and long-term social outcomes following pediatric traumatic brain injury. *Journal of the International Neuropsychological Society, 10*(3), 412–426.

Yeates, K. O., Taylor, H. G., Drotar, D., Wade, S., Stancin, T., & Klein, S. (1997). Preinjury family environment as a determinant of recovery from traumatic brain injury in school-age children. *Journal of the International Neuropsychological Society, 3*, 617–630.

Yeates, K. O., Taylor, H. G., Wade, S. L., Drotar, D., Stancin, T., & Minich, N. (2002). A prospective study of short- and long-term neuropsychological outcomes after traumatic brain injury in children. *Neuropsychology, 16*(4), 514–523.

CHAPTER 18

Interventions for Children with Neuropsychological Disorders

STEPHEN M. KANNE
MAUREEN O'KANE GRISSOM
JANET E. FARMER

Children with congenital and acquired brain disorders display a wide range of medical, cognitive, behavioral, emotional, social, and educational challenges that threaten to disrupt the course of normal development. Rapid technological and conceptual advances in the neurosciences show great potential to enhance our understanding of childhood brain disorders at the cellular, structural, and functional levels (Baron, 2004; Kolb, 2004). However, empirically based interventions that enhance the development of children with neurological impairments lag far behind.

In recent years, there has been a paradigm shift toward evidence-supported practices in psychology and in other health care fields (e.g., Chambless & Hollon, 1998; Kazdin & Weisz, 2003; Weisz, Hawley, Pilkonis, Woody, & Follette, 2000). This movement emphasizes treatments that have demonstrated efficacy as indicated by empirical evidence. These treatments are placed in a hierarchical framework based on an evaluation of the level of scientific rigor in available empirical studies. Many such hierarchies exist, all of which offer a system for classifying *levels of evidence* that separates research into categories defined by the quality of the methodology (e.g., Agency for Healthcare Research and Quality [AHRQ], 2002). These hierarchies can range from a few (e.g., three) to many more levels, and reflect the degree to which the methods are vulnerable to confounds and biases that interfere with the reliability and validity of the results. For example, the AHRQ recommends using five levels (see Table 18.1). Level 1 evidence includes randomized controlled trials (RCTs) and systemic reviews; Level 2 evidence includes cohort studies; and Level 3 evidence includes case–control studies (AHRQ, 2001).

TABLE 18.1. Levels of Evidence

Level	Type	Can include . . .
1a	Meta-analyses of multiple, well-designed studies	A systematic review that included at least one randomized controlled trial
1	Randomized controlled trials	Quasi-randomized processes
2	Nonrandomized controlled trials	Prospective studies with predetermined eligibility and outcome measures; quasi-experiments
3	Observational studies with controls	Retrospective, interrupted time series; case–control studies; cohort studies with controls; health services research adjusting for confounds
4	Observational studies without controls	Cohort studies without controls; case series

Note. Adapted from Agency for Healthcare Research and Quality (AHRQ, 2001).

Adhering to evidence-based practices and attending to levels of evidence may be especially important with regard to neuropsychological interventions. Unlike a clinical trial evaluating pharmaceutical treatment, interventions aimed at improving the outcomes of children with neurological conditions often involve cognitive and/or behavioral components that engender a range of additional confounds and obstacles (e.g., ethics of withholding treatment from a control group, recognizing experimenter bias, determining an appropriate comparison condition, defining the pivotal element of the intervention). Given the increased risk of experimental confounds and the prevalence of psychological interventions that have a popular following but no empirical support, the need for rigorous evidence becomes even more crucial. Thus, pediatric neuropsychologists interested in treatment should be aware of and attend to evidenced based treatments.

The purpose of this chapter is to provide an overview of the role of pediatric neuropsychologists in the design, implementation and evaluation of rehabilitation and educational treatments for children and youth. In addition, we provide examples of the state of the evidence from three diverse diagnostic groups: attention-deficit/hyperactivity disorder (ADHD), traumatic brain injury (TBI), and autism spectrum disorders (ASD). Finally, we address future directions for the field.

APPROACHES TO INTERVENTION

Professional practice in neuropsychology is grounded in an understanding of brain–behavior relationships, which provides an essential foundation for developing effective intervention programs for young people with neurological insults. Using standardized measures, neuropsychologists test hypotheses to clarify level of functioning and to describe a reliable and objective profile of each child's strengths and concerns (Baron, 2004). A thorough assessment not only includes estimates of cognitive and behavioral functioning, but also addresses how such factors as age, type of condition, persistent medical concerns, and environmental and cultural moderators either facilitate or interfere with maturation and recovery processes (Bernstein, 2000; Echemendia & Westerveld, 2006; Farmer & Deidrick, 2006; Taylor &

Alden, 1997). From the earliest writings of Luria (1963), a major goal of neuropsychological evaluation has been to identify interventions specifically tailored for each individual.

However, neuropsychologists often lack training in the design and implementation of interventions for children with brain-based impairments (Butler, 2006; Johnstone & Farmer, 1997). Historically, they have provided diagnostic and descriptive information about the nature and severity of cognitive impairments; assessed change in functioning over time; and provided recommendations to physicians, educators, family members, and others who support children in everyday settings. Others have proposed models that provide continual linkage between neuropsychological and other types of assessments and appropriate interventions (Teeter, 1997; Teeter & Semrud-Clikeman, 1995). For example, Teeter describes a staged model in which the first stages consist of structured behavioral and observational assessments with subsequent behavioral interventions. Later stages can include more extensive neuropsychological and medical evaluations that are used to develop more specific interventions. The assessment and consultation process in itself may have therapeutic effects. Parents report that such evaluations have value as a means of clarifying perceptions of their child, identifying ways to intervene at home and at school, and targeting other resources to support the child and family (Baron, 2004; Farmer & Brazeal, 1998).

In addition to consultation services, some pediatric neuropsychologists have delved further into direct treatment paradigms, working in rehabilitation or school settings to develop interventions that maximize functional child outcomes (Butler, 2006; D'Amato, Fletcher-Janzen, & Reynolds, 2005; Ylvisaker et al., 2005). Traditional cognitive rehabilitation therapies emphasize two approaches: (1) remediation strategies, which promote the acquisition of lost or delayed skills (deficits-focused); and (2) compensation strategies, which focus on the use of residual abilities and environmental supports to promote optimal functioning (strengths-focused). Intervention programs often combine these elements according to individual needs, and supplement cognitive interventions with behavioral management strategies. Factors that determine which approach to use include the individual's age and developmental level, severity of the brain insult, pattern of cognitive-behavioral strengths and weaknesses, and level of self-awareness (Lee & Riccio, 2005). Unlike adults, children and youth with central nervous system (CNS) impairments require a focus on strategies that promote the emergence of developmental milestones and the acquisition of many new skills (Ylvisaker, Chorazy, Feeny, & Russell, 1999). Ideally, interventions also must be sensitive to differing social and familial contexts and to the systems of care in which each child or youth is immersed (Farmer & Drewel, 2006).

Kolb (2004) proposes that rehabilitation researchers and practitioners develop new treatments based on a solid understanding of cortical plasticity and physiological processes associated with brain repair, such as neural sprouting, synaptogenesis, and reorganization of cortical maps. He points out that the capacity to change appears to be a fundamental characteristic of the CNS, and that such change is reflected in behavior. Thus, therapies that improve functional outcomes will be those that (1) stimulate morphological changes; (2) begin shortly after the injury occurs, to encourage optimal patterns of regeneration; (3) are comprehensive and multidimensional, addressing more than one aspect of recovery in a coordinated way; (4) include both behavioral and pharmacological therapies; and (5) vary according to such factors as age and gender. Technologies such as functional magnetic resonance brain imaging (fMRI), positron emission tomography, diffusion tensor imaging, and transcranial magnetic stimulation have the potential to identify changes in cerebral activation that are associated with improved outcomes following specific interventions, but this area of study is in its infancy.

The following sections present a brief overview of the types of cognitive, behavioral, and other interventions that have some empirical support for three different congenital or acquired brain disorders. Choosing these diverse disorders enables us to describe the commonalities and differences in various intervention approaches more clearly.

ATTENTION-DEFICIT/HYPERACTIVITY DISORDER

ADHD is a common childhood disorder estimated to affect between 4% and 12% of elementary school-age children. Depending on the diagnosed subtype, a different combination of inattention, hyperactivity, and impulsivity may be observed. The precise etiology of ADHD is still unclear, although evidence is consistent with biological rather than environmental causes. Numerous studies have supported a link between deficits seen in ADHD and specific regions of the brain, such as the frontal lobe, basal ganglia, and cerebellum (Barkley, 2002; see Willcutt, Chapter 14, this volume). Additional concerns outside the core deficits of ADHD have been noted in the areas of executive function, oppositional/ aggressive behavior, emotional regulation, social skills, memory, parent–child relationships, and academics (Barkley, 2002; Brown et al., 2001; Chhabildas, Pennington, & Willcutt, 2001; Klingberg et al., 2005; Willcutt, Pennington, & DeFries, 1999). Research also shows that children with ADHD have an increased risk of dropping out of school and experiencing social difficulties and substance abuse problems as adults (Barkley, 2002). This makes identification and treatment of ADHD a high priority, and neuropsychologists are often consulted to assess children with the disorder.

There is a vast literature in the area of intervention for children with ADHD. The major avenues of intervention include pharmacological, behavioral, or cognitive intervention; parent training; environmental modifications; or some combination thereof. Several research studies have attempted to address the question of which intervention or combination of interventions is most effective for treating children with ADHD. The 2007 American Academy of Child and Adolescent Psychiatry (AACAP) Practice Parameter relies heavily on the National Institute of Mental Health (NIMH) Multimodal Treatment Study of Children with ADHD (MTA) finding that pharmacological treatment is effective in treating the core symptoms of ADHD (Pliszka, 2007). However, the AACAP document maintains that in certain clinical situations (e.g., an ADHD diagnosis that is unclear, parental refusal of medication, extremely mild ADHD symptoms), behavior therapy alone may be the first step in treatment.

In 1998, Pelham, Wheeler, and Chronis concluded that only three validated interventions were effective as short-term treatments for ADHD: behavior modification, psychostimulants, and the combination of these two. This section explores results from subsequent major studies of cognitive intervention, behavioral intervention, and other approaches, with discussion of pharmacological intervention as it relates to these categories. Alternative approaches, such as electroencephalographic neurofeedback training, nutritional supplements, dietary management, hypnotherapy, relaxation training, guided imagery, and vision therapy, have also been investigated and have lower levels of evidence; therefore, they remain controversial and are not addressed in this section (Baydala & Wikman, 2001).

Cognitive Interventions

Numerous studies have attempted to remediate symptoms of inattention through laboratory-based attentional training activities. Unfortunately, such approaches are often plagued with conceptual and methodological concerns (Ponsford & Wilmott, 2004; Ylvisaker et al., 2005). However, a recent RCT (i.e., Level 1) involving children with ADHD found that computerized attention training was associated with improved performance in the areas of working memory and response inhibition, as well as improved parental ratings of attention and hyperactivity–impulsivity (Klingberg et al., 2005).

Riccio and French (2004) reviewed and critiqued attention training research by rating various cognitive intervention models (e.g., attention process training [APT], attention training system, and biofeedback) aimed at restoring attentional abilities for children with ADHD and other conditions that affect attention, such as TBI. Ratings were based on the methodology of the study (e.g., RCT, case report) and the results of the study (positive, negative, or inconclusive). The majority of studies were found lacking in some respect, in that they used case report, case series without controls, or nonrandomized trials. The authors determined that the evidence was insufficient to allow solid conclusions to be drawn about these interventions for attention deficits. APT received the highest rating for an intervention aimed at children, but still only received tentative support.

In addition to questions about short-term intervention effects, these studies did not report successful generalization to real-world activities. One problem, for example, is that real-world activities tend to be more complex than those in the training setting and take place under markedly different environmental conditions (Ponsford & Wilmott, 2004; Ylvisaker et al., 2005). Ponsford and Wilmott (2004) suggest that there may be ways to address this problem, such as the use of massed practice focusing on specific elements of more complex activities, until the activity becomes automatic and the demand on the controlled attention processing system is reduced. Clearly, attention interventions must focus on ways to transfer improvements to everyday settings for these interventions to have true utility.

Behavioral Interventions

The NIMH MTA followed 579 children with ADHD over 14 months and found that different treatments worked best for particular outcomes (Jensen et al., 2001). The study compared four conditions, including medication management, intensive behavioral treatment, a combination of these two interventions, and an untreated community control. The medication management and combination groups were found to be equally effective in decreasing the core ADHD symptoms of inattention, hyperactivity, and impulsivity. Both of these were superior to behavioral treatment alone or to the control condition. For selected outcomes outside the core symptoms of ADHD (e.g., oppositional/aggressive symptoms, internalizing symptoms, and academic functioning), the combination intervention was the only condition that evidenced better outcomes than the control condition. Thus these results indicate that medication alone improves the core ADHD symptoms; however, only the combination of medication and intensive behavioral treatment improves noncore ADHD symptoms.

Following the NIMH MTA's conclusion that behavioral intervention on its own is not sufficient to ameliorate the core symptoms of ADHD, Pelham et al. (2000) examined a subset of 60 unmedicated and 57 medicated children from the NIMH database who attended a summer program that consisted of an intensive behavioral intervention, in order to evaluate whether the intensity of treatment would affect the MTA findings. They found that the addition of medication resulted in only minimal incremental gains in functioning (assessed via a range of dependent variables, including peer sociometric ratings, parent satisfaction ratings, teacher and counselor ratings, and child self-perception ratings) when the behavioral intervention was "active and intensive" (p. 520). In addition to multiple methods of assessment, numerous symptoms (including both core and noncore symptoms) were assessed, and results indicated that the groups of medicated and unmedicated children receiving intensive behavioral intervention did not differ significantly on 81 out of 87 dependent measures (Pelham et al., 2000). Medication has been shown to enhance selective attention (Ponsford & Wilmott, 2004) and may increase an individual's ability to respond to behavioral treatments, but when the behavioral treatment is intensive, this boost may not be as necessary.

In school settings, antecedent controls and environmental modifications are commonly used by educators and are generally aimed at minimizing the effects of attentional and behavioral difficulties on the academic functioning of children with ADHD. There are many such modifications; they include such interventions as seating a child close to and in direct view of the teacher, reducing extraneous stimuli in the environment, and providing cues and prompts (Riccio & French, 2004). One study investigated choice making as a form of antecedent control for a 7-year-old boy with ADHD and found that when he was given a choice of assignments, his problematic behaviors decreased (Powell & Nelson, 1997). A meta-analysis by DuPaul and Eckert (1997) concluded that school-based interventions were effective in reducing problematic behavior (with effect sizes in the moderate to higher ranges), but effect sizes were smaller and frequently nonsignificant for academic outcomes. However, most studies included in the meta-analysis were not RCTs. This 1997 meta-analysis included between-subjects, within-subjects, and single-subject designs that assessed baseline data, allowing for estimation of effect sizes.

Other Interventions

In the past few years, behavioral parent training (BPT) has emerged as an empirically supported intervention for ADHD that can be delivered to individual parents or parent groups (Chronis, Chacko, Fabiano, Wymbs, & Pelham, 2004). Parents generally receive education about ADHD and behavior management principles. Then they learn to establish behavioral goals for the child with ADHD that can modified across time as goals are reached. However, such factors as parental mental health, age of the child, and the child's comorbid features may influence the degree to which BPT is appropriate and may affect parental adherence and child outcomes (Chronis et al., 2004). These methodological concerns were addressed in a recent RCT of BPT (twelve 120-minute sessions with six parents per group) conducted in the Netherlands (van den Hoofdakker et al., 2007). In conjunction with routine clinical care consisting of family support and (for some children in the study) medication management, BPT was helpful in improving noncore symptoms of ADHD (e.g., internalizing and externalizing problems), but it did not improve core symptoms or reduce parenting stress. This finding held both for children who were treated pharmacologically and for those who were not.

In sum, numerous interventions are available for ADHD, some with extensive empirical support (e.g., stimulant medication). However, it is still not completely clear which treatments or combination of treatments are most effective for which children. The brain's attentional system is complex and multidimensional, suggesting that a variety of rehabilitation methods will be required (Ponsford & Wilmott, 2004). Though the empirical basis for the use of stimulant medication is strong, the evidence supporting other interventions, such as behavioral approaches, has not been as well validated. Future research should continue to identify effective interventions and combinations of interventions, focus on provision of services in real-life settings, and improve research methodology through use of randomized control groups and diagnostically homogeneous groups (Riccio & French, 2004).

TRAUMATIC BRAIN INJURY

TBI is defined as any form of abrupt insult to the brain caused by an outside, mechanical impact, such as a blow to the head (Donders, 2006; see Yeates, Chapter 5, this volume). Annually, an average of approximately 18 per 10,000 children in the United States are hospitalized due to head injury (Kraus, 1995). Although it had previously been thought that a child's brain was less susceptible to damage than an adult's (the so-called "Kennard principle"), it is now clear that both immediate and long-term effects are often seen in children who sustain TBI during childhood (Taylor & Alden, 1997; Thomson & Kerns, 2000).

There is no universal profile of postinjury sequelae, but some of the more common difficulties following moderate to severe pediatric TBI include deficits in speed of information processing, learning/recall of complex new information, attention, executive function, adaptive behavior, and higher-order language skills (Brookshire, Levin, Song, & Zhang, 2004; Donders & Giroux, 2005; Wozniak et al., 2007; Yeates et al., 2005; Yeates & Taylor, 2005). The type and degree of deficit are typically related to the location and severity of the initial neurological insult. Children with TBI also exhibit more behavior problems than children with orthopedic injuries (Ganesalingam, Sanson, Anderson, & Yeates, 2006; Schwartz et al., 2003). Functional neuroimaging techniques have shed light on the pathophysiology of TBI (Munson, Schroth, & Ernst, 2006), but at the present time these techniques do not yield information that would translate easily into the design of interventions. Therefore, neuropsychologists must assess cognitive and behavioral functioning in children and adolescents who have sustained TBI, and plan interventions for use in residential, rehabilitation, and educational settings based on these data. The majority of intervention studies in the area of pediatric TBI tend to be cognitive or behavioral in nature, although there are also some package approaches and interventions aimed at assisting in the return to school and the family's coping with pediatric TBI (Ganesalingam et al., 2006).

Cognitive Interventions

In two recent reviews of intervention for children with TBI, Laatsch et al. (2007) reviewed available evidence regarding cognitive and behavioral interventions, and Limond and Leeke (2005) considered evidence in key areas of neuropsychological functioning: attention, memory, and executive functioning. The Limond and Leeke (2005) review uncovered no Level 1 RCTs, a limited number of studies that even included a control, and all but one study with a sample size of 10 or less. They identified only two published intervention studies that addressed attentional deficits following TBI, using Sohlberg and Mateer's (1989) APT method adapted for a pediatric sample (Sohlberg & Mateer, 1989; Thomson, 1995; Thomson & Kerns, 2000). Results of both Thomson studies suggested improvement in attention, with one study also suggesting gains in executive functioning after APT—an approach involving stepwise visual and auditory activities intended to assist in retraining attention and concentration, based on the notion that repeated activation of attentional systems may result in changes in capacity. However, neither study included a control group, making it difficult to establish solid support for the effect of the treatment on these areas of cognitive functioning in children.

The Laatsch et al. (2007) review identified one Level 1 study, that of Braga, Da Paz Júnior, and Ylvisaker (2005), which was an RCT conducted in Brazil to examine the effects of family-supported versus clinician-delivered rehabilitation. This study was directed at examining the context in which intervention took place, rather than the efficacy of a particular cognitive intervention, and is discussed below as a study of a comprehensive intervention program. In the area of memory functioning, the Limond and Leeke (2005) and Laatsch et al. (2007) reviews identified a few isolated studies of interventions aimed at the remediation of memory deficits in children with TBI. For instance, elaborate encoding strategies have been shown to result in significant effects on learning and recall of the definitions of age-appropriate words (Frazen, Roberts, Schmidts, Verduyn, & Manshadi, 1996; Oberg & Turkustra, 1998).

In the area of executive dysfunction, there was a similar paucity of intervention studies (Limond & Leeke, 2005). However, a study by Suzman, Morris, Morris, and Milan (1997) incorporated a combined package of (1) self-instruction training (self-directed statements used to guide oneself through the problem-solving process); (2) self-regulation training (establishment of a goal, monitoring one's own progress toward the goal, and rewarding oneself when the goal is reached); (3) metacognitive training (assistance in how to identify what steps to take when facing a particular problem); (4) attribution training (identification of the relationship between effort and successful performance); and (5) reinforcement for successful problem solving, as well as for appropriate use of the strategies described above. This treatment package resulted in improved performance on standardized problem-solving measures, a decrease in the number of errors on a computerized problem-solving task, and improvement in the problem-solving ability of five participants with moderate to severe TBI (Suzman et al., 1997). Others have found that direct instruction (an approach incorporating task analysis, modeling, and shaping) resulted in improved task performance and some degree of generalization to academic functioning in such areas as math facts, basic reading skills, spelling, reasoning skills, and keyboarding (Glang, Singer, Cooley, & Tish, 1992). The Glang et al. study consisted of three case studies with outcome measures that were not standardized, but instead were measures of percent correct from the instructional programs described. Overall, reviews indicate that there are few intervention studies in the area of cognitive intervention for children and adolescents with TBI, and that the existing studies suffer from methodological flaws, such as lack of control groups and small sample size.

Behavioral Interventions

Behavioral interventions for children and adolescents with TBI are generally directed at decreasing challenging behaviors and improving academic behaviors, according to a review by Gurdin, Huber, and Cochran (2005). Nine intervention studies that took place in rehabilitation or therapeutic settings were generally conducted during other therapy sessions (e.g., speech–language, occupational, or physical therapies), and included various reinforcement procedures with the goal of assisting children and adolescents to attain their therapeutic goals and return home. Two of the nine identified studies in this area suggested that combining reinforcement with behavioral procedures such as antecedent control and shaping may reduce noncompliant behavior and increase the likelihood of reaching therapeutic goals (Hegel, 1988; Silver & Stelly-Seitz, 1992). However, this base of research support is again limited by the lack of Level 1 RCT support. The majority of the studies reviewed were single-subject designs or included a sample of fewer than 10 participants with no control group. At the time of the Laatsch et al. (2007) review, which covered both cognitive and behavioral intervention studies, still no Level 1 or Level 2 studies assessing behavioral intervention had been identified in the pediatric TBI literature.

Use of functional analysis strategies to determine variables maintaining problematic behaviors for children with TBI, combined with functional communication training and response extinction, was also supported as a method of decreasing aggressive and self-injurious behaviors for children with TBI (Treadwell & Page, 1996). Other studies have reported the use of differential reinforcement and other operant techniques to decrease maladaptive behaviors during rehabilitation (Slifer, Cataldo, & Kurtz, 1995; Slifer et al., 1997).

In general, studies that took place in school or residential settings analyzed antecedent conditions to determine the function of particular behaviors in children and adolescents with TBI (e.g., aggressive behavior helped children avoid cognitively challenging work) and provided them with cognitive-behavioral supports that addressed deficits in executive functioning (e.g., plan–do–review routines). One recent intervention study found that a behavioral intervention package including classroom rules, a token economy with response cost, and the use of "mystery motivators" was successful in reducing problematic behavior (Mottram & Berger-Gross, 2004). Again, however, it must be noted that these studies were based on small sample sizes with no control groups.

Ylvisaker et al. (2005), reviewing 20 years of rehabilitation and community supports for children and youth with TBI, advocated for comprehensive intervention programs rather than isolated cognitive or behavioral interventions. They noted the inseparability of cognition, executive functioning, and behavioral issues following brain injury, and provided initial evidence for the efficacy of flexible, multicomponent treatment paradigms as opposed to cognitive exercises and other decontextualized interventions. This integrated program for children with TBI included positive behavioral supports with antecedent controls, an emphasis on organizational and metacognitive strategies, and contextual interventions using everyday events to enhance cognitive processing and improve functional outcomes. Since that review, one RCT comparing clinician-delivered care (n = 34) and family-supported intervention (n = 38) in Brazilian children ages 5–12 who had sustained TBI has been published (Braga et al., 2005). The study followed children for 1 year, and findings supported the suggestion above that contextual interventions resulted in better cognitive and physical outcomes (as measured by the Wechsler Intelligence Scale for Children—Third Edition and the Substance Abuse Recovery and HIV/AIDS [SARAH] Scale of Motor Development).

In considering specific cognitive and behavioral rehabilitation strategies in such programs, Ylvisaker and Szekeres (1998) have described key issues for children and youth. These take into account remediation and compensation strategies, as well as the critical element of support for normal developmental progressions. Their 12 cardinal rules for cognitive rehabilitation following TBI are presented in Table 18.2, but these are also likely to apply to children and youth with many other neurological conditions. Because of the similarities in cognitive challenges across diagnostic groups, Ylvisaker et al. (2005) have also recommended the use of research-based instructional strategies originally developed for students with learning difficulties for reasons other than TBI. These strategies include appropriate pacing; facilitation of high rates of success (e.g., through environmental structuring and errorless learning paradigms); task analysis and advance organizers; frequent practice and review; initial instruction to the point of mastery; support for transfer of training/generalization; flexible teaching strategies shaped by ongoing assessment; and curriculum modifications tailored to the individual.

Finally, in their review of the literature regarding behavioral management, Ylvisaker et al. (2005) found emerging evidence for use of positive behavioral supports for children with neurological conditions, as opposed to traditional applied behavior analysis (ABA). Positive behavioral supports target meaningful lifestyle change rather than changes in individual behaviors; use of antecedent controls rather than heavy reliance on contingency manage-

---

TABLE 18.2. Twelve Key Issues for Cognitive Rehabilitation in Children with Neurological Conditions

1. Follow normal progressions in cognitive development (e.g., from surface to depth, concrete to abstract).
2. Build a knowledge base by helping the child to acquire meaningful new content.
3. Target the efficiency of cognitive processing.
4. Teach organizing strategies that increase memory capacity in real-life settings until they become habituated.
5. Use an approach balanced among targeted cognitive activities, compensation strategies, and environmental structuring based on each child's short- and long-term goals.
6. Support generalization of new learning to real-world tasks.
7. Provide services in a meaningful context to support daily living, academic, social, vocational, and recreational goals.
8. Consider the importance of motivation and executive functioning, and actively teach strategies to enhance performance as well as new learning.
9. Integrate and organize training activities over time, and avoid setting too many goals at once.
10. Teach all adults to be cognitive coaches and to engage in effective behavior management strategies.
11. Provide a high level of support initially, and reduce it only as a child is able to succeed.
12. Teach adults the link between cognitive impairments and behavior problems in children with brain insults.

Note. Adapted from Ylvisaker and Szekeres (1998). Copyright 1998 by Elsevier. Adapted by permission.

ment; behavior change in natural settings and through everyday activities rather than in clinics; and use of natural change agents (e.g., parents or teachers) in consultation with behavior specialists. Their recommended interventions have the potential advantage of supporting generalization of new learning and maintenance of behavioral improvements.

Other Interventions

Researchers have recently turned their attention to interventions with the families of children who have sustained TBI, now that research has found such systems to have an impact on child outcomes following neurological insults (Farmer & Drewel, 2006; Hibbard, Martin, Cantor, & Moran, 2006; Wade, 2006; Ylvisaker et al., 2005). Family-centered care values the family as the constant in a child's life, insists on collaboration and open communication between family members and healthcare professionals, encourages family-to-family supports, and designs systems of care to be responsive to family needs. Research has shown that this approach results in increased family satisfaction with care, parental well-being, family adjustment, and parental self-efficacy, as well as improvements in child academic achievement and ratings of self-worth (Naar-King & Donders, 2006; Wade, 2006).

As an example of parent-focused interventions, Wade, Michaud, and Brown (2006b) conducted an RCT to test a seven-session problem-solving intervention with 32 families of children with TBI. Based on parental report, children in the problem-solving group (as opposed to the usual-care group) showed greater improvement in the areas of withdrawal, anxious/depressive symptoms, and internalizing symptoms. Wade, Carey, and Wolfe (2006a) subsequently modified this intervention by making it an online family problem-solving therapy, which included problem-solving training in addition to training in other skills (such as antecedent behavior management) that are appropriate for pediatric TBI. Both of the Wade et al. studies included random assignment to conditions and had larger sample sizes than studies previously discussed.

In sum, cognitive and behavioral interventions hold promise in addressing many of the postinjury sequelae of pediatric TBI both in rehabilitation settings and at school, especially when these strategies can be integrated into a comprehensive treatment program. Traditional methods of intervention tend to address specific deficits, whereas more recent methods pursue a more comprehensive approach that builds on existing strengths. However, more research is needed to establish the effectiveness of these interventions in comparison to control groups, to increase sample sizes, and to identify ways to generalize learned skills to novel tasks and environments. Some of the recent research in the area of family-level interventions appears to better address these methodological concerns and has garnered support for family-level training in problem solving and the use of interventions in natural settings.

Based on the results of what would be considered Level 1 and Level 2 studies, Laatsch et al. (2007) have derived evidence-based recommendations. They concluded that professionals working with the pediatric TBI population should consider attention remediation strategies to enhance the recovery process, and that family members of the affected child or adolescent should be considered for active involvement as providers in the treatment plan. Recommendations regarding specific strategies to address the other areas above could not be made, based on the research evidence available at the time of the 2007 review.

AUTISM SPECTRUM DISORDERS

ASD involve impairments in communication and social skills, together with characteristic behaviors. Recent estimates of the prevalence of ASD have ranged as high as 1 per 150 (Chakrabarti & Fombonne, 2005; Charman, 2002; Fombonne, 2005; Yeargin-Allsopp et al., 2003), making these the second most common developmental disability (behind intellectual impairment), with increases in both incidence (Rutter, 2005) and prevalence (Fombonne, 2005); however, some researchers believe that methodological factors could account for much of the increase in prevalence (see Ozonoff, Chapter 15, this volume, for a discussion). With more children being identified as possibly having ASD, neuropsychologists are being asked more frequently to assess their behavioral and cognitive functioning. ASD are regarded as heterogeneous, genetically based neurological disorders involving both structural and functional changes in the brain. Research has identified a range of structural abnormalities in the brains of individuals with ASD, including differences in total brain volume, corpus callosum, left planum temporale, left inferior prefrontal gyrus, anterior cingulated cortex, hippocampus, amygdala, and cerebellum (see Minshew, Sweeney, Bauman, & Webb, 2005). Imaging studies (e.g., fMRI) have found differences in the brain areas associated with language (responding to vocal vs. nonvocal sounds, sentence comprehension—e.g., superior temporal sulcus), face perception (e.g., fusiform gyrus, amygdala), social cognition (e.g., dorsomedial prefrontal cortex), and executive functioning (e.g., dorsolateral prefrontal cortex) between individuals with ASD and typical controls (Schultz & Robins, 2005). No consistent pattern of neurological insult has been identified among those with ASD, underscoring the heterogeneity in ASD (cf. Volkmar, Lord, Bailey, Schultz, & Klin, 2004).

Several theories have evolved that attempt to explain the behavioral and functional difficulties associated with ASD. For example, some posit that deficits in executive functioning can account for many of the difficulties observed in ASD, such as problems with planning effectively or thinking abstractly (e.g., Ozonoff & Jensen, 1999). However, executive functioning deficits are seen in disorders that do not share the other features of ASD, and they do not account for all of the difficulties observed. To better account for the core symptoms of ASD, many variants of social-cognitive theories have arisen. These include the ability of children to take the perspective of others—an ability termed *theory of mind* (Baron-Cohen, Leslie, & Frith, 1985)—and the development of basic social-communicative skills such as joint attention (Mundy & Burnette, 2005). The *central coherence theory* (Frith, 2006) attempts to account for a specific pattern of difficulties that many individuals with ASD demonstrate, wherein they appear to focus on details and overlook the broader picture or overarching context.

Given the immense variety of behavioral and cognitive manifestations with which ASD can present, one can also appreciate the challenges in finding an effective treatment or intervention for the disorder. As Sigman, Spence, and Wang (2006) note,

> . . . significant progress has been made in identifying the core deficits in autism, arriving at criterion for the diagnosis, and in creating and testing diagnostic instruments that are reliable and valid. In contrast, less progress has been made in identifying the causes of autism or in creating and, particularly, in testing interventions aimed at the remediation of the deficits in autism. This is true for the amelioration of both the core deficits and associated symptoms manifested by individuals with autism. (p. 343)

Although numerous studies have been conducted exploring many different interventions, this research has problems with methodology and other design issues, such as randomized assignment. This led the Committee on Educational Interventions for Children with Autism to conclude in 2001 that the extant literature examining the efficacy of treatment does not meet required standards (National Research Council, 2001).

Cognitive Interventions

Several developmentally based programs have arisen to address concerns related to ASD, such as the Treatment and Education of Autistic and related Communcation-handicapped CHildren (TEACCH) program out of North Carolina and the Denver model, and these have enjoyed some empirical support. As Ozonoff, South, and Provencal (2005) note, these approaches tend to address social and communication difficulties and often take a more comprehensive approach involving other contexts (such as the school), but can also employ techniques that are behavioral and/or cognitive in nature. For example, the TEACCH program targets specific cognitive domains for improvement, such as executive, language, and visual–spatial skills; breaks down complex tasks into component parts; and then teaches necessary skills in order of increasing complexity, while also emphasizing compensatory strategies. Note that, of these types of programs, only the TEACCH program has published a controlled outcome study (Rogers, 1998).

Behavioral Interventions

Early and intense ABA therapy (e.g., Green, 1996) is the one intervention consistently cited as having the most empirical support (Clark, Tuesday-Heathfield, Olympia, & Jenson, 2006). O. Ivor Lovaas, while working with the Early Autism Project at UCLA, developed a program wherein children who participated in a one-on-one operant-style paradigm made remarkable progress in a number of important areas (Lovaas, 1987). However, this type of therapy has also garnered some criticism because of its strict discrete-trial approach and its difficulties in generalizing the skills learned to other contexts. Pivotal response treatment (PRT), another behavioral approach, identifies a behavior or response (e.g., being motivated to respond to social stimuli) that affects a wide range of other behaviors, so that changing this pivotal area has a widespread impact on an individual's functioning (Burke & Cerniglia, 1990; Koegel, Koegel, Harrower, & Carter, 1999). Koegel and others have conducted several studies that examine the efficacy of a PRT approach, some of which used random assignment to groups and/or multiple-baseline designs (see Koegel, Koegel, & Brookman, 2003, for a review).

Other Interventions

Other types of interventions have been developed specifically to target the core social and communicative difficulties in ASD. These interventions have obtained some empirical support, though without the same level of scientific rigor as that for the behavioral approach (Clark et al., 2006; Myers, Johnson, & U.S. Council on Children with Disabilities, 2007). With regard to social interaction deficits, these include peer-mediated interventions (e.g., prompting and reinforcing peers to initiate), related skills interventions (e.g., teaching communication and play skills), structured environment interventions (e.g., creating structured play groups), and direct skills interventions (e.g., self-monitoring of behaviors). For functional communication deficits, ABA interventions have been successful, as have functional equivalence training programs (e.g., teaching and reinforcing communication skills to replace problem behavior) and alternative communication interventions (e.g., picture exchange communication systems, sign language). Occupational therapy has been used to address and promote adaptive skills. Shaping and extinction have been successful in addressing aggressive and/or self-stimulatory behaviors, as have differential reinforcing, communication interventions (e.g., verbal directives such as "stop") and aversive interventions (e.g., time out, response cost, overcorrection). Note that many of these interventions continue to rely on behavioral principles (e.g., reinforcement, shaping). Also, pharmacological interventions, such as the use of risperidone, have been receiving more attention and have demonstrated some success (Clark et al., 2006). However, despite having supporters with compelling testimonials, interventions such as Vitamin B, sensory integration, secretin, facilitated communication, and auditory integration have little to no rigorous empirical support.

In sum, the heterogeneity of ASD has made it difficult to develop effective interventions to address these disorders in all of their manifestations. Moreover, although many different therapies exist and may have garnered a degree of "grassroots" support, not many have been subjected to sound and rigorous methodological assessment of their efficacy—which is essential to promoting and extending their use. Intense behavioral interventions have the most empirical support, with pharmacological approaches (e.g., risperidone) and developmental approaches such as TEACCH and the Denver model also receiving some empirical substantiation. However, at the time Lord et al. (2005) reviewed the literature, there were only three published studies using RCT to examine treatment outcome after psychosocial intervention (i.e., a parent training intervention, a caregiver-based intervention in day care centers, and a study of the Lovaas treatment model), leading to their recommendation that RCTs investigating the efficacy of psychosocial treatment should have the highest priority.

Neuropsychologists are often called upon to assess individuals with ASD, and can contribute much to the understanding of these individuals' cognitive and neuropsychological abilities. Given the broad impact that an ASD has on an individual's development and cognitive skills, a neuropsychological approach can be informative in guiding interventions across a variety of settings. As the understanding of the brain basis for social behaviors expands, neuropsychologists can play an important role in developing the tools needed to measure these skills in a standardized manner. The strong emphasis on the individual's behavioral presentation and history, upon which the current manner of diagnosing an ASD ultimately relies, suggests that neuropsychologists need to become increasingly adept at assessing areas outside traditional cognitive domains.

SUMMARY AND FUTURE DIRECTIONS

This survey of interventions for children and youth with neurological conditions is notable for the similarities in approach to treatment across disability types, and yet it is also remarkable for the limited cross-fertilization of intervention approaches (Butler, 2006; Ylvisaker et al., 2005). In general, common approaches include memory and attention training, specialized instruction for academic learning, metacognitive and organizational strategies, use of positive behavioral supports and environmental structure, emphasis on functional outcomes in real-life situations, and interventions with families and other social/peer contexts. As noted, maintaining attention to evidence-based practices and continuing to conduct studies that meet criteria for the highest levels of evidence will be especially important with regard to neuropsychological interventions. Key issues for advances in intervention research include the following:

1. *Methodological improvements.* Studies are limited by such methodological challenges as small sample size, lack of comparison groups, poor definition of groups, and lack of standardized treatment strategies. Furthermore, methods of matching treatment to an individual child are lacking. These limitations create difficulties in assessing the efficacy of treatment interventions, and also enhance the opportunity for less effective or even harmful interventions to remain viable options for families. Thus there is a great need to study interventions with more rigorous attention to methodology that aspires to meet evidence-based criteria for the highest level of evidence, whenever possible.

2. *Theoretical framework.* There is a need for a unifying theoretical base for intervention programs that would operate and guide practice across presenting disorders. One promising model is the World Health Organization (2001) framework for health and disability. This framework proposes that outcomes are multiply determined by the nature of physical, cognitive, and behavioral impairments; resulting level of functioning; and ability to participate in social roles. It underscores the need to consider these factors in the context of individual differences and environmental influences. This framework has the potential to promote understanding of common approaches to intervention across disability types, and yet it also allows for the development of specific interventions for unique aspects of each child's disability and environmental context.

3. *Developmental perspective.* Treatment interventions must differ according to age and developmental level. Although this seems like a fundamental premise in pediatric neuropsychology, few studies have examined ways to enhance cognitive and behavioral functioning at different ages or developmental levels. Nor have there been enough studies that examine the longitudinal course of recovery over time or the interventions that sustain positive outcomes from childhood to adulthood and beyond.

4. *Psychological adjustment.* Interventions to promote adjustment to disability will be necessary for many children and youth, given the high rate of depression and similar concerns in this group (Wallander & Varni, 1998). Such interventions are essential for supporting motivation to engage in rehabilitation and educational treatments. Neuropsychologists, with their unique training that combines knowledge of psychosocial interventions and therapeutic techniques with knowledge regarding the impact of brain disorders on functioning, are well positioned to develop interventions that address psychological concerns.

5. *Comprehensive and coordinated care.* Children with neurological conditions often receive services not only from pediatric neuropsychologists, but also from numerous other professionals (e.g., educators, community agencies, therapists, primary and specialty physicians) in a variety of settings. For optimal outcomes, children need comprehensive and coordinated care from an interdisciplinary team in their home community (Farmer, Clark, & Marien, 2003). Pediatric neuropsychologists, with their broad focus on child and family

strengths and concerns, are well suited to play a leadership role on these teams and to help coordinate each child's care across disciplines and settings.

6. *Family-centered care.* As several lines of research have demonstrated (Wade, 2006), the role of the family in supporting and maintaining care for the individual with a disability is very important. Moreover, the entire family is affected when a child or youth experiences a disability. This observation often leads a pediatric neuropsychologist to make recommendations regarding the need for family counseling or support services. Successful interventions should include provisions for family-centered care.

7. *Integration of neuroscience with treatment modalities.* As the current survey of interventions for three common diagnostic groups has made clear, rarely is a clear link drawn between intervention approach and underlying cerebral injury or preserved brain functioning (Ponsford, 2004). As we learn more about cortical plasticity, especially in the developing brain, and as science better identifies the brain mechanisms underlying many of the disorders with which pediatric neuropsychologists are confronted, more specific interventions firmly grounded in neuroscience can be designed and implemented (Kolb, 2004).

8. *Public policy.* Effective interventions have no utility if families cannot access them. There must be policies in place that encourage the translation of new treatments into practice through well-funded internship and postdoctoral training programs, as well as continuing education initiatives. In addition, access to services must be encouraged through adequate health insurance coverage, enhanced public agency funding, and seamless systems of care.

Pediatric neuropsychology is still in its infancy, especially in regard to interventions that support optimal child development. We are likely to make strides in our understanding of various disorders, including their underlying pathophysiology and impact on children's functioning. Translating this knowledge into effective interventions that successfully address cognitive, behavioral, and psychosocial concerns should be a top priority.

REFERENCES

Agency for Healthcare Research and Quality (AHRQ). (2001). *Making health care safer: A critical analysis of patient safety practices* (Evidence Report/Technology Assessment No. 43, AHRQ Publication No. 01-E058). Rockville, MD: Author. (Available at *www.ahrq.gov/clinic/ptsafety*)

Agency for Healthcare Research and Quality (AHRQ). (2002). *Systems to rate the strength of scientific evidence. Summary* (Evidence Report/Technology Assessment No. 47, AHRQ Publication No. 02-E015). Rockville, MD: Author. (Available at *www.ahrq.gov/clinic/epcsums/strengthsum.htm*)

Barkley, R. A. (2002). Consensus statement on ADHD. *European Child and Adolescent Psychiatry, 11*, 96–98.

Baron-Cohen, S., Leslie, A. M., & Frith, U. (1985). Does the autistic child have a "theory of mind"? *Cognition, 21*, 37–46.

Baron, I. S. (2004). *Neuropsychological evaluation of the child.* New York: Oxford University Press.

Baydala, L., & Wikman, E. (2001). The efficacy of neurofeedback in the management of children with attention deficit/hyperactivity disorder. *Paediatrics Child Health, 6*(7), 451–455.

Bernstein, J. H. (2000). Developmental neuropsychological assessment. In K. O. Yeates, M. D. Ris, & H. G. Taylor (Eds.), *Pediatric neuropsychology: Research, theory, and practice* (pp. 405–438). New York: Guilford Press.

Braga, L. W., Da Paz Júnior, A. C., & Ylvisaker, M. (2005). Direct clinician-delivered versus indirect family-supported rehabilitation of children with traumatic brain injury: A randomized controlled trial. *Brain Injury, 19*(10), 819–831.

Brookshire, B., Levin, H. S., Song, J., & Zhang, L. (2004). Components of executive function in typically developing and head-injured children. *Developmental Neuropsychology, 25*(1–2), 61–83.

Brown, R. T., Freeman, W., Perrin, J. M., Stein, M. T., Amler, R. W., Feldman, H. M., et al. (2001). Prevalence and assessment of attention-deficit/hyperactivity disorder in primary care settings [Electronic version]. *Pediatrics, 107*, e43. Retrieved from *pediatrics.aappublications.org/cgi/content/full/107/3/e43*

Burke, J. C., & Cerniglia, L. (1990). Stimulus complexity and autistic children's responsivity: Assessing and training a pivotal behavior. *Journal of Autism and Developmental Disorders, 20*(2), 233–253.

Butler, R. W. (2006). Cognitive and behavioral rehabilitation. In J. E. Farmer, J. Donders, & S. Warschausky (Eds.), *Treating neurodevelopmental disabilities* (pp. 186–207). New York: Guilford Press.

Chakrabarti, S., & Fombonne, E. (2005). Pervasive developmental disorders in preschool children: Confirmation of high prevalence. *American Journal of Psychiatry, 162*(6), 1133–1141.

Chambless, D. L., & Hollon, S. D. (1998). Defining empirically supported therapies. *Journal of Consulting and Clinical Psychology, 66*(1), 7–18.

Charman, T. (2002). The prevalence of autism spectrum disorders: Recent evidence and future challenges. *European Child and Adolescent Psychiatry, 11*(6), 249–256.

Chhabildas, N., Pennington, B. F., & Willcutt, E. G. (2001). A comparison of the neuropsychological profiles of the DSM-IV subtypes of ADHD. *Journal of Abnormal Child Psychology, 29*, 529–540.

Chronis, A. M., Chacko, A., Fabiano, G., Wymbs, B. T., & Pelham, W. E. (2004). Enhancements to the behavioral parent training paradigm for families of children with ADHD: Review and future directions. *Clinical Child and Family Psychology Review, 7*(1), 1–27.

Clark, E., Tuesday-Heathfield, L., Olympia, D., & Jenson, W. (2006). Empirically based interventions for children with autism. In J. Farmer, J. Donders, & S. Warschausky (Eds.), *Treating neurodevelopmental disabilities* (pp. 249–268). New York: Guilford Press.

D'Amato, R. C., Fletcher-Janzen, E., & Reynolds, C. R. (2005). *Handbook of school neuropsychology.* Hoboken, NJ: Wiley.

Donders, J. (2006). Traumatic brain injury. In J. Farmer, J. Donders, & S. Warschausky (Eds.), *Treating neurodevelopmental disabilities* (pp. 23–41). New York: Guilford Press.

Donders, J., & Giroux, A. (2005). Discrepancies between the California Verbal Learning Test: Children's Version and the Children's Category Test after pediatric traumatic brain injury. *Journal of the International Neuropsychological Society, 11*(4), 386–391.

DuPaul, G. J., & Eckert, T. L. (1997). The effects of school-based interventions for attention deficit disorder: A meta-analysis. *School Psychology Review, 26*(1), 5–27.

Echemendia, R. J., & Westerveld, M. (2006). Cultural perspectives in pediatric rehabilitation. In J. E. Farmer, J. Donders, & S. Warschausky (Eds.), *Treating neurodevelopmental disabilities* (pp. 289–308). New York: Guilford Press.

Farmer, J. E., & Brazeal, T. J. (1998). Parent perceptions about the process and outcomes of child neuropsychological assessment. *Applied Neuropsychology, 5*(4), 1994–1201.

Farmer, J. E., Clark, M. J., & Marien, W. E. (2003). Building systems of care for children with chronic health conditions. *Rehabilitation Psychology, 48*(4), 242–249.

Farmer, J. E., & Deidrick, K. K. (2006). Introduction to childhood disability. In J. E. Farmer, J. Donders, & S. Warschausky (Eds.), *Treating neurodevelopmental disabilities* (pp. 3–19). New York: Guilford Press.

Farmer, J. E., & Drewel, E. (2006). Systems intervention for comprehensive care. In J. E. Farmer, J. Donders, & S. Warschausky (Eds.), *Treating neurodevelopmental disabilities* (pp. 269–288). New York: Guilford Press.

Fombonne, E. (2005). The changing epidemiology of autism. *Journal of Applied Research in Intellectual Disabilities, 18*(4), 281–294.

Frazen, K. M., Roberts, M. A., Schmidts, D., Verduyn, W., & Manshadi, F. (1996). Cognitive remediation in pediatric brain injury. *Child Neuropsychology, 2*, 176–184.

Frith, U. (2006). *Autism: Understanding the enigma.* Oxford: Blackwell.

Ganesalingam, K., Sanson, A., Anderson, V., & Yeates, K. O. (2006). Self-regulation and social and behavioral functioning following childhood traumatic brain injury. *Journal of the International Neuropsychological Society, 12*(5), 609–621.

Glang, A., Singer, G., Cooley, E., & Tish, N. (1992). Tailoring direct instruction techniques for use with elementary students with TBI. *Journal of Head Trauma Rehabilitation, 7*, 92–108.

Green, G. (1996). Early behavioral intervention for autism: What does research tell us. In C. Maurice (Ed.), *Bahavioral interventions for young children with autism: A manual for parents and professionals* (pp. 29–44). Austin, TX: PRO-ED.

Gurdin, L. S., Huber, S. A., & Cochran, C. R. (2005). A critical analysis of data-based studies examining behavioral interventions with children and adolescents with brain injuries. *Behavioral Interventions, 20*(1), 3–16.

Hegel, M. T. (1988). Application of a token economy with a non-compliant closed head-injured male. *Brain Injury, 2*, 333–338.

Hibbard, M. R., Martin, T., Cantor, J., & Moran, A. I. (2006). Students with acquired brain injury: Identification, accommodations, and transactions in the schools. In J. E. Farmer, J. Donders, & S. Warschausky (Eds.), *Treating neurodevelopmental disabilities* (pp. 208–233). New York: Guilford Press.

Jensen, P. S., Hinshaw, S. P., Swanson, J. M., Greenhill, L. L., Conners, C. K., Arnold, L. E., et al. (2001). Finding from the NIMH Multimodal Treatment Study of ADHD (MTA): Implications and applications for primary care providers. *Journal of Developmental and Behavioral Pediatrics, 22*(1), 60–73.

Johnstone, B., & Farmer, J. E. (1997). Preparing neuropsychologists for the future: The need for additional training guidelines. *Archives of Clinical Neuropsychology, 12*, 523–530.

Kazdin, A. E., & Weisz, J. R. (2003). *Evidence-based psychotherapies for children and adolescents.* New York: Guilford Press.

Klingberg, T., Fernell, E., Olesen, P., Johnson, M., Gustafsson, P., Dahlstrom, K., et al. (2005). Computerized training of working memory in children with ADHD: A randomized, controlled trial. *Journal of the American Academy of Child and Adolescent Psychiatry, 44*(2), 177–186.

Koegel, L. K., Koegel, R. L., Harrower, J. K., & Carter, C. M. (1999). Pivotal response intervention: I. Overview of approach. *Journal of the Association for Persons with Severe Handicaps, 24*(3), 174–185.

Koegel, R. L., Koegel, L. K., & Brookman, L. I. (2003). Empirically supported pivotal response interventions for children with autism. In A. E. Kazdin & J. R. Weisz (Eds.), *Evidence-based psychotherapies for children and adolescents* (pp. 341–357). New York: Guilford Press.

Kolb, B. (2004). Mechanisms of cortical plasticity after neuronal injury. In J. Ponsford (Ed.), *Cognitive and behavioral rehabilitation: From neurobiology to clinical practice* (pp. 30–58). New York: Guilford Press.

Kraus, J. F. (1995). Epidemiological features of brain injury in children: Occurrence, children at risk, causes, and manner of injury, severity and outcomes. In S. Broman & M. Michel (Eds.), *Traumatic head injury for children* (pp. 22–39). New York: Oxford University Press.

Laatsch, L., Harrington, D., Hotz, G., Marcantuono, J., Mozzoni, M. P., Walsh, V., et al. (2007). An evidence-based review of cognitive and behavioral rehabilitation treatment studies in children with acquired brain injury. *Journal of Head Trauma Rehabilitation, 22*(4), 248–256.

Lee, H. S., & Riccio, C. A. (2005). Test review: Delis–Kaplan Executive Function System. *Journal of Clinical and Experimental Neuropsychology, 27*(5), 599–609.

Limond, J., & Leeke, R. (2005). Practitioner review: Cognitive rehabilitation for children with acquired brain injury. *Journal of Child Psychology and Psychiatry, 46*(4), 339–352.

Lord, C. A., Wagner, A., et al. (2005). Challenges in evaluating psychosocial interventions for autistic spectrum disorders. *Journal of Autism and Developmental Disorders, 35*(6), 695–708.

Lovaas, O. I. (1987). Behavioral treatment and normal educational and intellectual functioning in young autistic children. *Journal of Consulting and Clinical Psychology, 55*, 3–9.

Luria, A. R. (Ed.). (1963). *Restoration of function after brain injury.* New York: Macmillan.

Minshew, N., Sweeney, J., Bauman, M., & Webb, S. (2005). Neurologic aspects of autism. In F. Volkmar,

R. Paul, A. Klin, & D. Cohen (Eds.), *Handbook of autism and pervasive developmental disorders* (3rd ed., Vol. 1, pp. 473–514). Hoboken, NJ: Wiley.

Mottram, L., & Berger-Gross, P. (2004). An intervention to reduce disruptive behaviors in children with brain injury. *Pediatric Rehabilitation, 7*(2), 133–143.

Mundy, P., & Burnette, C. (2005). Joint attention and neurodevelopmental models of autism. In F. Volkmar, R. Paul, A. Klin, & D. Cohen (Eds.), *Handbook of autism and pervasive developmental disorders* (3rd ed., Vol. 1, pp. 650–681). Hoboken, NJ: Wiley.

Munson, S., Schroth, E., & Ernst, M. (2006). The role of functional neuroimaging in pediatric brain injury. *Pediatrics, 117*, 1372–1381.

Myers, S. M., Johnson, C. P., & U.S. Council on Children with Disabilities. (2007). Management of children with autism spectrum disorders. *Pediatrics, 120*(5), 1162–1182.

Naar-King, S., & Donders, J. (2006). Pediatric family-centered rehabilitation. In J. E. Farmer, J. Donders, & S. Warschausky (Eds.), *Treating neurodevelopmental disabilities* (pp. 149–169). New York: Guilford Press.

National Research Council. (2001). *Educating children with autism: Committee on Educational Interventions for Children with Autism.* Washington, DC: National Academy Press.

Oberg, L., & Turkustra, L. S. (1998). Use of elaborative encoding to facilitate verbal learning after adolescent traumatic brain injury. *Journal of Head Trauma Rehabilitation, 13*, 44–62.

Ozonoff, S., & Jensen, J. (1999). Brief report: Specific executive function profiles in three neurodevelopmental disorders. *Journal of Autism and Developmental Disabilities, 29*, 171–177.

Ozonoff, S., South, M., & Provencal, S. (2005). Executive functions. In F. R. Volkmar, R. Paul, A. Klin, & D. Cohen (Eds.), *Handbook of autism and pervasive developmental disorders* (3rd ed., Vol. 1, pp. 606–627). Hoboken, NJ: Wiley.

Pelham, W. E., Wheeler, T., & Chronis, A. (1998). Empirically supported treatments for attention deficit hyperactivity disorder. *Journal of Clinical Child Psychology, 27*(2), 190–205.

Pelham, W. E., Jr., Gnagy, E. M., Greiner, A. R., Hoza, B., Hinshaw, S. P., Swanson, J. M., et al. (2000). Behavioral versus behavioral and pharmacological treatment in ADHD children attending a summer treatment program. *Journal of Abnormal Child Psychology, 28*(6), 507–525.

Pliszka, S. (2007). Practice parameter for the assessment and treatment of children and adolescents with attention-deficit/hyperactivity disorder. *Journal of the American Academy of Child and Adolescent Psychiatry, 46*(7), 894–921.

Ponsford, J. (Ed.). (2004). *Cognitive and behavioral rehabilitation: From neurobiology to clinical practice.* New York: Guilford Press.

Ponsford, J., & Wilmott, C. (2004). Rehabilitation of nonspatial attention. In J. Ponsford (Ed.), *Cognitive and behavioral rehabilitation: From neurobiology to clinical practice* (pp. 59–99). New York: Guilford Press.

Powell, S., & Nelson, B. (1997). Effects of choosing academic assignments on a student with attention deficit hyperactivity disorder. *Journal of Applied Behavior Analysis, 30*, 181–183.

Riccio, J., & French, C. L. (2004). The status of empirical support for treatments of attention deficits. *The Clinical Neuropsychologist, 18*, 528–558.

Rogers, S. (1998). Neuropsychology of autism in young children and its implications for early intervention. *Mental Retardation and Developmental Disabilities Research Reviews, 4*, 104–112.

Rutter, M. (2005). Incidence of autism spectrum disorders: Changes over time and their meaning. *Acta Paediatrica, 94*(1), 2–15.

Schultz, R., & Robins, D. (2005). Functional neuroimaging studies in autism spectrum disorders. In F. Volkmar, R. Paul, A. Klin, & D. Cohen (Eds.), *Handbook of autism and pervasive developmental disorders* (3rd ed., Vol. 1, pp. 515–333). Hoboken, NJ: Wiley.

Schwartz, L., Taylor, H. G., et al. (2003). Long-term behavior problems following pediatric traumatic brain injury: Prevalence, predictors, and correlates. *Journal of Pediatric Psychology, 28*(4), 251–263.

Sigman, M., Spence, S., & Wang, T. (2006). Autism from developmental and neuropsychological perspectives. *Annual Review of Clinical Psychology, 2*, 327–355.

Silver, B. V., & Stelly-Seitz, C. (1992). Behavioral treatment of adipsia in a child with hypothalamic injury. *Developmental Medicine and Child Neurology, 34*(6), 534–546.

Slifer, K. J., Cataldo, M. D., & Kurtz, P. F. (1995). Behavioral training during acute brain trauma rehabilitation: An empirical case study. *Brain Injury, 9*(6), 585–593.

Slifer, K. J., Tucker, C. L., Gerson, A. C., Sevier, R. C., Kane, A. C., Amari, A., et al. (1997). Antecedent management and compliance training improve adolescents' participation in early brain injury rehabilitation. *Brain Injury, 11*(12), 877–889.

Sohlberg, M. M., & Mateer, C. A. (1989). *Introduction to cognitive rehabilitation: Theory and practice.* New York: Guilford Press.

Suzman, K. B., Morris, R. D., Morris, M. K., & Milan, M. A. (1997). Cognitive behavioral remediation of problem solving deficits in children with acquired brain injury. *Journal of Behavior Therapy and Experimental Psychiatry, 28*, 203–212.

Taylor, H. G., & Alden, J. (1997). Age-related differences in outcomes following childhood brain insults: An introduction and overview. *Journal of the International Neuropsychological Society, 3*, 555–567.

Teeter, P. A. (1997). Neurocognitive interventions for childhood and adolescent disorders. In C. R. Reynolds & E. Fletcher-Janzen (Eds.), *Handbook of clinical child neuropsychology* (2nd ed., pp. 387–417). New York: Plenum Press.

Teeter, P. A., & Semrud-Clikeman, M. (1995). Integrating neurobiological, psychosocial, and behavioral paradigms: A transactional model for the study of ADHD. *Archives of Clinical Neuropsychology, 10*(5), 433–461.

Thomson, J. B. (1995). Rehabilitation of high school aged individuals with TBI through use of an attention-training program. *Journal of the International Neuropsychological Society, 1*, 149.

Thomson, J. B., & Kerns, K. A. (2000). Cognitive rehabilitation of the child with mild traumatic brain injury. In S. Raskin & C. Mateer (Eds.), *Neuropsychological management of mild traumatic brain injury* (pp. 233–253). New York: Oxford University Press.

Treadwell, K., & Page, T. J. (1996). Functional analysis: Identifying the environmental determinants of severe behavioral disorders. *Journal of Head Trauma Rehabilitation, 11*(1), 62–74.

van den Hoofdakker, B. J., van der Veen-Mulders, L., et al. (2007). Effectiveness of behavioral parent training for children with ADHD in routine clinical practice: A randomized controlled study. *Journal of the American Academy of Child and Adolescent Psychiatry, 46*(10), 1263–1271.

Volkmar, F. R., Lord, C., Bailey, A., Schultz, R. T., & Klin, A. (2004). Autism and pervasive developmental disorders. *Journal of Child Psychology and Psychiatry, 45*(1), 135–170.

Wade, S. L. (2006). Intervention to support families of children with traumatic brain injuries. In J. Farmer, J. Donders, & S. Warschausky (Eds.), *Treating neurodevelopmental disabilities* (pp. 170–185). New York: Guilford Press.

Wade, S. L., Carey, J., & Wolfe, C. R. (2006a). An online family intervention to reduce parental distress following pediatric brain injury. *Journal of Consulting and Clinical Psychology, 74*(3), 445–454.

Wade, S. L., Michaud, L. M., & Brown, T. M. (2006b). Putting the pieces together: Family intervention to improve child outcomes following traumatic brain injury (TBI). *Journal of Head Trauma Rehabilitation, 21*, 57–67.

Wallander, J. L., & Varni, J. W. (1998). Effects of pediatric chronic physical disorders on child and family adjustment. *Journal of Child Psychology and Psychiatry, 39*(1), 29–46.

Weisz, J. R., Hawley, K. M., Pilkonis, Woody, & Follette. (2000). Stressing the (other) three Rs in the search for empirically supported treatments: Review procedures, research quality, relevance to practice and the public interest. *Clinical Psychology: Science and Practice, 7*(3), 243–258.

Willcutt, E. G., Pennington, B. F., & DeFries, J. C. (1999). Twin study of the etiology of comorbidity between reading disability and attention-deficit/hyperactivity disorder. *American Journal of Medical Genetics, 96*, 293–301.

World Health Organization. (2001). *World Health Report 2001, Mental Health: New Understanding, New Hope.* Geneva: World Health Organization.

Wozniak, J. R., Krach, L., Ward, E., Mueller, B. A., Muetzel, R., Schnoebelen, S., et al. (2007). Neurocognitive and neuroimaging correlates of pediatric traumatic brain injury: A diffusion tensor imaging (DTI) study. *Archives of Clinical Neuropsychology, 22*(5), 555–568.

Yeargin-Allsopp, M., Rice, C., Karapurkar, T., Doernberg, N., Boyle, C., & Murphy, C. (2003). Prevalence of autism in a U.S. metropolitan area. *289*(1), 49–55.

Yeates, K. O., Armstrong, K., Janusz, J., Taylor, H. G., Wade, S., Stancin, T., et al. (2005). Long-term attention problems in children with traumatic brain injury. *Journal of the American Academy of Child and Adolescent Psychiatry, 44*(6), 574–584.

Yeates, K. O., & Taylor, H. G. (2005). Neurobehavioural outcomes of mild head injury in children and adolescents. *Pediatric Rehabilitation, 8*(1), 5–16.

Ylvisaker, M., Adelson, P. D., Braga, L. W., Burnett, S. M., Glang, A., Feeney, T., et al. (2005). Rehabilitation and ongoing support after pediatric TBI: 20 years of progress. *Journal of Head Trauma Rehabilitation, 20,* 95–109.

Ylvisaker, M., Chorazy, A. J. L., Feeny, T. J., & Russell, M. L. (1999). Traumatic brain injury in children and adolescents: Assessment and rehabilitation. In M. Rosenthal, E. R. Griffith, J. S. Kreutzer, & B. Pentland (Eds.), *Rehabilitation of the adult and child with traumatic brain injury* (pp. 356–392). Philadelphia: Davis.

Ylvisaker, M., & Szekeres, S. F. (1998). A framework for cognitive rehabilitation. In M. Ylvisaker (Ed.), *Traumatic brain injury rehabilitation* (pp. 125–158). Newton, MA: Butterworth-Heinemann.

Index

Page numbers followed by an *f* or *t* indicate figures or tables.